AF710035

UROLITHIASIS
A Medical and Surgical Reference

MARTIN I. RESNICK, M.D.

Professor and Chairman, Division of Urology,
Case Western Reserve University School of Medicine,
Cleveland, Ohio

CHARLES Y.C. PAK, M.D.

University Distinguished Chair in Mineral Metabolism,
University of Texas Southwestern Medical School,
Dallas, Texas

1990

W.B. SAUNDERS COMPANY

Harcourt Brace Jovanovich, Inc.

Philadelphia, London, Toronto, Montreal, Sydney, Tokyo

W. B. SAUNDERS COMPANY
Harcourt Brace Jovanovich, Inc.

The Curtis Center
Independence Square West
Philadelphia, PA 19106

Library of Congress Cataloging-in-Publication Data

Resnick, Martin I.

Urolithiasis : a medical and surgical reference / Martin I. Resnick, Charles Y. C. Pak.

p. cm.

1. Urinary organs—Calculi. 2. Urinary organs—Calculi—Surgery. I. Pak, Charles Y. C. II. Title. [DNLM: 1. Kidney Calculi—surgery. 2. Lithotripsy. 3. Ureteral Calculi—surgery. WJ 356 R434u]

RC916.R48 1990 616.6′22—dc20 90-8333

DNLM/DLC

ISBN 0–7216–2439–1

Acquisition Editor: William Lamsback
Manuscript Editor: Bonnie Boehme
Production Manager: Frank Polizzano
Indexer: Susan Thomas

UROLITHIASIS ISBN 0–7216–2439–1

Copyright © 1990 by W. B. Saunders Company.

All rights reserved. No part of this publication may be reproduced or transmitted in any form or by any means, electronic or mechanical, including photocopy, recording, or any information storage and retrieval system, without permission in writing from the publisher.

Printed in the United States of America.

Last digit is the print number: 9 8 7 6 5 4 3 2 1

Dedicated to
Birdwell Finlayson, M.D., Ph.D.
We all miss him.

Contributors

MALACHY J. GLEESON, M.Ch., F.R.C.S.I.
Postdoctorate Fellow, Baylor College of Medicine, Houston, Texas; Registrar in Urology, St. James's Hospital, Dublin, Ireland

DONALD P. GRIFFITH, M.D.
Professor of Urology, Baylor College of Medicine, Houston, Texas

JOHN L. MEYER, Ph.D.
Grants Review Branch, National Cancer Institute, National Institutes of Health, Bethesda, Maryland

J. PATRICK SPIRNAK, M.D.
Assistant Professor of Urology, Case Western Reserve University School of Medicine; Director of Urology, Metrohealth Medical Center, Cleveland, Ohio

Preface

We have witnessed a significant change in the management of patients with urolithiasis during the last decade. There have been major innovations involving introduction of percutaneous techniques and the development of extracorporeal shock wave lithotripsy which for practical purposes have replaced open surgical procedures. Additionally, the development of ureteroscopy with refinement of instrumentation and stone fragmenting devices has allowed for safer, improved management of many ureteral stones. These changes have greatly benefitted the stone-forming patient; it is very likely that further developments and refinements in this new technology will follow.

Unfortunately, those advances related to the removal and fragmentation of stones have not necessarily been paralleled by advances in understanding of the disease and in its prevention. In the early and mid 1970s significant information was gained regarding the etiology and pathogenesis of urolithiasis. Associated with these advances was the introduction of treatment and therapeutic programs. Knowledge gained from research has continued, but these developments have oftentimes been overshadowed by the more dramatic improvements in technology. It is important to remember that in most instances the cause of stone disease can be identified and this information may be applied in a rational manner to reduce or prevent recurrences. All too often physicians are remiss in applying these principles after the stone has been removed.

In *Urolithiasis* we attempt to address the current methods of treating all aspects of urolithiasis. Principles of patient evaluation and medical management are detailed, as are the newer interventional and technological developments. The monograph is meant to be a practical one, and although areas of research and further development are discussed, most of the emphasis relates to clinical and practical care. The editors hope that readers of this text will find the material useful in the management of their patients with urolithiasis.

The editors would like to express their appreciation to William J. Lamsback of W.B. Saunders Company, who was most supportive in the development of this monograph. Additionally, the editors are most appreciative to Drs. Griffith, Meyer, and Spirnak, who wrote important chapters in the book. Finally our thanks go to Ms. Barbara Goldberg, Faye Britton, and Jan LeMaire, who have been very helpful in collating all manuscripts and maintaining a friendly dialogue with the contributing authors and publisher.

M. I. Resnick
C. Y. C. Pak

Contents

1 Introduction

Charles Y.C. Pak
Martin I. Resnick

Urolithiasis has plagued humans since antiquity. Ancient Babylonians and Egyptians were familiar with stones of the urinary tract.[1] Bladder stones have been discovered in Egyptian mummies.[2] Hippocrates attributed stone formation to dehydration and cystitis.[3] Some of the notable figures in history who suffered from stones include Pliny, Sir Walter Scott, Benjamin Franklin, Napoleon, and Lyndon B. Johnson.

Until about 20 years ago, the progress in the pathophysiologic elucidation and management of urolithiasis was slow. For most forms of stone disease, the cause of stone formation was largely shrouded in mystery. The diagnosis of stone disease was mainly based on stone composition. Preventive treatment options were few. Stone removal often involved invasive open surgery with considerable morbidity and long recovery. Too often, no serious evaluation or prophylactic program was offered after such a surgery, leaving the patient exposed to repeated stone recurrences or operations.

During the past 20 years, some of the most notable advances in medicine have occurred in the study and treatment of stones. Much is now known regarding the physicochemical background for the crystallization of stone salts in urine. Many environmental and metabolic disturbances leading or contributing to stone formation have been identified. It is now possible to diagnose the cause of stone disease in more than 95 per cent of patients. With a variety of treatment programs, stone formation can be halted or retarded in most patients with recurrent calculi. A most dramatic and miraculous achievement has resulted from the recent introduction of percutaneous lithotripsy and extracorporeal shock wave lithotripsy (ESWL). Most stones can now be removed with greater ease and less morbidity, often without surgery. It is the object of this book to review this progress.

CHANGING EPIDEMIOLOGY OF STONE DISEASE

The trend in the location and type of urinary stones has changed with the advance of civilization. Before industrialization, stones located in the bladder were common.[4] Even today, bladder stones are prevalent in developing countries.[5] Moreover, stones composed of uric acid and struvite were frequently encountered.

In the United States and developed countries today, bladder stones have become rare. The most common stones now are those that originate in the kidneys and are composed predominantly of calcium oxalate. The frequency of stone disease appears to be increasing in the United States.[6] The incidence of stone disease is estimated to be 0.1 to 0.3 per cent; that is, 240,000 to 720,000 Americans suffer from stone episodes yearly. The prevalence of stone disease is 5 to 10 per cent; in other words, 12 to 24 million Americans will develop stones in their lifetime.

Whereas some forms of stone disease have a genetic basis, others show strong dependence on environmental or nutritional factors for their origin. Thus, the incidence of stone disease has shown positive correlation with the consumption of beef[7] or refined sugars.[8] The occurrence of stone disease was less common during both world wars. "White collar" workers and those in a high social economic class are more likely to form stones than are "blue collar" workers.

It has been suggested that the southeastern United States is a "stone belt," with a high concentration of stone disease.[9] A recent study, however, has disclosed that stone-forming patients residing in the stone belt carried environmental and metabolic risk factors identical in severity and frequency with those in patients residing elsewhere in the United States.[10] This lack of regional heterogeneity may reflect an increasing mobility of the population, the wide dissemination of various food products throughout the year and across the country, and the availability of air conditioning, resulting in less sweating.

IDENTIFICATION OF METABOLIC AND ENVIRONMENTAL RISK FACTORS

Many biochemical abnormalities in urine have been identified among patients with recurrent nephrolithiasis.[11] Because of their presumed etiologic role in stone formation, they have been called risk factors. Some of them are entirely environmental or nutritional in origin. Others, while affected by environmental and nutritional influences, may have a metabolic basis (i.e., due to a fundamental metabolic defect). The environmental risk factors include low urine volume, high urinary sodium, high urinary sulfate, high urinary phosphate, and low urinary magnesium. The metabolic risk factors are represented by hypercalciuria, hyperoxaluria, hyperuricosuria, hypocitraturia, and high or low urinary pH.

Attempts have been made to rate different risk factors according to their presumed role in stone formation.[12] One attempt[12] based its analysis on the frequency distribution of each variable in the stone-forming population and in the control population. Important risk factors were low urine volume, hyperuricosuria, and hyperoxaluria. Hypercalciuria was considered less of a risk than hyperoxaluria. In contrast, another study based on a discriminant analysis of results of treatment disclosed that hypercalciuria was the most important contributing factor to continued stone formation.[13]

Such a discrepancy is not unexpected. Stone disease is not a homogeneous entity but, rather, is the result of various causes with differing presentations.

Moreover, several abnormalities or risk factors are usually present in the same patient.

ADVANCES IN DIAGNOSTIC DIFFERENTIATION

Reliable diagnostic protocols have been introduced, based largely on underlying metabolic derangements.[14] The classification schemes have been refined by further categorization of principal derangements and recognition of additional risk factors.[15]

With use of the updated protocol, it is now possible to diagnose the cause of stone disease in more than 95 per cent of patients with recurrent renal calculi.[16] Table 1–1 presents various diagnostic categories and their relative frequency from the experience at Dallas.

EFFICACY OF CURRENT PROPHYLACTIC PROGRAMS

Many reports indicate that the recurrent formation of renal stones may be inhibited in a majority of patients by using a variety of treatment programs.[17–20] This progress has been possible because of advances in pathophysiologic elucidation and in diagnostic differentiation, as well as the development of new drugs capable of correcting much of the abnormal metabolic picture. The beneficial response to a conservative program, or the "stone clinic effect" on stone formation, is well known.[21] However, the following lines of evidence support the positive effect of specific medical treatment provided. In eight clinical trials of thiazide in patients with idiopathic calcium nephrolithiasis, stone recurrence

TABLE 1–1. DIAGNOSTIC CATEGORIES OF NEPHROLITHIASIS

Category	Per Cent*
Absorptive hypercalciuria	20–40
Type I	
Type II	
Renal hypercalciuria	5–8
Primary hyperparathyroidism	3–5
Unclassified hypercalciuria	15–25
Renal phosphate leak	
Fasting hypercalciuria	
Hyperoxaluric calcium nephrolithiasis	2–15
Enteric hyperoxaluria	
Primary hyperoxaluria	
Dietary hyperoxaluria	
Hyperuricosuric calcium nephrolithiasis	10–40
Hypocitraturic calcium nephrolithiasis	10–50
Distal renal tubular acidosis	
Chronic diarrheal syndrome	
Idiopathic	
Gouty diathesis	15–30
Cystinuria	<1
Infection stones	1–5
Hypomagnesiuric calcium nephrolithiasis	5–10
Low urine volume	10–50
No disturbance and miscellaneous causes	<3

The range in percentage for each diagnosis represents approximate estimates based on experience in Dallas, from sole occurrence to combined occurrence with other abnormalities.

rates during thiazide treatment were compared with either a parallel placebo control or a pretreatment period.[22] In most of the trials, the remission rate and the reduction in group stone formation rate were lower in the group receiving thiazide. Among patients with mild-to-moderate stone disease (one stone per year or less), potassium citrate therapy reduced the stone formation rate from 0.52 to 0.02 per patient-year and produced a remission rate of 96 per cent and a reduction in the group stone formation rate of 96 per cent.[23] In contrast, a review of 11 conservative or placebo trials disclosed a much less favorable response, with a reduction in stone formation rate from 0.54 to 0.25 stone per patient-year, a remission rate of 61 per cent, and a decline in the group stone formation rate of 54 per cent. This finding supported the superior clinical response of medical therapy (the response with potassium citrate versus that with conservative or placebo trials) among patients with stone disease of comparable severity. Moreover, in patients with hypercalciuric nephrolithiasis who continued to form stones while on thiazide therapy, the replacement of potassium chloride by potassium citrate produced an inhibition of stone formation in most patients.[24]

However, it is not known whether a rigorous selective treatment program is more effective than a less selective one. In a recent study,[25] chlorthalidone was found to be more effective than a placebo in inhibiting new stone formation in patients with idiopathic calcium oxalate nephrolithiasis, noncategorized with regard to the cause of hypercalciuria and without classification into normal or excessive renal excretion of calcium or uric acid. However, a study at Dallas indicated that a more selectively applied potassium citrate therapy in patients with hypocitraturia provided a better clinical response than that in those patients with normocitraturic calcium nephrolithiasis.[26] Thus, in the hypocitraturic group, the stone formation rate declined from 4.14 to 0.4 stones per patient-year following potassium citrate treatment, 82.3 per cent of patients had remission, and the group stone formation rate declined by 90.3 per cent. In contrast, the normocitraturic group showed a reduction in the stone formation rate from 3.33 to 0.75 stones per patient-year, a remission rate of 74 per cent, and a decline in the group stone formation rate of 77.5 per cent. The less favorable response in the normocitraturic group probably reflected the presence of other metabolic abnormalities not corrected by potassium citrate therapy.

ADVANCES IN THE REMOVAL OF STONES

The treatment of both renal and ureteral stones has undergone significant changes over the past several decades. Although surgical techniques improved in the first half of the century, much of the progress since the 1950s has related to the improvement in preoperative care, the development of appropriate antibiotics, the advent of new technologic techniques related to microsurgical instrumentation, and the introduction of fine absorbable suture material. In addition, more effective anesthetic agents and better management of cardiorespiratory problems in the preoperative and postoperative periods contributed to the improved outcome of surgery. In the late 1960s and early 1970s, many open surgical procedures, particularly anatrophic nephrolithotomy, were perfected. Improved results after the removal of all types of stones were thus realized. Percutaneous techniques were developed in the late 1970s, and ESWL became a reality in the 1980s. These two techniques used either alone or in combination have been successfully employed in the treatment of many stones. Technologic developments had an effect on the management of ureteral stones as well. Percutaneous techniques were used for removing these stones in an antegrade fashion, and ESWL has become a useful adjunct in fragmenting them as well. Finally, technologic advances and improvement in optical systems permitted the development of ureteroscopes, which allowed for the manipulation, fragmentation, and removal of ureteral stones, in a more controlled and safe manner.

Although the procedures have changed over the years, the objectives have remained unchanged. These goals include removal of all stones, improvement of intrarenal drainage with reconstruction of the collecting system when necessary, preservation of maximal renal function, and, when present, eradication of upper urinary tract infection to reduce the rate of stone recurrence. Today, most small renal stones can be treated with ESWL or percutaneous nephrostolithotomy, and most ureteral stones can be managed with ureteroscopy or ESWL. The role of open surgery is certainly reduced.

Surgery

Open surgical techniques for the removal of intrarenal stones were described by Hippocrates. In most instances, they were carried out because of the development of perirenal abscess, hydronephrosis, or urinary obstruction. It was not until the 1880s that procedures were performed for the removal of stones in kidneys free of these problems.[27-29] Developments over the ensuing 50 years were significant, particularly as related to an improved understanding of renal anatomy and surgical techniques.[30, 31] Progress continued and culminated with the description of anatrophic nephrolithotomy by Smith and Boyce in 1968.[32] Advances were also made during this time in the surgical removal of ureteral stones, resulting in high rates of success and minimal morbidity.

Percutaneous Nephrostolithotomy

Percutaneous nephrostolithotomy was the natural extension of the development of percutaneous drainage of the kidney. The first percutaneous tract designed for the removal of stones was created in 1976, and from that time to the present, the rapid development of new techniques and instruments has made this procedure an essential component of the urologic surgeon's armamentarium. When utilized for the removal of small renal pelvic stones, the technique is most effective, and success rates of greater than 95 per cent have been reported.[33] These techniques have also been applied for the removal of ureteral stones and have been found to be more effective in the extraction of those located in the upper third compared with the lower third.

Extracorporeal Shock Wave Lithotripsy

The development of ESWL has revolutionized the removal of all types of urinary calculi. Stones less than 2 cm in size that are located in the renal pelvis can be effectively treated with this technique, with minimal complications and morbidity. With further experience, stones of various sizes and those located in all portions of the ureter have been successfully treated. This technology has also been applied to biliary stones, and if the experience in the urinary tract is any indication, this form of therapy will have a significant impact on this type of stone disease as well.

Ureteroscopy

In the 1960s, several reports detailed the development of the ureteroscope, but it was not until the late 1970s and early 1980s that specialized instruments were introduced.[34–37] With continuing developments in instrumentation, stones are extracted intact or fragmented by a variety of newly developed techniques.[38–40]

Many new approaches are available for the management of patients with urinary calculi. Further study and experience will define the advantages of each of these new techniques as they relate to a particular stone. The reduction in cost and recuperative time is often associated with the requirement for multiple procedures, particularly with large stones. Both the advantages and the disadvantages of these new approaches remain to be fully defined. In addition, more information is required on both the systemic and the local effects of these new forms of treatment, particularly ESWL, as any adverse finding will have a significant impact on its use in the future. At the current time, a variety of approaches are available, and no single one can be considered correct in all instances. In consultation with the patient, the urologic surgeon must decide on the best technique based on the clinical findings and his or her own expertise.

NEED FOR INTEGRATED MEDICAL AND SURGICAL APPROACHES

Despite dramatic progress in both medical and "surgical" areas, there has been an unfortunate tendency to promote one approach while disparaging or ignoring the other. It should be clear that the two approaches are complementary and that the ultimate control of nephrolithiasis requires a conscientious application of both approaches.[16, 26] The objectives of the two approaches are fundamentally different, since the goal of medical treatment is the prevention of recurrent

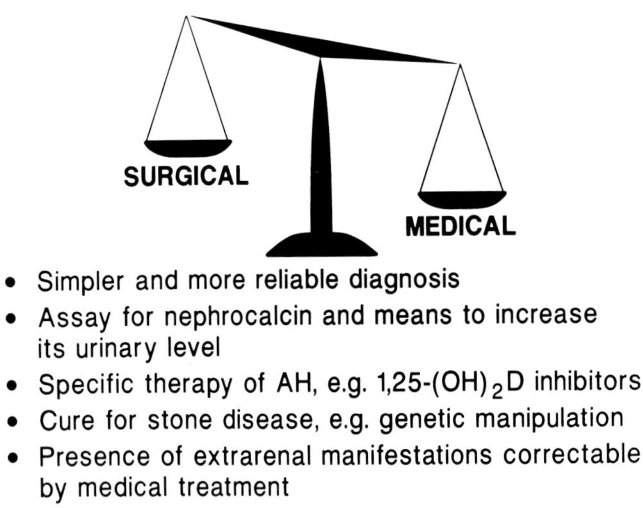

FIGURE 1–1. Factors favoring medical preventive program.

stone formation, whereas that of the surgical approach is the removal of existing stones. Both goals must be satisfied.

Arguments for the continued application of the medical prophylactic program were set forth at a recent National Institutes of Health (NIH)—sponsored Consensus Conference on Nephrolithiasis. Justifications for the medical approach were the inhibition of recurrent stone formation and spontaneous stone passage, the reduced need for stone removal, the correction of nonrenal manifestations of the underlying stone disease, and cost effectiveness.[26]

Despite the potential advantages of the medical approach, certain inherent problems of the medical treatment program should not be overlooked. To be effective, the medical prevention program requires rigid compliance by the patient and constant surveillance by the physician. It demands commitment by the patient to adhere to the chosen program on a daily continuing basis for an extended period of many years. Regular follow-up evaluation by the physician is critical to ensure that the response is appropriate. Moreover, all medical treatments have certain hazards, especially if they are misused. Finally, there is no cure for stone disease obtainable by the current medical prophylactic program.

It is expected that continued improvements will be made in surgical removal techniques and in medical approaches regarding efficacy, facility, safety, and cost. It may be presumed that the need for a medical approach would be greater with the development of a simpler and more reliable diagnosis, an assay for nephrocalcin and a means to increase its urinary level, a specific therapy for absorptive hypercalciuria (e.g., 1,25-$(OH)_2$ vitamin D inhibitors), and a cure for stone disease (e.g., by genetic manipulation), as well as with the presence of extrarenal manifestations correctable by medical treatment (Fig. 1–1). On the other hand, the surgical approach would be reinforced by improvements in methods of stone removal that have a higher success rate and are less invasive and that are easier, safer, and cheaper to apply (Fig. 1–2). It is critical that the need for medical and surgical treatments be continually reappraised to accommodate these changing trends.

Overall Aims of the Book

The main objective of this book is to highlight the advances made in the medical and surgical approaches to stone disease. The underlying thesis is the conviction that the two approaches are complementary.

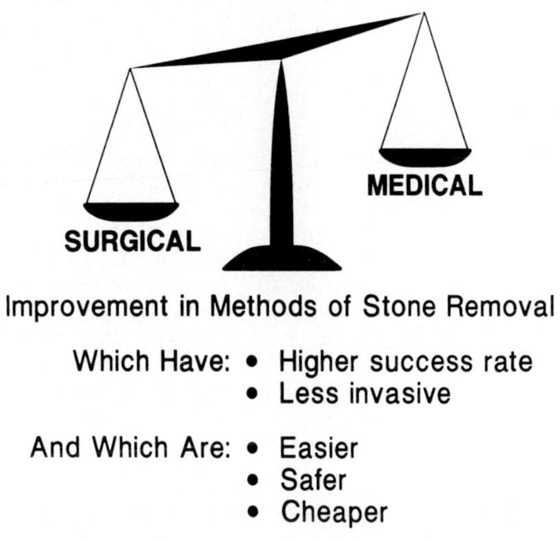

FIGURE 1–2. Factors favoring "surgical" removal of stones.

The physicochemistry of stone formation is discussed first (in Chapter 2) from a fresh perspective to facilitate the understanding of pathogenetic mechanisms, to be described in subsequent chapters. In succeeding chapters (Chapters 3 to 10), the main disorders of stone disease (as outlined in Table 1–1) are discussed in detail from the perspective of pathogenesis, diagnosis, and management. Chapters 11 and 12 give practical guidelines in the medical diagnosis and management of stone disease in general.

The remaining portion of the book addresses the specific interventional approaches utilized for managing stones in the urinary tract. Rather than being devoted to a particular stone type, each chapter instead deals with a technologic application or procedure. Each is described, and the approach is outlined. Specific chapters focus on chemolysis (Chapter 13), surgery of the kidney and ureteral stones (Chapter 14), ureteroscopic techniques (Chapter 15), percutaneous management (Chapter 16), and ESWL (Chapter 17). These chapters explain the technical aspects of the procedure, review results and complications, and address their future role.

REFERENCES

1. Atsmon A, de Vries A, Menachem F: Historical notes. *In* Uric Acid Lithiasis. New York, Elsevier, 1963, pp 1–13.
2. Kittredge WE, Downs R: The role of gout in the formation of urinary calculi. J Urol 67:841, 1952.
3. Hippocrates: On Airs, Waters and Places. *In* The Genuine Works of Hippocrates: Translated from the Greek with a Preliminary Discourse and Annotations by Francis Adams. Vol I, Number 9. New York, William Wood & Company, 1948, pp 165–166.
4. Thorwald J: Stones. *In* The Century of the Surgeon. New York, Pantheon Books, 1957, pp 24–64.
5. Valyasevi A, Dhanamitta S, Van Reen R: Studies of bladder stone disease in Thailand. XVI. Effect of 4-hydroxy-L-proline and orthophosphate supplementations on urinary composition and crystalluria. Am J Clin Nutr 26:1207–1211, 1973.
6. Frangos DN, Rous SN: Incidence and economic factors in urolithiasis. *In* Stone Disease: Diagnosis and Management. Orlando, FL, Grune & Stratton, 1987, pp 3–10.
7. Robertson WG, Peacock M, Heyburn PJ, et al: The risk of calcium stone formation in relation to affluence and dietary animal protein. *In* Brockis JG, Finlayson B (eds): Urinary Calculus. Littleton, MA, PSG Publishing Company, 1981, pp 3–12.
8. Thom JA, Morris JE, Bishop A, Blacklock NJ: Effect of dietary sucrose on urinary calcium oxalate activity product. *In* Brockis JG, Finlayson B (eds): Urinary Calculus. Littleton, MA, PSG Publishing Company, 1981, pp 103–115.
9. Holmes RJ, Coplan MM: A study of the geographic incidence of urolithiasis with consideration of etiological factors. J Urol 23:477–489, 1930.
10. Harvey JA, Hill KD, Pak CYC: Similarity of urinary risk factors among stone-forming patients in five regions of the United States. J Lithotripsy Stone Disease. (Accepted).
11. Pak CYC, Skurla C, Harvey J: Graphic display of urinary risk factors for renal stone formation. J Urol 134:867–870, 1985.
12. Robertson WG, Peacock M, Heyburn PJ, et al: A risk factor model of stone-formation: Application to the study of epidemiological factors in the genesis of calcium stones. *In* Smith LH, Robertson WG, Finlayson B (eds): Urolithiasis. New York, Plenum Publishing, 1981, pp 303–307.
13. Strauss AL, Coe FL, Deutsch L, Parks JH: Factors that predict relapse of calcium nephrolithiasis during treatment. Am J Med 72:17–24, 1982.
14. Pak CYC, Britton F, Peterson R, et al: Ambulatory evaluation of nephrolithiasis: Classification, clinical presentation and diagnostic criteria. Am J Med 69:19–30, 1980.
15. Nicar MJ, Skurla C, Sakhaee K, Pak CYC: Low urinary citrate excretion in nephrolithiasis. Urology 21:8–14, 1983.
16. Pak CYC: Medical management of nephrolithiasis: Update 1987. J Urol 140:461–467,1988.
17. Ettinger B, Tang A, Citron JT, et al: Randomized trial of allopurinol in the prevention of calcium oxalate calculi. N Engl J Med 315:1386–1389, 1986.
18. Yendt ER, Cohanim M: Prevention of calcium stones with thiazides. Kid Int 13:397–409, 1978.
19. Coe FL, Kavalach AG: Hypercalciuria and hyperuricosuria in patients with calcium nephrolithiasis. N Engl J Med 291:1344–1350, 1974.

20. Pak CYC, Fuller C, Sakhaee K, et al: Long term treatment of calcium nephrolithiasis with potassium citrate. J Urol 134:11–19, 1985.
21. Hosking DH, Erickson SB, Van Den Berg CJ, et al: The stone clinic effect in patients with idiopathic calcium urolithiasis. J Urol 130:1115–1118, 1983.
22. Coe FL, Parks JH: Nephrolithiasis: Pathogenesis and Treatment. 2nd ed. Chicago, Year Book Medical Publishers, 1988.
23. Preminger GM, Harvey JA, Pak CYC: Comparative efficacy of "specific" potassium citrate therapy vs. conservative management in nephrolithiasis of mild-moderate severity. J Urol 134:658–661, 1985.
24. Pak CYC, Peterson R, Sakhaee K, et al: Correction of hypocitraturia and prevention of stone formation by combined thiazide and potassium citrate therapy in thiazide-unresponsive hypercalciuric nephrolithiasis. Am J Med 79:284–288, 1985.
25. Ettinger B, Citron JT, Livermore B, Dolman L: Chlorthalidone reduces calcium oxalate calculous recurrence but magnesium hydroxide does not. J Urol 139:679–684, 1988.
26. Pak CYC: Role of medical prevention. J Urol 141:798–801, 1989.
27. Hippocrates, quoted by Murphy LJT: The History of Urology. Springfield, IL, Charles C Thomas, 1972, p 220
28. Bell B, cited by Mathe CP: History of Urology. Vol I. Baltimore, The Williams & Wilkins Company, 1933, p 289.
29. Morris H: A case of nephrolithotomy or the extraction of a calculous from an undilated kidney. Trans Clin Soc Lond 14:31, 1981.
30. Brodel M: The intrinsic blood vessels of the kidney and their significance in nephrotomy. Bull Johns Hopkins Hosp 12:10, 1901.
31. Moore JE, Corbett JF: The damage done to the kidney by operation. Ann Surg 53:373, 1911.
32. Smith MJ, Boyce WH: Anatrophic nephrotomy and plastic calyorrhaphy. J Urol 99:521, 1968.
33. Segura JW, Patterson BE, LeRoy AJ, et al: Percutaneous removal of kidney stones: Review of 1000 cases. J Urol 134:1077, 1985.
34. Marshall VF: Fiberoptic in urology. J Urol 91:110, 1964.
35. Takagi T, Takayasu H, Go T, Aso Y: Fiberoptic pyeloureteroscope. Surgery 70:661, 1971.
36. Ryan ES, Kyker JS, Schoenberg HW: Transurethral ureteroscopy in women: A real addition to the urologic armamentarium. J Urol 119:35, 1978.
37. Huffman JL, Bagley DH, Lyon ES: Extending cystoscopic techniques into the ureter and renal pelvis—experience with ureteroscopy and pyeloscopy. JAMA 250:2004, 1983.
38. Huffman JL, Bagley DH, Schoenberg HW, et al: Transurethral removal of large ureteral and renal pelvic calculi using ureteroscopic ultrasonic lithotripsy. J Urol 130:31, 1983.
39. Watson G, Murray S, Dretler SP, et al: The pulsed dye laser for fragmenting ureteral urinary calculi. J Urol 138:195, 1987.
40. Green DF, Lytton B: Early experience with direct vision electrohydraulic lithotripsy of ureteral calculi. J Urol 133:767, 1985.

2

Physicochemistry of Stone Formation

John L. Meyer

In its simplest form, the initiation and growth of urinary calculi involve a chemical precipitation of dissolved ions or molecules from a solution that has become supersaturated with respect to those components as the glomerular filtrate traverses the nephron. To understand how this can occur from a physicochemical point of view, one must first understand in general terms how the degree of supersaturation or undersaturation of a given solution (urine) influences the probability that a urinary stone will form or, if already present, dissolve.

A relatively simple diagram (Fig. 2–1) depicts the states of saturation of any solution, and an understanding of the concepts, probabilities, and predictions it conveys is crucial for the following discussion and, ultimately, for an understanding of what role the chemistry of urine plays in the formation of calculi. Before this diagram is discussed in some detail, however, one must consider the actual crystalline components that will be encountered in the various stone disease states. These components have been well known for a number of years, particularly through the pioneering work of Prien.[1] The principal ones are calcium oxalate monohydrate ($CaOx \cdot H_2O$, whewelite), calcium oxalate dihydrate ($CaOx \cdot 2H_2O$, weddelite), calcium phosphate ($Ca_5(PO_4)_3OH$, apatite), magnesium ammonium phosphate ($Mg(NH_4)(PO_4)$, struvite), uric acid, and cystine.

STATES OF SATURATION

Figure 2–1 illustrates three general conditions for a solution containing ions or molecules of sparingly soluble crystalline materials. The diagram is constructed with increasing "concentration product" from bottom to top. Concentration product refers to a mathematical expression that can be related to the solubility product of the stone component under consideration. For example, the concentration product expression for hydroxyapatite (chemical formula above), the

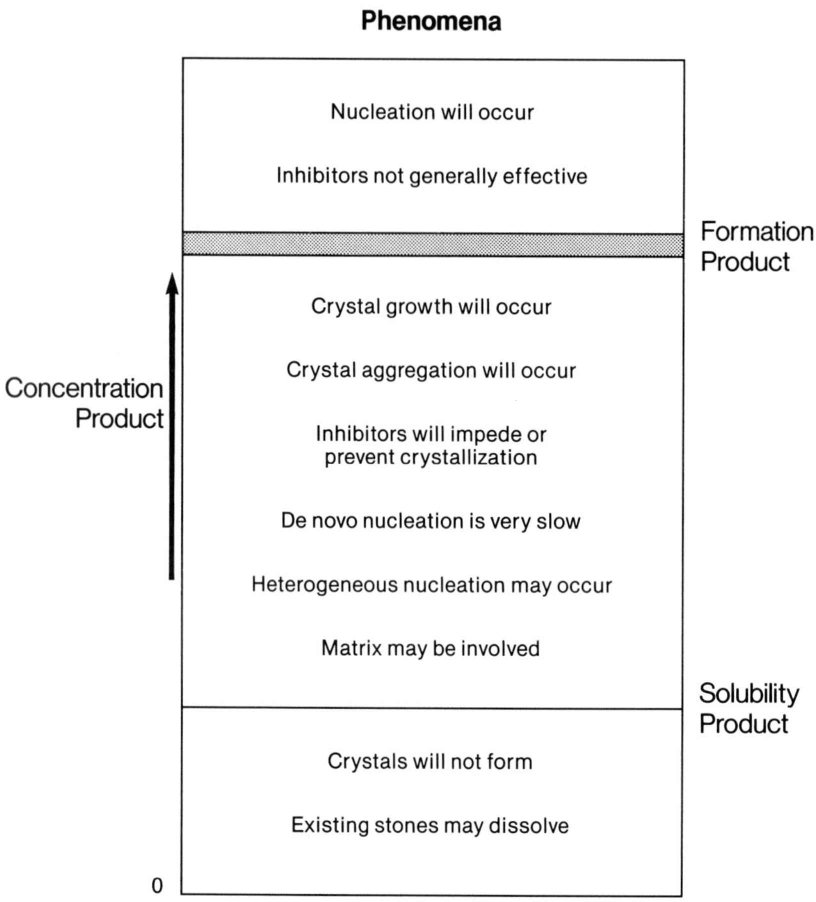

FIGURE 2–1. States of saturation. Listed are solid-solution phenomena that are likely to occur at a given range of concentration products. Three general situations are considered: (1) concentrations less than the solubility product (undersaturation), (2) concentrations that are metastable with respect to de novo precipitation (between the solubility product and the formation product), and (3) concentrations that are greater than the formation product (unstable).

mineral prototype for the apatites formed in biologic systems, is

$$CP = [Ca^{2+}]^5[PO_4^{3-}]^3[OH^-] \quad (1)$$

Similarly, the expression for a simple molecular crystalline material, such as fully protonated uric acid (HU), is

$$CP = [HU] \quad (2)$$

On the right-hand side of the diagram, the relative positions of the "solubility product" and the "formation product" for each of the stone components are indicated. Units and numerical values are not included in the diagram, since they are different for each of the stone components; however, the general features of Figure 2–1 apply to all the crystalline materials. The solubility product, K_{sp}, is the concentration product at which dissolved and crystalline components are in equilibrium with each other at a given set of conditions. The formation product, K_f, is the concentration product at which the stone component will begin to precipitate (at a kinetically significant rate) in the absence of preformed crystalline material. The solubility product is an invariant constant for a pure crystalline material, at a given temperature. The formation product is much more difficult to reproduce experimentally, probably because it is dependent upon the kinetics of initial phase separation rather than the thermodynamic properties of solid-solution equilibrium, and this is indicated in the diagram by a shaded area.

Strictly speaking, the ionic "activities," not concentrations of the dissolved species, govern the solubility principles described here. Ionic activities are influenced by the presence of other ions in solution (ionic strength) and by the presence of other species that form complex ions, thereby reducing their "free" concentrations in solution. These considerations do not detract from the qualitative discussions that follow. In this chapter, qualitative comparisons are used to focus on the chemistry of the stone-forming process of each of the crystalline components and the effects of metabolic intervention on the propensity for further stone growth. For those interested in how the true thermodynamics of the urinary system can be determined from chemical analysis, an appendix describing computational procedures is provided at the end of the chapter.

The solubility product and the formation product are the concentration terms that differentiate the three major states of saturation in urine. At concentration products below K_{sp}, it is impossible for crystals to form under any circumstances. Crystals added to such a solution would dissolve until the solution becomes saturated. Thus, it is theoretically possible to dissolve stones already present, assuming that the urine can be made undersaturated with respect to that crystalline phase and that the undersaturated urine is not prevented from coming in contact with the existing stone. At concentration products greater than K_f, nucleation, the initial formation of a new crystalline phase, will occur. Under these conditions, the driving force for the formation of the solid phase is so great that little, if anything, can be done to stop it. Thus, in urinary infections, the rise in pH, coupled with the high concentrations of ammonium ion (discussed in more detail further on), causes the ion product [Mg] [NH_4] [PO_4] to become so much greater than K_{sp} that struvite stone formation is uncontrollable in many instances until the infection can be brought under control.

The region of most interest from a chemical point of view is the urinary concentration range between the saturated state (K_{sp}) and the "unstable" state (greater than K_f), where crystallization cannot be prevented. This "metastable" state also happens to be of the most interest from a biologic and medical point of view, since the urines of *both* normal and stone-forming subjects seem often to have concentration products in that range for the most common urinary calculi components.[2] This is also the region in which there is more biologic control of the factors that influence stone formation and growth and in which therapeutic interventions seem to be most beneficial. In this region, there is a precarious balance between forces that would accelerate the stone-forming process and those that would delay or prevent it. In this concentration product range, the ability of urine to engage in the heterogeneous nucleation of new crystalline phase and the crystal growth or aggregation of existing crystals is counterbalanced by the presence of specific inhibitors. The relative importance of each of these opposing forces may indeed presage the formation of a new stone in a given urinary system.

Before each of these factors that influence the probability of forming a stone is described, the phenomena operative in the metastable concentration range will be looked at in greater detail. The energetics of this range allow for the crystal growth on existing crystals but not for the de novo formation of crystals in the time it takes for filtered urine to reach the bladder. However, there would appear to be three different situations allowing for the appearance of crystalline phase in this region. First, local nephron or upper urinary tract concentration products may exceed K_f for a period long enough for significant nucleation to occur. This situation could not be detected by "average" bladder concentrations. Second, there may be anatomic regions within the kidney that allow for stasis of the metastable urine. Any metastable solution, given enough time, will form nuclei, which will then undergo crystal growth. Again, nucleation is a kinetic, not a thermodynamic, phenomenon. Finally, urine contains a number of microscopic impurities that would aid in the nucleation process. It has been shown theoretically and experimentally that there are a number of potential urinary constituents that would allow the crystal lattice ions of a given urinary stone crystal (e.g., calcium and oxalate ions) to nucleate at a concentration product much less than the K_f determined in pure solutions. The mechanism would appear to be the absorption of the crystal lattice components, first in a two- and then in a three-dimensional array in a geometric arrangement similar to that of the native crystal. In this way, the high energies required for nucleation in a "homogeneous" solution are circumvented. In general, the closer the fit of the molecular dimensions of the impurity to that of the lattice dimensions of the newly formed stone crystal, the more effective the induced nucleation will be. The generic name for this process is "heterogeneous" nucleation. In special cases in which the fit is so precise that the newly formed phase overgrows the substrate, the term is "epitaxial" nucleation.

There is another common component of urinary stones that may play a role here, and that is the ubiquitous organic matrix. It has been well known and well characterized for a number of years.[3] Since the matrix is structurally integrated within the stone, is of relatively constant chemical composition, and is found as a constant percentage by weight (depending on the stone material), it is tempting to conclude that its architecture is essential for stone growth. It is entirely possible that stone matrix acts as a nucleation site, as described above; however, there is little experimental evidence to support this hypothesis. It is perhaps just as likely that the stone matrix is a product of nonspecific adsorption of certain common urinary constituents unrelated to the stone-forming process. In fact, the opposite argument could be made that the presence of a mucoprotein coat impedes the further growth of the stone and any possible dissolution of a stone from an undersaturated urine. In any event, stone matrix remains a scientific curiosity and merits further study.

By whatever mechanism, the crucial event that must occur for stones to form in human urine is nucleation. This event by itself is not enough, however, since nuclei are very small in comparison to the diameter of the nephron and should be washed harmlessly into the urine. Crystal growth alone will not allow the initially formed nuclei to become large enough to get lodged in the urinary tract in the time scale required for filtered urine to reach the bladder. If enough nuclei are formed and continue to grow, they will, if unhindered, "aggregate" into larger particles, which have a greater probability of becoming trapped in the kidney. Alternatively, the individual nuclei and aggregates may adhere to membrane walls or be deposited in some anatomic structure within the kidney and continue to grow and aggregate as the supersaturated urine flows past until they are too large to pass the kidney.

Given the clinical analytical data that urine is often supersaturated with respect to the most common stone components,[2] the fact that there are a number of predisposing factors that allow for the formation of stone crystals in urine, and the relatively long life (number of opportunities to initiate stone growth) of the human population, the real question would appear not to be what causes stone growth but, perhaps more important, why everyone does not form stones. One answer to this question may be that there are a number of substances in human urine that act rather specifically and at very low concentrations to inhibit the growth and aggregation of stone crystals. These "inhibitors" are quite specific to the type of crystals they affect, and pertinent examples will be given further on. The mechanism of action appears to be the adsorption of the inhibitors to specific growth sites on the crystal surfaces, which are thought to be dislocations in the crystal lattice. This adsorption prevents the further deposition of crystal lattice ions and prevents the crystals from "sticking" together in an aggregation process. These growth sites constitute only a small fraction of the total surface; therefore, only a small concentration of a specific inhibitor is required to adsorb at these sites and prevent crystal growth and aggregation over the entire crystal. As mentioned previously, the stone matrix may play a role here, perhaps in a rather nonspecific fashion, by serving as a diffusion barrier for ions entering and leaving the stone crystal lattice.

Figure 2–2 illustrates this phenomenon in a schematic fashion. Under normal crystal growth conditions, lattice ions such as calcium and oxalate adsorb to preformed calcium oxalate crystals and migrate toward the energetically favorable sites on the surface, where they are incorporated into the crystal lattice. Adsorption of inhibitor molecules (indicated by spheres in this figure) effectively "hides" the growth sites, and the adsorbed ions are left to migrate randomly across the surface, unable to add to the crystal mass. Adsorption of inhibitors will also tend to change the surface charge, affecting the attractive forces between crystals, resulting in altered degrees of aggregation.

The difference between a stone-forming urine and a normal urine, therefore, may be dependent on whether the stone-promoting potential (as indicated in Fig. 2–1) or the stone-inhibiting ability of the urinary components is dominant. Somewhat successful predictors of stone disease have been developed on this basis.[4, 5] From a therapeutic point of view, a general strategy would be to reduce the risk factors and increase the number and concentration of inhibitors. In practice, it appears that the most important intervention is to lower the supersaturation. As mentioned earlier, stone formation *cannot* occur from an

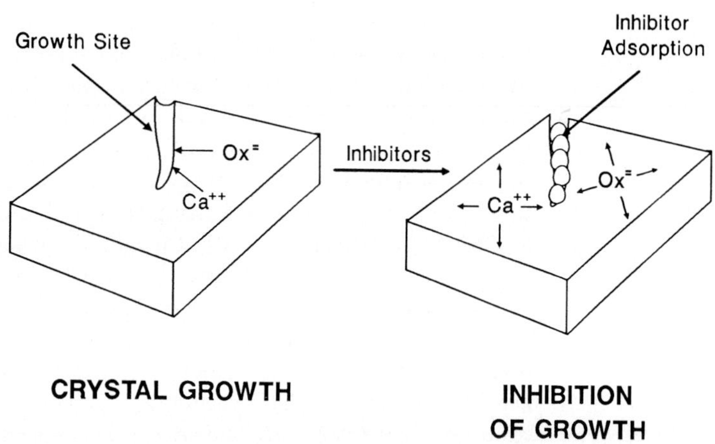

FIGURE 2–2. Crystal growth inhibition. Inhibitor molecules (spheres) selectively adsorb at growth sites on crystal surfaces. Adsorbed lattice ions, such as calcium and oxalate, instead of being incorporated into the crystal at these dislocations, migrate randomly across the surface.

undersaturated solution, and under favorable conditions dissolution of existing stones can occur.

Dissolution can be accomplished by a number of strategies from a chemical point of view. The simplest is dilution (increased fluid intake). Other viable approaches include the following:

1. Decreased ingestion or decreased intestinal absorption, or both, by binding agents or transport blockers.
2. Decreased metabolic production by enzymatic and hormonal interactions.
3. Decreased renal clearance by agents that enhance tubular reabsorption or decrease tubular secretion.
4. Administration of agents (such as citrate ion) that form complexes with stone components, thereby reducing the free ionic activity.
5. Affecting the pH of urines containing substances whose free concentrations are sensitive to acid-base reactions in the urinary pH range.

All of the above interventions have been successful to a greater or lesser degree, and specific examples will be given further on.

More problematic, however, is any attempt to increase the inhibitory power of human urine. Attempts to increase the natural inhibitors in urine have met with limited success, and these substances cannot, in general, be given as oral drugs, since they are readily metabolized in the gut. A number of potent inhibitors of crystal growth and aggregation have been synthesized that are not subject to enzymatic degradation; however, they also appear to affect bone metabolism (e.g., calcium phosphate is present in stones and bone) and produce undesirable side effects.

INDIVIDUAL STONE COMPONENTS

Following the preceding discussion, the focus is now on each of the common urinary stone components and on their individual solid-solution chemistry. An attempt is made to understand why they form solid concretions in urine and to devise therapeutic strategies, from a solution chemist's point of view, to prevent the formation of new stones or to treat existing ones. In the not so rare event that stones of mixed composition are under consideration, an understanding of the overall chemistry of human urine should allow for a judicious compromise among alternate approaches.

In the treatment of urolithiasis, the most important consideration is the composition of the stones. As shall be seen further on, an attempt to alter the urine chemistry to prevent the formation of one kind of calculus could result in the calamitous formation of another solid concretion. The general approach in the following paragraphs is to determine how to alter clinically the urine chemistry of stone formers first to prevent the precipitation of new material and possibly dissolve some or all of any existing stones. Each of the crystalline materials found to exist to any significant extent in human urinary calculi is discussed.

Calcium Phosphate. The discussion begins with the solid phase with perhaps the most complicated solid-solution chemistry. The various calcium phosphate phases are also among the most common and are found in greater or lesser amounts in a high percentage of human calculi. "Pure" calcium phosphate stones are relatively rare, however, accounting for only a few per cent of most populations. The most common form is termed "apatitic," with an x-ray diffraction pattern similar to that of the well-defined hydroxyapatite, $Ca_5(PO_4)_3OH$. The apatite lattice easily picks up impurities such as carbonate. This ion readily substitutes for phosphate in urines containing high concentrations of carbonate ion, and this material is usually referred to as carbonate apatite. A rare form of solid calcium phosphate in calculi is brushite, $CaHPO_4 \cdot 2H_2O$, which forms from more acidic urine, high in calcium and phosphate concentration, such as that found in renal tubular acidosis.

Whatever the actual composition of the calcium phosphate phase, a similar approach would be used to increase its solubility, since the same chemical principles apply to all phases, pure or impure. The attempt is to reduce the relative saturation of the stone former's urine with respect to calcium phosphate. The relative saturation ratio or concentration product ratio (CPR) can be defined as the ratio of the concentration product for a given urine to that of the solubility product (in this case for hydroxyapatite):

$$\mathrm{CPR} = \frac{[\mathrm{Ca}^{2+}]^5[\mathrm{PO_4}^{3-}]^3[\mathrm{OH}^-]}{K_{sp}} \tag{3}$$

Any reduction in the magnitude of the numerator will make the urine in question less saturated with respect to calcium phosphate and thus reduce the likelihood for the precipitation of solid phase. Thus, from a chemical point of view, any reduction in free calcium ion, Ca^{2+}, free trivalent phosphate ion, PO_4^{3-}, or hydroxide ion, OH^-, will result in a more stable urine.

The total urinary calcium concentration can be reduced by either decreasing the filtered load or increasing tubular reabsorption by the therapeutic means described in the other chapters of this book. The free calcium concentration is dependent on the total urinary concentration but also on the presence of complexing agents, which form stable ion pairs. These include carbonate, phosphate, sulfate, and oxalate species, and, most important, citrate ion. Citrate forms the strongest complexes with calcium and is perhaps the most easily controlled by exogenous means. This reduction in free calcium ion concentration may form the basis for the successful treatment of patients with calcium urolithiasis with citrate salts.[6] Because the free calcium concentration in Equation 3 is raised to the power of 5, decreases in this factor result in marked reductions in the relative saturation of the solution.

The normal urinary concentration of total phosphate ion is relatively high and not easily subject to wide variation by intervention. Although complexes are formed between phosphate ions and calcium and magnesium ions, these are not particularly significant in reducing free phosphate ion concentration. The urinary variable that has the greatest impact on the free trivalent phosphate ion concentration is the pH of the solution. This is because the PO_4^{3-} concentration is dependent upon the position of the acid-base equilibria of the two principal phosphate species that exist in the normal urinary pH range, HPO_4^{2-} and $H_2PO_4^-$.

$$H_2PO_4^- = HPO_4^{2-} + H^+ \tag{4}$$

$$HPO_4^{2-} = PO_4^{3-} + H^+ \tag{5}$$

According to the equilibria above, an increase in hydrogen ion concentration will shift both equations to the left, resulting in a lower free PO_4^{3-} concentration. Thus, a decrease by one pH unit (a 10-fold increase in H^+ concentration) results in a corresponding 10-fold decrease in free PO_4^{3-} concentration, with no change in urine phosphate. Since it is the PO_4^{3-} species that appears in the concentration product expression, raised to the power of 3, a 30-fold decrease in CPR results. This, coupled with the fact that OH^- also appears in the expression (inversely proportional to H^+ concentration), results in a 40-fold decrease in CPR. This observation explains why the solubility of the calcium phosphates is extremely sensitive to pH. Therefore, low urinary pH tends to preclude the formation of calcium phosphate as a major or minor component of urinary calculi, whereas high urinary pH is a definite risk factor for calcium phosphate precipitation. The common occurrence of apatite accompanying struvite in the high-pH milieu of infected stones is support for this view.

Of potential importance in the pathogenesis of human urinary stones is the presence of specific inhibitors of crystal growth and aggregation of calcium phosphate. These tend to be low molecular weight materials, with the majority of the inhibitory potential being ascribed to pyrophosphate, citrate, and magnesium ions and to an as yet unidentified anionic material.[7] It is possible that other low molecular weight materials, such as trace metal ions, may play a role in certain instances.[8, 9] The overall importance of these inhibitors is uncertain at present. The effectiveness of phosphate and citrate therapy for calcium stones may be partially attributable, however, to the accompanying increases in the calcium phosphate inhibitors pyrophosphate and citrate, respectively. This feature is in addition to their ability to reduce the concentration of free calcium ion in urine by complexation or intestinal binding.

Finally, there is little evidence that heterogeneous nucleation is important for the formation of calcium phosphate phases in urine. Matrix may play a role here, but the evidence is inconclusive. Although apatite is often found near the center of mixed calculi[1] (suggesting a role in nucleating other phases), there is little evidence to suggest that other urinary components can facilitate the separation of calcium phosphate phases.

Uric Acid. The solid-solution chemistry of uric acid and cystine is relatively simple, compared with that of the calcium phosphates, since these components precipitate as the uncharged free acid. Although uric acid has two potentially dissociable protons, only the first is of importance in the urinary pH range, and free, undissociated uric acid will be designated HU. The proton dissociation equilibrium is

$$HU = U^- + H^+ \qquad (6)$$

and the CPR is defined by

$$CPR = \frac{[HU]}{K_{sp}} \qquad (7)$$

Since uric acid does not appear to form stable ion pairs with other urine components and since neither natural inhibitors nor heterogeneous nucleators seem to influence the formation of solid uric acid, the only parameters that are important in the physicochemistry of uric acid stone disease are total urinary urate and pH. As with phosphate, a decrease in urinary pH (increase in H^+ concentration) results in a shift of the equilibrium to the left, resulting in a greater HU concentration. HU, however, is the insoluble form of uric acid, and a decreased pH creates a more supersaturated solution (greater CPR) and an increased risk for uric acid stone disease.

The solubility of pure uric acid is about 43 mg/liter, and it has a first acid dissociation constant with a pK of 5.5.[10] In other words, only 43 mg of the undissociated uric acid, HU, will remain in solution in 1 liter of urine in a stable state. In addition, the value given for the pK suggests that at a pH of 5.5 (equal to the pK) 50 per cent of the total urate in urine would exist as the insoluble HU form of uric acid. Therefore, a urinary pH of 5.5 would support a stable uric acid concentration of 86 mg/liter (43 mg/liter of HU + 43 mg/liter of soluble U^-). The relationship between pK and pH is such that for every one pH unit there is about a 90 per cent change in the HU/U^- ratio. For example, at a pH of 6.5 (one pH unit higher than the pK), a much smaller percentage of the total urate in urine exists in the insoluble HU form, meaning that 472 mg/liter could remain in an undersaturated state (43 mg/liter of HU plus 430 mg/liter of U^-, a 1:10 ratio). Thus, it is clear that the tendency to form uric acid stones can be reversed by simple manipulation of urinary pH, since the solubility of uric acid is so sensitive to pH.

There are two possible complications introduced by an increase in urinary pH in this system that should be considered regardless of the effect of urinary pH on the metabolism and transport of other urinary components. First, if the pH remains too high, as discussed previously, there is an increased risk for the formation of solid calcium phosphate. Second, some salts of the more soluble urate ion, U^-, are also sparingly soluble, such as sodium urate formed in gout. Such salts are rarely found in urine, however.

This discussion would suggest that the approaches to be used to decrease the solubility of uric acid in a stone-forming urine would be a reduction in systemic uric acid concentration by dietary or enzymatic means (such as allopurinol), or both, coupled with modest increases in urinary pH.

CYSTINE. The solid-solution chemistry of cystine is very similar to that of uric acid, in principle, except that the first pK for cystine is much larger, 8.0. The acid dissociation of cystine (H_2CSSC) can be represented by the following:

$$H_2CSSC = HCSSC^- + H^+ \tag{8}$$

and the CPR can be shown by

$$CPR = \frac{[H_2CSSC]}{K_{sp}} \tag{9}$$

As with uric acid, cystine does not form significant concentrations of ion pairs with other urine components and neither inhibitors nor heterogeneous nucleators appear to be a factor in its stone-forming chemistry. As opposed to uric acid, which would appear to be a threat to the general population, particularly those individuals with consistently acid urines, cystine stone formation occurs only in those patients with a genetic defect resulting in cystinuria. The physicochemical approach used to reduce the propensity for urine cystine precipitation, as noted above for uric acid, would be to increase urinary pH or reduce the urine concentration of cystine or both. This approach is not as easily accomplished for cystine as it is for uric acid, however. First, the pH must be increased to a much higher value to effect a significant change in solubility (because of the higher pK). This much higher pH results in a much greater risk for the formation of apatitic compounds. Second, since cystine is an essential metabolite (as opposed to uric acid), enzymatic interventions cannot be used to reduce its filtered load. Instead, other approaches must be used, such as administering sulfur-containing compounds that compete with the monomer cysteine to form more soluble disulfide compounds with cysteine than the stone-forming cystine. Some of these compounds produce significant side effects, however.

Calcium Oxalate. Calcium oxalate is the most common major urinary stone component, and most clinical attention is directed toward this crystalline material. Although two distinct crystallographic forms, the monohydrate and dihydrate, are commonly found in stones, the chemical approaches to reduce the likelihood of calcium oxalate urolithiasis are essentially the same for both crystal forms. In practical terms, the only difference between the two is that the dihydrate is slightly more soluble and often is the first precipitable phase. The CPR for both substances is

$$CPR = \frac{[Ca^{2+}][Ox^{2-}]}{K_{sp}} \tag{10}$$

where Ox^{2-} is the abbreviation for the oxalate ion $C_2O_4^{2-}$. Oxalic acid is a relatively strong acid, with the second acid dissociation reaction having a pK of about 4. This equilibrium is illustrated by the following equation:

$$HOx^- = Ox^{2-} + H^+ \tag{11}$$

Such a low pK for the above reaction results in the situation that changes in urinary pH within the range available by common therapeutic means will have little effect on the free concentration of Ox^{2-} and thus on the CPR. In fact, any attempt to maintain a low enough pH (less than 5) to affect the above equilibrium significantly would create a risk factor for uric acid urolithiasis.

The CPR for calcium oxalate is a simple expression involving free Ca^{2+} and Ox^{2-}. Since it is not practical to affect solubility by manipulating urinary pH, the only available means to reduce the driving force for stone formation, the CPR, is a reduction in free calcium and oxalate concentrations. As discussed previously for calcium phosphate, calcium delivery to the upper urinary tract can be reduced by decreased intestinal absorption (indigestible calcium binders, such as cellulose phosphate, or the formation of insoluble precipitates, as in inorganic phosphate therapy) or by decreased renal clearance (thiazides). This topic is discussed in Chapter 3. The administration of strong chelating agents, such as citrate ion, should also be effective in reducing the free calcium concentration in the total urinary load.

Reductions in free oxalate concentrations are not as easy to conceptualize, since a common source does not exist for this stone component. Urinary oxalate results from both dietary and metabolic components. Complicating the issue is the fact that urinary oxalate is normally excreted at only about one-tenth the concentration of calcium and that the analytical methodology for oxalate, particularly free oxalate, is not as precise as that available for calcium. Nonetheless, a few general strategies can be employed to reduce the urinary concentration of oxalate. For the hyperabsorptive states, binding agents have been tried with some success. One of these, oral calcium, would seem to be of limited success from a physicochemical point of view, since urinary calcium, the other term in the CPR (Equation 10), would be expected to increase. The argument has been made, however, that stone formation is more sensitive to the urine oxalate concentration than the filtered load of calcium. The overproduction of oxalate can also be treated, in principle, by affecting the metabolic pathways for oxalic acid formation. Agents such as pyridoxine have been used for this purpose.[11] The primary complexing agents in urine for oxalate are divalent calcium and magnesium ions. Reduction of free oxalate ion by increasing their concentrations would not seem to be of much practical importance, however.

From a chemical point of view, the simplest and apparently an effective means of reducing the CPR of calcium oxalate (at least for the "normal" calciuric and oxaluric states, in which it is not clear which of the lattice ions is posing the greatest threat for stone formation) is increasing fluid intake, thereby reducing the concentration of both terms that appear in the CPR and thus the tendency to precipitate calcium oxalate. As noted previously, many of the therapeutic interventions that reduce oxalate concentration increase calcium ion concentration and vice versa. The physicochemistry of urine dictates that all parameters should be considered before a single therapeutic approach is attempted with the sole purpose of reducing the concentration product of calcium oxalate in urine.

The precipitation of calcium oxalate is strongly influenced by factors other than the state of saturation of the solution. There are a number of substances present in normal urine, often in lesser concentrations in stone-forming urine, that are known to inhibit the growth and aggregation of calcium oxalate. Most of these are not ordinarily dialyzable, as they have molecular weights greater than 10,000. There is some low molecular weight activity, however, mostly attributable to pyrophosphate and citrate ion. As for calcium phosphate, part of the effectiveness of inorganic phosphate and citrate therapy can be assigned to increased concentrations of these species in urine as calcium oxalate crystallization inhibitors. The majority of the activity consists of high molecular weight anionic substances, however, that are effective in inhibiting calcium oxalate at very low concentrations. Classes of molecules that have been identified in human urine include glycosaminoglycans[12] (such as chondroitin sulfate), ribonucleic acid (RNA) fragments,[13] and a group of well-characterized glycoproteins.[14] The relative importance of each of these high molecular weight inhibitors is uncertain at present, but each of them has the potential to affect calcium oxalate crystallization significantly. It may be important that some stone formers' urines contain a lower concentration of inhibitor. However, since inhibitors function by adsorption to crystal surfaces, it is possible that the decreased urine concentration merely reflects the reduction of normal concentrations of inhibitor by adsorption on actively growing stone surfaces.

As presented earlier, it is difficult, from a physicochemistry approach, to verify whether supersaturation or inhibition (Fig. 2–1) is dominant in controlling calcium oxalate crystal growth and aggregation in urine and, presumably, calcium oxalate urolithiasis. Attempts have been made to combine the two measurements in various ways in a rational approach to consider both variables in conjunction with various metabolically defined disease states with success.[4, 5] In these studies, a concentration product term, such as the CPR, is combined with an inhibitor-sensitive term, such as the formation product ratio (FPR). The FPR is discussed in more detail later in the chapter. The consideration of the two terms together tends to differentiate more clearly normal urines from those with a propensity for stone formation.

There is a final complicating factor, essentially unique to calcium oxalate, that makes it more difficult to predict whether calcium oxalate stones will form, and that is the potential presence in urine of a number of effective heterogeneous nucleating agents. Given the data that the urines of both normal subjects and patients with stones are often supersaturated with respect to calcium oxalate[2] and that it is difficult (from a solution chemistry approach) to ensure that an undersaturated urine can be maintained indefinitely by metabolic manipulations, heterogeneous nucleation may be the driving force that alters a "metastable" urine so that it becomes an "unstable" urine allowing the nucleation of the first calcium oxalate crystals. As discussed, once the first nuclei are formed, crystal growth and aggregation processes can occur at the much lower concentrations present in the metastable state (as shown in Fig. 2–1).

There is only circumstantial evidence that this phenomenon actually occurs in vivo, however. First, there is ample evidence, in vitro, that substances such as apatite, brushite, and uric acid can reduce the time required for nucleation from a metastable solution of calcium oxalate (see further on). Second, careful inspection of human calculi containing calcium oxalate often reveals the presence of other phases, particularly calcium phosphate and uric acid. In this regard, it may be of interest that intranephronic calculosis (calcium phosphate) has been consistently observed in the kidneys of calcium oxalate stone formers, but not in non–stone formers or patients with other forms of stone disease.[15] Furthermore, there appears to be a link between hyperuricosuria and the incidence of calcium oxalate stone disease. Treatment by agents that reduce urine uric acid concentration, such as allopurinol, appears to be beneficial.[16, 17] A direct cause and effect relationship has yet to be established; however, it is tempting to conclude that the patients with calcium oxalate stones and hyperuricosuria form uric acid or urate crystals that serve as the heterogeneous nucleating sites.

STRUVITE. As with cystine stones, there is only one situation in which struvite (magnesium ammonium phosphate) is formed in human urine, and that is accompanying urinary tract infection. Only under this condition are the ionic components that contribute to the CPR,

$$CPR = \frac{[Mg^{2+}][NH_4^{+}][PO_4^{3-}]}{K_{sp}} \tag{12}$$

formed in sufficiently high concentrations to result in the precipitation of struvite. The ion unique to struvite stones is the ammonium ion, generated as ammonia by the urease enzyme, which is produced by the infection. The production of ammonia is especially harmful; not only does it supply the crucial ion needed for the CPR to be at the supersaturated level (NH_4^+) but also it reacts with available hydrogen ion by the following reaction to increase the pH of the solution.

$$NH_3 + H^+ = NH_4^+ \tag{13}$$

This decrease in hydrogen ion concentration increases the free trivalent phosphate concentration (see Equation 5), which also increases the magnitude of the CPR, in turn causing the urine to become unstable and allowing stone formation to occur. The high pH brought about by the production of ammonia is also ideal for the precipitation of apatites, and mixed struvite-apatite infection stones are common.

The appearance of significant concentrations of ammonium ion, coupled with the high pH, is such an overwhelming predisposing factor for stone formation that other considerations, such as complexing agents, inhibitors, or heterogeneous nucleators, appear to play little, if any, role in the overall process. In fact, the stone-forming process can be slowed or stopped even if the infection continues by merely preventing the metabolism of urea with urease inhibitors.[18] The production of ammonia is curtailed, and the two essential ingredients for struvite precipitation, ammonium ion and high pH, are eliminated, and thus struvite formation is impossible. This circumstance allows time for the physician to treat the infection without the complication of new calculi formation. In addition, the maintenance of a low urine pH and ammonium ion concentration results in an undersaturated solution, which would permit, under favorable conditions, the dissolution of any stone material that may have formed before treatment could begin.

Historical Perspective. The physicochemical phenomena described in Figure 2–1 and the solid-solution chemistry for each of the urinary stone components had been known for a number of years before this knowledge was applied to the study of urolithiasis. A number of pioneers in this field had the foresight to apply the chemical principles developed in "pure" systems to the exceedingly complex system of human urine. The essential beginnings of much of what is known today was developed by these medical scientists in the late 1950s to the middle 1960s. This chapter represents an amplification of these early theories and observations, building upon more modern results and methodologies as well.

The ability of human urine to exist in a metastable supersaturated state was recognized by Vermeulen and his coworkers[19] when they made the observation that solid concretions grown in vitro from urine on a suitable substrate had many of the features of urinary calculi. They were able to predict correctly that the appropriate changes in concentration, complexing agents, and pH, as discussed previously, could and would markedly affect the ability of urine to form precipitates. Thus, it was proved that the chemistry so well known in simple systems could be applied to an understanding of a complicated disease process in vivo.

The fact that human urine contains substances that affect crystallization other than those that influence the supersaturation, as proposed by Vermeulen, was suggested by the pioneering observations of John Eager Howard and colleagues.[20] He noted that urines from normal subjects and patients who had previously had stones but who were no longer making stones were unable to calcify rachitic rat cartilage, whereas similar, isotonic urines from patients with metabolically active stone disease calcified the cartilage readily. He termed these "good" and "evil" urines, respectively. A similar situation appeared to occur in uremic bone disease, in which the substances (now known as crystal growth inhibitors) that caused the "good" urines were no longer removed from the serum via the kidney, became concentrated, and interfered with normal bone (calcium phosphate) metabolism. It is now believed that the components contributing to "good" urines are pyrophosphate, citrate, and magnesium ions and an unidentified low molecular weight component. This last species was tentatively identified as phosphocitrate by Howard and his coworkers.[21] It should be noted that the early studies focused on inhibitors of calcium phosphate crystallization, but similar principles were applied in later years to the study of other classes of inhibitors, such as the high molecular weight anionic substances noted previously, which seem to be so important for regulating calcium oxalate stone formation.

If inhibitors of crystal growth are present in urine, it would seem possible that promoters of the crystallization process would also be present in such a complex mixture. Studies of such promoters historically have centered on two types of substances, both of which would accelerate the stone-forming process by acting as nidi for heterogeneous nucleation. The first substance studied in detail is the organic matrix, present as an architecturally defined component of *all* calculi. The most comprehensive and careful studies on the organic matrix present in human stones were carried out by William Boyce and colleagues at Bowman-Gray.[3] Although slight variations were noted in the chemical composition and per cent abundance by weight for each of the different types of stone components, the organic matrix appeared to be remarkably similar in all settings. Since it became clear early on that apparently similar individuals with similar urine chemistries had markedly different stone formation potentials, it was tempting to conclude that stone formers producd a matrix that served as a nidus that induced crystallization from an otherwise metastable supersaturated urine. Ultrastructural examination of stones reinforced the intimate and interrelated nature of matrix and crystalline phase. Unfortunately, attempts to support this concept in vitro using demineralized stone matrix as a substrate for controlled heterogeneous nucleation have yielded equivocal results. Thus, the role of matrix in the stone-forming process remains an intellectual curiosity.

The second type of substance that showed promise as a "promoter" of stone formation was a different crystalline phase, which could act as a substrate for heterogeneous nucleation. Kathleen Lonsdale proposed in 1968[22] that epitaxy or, more generally, heterogeneous nucleation was likely to occur among the crystallographically defined urinary stone components based upon the excellent matching of their lattice dimensions. She deemed that there were too many close fits to be purely coincidental and that epitaxy must play a role in urolithiasis. Subsequent in vitro studies have proved her correct. However, the ability of one crystalline material to nucleate another effectively is not as universal as predicted by crystal lattice dimensions alone, and other factors must be operative. Nevertheless, it has been shown that pure crystals of some stone components can induce nucleation at a supersaturation much below its normal formation product for "spontaneous" nucleation (see discussion further on). Thus, the potential exists for this mechanism in human urine, although it has not been specifically proved to occur in vivo. Perhaps the most likely candidate for epitaxial nucleation is calcium oxalate, since a number of stone crystals are known to nucleate this material in vitro and there is a rather high percentage of idiopathic calcium oxalate stone formers for whom the other known causes of calculi production have been ruled out.

TECHNICAL ASPECTS

The discussions and conclusions of the preceding sections have relied extensively upon experimental results obtained in actual or simulated urines in an attempt to verify which of the chemical principles known to be relevant for pure solutions are important in controlling urinary stone formation. As discussed earlier, the likelihood of a given urine to produce calculi would seem to be dependent on the delicate balance between the tendency to precipitate dissolved stone components and the ability of human urine to counteract this process. To determine experimentally the relative magnitude of each of these opposing forces, and thus gain insight into the stone-forming process, a number of methodologies have been described to address this problem. These are summarized here. An exhaustive review is not presented but, rather, selective techniques are chosen that illustrate a spectrum of the types of experimental approaches that have been and can be used.

SUPERSATURATION. Stone formation and growth are thermodynamically impossible unless the glomerular filtrate and subsequent intranephron solutions become supersaturated with respect to the stone material. The greater the supersaturation, the greater the driving force for precipitation and the greater the probability for stone initiation and growth. The supersaturation of a given freshly voided urine (which is assumed to be the same as that of the upper urinary tract, where stone initiation actually occurs) either can be calculated *ab initio* or can be determined experimentally.

Insight into the mathematical procedure, which requires chemical analysis of all major urine components, is presented in the appendix to this chapter. Computer programs have been written to perform the calculations. A good example is the EQUIL program written by Finlayson.[23]

The principle underlying the experimental procedure for determining relative supersaturation (or undersaturation) is to equilibrate a freshly voided urine at body temperature with pure crystals of the stone material under investigation until the urine becomes saturated with respect to that phase. For example, a urine supersaturated with respect to calcium oxalate would be continually mixed with synthetic crystals of calcium oxalate monohydrate until the calcium and oxalate concentrations stabilized in solution.[24] If the urine were supersaturated, calcium and oxalate concentrations would decrease until saturation was attained. An undersaturated urine would be identified by an increase in the lattice ions, as the added crystals would dissolve to reach the stable state. A relative CPR could then be calculated by dividing the products of the total calcium, T_{Ca}, and oxalate, T_{Ox}, concentrations obtained before and after the equilibration step.

$$\text{CPR} = \frac{T_{Ca} \times T_{Ox} \text{ (urine)}}{T_{Ca} \times T_{Ox} \text{ (saturated)}} \tag{14}$$

The CPR obtained in this manner approximates a true free CPR, since the concentrations of ion pairs formed with Ca^{2+} and Ox^{2-} tend to cancel out between the numerator and the denominator. The CPR calculated in this manner also approximates an activity product ratio (APR), since the activity coefficients (see the appendix to the chapter) also tend to cancel out. Potential pitfalls in this type of measurement include the possibility that a saturated state is not attained during the equilibration step (owing to the presence of crystal growth inhibitors) or that during the long reaction times required (up to 2 days) biochemical changes occur in the urine that affect its composition.

Inhibition. The measurement of the amount of inhibition in a given urine is essentially a measurement of the kinetics of the approach to saturation once the solution has been induced to begin crystallization. The solution may be whole urine, diluted urine, or whole urine modified so that its supersaturation is either a well-defined constant value that remains metastable or sufficiently supersaturated so that spontaneous nucleation occurs.

A relatively simple and straightforward method to determine the inhibitory potential of a given urine is to measure its FPR. This measurement is accomplished by adding successively larger concentrations of a stone component—for example, oxalate ion—to aliquots of a urine, letting the samples equilibrate for a fixed period and noting the minimal concentration required for visible nucleation and crystal growth to occur.[24] The higher the concentration required to induce precipitation, the greater the amount of crystallization inhibitor that must be present to balance the driving force for the separation of the solid phase (supersaturation). The actual driving force present can then be calculated by measuring the concentration product after the sample approaches equilibrium (saturation). The calculation is essentially identical with that for the CPR given earlier.

$$\text{FPR} = \frac{T_{Ca} \times T_{Ox} \text{ (formation)}}{T_{Ca} \times T_{Ox} \text{ (saturation)}} \tag{15}$$

Perhaps the most precise measurements of the amount of total inhibition present in urine are those conducted on diluted urines. Dilution presents two advantages. First, the supersaturation of the solution can be carefully controlled so that comparisons can be readily made between different sources of urine. It is difficult to ensure a constant supersaturation in whole urines because of the uncertainties posed by such a complex mixture. Estimates could be made, based upon the computational and experimental methods discussed earlier, but this approach is rather time consuming and tedious, particularly if one wants to screen large numbers of urine samples. The addition of a few per cent urine to a defined in vitro system is convenient and precise. Second, the amount of inhibitor present in whole urine, at least for calcium oxalate and phosphate crystallization, is so great (in normal urines) that the rate of approach to equilibrium is very slow. Dilution allows multiple measurements of inhibitor activity in a realistic time scale. The disadvantage of diluted urine measurements is that the inhibitors are not being evaluated in their natural state and that extrapolation back to whole-urine conditions may lead to erroneous conclusions.

The general technique for determining inhibitor activity in diluted urine is to prepare a metastable supersaturated solution by the careful addition of dissolved stone components to a container maintained at a constant temperature, add a known amount of inhibitor or urine, establish that spontaneous nucleation is not occurring, and add seed crystals of the solid phase. For example, a solution of a soluble oxalate salt could be added dropwise with constant stirring to a solution containing calcium ion until the desired supersaturation is attained, and then seed crystals of calcium oxalate monohydrate could be added to induce the crystallization of calcium oxalate (Fig. 2–3). The kinetics of such a reaction can be monitored by measuring the solution concentration of calcium or oxalate ion, or both, as the precipitation proceeds. The rate laws for the crystal growth of each of the stone materials have been determined, and the reduction in rate constant induced by the inhibition of crystal growth can be quantified.[25] For calcium oxalate, the rate law is

$$\text{Rate} = k[Ca^{2+}][Ox^{2-}] \qquad (16)$$

where k is the rate constant and the terms in the brackets are the free concentrations (or activities) of the lattice ions. Since crystal growth inhibition is an adsorption process, inhibition rate data can be plotted in the form of an adsorption isotherm, such as that proposed by Langmuir, and the resulting linear plot can be used to obtain quantitative data concerning urinary inhibitors.[25]

The mathematical treatment above is for estimating crystal growth inhibition. The same experimental design can also be used to measure aggregation. In this case, it is the increasing size of the particles that is of interest, and these can be monitored by a number of techniques, the most common being with a Coulter counter.[26]

The study of crystallization inhibitors in whole urine is more difficult, but the uncertainty of how a diluted set of urine inhibitors differs from their natural setting is eliminated to a certain extent. However, the urine must still be treated in some fashion to ensure that a supersaturated state is achieved. The only way inhibitory activity can be identified and measured is by its action on the kinetics of a crystallization process, by nucleation, crystal growth, or aggregation. Once all urinary inhibitors have been identified and their individual effectiveness and synergism with other urine components quantified, a simple analytical measurement for inhibitor molecules should suffice for the characterization of total urine inhibition. Until that time, whole-urine inhibition must be measured independently for each urine sample.

There are two ways to increase whole-urine supersaturation: addition of

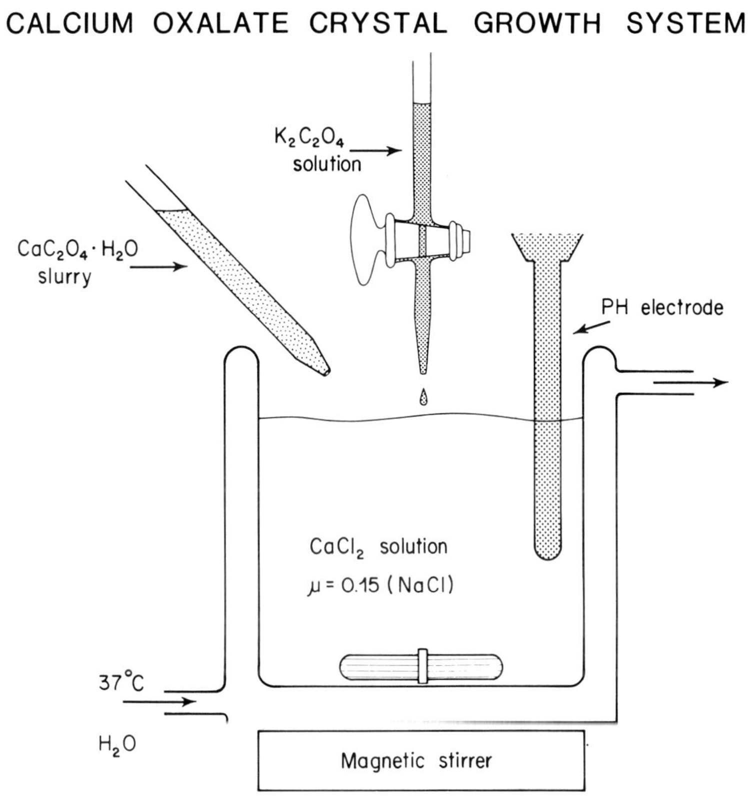

FIGURE 2–3. A typical in vitro crystal growth system. The concentration product for a given stone crystal, such as calcium oxalate, is increased slowly to avoid spontaneous nucleation, at a fixed temperature and pH to a metastable supersaturation. Crystal growth and aggregation are initiated by the addition of the appropriate seed crystals. The effect of inhibitors is noted by adding them to the system before the seed crystals. A constant ionic strength (μ) is desirable. (From Smith LH, Meyer JL; Urinary inhibitors of calcium oxalate crystal growth. *In* Finlayson B, Thomas WC [eds]: Colloquium on Renal Lithiasis. Gainesville, FL, The University Presses of Florida, 1976; with permission.)

soluble stone-forming components or removal of the solvent phase to concentrate the urine. The latter has been used in a semiquantitative manner to assess the number and types of crystals formed from urines, using osmolality as the standardizing feature.[27] Interesting results can be obtained, but osmolality alone does not ensure that solutions with similar potentials for stone formation (i.e., supersaturation) are being compared.

A similar potential problem exists for the whole-urine assays in which additional crystallizing salts are added to the urine before the introduction of seed crystals to measure the rate of crystallization. A rather ingenious tactic has been developed to circumvent this issue, at least for calcium phosphate inhibition, by Fleisch and coworkers.[28] This technique involves first equilibrating a sample of urine with dicalcium phosphate dihydrate (brushite), a calcium phosphate phase more soluble than hydroxyapatite, at a fixed pH and then adjusting other samples of that urine to have the same equilibrated concentration of calcium and phosphate. In this manner, all samples to be tested would have the same relative supersaturation with respect to hydroxyapatite. The relatively large amount of inhibitor usually present in whole urine is then "titrated" by adding successively larger amounts of apatite seed crystals to different tubes containing the adjusted urine and measuring the amount of precipitation in a set period. This approach has been proved to be a highly reproducible technique and has more recently been applied to the quantification of calcium phosphate inhibitors in blood.[29]

Heterogeneous Nucleation. The experimental design for the detection of heterogeneous nucleation or any other phenomenon that would increase the rate of crystallization of stone components is essentially the same as described previously for inhibition studies.[30] In each case, the first step is to prepare a metastable supersaturated solution of a stone material phase (see Fig. 2–3) and then inoculate the solution with a substance believed to accelerate the crystallization process. For example, stable supersaturated solutions of calcium oxalate that are seeded with apatite crystals become unstable, nucleate upon the calcium phosphate solid phase, and then undergo crystal growth until saturated conditions are attained (Fig. 2–4). Uric acid crystals added to a similarly supersaturated solution also appear to nucleate calcium oxalate, as indicated by the solution chemistry and by morphologic examination of the solid phases (Fig. 2–5). This general experimental design has been used to test many of the potential relationships proposed by Lonsdale[22] and others for the various stone crystals. There has been little success, however, with other urine constituents, such as the stone organic matrix or the various macromolecules, and the role of other urinary stone promoters is still open to question.

CONCLUSION

Some diagrams may serve to illustrate some of the most important concepts discussed in this chapter. Figure 2–6 illustrates the principal crystallization phenomena that occur in urine and that play a greater or lesser role in the formation of all the solid phases that make up the human urinary stone. The

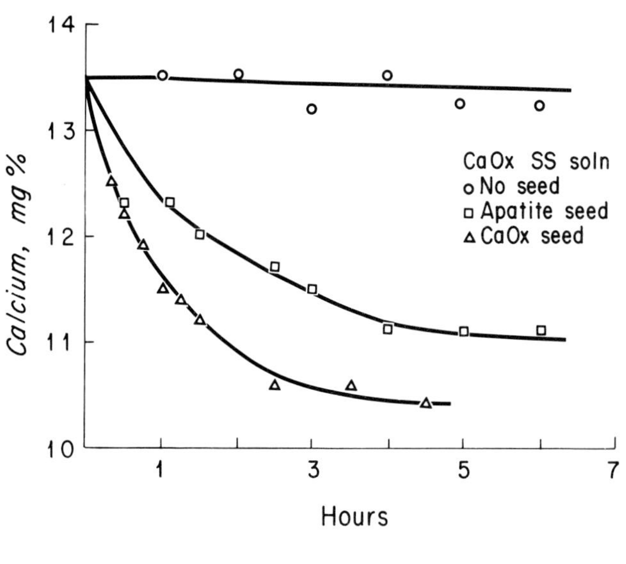

FIGURE 2–4. Heterogeneous nucleation. Apatite seed crystals added to a metastable calcium oxalate solution induce the crystallization of calcium oxalate, as measured by the decrease in calcium concentration in the solution. Results from a calcium oxalate–seeded crystal growth experiment are included for comparison. (From Smith LH, Meyer JL: Urinary inhibitors of calcium oxalate crystal growth. *In* Finlayson B, Thomas WC [eds]: Colloquium on Renal Lithiasis. Gainesville, FL, The University Presses of Florida, 1976; with permission.)

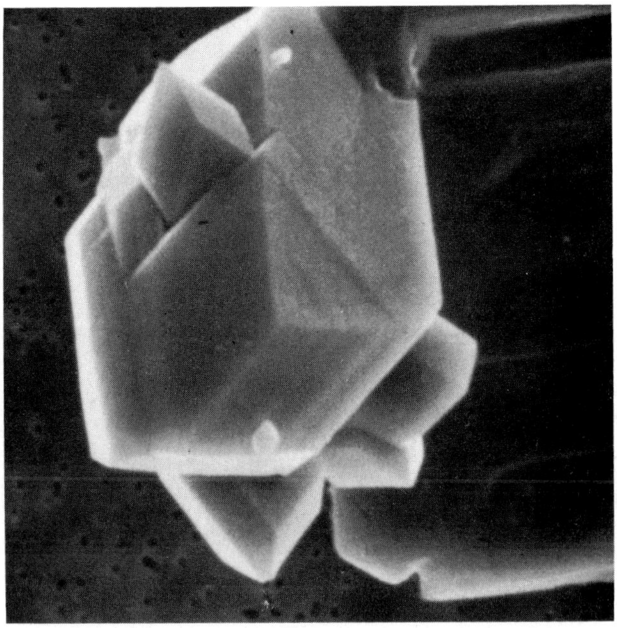

FIGURE 2–5. Crystals of calcium oxalate nucleated by a uric acid crystal (flat, platy morphology). (From Meyer JL, et al: The epitaxially induced crystal growth of calcium oxalate by crystalline uric acid. Invest Urol 14:115–119, 1976. Copyright © 1976 by The Williams & Wilkins Co.)

essential requirement for all processes is a supersaturated urine. Once that condition is met, the growth of stone crystals will occur (Fig. 2–6*A*). Growth is modulated by a number of natural components, such as inhibitors and matrix. The production of the initial crystal phase itself, however, is tenuous and is greatly dependent on a number of factors (Fig. 2–6*B*). First, the nuclei must reach a stable critical size before they can exist as an independent entity. A concentration product of the free ions must become large enough so that the rate of formation of the initial crystals (nucleation) exceeds that for dissolution of the very small particles. This concentration product, usually envisioned as the formation product, K_f, (see Fig. 2–1) is dependent on a number of situations, such as the presence of complexing agents, which lower the free concentrations.

Competing with the homogeneous nucleation process is the initial production of stone crystals by heterogeneous nucleation, which can occur under the proper conditions at much lower supersaturation. Two situations, known to occur in vitro, are shown (Fig. 2–6*C*). Calcium oxalate is nucleated by uric acid crystals (see Fig. 2–5) and by calcium phosphate crystals (see Fig. 2–4). However, the initial formation of each of these seed crystals is governed by the same principles described for homogeneous nucleation earlier. Urinary pH is especially important, since the solubility of both uric acid and apatite is extremely sensitive to this variable. Inhibitors are again included, since they affect this as well as the other crystallization processes.

A final, very important, phenomenon is crystal aggregation (Fig. 2–6*D*). Without aggregation, the relatively small crystal nuclei formed in the upper urinary tract would likely be washed out without incident in the urine. As for the other crystallization processes, this equilibrium occurs with aggregation and disaggregation in concert. Along with the ubiquitous inhibitors, it is likely that there are promoters (matrix?) that influence the final amount of aggregated crystals.

Human urine maintains a curious balance between those forces that would

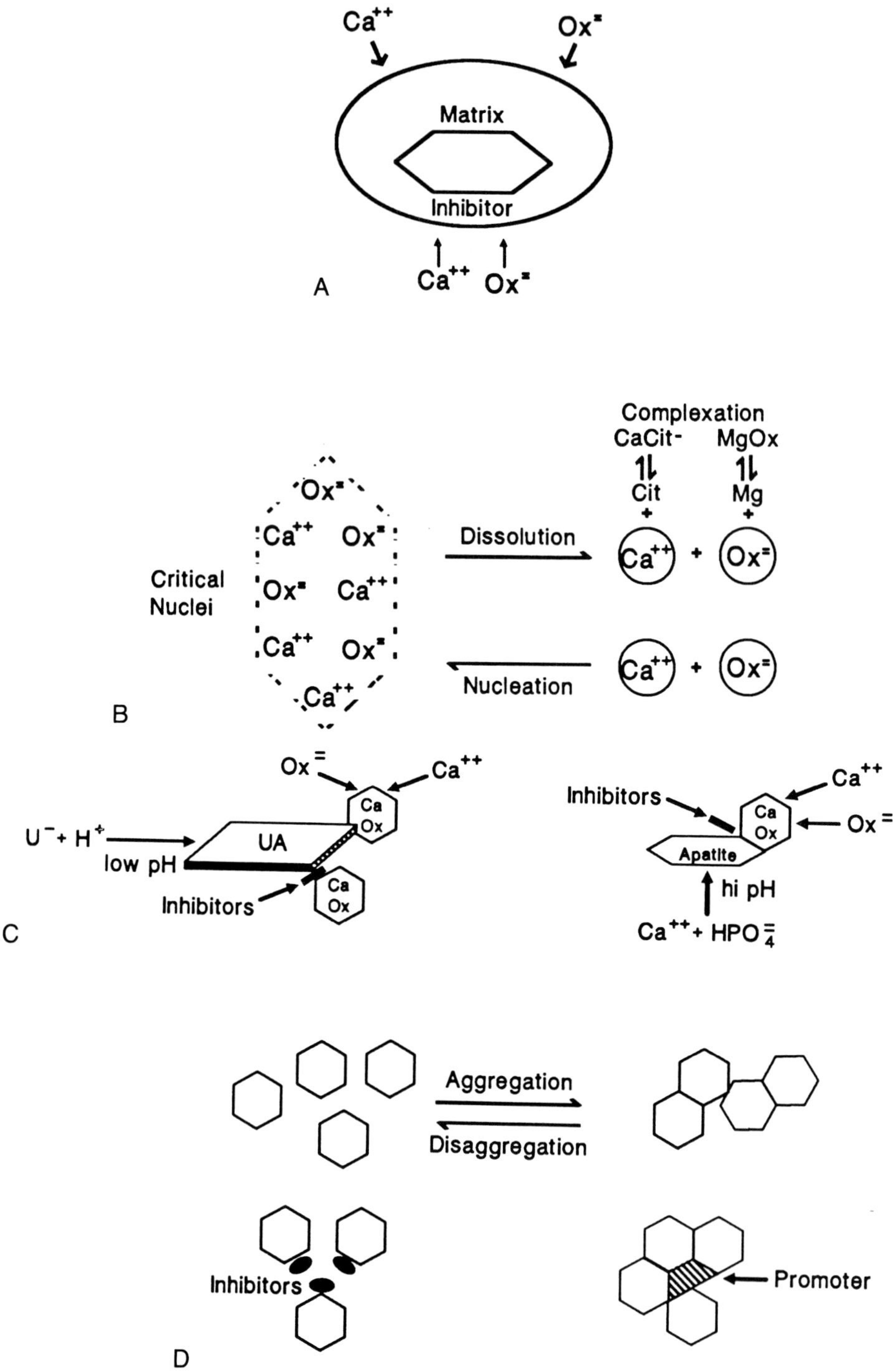

FIGURE 2–6. Diagram showing a collage of crystallization phenomena occurring in a supersaturated solution. Depicted are a number of events accompanying crystal growth (*A*), homogeneous nucleation (*B*), heterogeneous nucleation (*C*), and aggregation (*D*).

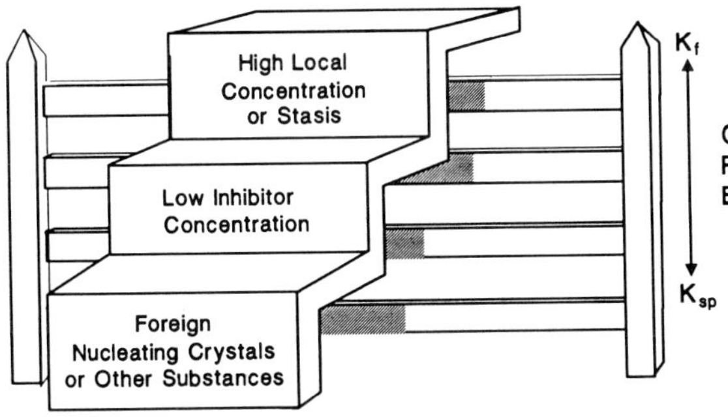

FIGURE 2–7. Diagram illustrating the barrier to de novo crystallization and the steps that can and do occur to aid in nucleating crystalline phase from an otherwise metastable supersaturated urine.

precipitate a stone and those that strive to prevent it. A natural barrier exists in urine that limits the initial formation of stone crystals. This concept is depicted in Figure 2–7 as a fence that must be crossed, and the magnitude of that barrier (the height of the fence) is the concentration of stone components necessary to form the first crystalline phase. Chemically speaking, this is the operational formation product. Present in urine are opportunities to decrease or circumvent this barrier, however, and this is illustrated by steps used to cross the fence. Locally high concentrations, low urine inhibitor concentrations, and the presence of foreign nucleating substances all help to facilitate the production of stone crystals.

If and when this barrier is crossed and crystals are formed in metastable urine, compensating barriers are already in place or can be constructed by appropriate medical intervention to control or prevent the stone-forming process, as shown in Figure 2–8. The formation of a human stone involves both the growth of nucleated crystals and their aggregation to form particles large enough to become trapped in the urinary tract. The means of slowing this process include a lowering of urinary supersaturation, and thus the driving force for crystallization, and the presence of natural or therapeutic inhibitors of crystal growth or

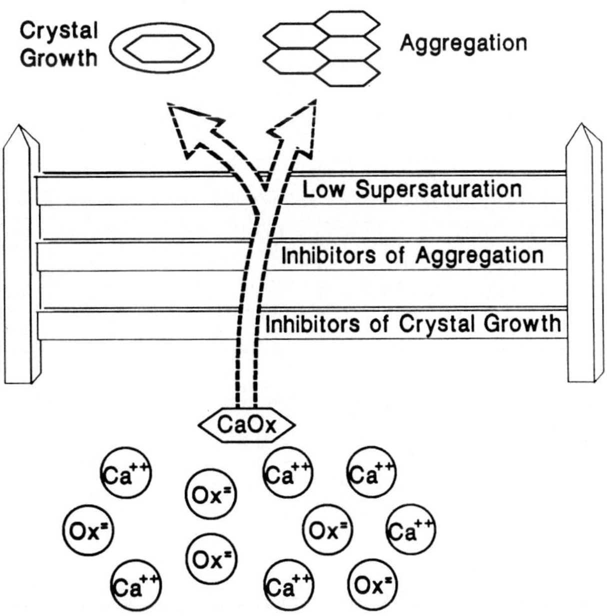

FIGURE 2–8. Diagram illustrating some of the barriers that exist naturally in human urine or that can be introduced therapeutically to prevent or slow the processes of crystal growth and aggregation that lead to stone disease.

aggregation. The urine of "normal" individuals would appear to be usually undersaturated or only slightly supersaturated and to have an abundance of crystallization inhibitors. The goal for the medical management of stone disease, therefore, would seem to be the attempt to build the barrier to future stone growth as large as possible.

An attempt has been made to describe a very complex medical problem, the prevention and treatment of human urinary calculi, in terms of a few relatively simple physicochemical principles. Unfortunately, although the chemistry of the stone-forming process in vitro is relatively straightforward, the management of patients is not. It is hoped, however, that some additional insight into the treatment of patients has been gained from this discussion focusing on the chemistry of urine.

APPENDIX. In this section, the procedure for calculating the free ionic activities of all the principal species in urine is described. The substances considered are either those that are directly involved in the stone-forming process or those that have a significant effect on the ionic strength of urine. The ions and their ion pairs that are of importance in establishing the ionic environment and thus the thermodynamic stability of urine are indicated in Table 2–1. Most of the crystallization inhibitors discussed in the chapter do not appear in the table because their normal concentrations are not sufficient to affect the free ionic activities of the other substances, even though they are capable of modulating crystal growth.

The first parameter that needs to be defined is the ionic strength of the solution. This is a relatively simple calculation in which the concentration of all the charged species, positive and negative, are summed and divided by 2. The concentration of ions with a charge greater than 1 is multiplied by the square of the charge. The working equation is

$$I = 1/2\ \Sigma\ z^2C \tag{17}$$

where I is the ionic strength, z the charge of each ion, and C its molar concentration.

Once an initial estimate of the ionic strength is calculated, activity coefficients for the ionic species can be estimated by an extended version of the Debye-Huckel equation.[31]

$$-\log f_z = Az^2\ [\sqrt{I}/(1 + \sqrt{I}) - 0.3I] \tag{18}$$

The term f_z represents the activity coefficient of an ion of charge + or −z, and A is a temperature-dependent coefficient that has the value of 0.5209 at 37°C.

Table 2–1 shows the free ions and ion pairs that make up the majority of

TABLE 2–1. PRINCIPAL IONIC SPECIES IN URINE

CATIONS	ANIONS	CA ION PARIS	MG ION PARIS
Na^+	Cl^-	$CaCO_3$	$MgCO_3$
K^+	CO_3^{2-}	$CaHCO_3^-$	$MgHCO_3^+$
NH_4^+	HCO_3^-	$CaHPO_4$	$MgHPO_4$
Ca^{2+}	HPO_4^{2-}	$CaH_2PO_4^+$	$MgH_2PO_4^+$
Mg^{2+}	$H_2PO_4^-$	$CaSO_4$	$MgSO_4$
	SO_4^{2-}	CaHCit	MgHCit
	$HCit^{2-}$	$CaCit^-$	$MgCit^-$
	Cit^{3-}	CaC_2O_4	MgC_2O_4
	$C_2O_4^{2-}$		
	U^-		

the charged species found in urine. Their calculated free concentrations are dependent on the computed f_z terms. For example, the concentration of the complex formed between calcium ion and trivalent citrate ion (Cit^{3-}) is calculated from the equilibrium constant

$$K = \frac{[CaCit^-]f_1}{[Ca^{2+}][Cit^{3-}]f_2f_3} \tag{19}$$

for the equilibrium

$$Ca^{2+} + Cit^{3-} = CaCit^- \tag{20}$$

Similarly constructed equilibrium constant expressions are obtained for the other ion pairs in the table. An activity coefficient of 1 is assumed for uncharged ion pairs and other urine constituents.

A number of mathematical procedures could be used to solve for the free ionic concentrations of the substances in Table 2–1. A direct algebraic solution of simultaneous equations is possible but very cumbersome. With access to a high-speed computer, the method of choice for most investigators is an iterative procedure using mass balance equations. These are particularly well conditioned for an iterative approach and converge very rapidly to a fixed value. An example of this type of mass balance equation, for free calcium ion concentration, is given below. What is required are analytical measurements of the total concentrations of the major constituents, such as calcium, T_{Ca}, in the urine.

$$\begin{aligned} T_{Ca} = {} & [Ca^{2+}] + [CaHCO_3^+] + [CaCO_3] + [CaHPO_4] \\ & + [CaH_2PO_4^+] + [CaSO_4] + [CaHCit] + [CaCit^-] \\ & + [CaC_2O_4] \end{aligned} \tag{21}$$

Equilibrium constant expressions, such as that for the CaCit– ion pair, are then substituted for each of the species, common cations and anions are factored out, and the equation is rearranged to yield an expression for the free calcium ion concentration.

$$\begin{aligned} [Ca^{2+}] = {} & T_{Ca}/(1 + [HCO_3^-]B + [HPO_4^{2-}]C + [SO_4^{2-}]D \\ & + [Cit^{3-}]E + [C_2O_4^{2-}]F) \end{aligned} \tag{22}$$

The terms B, C, D, E, and F are the activity coefficients and equilibrium constants that are relevant for each of the species. Also included is the hydrogen ion concentration when multiple protonated species are present at urinary pH, such as the carbonate, phosphate, and citrate ions. Similar equations can be derived for all the other species in Table 2–1, which exist in multiple forms in urine. In practice, a reasonable initial value for the free concentration of each of the ions, such as the total concentration, is substituted, and the iteration is allowed to proceed. Each iteration results in slightly different calculated free ion concentrations, until convergence is obtained; therefore, the ionic strength and activity coefficients must also be recalculated after each iteration. Generally, no more than three or four calculation passes are required to achieve a tenth of a per cent or better convergence. Once the free concentrations of each of the urine species are known, along with their activity coefficient for the particular urine solution, thermodynamic calculations such as activity products and APRs can be performed.

REFERENCES

1. Prien EL, Frondel C: Studies in urolithiasis. I. The composition of urinary calculi. J Urol 57:949–991, 1947.

2. Robertson WG, Peacock M, Nordin BEC: Activity products in stone-forming and non–stone-forming urine. Clin Sci 34:579–594, 1968.
3. Boyce WH: Organic matrix of human urinary concretions. Am J Med 45:673–683, 1968.
4. Pak CYC, Galosy RA: Propensity for spontaneous nucleation of calcium oxalate: Quantitative assessment by urinary FPR-APR discriminant score. Am J Med 69:681–689, 1980.
5. Robertson WG, Peacock M, Marshall RW, et al: Saturation-inhibition index as a measure of the risk of calcium oxalate stone formation in the urinary tract. N Engl J Med 294:249–252, 1976.
6. Pak CYC, Fuller C: Idiopathic hypocitraturic calcium-oxalate nephrolithiasis successfully treated with potassium citrate. Ann Intern Med 104:33–37, 1986.
7. Smith LH, Meyer JL: Urinary inhibitors of calcium oxalate crystal growth. *In* Finlayson B, Thomas WC (eds): Colloquium on Renal Lithiasis. Gainesville, FL, The University Presses of Florida, 1976, pp 112–118.
8. Meyer JL, Thomas WC: Trace metal–citric acid complexes as inhibitors of calcification and crystal growth. I. Effects of Fe(III), Cr(III) and Al(III) complexes on calcium phosphate crystal growth. J Urol 128:1372–1375, 1982.
9. Meyer JL, Angino EE: The role of trace metals in calcium urolithiasis. Invest Urol 14:347–350, 1977.
10. Finlayson B, Smith A: Stability of first dissociable proton of uric acid. J Chem Eng Data 19:94–97, 1974.
11. Yendt ER, Cohanim M: Response to physiologic dose of pyridoxine in Type 1 primary hyperoxaluria. N Engl J Med 314:953–957, 1985.
12. Ryall LR, Harnett RM, Marshall VR: The effect of urine, pyrophosphate, citrate, magnesium and glycosaminoglycans on the growth and aggregation of calcium oxalate crystals in vitro. Clin Chim Acta 112:349–356, 1981.
13. Schrier EE, Rubin JL, Lee KE, et al: Characterization of the calcium oxalate crystal growth inhibitors in human urine. *In* Smith LH, Robertson WG, Finlayson B (ed): Urolithiasis: Clinical and Basic Research. New York, Plenum, 1981, pp 579–588.
14. Nakagawa Y, Abram V, Kezdy FL, et al: Purification and characterization of the principal inhibitor of calcium oxalate crystal growth in human urine. J Biol Chem 258:12594–12600, 1983.
15. Malek RS, Boyce WH: Intranephronic calculosis: Its significance and relationship to matrix in nephrolithiasis. J Urol 109:551–555, 1973.
16. Coe FL: Hyperuricosuric calcium oxalate nephrolithiasis. Kid Int 13:418–426, 1978.
17. Coe FL, Raisen L: Allopurinol treatment of uric-acid disorders in calcium-stoneformers. Lancet 1:129–131, 1973.
18. Griffith DP, Gibson JR, Clinton CW, Musher DM: Acetohydroxamic acid: Clinical studies of an urease inhibitor in patients with staghorn renal calculi. J Urol 119:9–15, 1978.
19. Vermeulen CW, Lyon ES: Mechanism of genesis and growth of calculi. Am J Med 45:684–692, 1968.
20. Howard JE: Urinary stone. Can Med Assoc J 86:1001–1007, 1962.
21. Howard JE: Studies on urinary stone formation: A saga of clinical investigation. Johns Hopkins Med J 139:239–252, 1976.
22. Lonsdale K: Epitaxy as a growth factor in urinary calculi and gallstones. Nature 217:56–58, 1968.
23. Finlayson B: Calcium stones: Some physical and clinical aspects. *In* David DS (ed): Calcium Metabolism in Renal Failure and Nephrolithiasis. New York, John Wiley & Sons, 1977, pp 337–382.
24. Nicar MJ, Hill K, Pak CYC: A simple technique for assessing the propensity for crystallization of calcium oxalate and brushite in urine from the increment in oxalate or calcium necessary to elicit precipitation. Metabolism 32:906–910, 1983.
25. Meyer JL, Smith LH: Growth of calcium oxalate crystals. II. Inhibition by natural urinary crystal growth inhibitors. Invest Urol 13:36–39, 1975.
26. Robertson WG, Peacock M, Nordin BEC: Inhibitors of the growth and aggregation of calcium oxalate crystals in vitro. Clin Chim Acta 43:31–37, 1973.
27. Hallson PC, Rose GA: A new urinary test for stone "activity." Br J Urol 50:442–448, 1978.
28. Bisaz S, Felix R, Neuman WF, Fleisch H: Quantitative determination of inhibitors of calcium phosphate precipitation in whole urine. Miner Electrolyte Metab 1:74–83, 1978.
29. Meyer JL, Fleisch H: Calcification inhibitors in rat and human serum and plasma. Biochim Biophys Acta 799:115–121, 1984.
30. Meyer JL, Bergert JH, Smith LH: Epitaxial relationships in urolithiasis: The calcium oxalate monohydrate-hydroxyapatite system. Clin Sci Mol Med 49:369–374, 1975.
31. Davies CW: Ion Association. London, Butterworth's, 1962.

3

Hypercalciuric Calcium Nephrolithiasis

Charles Y.C. Pak

Hypercalciuria has long been associated with nephrolithiasis.[1] It is one of the most common metabolic derangements identified, occurring in approximately 50 per cent of patients with stones. Extensive studies have been conducted on the pathophysiologic elucidation and treatment of hypercalciuria, clearly more so than with any other derangement.[2–6] This commitment does not necessarily reflect recognition of any special pathogenetic importance of hypercalciuria over other derangements. It more likely is the result of a general interest in calcium metabolism and the availability of reliable methods for investigation.

Despite the ongoing controversy, the following conclusions may be drawn. First, the hypercalciuria of nephrolithiasis is heterogeneous in origin.[7] No single scheme could explain the pathogenesis of hypercalciuria encountered in stone-forming patients. Second, the diagnosis of different forms of hypercalciuria can be made with increasing facility.[8] Third, many treatment programs have been formulated that have been shown to retard the rate of new stone formation in patients with hypercalciuric calcium nephrolithiasis.[9, 10] Some of these treatments are directed at the correction of the underlying pathophysiologic derangement responsible for the hypercalciuria; others are not. There is currently no evidence that the former "specific" or "selective" therapies are more effective in preventing new stone formation than the latter "nonselective" or "random" programs.[11]

It is this uncertainty that has fueled the argument against an extensive evaluation and investigation of hypercalciuric nephrolithiasis. However, the position for limited involvement could be opposed on the following grounds. The current therapeutic program for hypercalciuric nephrolithiasis is far from complete. There is no treatment, for example, that corrects the basic underlying defect in classic absorptive hypercalciuria (to be discussed further on). Continuing exploration and elucidation of the pathophysiology of hypercalciuria could lead to the development of new effective treatment programs. Because of the ubiquitous nature of calcium, treatments directed at the correction of hypercalciuria could adversely affect the metabolism of tissues outside the kidney. It is logical to assume that nonspecific treatments rather than specific treatments would be more likely to cause nonrenal complications.[12] Among drugs already available in the marketplace, some are clearly contraindicated for certain forms of hypercalciuria because of probable ineffectiveness or potential complications—for example, sodium cellulose phosphate in renal hypercalciuria (to be discussed later). A careful differentiation among hypercalciurias could prevent the misuse of drugs.

This discussion of hypercalciuria is undertaken with the basic assumption that the hypercalciuria of nephrolithiasis is heterogeneous in origin and thus requires differentiation and selective treatment. This chapter first presents a brief historical perspective and the pathogenetic importance of hypercalciuria in stone formation. A detailed discussion of pathophysiology, diagnosis, and treatment is then provided.

HISTORICAL CONSIDERATIONS

The association of hypercalciuria with calcium nephrolithiasis was first recognized by Flocks in 1939.[1] In 1953, Albright and colleagues described a group of patients with hypercalciuria, normocalcemia, and a history of recurrent passage of calcium-containing renal stones.[13] The term "idiopathic hypercalciuria" was used to denote this condition, since the exact cause of hypercalciuria was not known. However, noting a history of urinary tract infection in some of their patients, these investigators suggested that the cause of hypercalciuria was a decreased renal tubular reabsorption of calcium, consequent to tubular damage by pyelonephritis. In 1958, Henneman and associates found intestinal hyperabsorption of calcium in some of their hypercalciuric patients.[14]

Subsequently, many conflicting reports have appeared, supporting either the primacy of "renal leak" or an intestinal hyperabsorption of calcium. In 1972, Nordin and coworkers reported normal fasting urinary calcium and exaggerated calcium excretion during a high calcium intake in the setting of normocalcemia in stone-forming patients with hypercalciuria.[2] They introduced the term "absorptive hypercalciuria" to indicate that the principal defect was intestinal hyperabsorption of calcium. In 1973, Coe and colleagues found parathyroid stimulation in many of their hypercalciuric patients with nephrolithiasis and suggested that an underlying renal calcium leak had caused secondary hyperparathyroidism.[15] In 1974, Pak and associates suggested that the hypercalciuria of nephrolithiasis was heterogeneous in origin and that absorptive hypercalciuria was the major variant.[3] They introduced the terms "renal hypercalciuria" and "resorptive hypercalciuria" to describe the renal calcium leak and excessive bone resorption that occur in primary hyperparathyroidism, respectively, constituting remaining variants. Since then, Shen and coworkers[4] and Lemann and colleagues[16] suggested that absorptive hypercalciuria resulted from renal phosphate leak, leading to stimulated renal synthesis of 1,25-$(OH)_2$vitamin D and intestinal calcium absorption. In contrast, Broadus and associates suggested that a primary overproduction of 1,25-$(OH)_2$vitamin D was responsible for the intestinal hyperabsorption of calcium.[5] In 1982, Coe and associates presented a potentially unifying scheme, in which afflicted subjects were assumed to suffer from multiple disturbances in renal tubular function, characterized by varying degrees of calcium leak, a disturbance in phosphate transport, and accelerated 1,25-$(OH)_2$vitamin D synthesis.[17] In 1981, Buck and associates suggested that an excessive production of prostaglandin E_2 might account for the hypercalciuria.[18] Recently, the occurrence of absorptive hypercalciuria was supported by the finding of a similar biochemical and physiologic picture in inbred hypercalciuric rats[19] and by the confirmation of persistent intestinal hyperabsorption of calcium and calcium retention during thiazide therapy.[20]

This chapter attempts to present an integrated view of hypercalciuria, incorporating many of the above-mentioned schemes.

PATHOGENETIC ROLE OF HYPERCALCIURIA IN STONE FORMATION

Hypercalciuria could cause or contribute to calcium stone formation by two mechanisms. First, it increases the saturation of urine with respect to stone-forming calcium salts.[2] It was initially suggested that hyperoxaluria was more effective than hypercalciuria in augmenting the urinary saturation of stone-forming calcium salts.[2] Because of the prominent complexation of oxalate by calcium, the rise in ionic calcium concentration from hypercalciuria was believed to be opposed by a decline in ionic oxalate concentration. However, a reexamination of the problem using a different computer program for the computation of soluble complexes has disclosed an equivalent action of calcium and oxalate.[21] Within the range of concentrations encountered in urine, the rise in calcium concentration was as effective as the increase in oxalate concentration in raising the urinary saturation of calcium oxalate. This computer program has been validated by the close correspondence of calculated ionic calcium concentration to the experimentally derived value (by ion-selective electrode), lending support to the preceding conclusion.

The urinary environment has been extensively examined for urinary saturation with respect to stone-forming calcium salts by using the activity product ratio (or concentration product ratio).[22] These semiempirical methods probably represent the most reliable approaches to the measurement of urinary saturation. These studies have disclosed that the urinary saturation of calcium oxalate and calcium phosphate was directly correlated with urinary calcium concentration (Fig. 3–1). Moreover, the urinary environment of patients with hypercalciuric nephrolithiasis was typically supersaturated with respect to these salts.[22] Although the urinary environment of normal subjects without stones was also sometimes supersaturated, it was to a lesser degree than in the hypercalciuric stone-forming population. Finally, induced hypercalciuria from a high calcium intake often increases the urinary saturation of stone-forming salts, since the opposing effect of the fall in urinary oxalate from intestinal oxalate binding by calcium is relatively modest or nonexistent[23] (Fig. 3–2).

The second mechanism for the pathogenetic role of hypercalciuria is less well appreciated. Hypercalciuria may reduce the inhibitor activity in urine against the crystallization of stone-forming calcium salts by binding negatively charged inhibitors and inactivating them. Thus, Zerwekh and colleagues recently reported that the inhibitor against the spontaneous nucleation of calcium oxalate exhibited by citrate and chondroitin sulfate was reduced by calcium.[24] This attenuation of inhibitor activity apparently is not universal, since calcium was shown to augment the inhibitor activity expressed by urinary glycopeptides. Despite a need for further clarification, their study suggests that calcium under certain circumstances could contribute to renal stone formation by inactivated

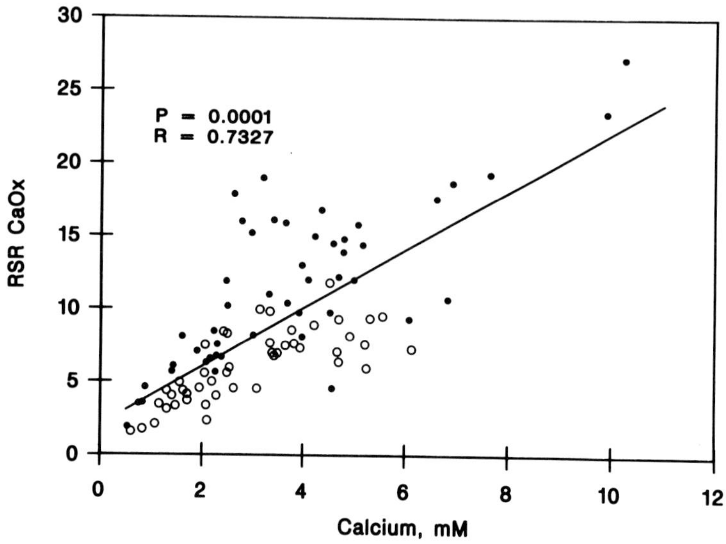

FIGURE 3–1. Dependence of urinary saturation of calcium oxalate and brushite on urinary calcium concentration. RSR = relative saturation ratio.

inhibitors. This conclusion is supported by the finding of a low limit of metastability (formation product) in the urine of some hypercalciuric stone-forming patients[22] and a reduction in formation product upon the addition of calcium in vitro to certain urine samples.[24]

The causal role of hypercalciuria in stone formation is further supported by the amelioration of stone disease upon correction of hypercalciuria with thiazide[9] or sodium cellulose phosphate.[10]

COEXISTENCE OF OTHER DERANGEMENTS

In many patients with hypercalciuric nephrolithiasis, hypercalciuria coexists with other abnormalities. Among 3473 stone-forming patients from various parts of the United States who had submitted a 24-hour urine sample for the Stone Risk Profile,[25] hypercalciuria (>250 mg/day) was disclosed in 40.6 per cent of patients. Among these hypercalciuric patients, 25 per cent had hyperuricosuria (>700 mg/day), 23 per cent had hyperoxaluria (>45 mg/day), 17 per cent had hypocitraturia (<320 mg/day), 17 per cent had low urinary pH (<5.5), 69 per cent had low urine volume (<2 liters/day), 38 per cent had high urinary sodium (>200 mEq/day), and 3 per cent had low urinary magnesium (<60 mg/day).

The coexistence of these abnormalities suggests that they may be environmental or nutritional in origin, since a single abnormality is more likely to ensue from a genetic defect. For example, a diet high in animal protein might augment calcium and uric acid excretion while reducing citrate excretion and pH.[26] An exaggerated sodium intake may augment calcium excretion[27] and sometimes lower citrate excretion. These remarks emphasize the potentially important role of environmental and nutritional factors in stone formation.

However, the frequent association of hypercalciuria with other derangements does not exclude the metabolic or genetic etiology of hypercalciuria. Hypercalciuria often persists during maintenance on a standard diet. Dietary manipulation is often ineffective in controlling hypercalciuria. The co-occurrence of various derangements could also be explained by the following:

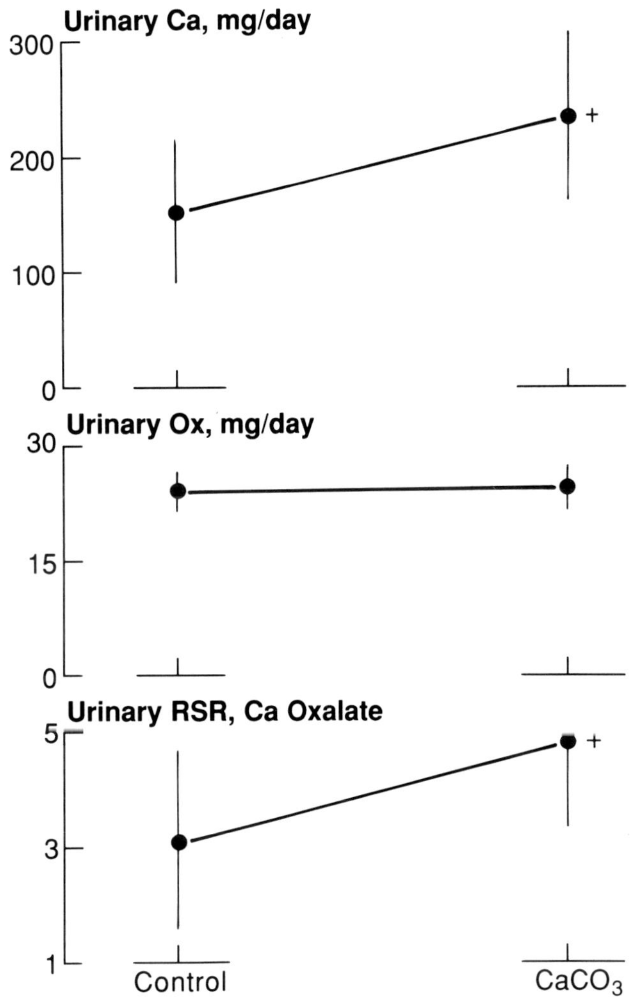

FIGURE 3–2. Effect of calcium carbonate supplementation (200 mg Ca four times a day) on urinary calcium, oxalate, and relative saturation ratio (RSR) of calcium oxalate. RSR is a measure of saturation in which a value greater than 1 indicates supersaturation. + = $p < .001$.

1. Superimposition of a dietary or environmental aberration on an underlying metabolic abnormality.
2. Coexistence of separate metabolic abnormalities in the same patient (e.g., distal renal tubular acidosis causing hypercalciuria and hypocitraturia).[28]
3. Hypercalciuria of metabolic origin causing other derangements (e.g., increased intestinal calcium absorption, leaving less calcium remaining in the gut to bind oxalate, thus resulting in hyperoxaluria).

PATHOGENESIS OF HYPERCALCIURIA

A brief review of the physiologic handling of calcium and calcium homeostasis is indicated to understand more fully the pathophysiology of hypercalciuria.

Renal Handling of Calcium[29]

Under normal circumstances, approximately 8 grams of calcium is filtered by the kidneys each day. Approximately 65 per cent of filtered calcium is reabsorbed in the proximal tubule by both paracellular (diffusion and solvent drag) and transcellular (active) transport. In the loop of Henle, an additional 25 per cent is reabsorbed by passive diffusion. The final regulation, accounting for 7.5 per cent of the filtered load, takes place in the distal tubule by an active transcellular transport, which occurs independently of sodium reabsorption. Thus, only about 2.5 per cent of the filtered load of calcium is excreted in urine, normally amounting to 200 mg/day.

Many factors affect the renal tubular reabsorption of calcium (Fig. 3–3). The expansion of extracellular fluid volume (e.g., following sodium load) augments calcium excretion by inhibiting the proximal tubular reabsorption of calcium; the contraction of the extracellular fluid volume (e.g., dehydration) does the opposite. Acetazolamide also retards the proximal tubular reabsorption of calcium. Furosemide and ethacrynic acid inhibit calcium reabsorption in the thick ascending loop of Henle. This effect is opposed by the indirect enhancement of the proximal tubular reabsorption of calcium, which occurs from natriuresis and extracellular fluid volume contraction.

Thiazide augments calcium excretion by directly augmenting calcium reabsorption in the distal convoluted tubule and by indirectly enhancing calcium reabsorption in the proximal tubule (from natriuresis and volume contraction). Amiloride increases reabsorption of calcium in the distal convoluted tubule at a site distal to thiazide action. Parathyriod hormone augments calcium reabsorption

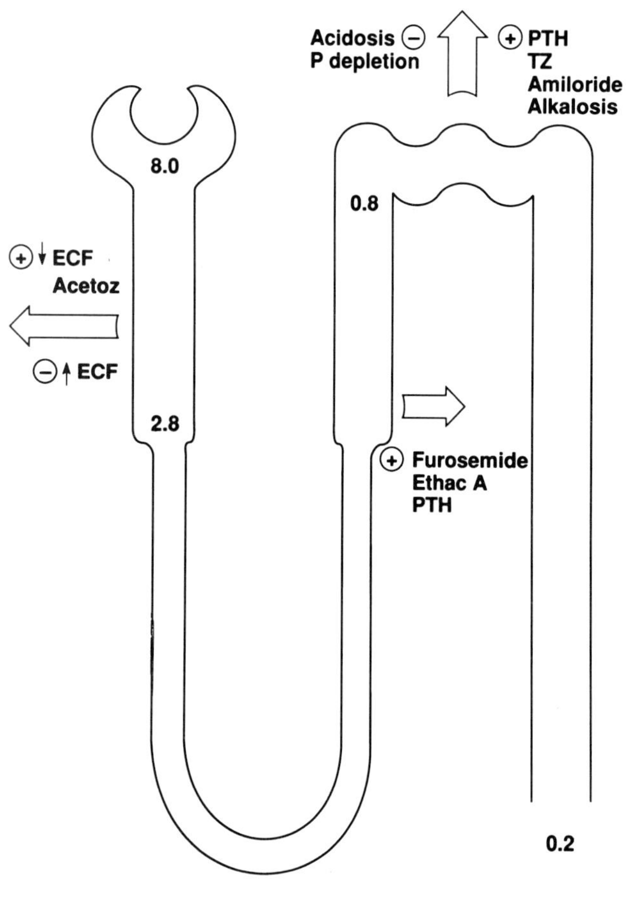

FIGURE 3–3. Sites of calcium absorption in the nephron. Enhancement of calcium reabsorption is indicated by ◯+ and inhibition by ⊖. Numbers within the lumen indicate the amount of calcium in grams per day handled normally each day. ECF = extracellular fluid; Ethac A = ethacrynic acid; PTH = parathyroid hormone; Acetoz = acetazolamide; TZ = thiazide.

in the distal tubule; it also enhances calcium reabsorption in the thick ascending loop of Henle, though to a minor extent. Alkalosis increases calcium reabsorption in the distal convoluted tubule; acidosis has the opposite action. Phosphorus depletion impairs calcium reabsorption in the late distal tubule.

Intestinal Absorption of Calcium

Calcium absorption occurs actively as well as passively (Fig. 3–4).[30] The active transport occurring transepithelially is rate limiting and is dependent on 1,25-$(OH)_2$vitamin D.[31] The binding of 1,25-$(OH)_2$vitamin D to the cytosolic-nuclear receptor results in an elaboration of messenger RNA (mRNA) for the synthesis of calcium-binding protein (CaBP) as well as certain enzymes involved in calcium transport (e.g., calcium–adenosine triphosphatase [Ca-ATPase]). The translocation of calcium from the mucosal to the serosal side may be mediated by CaBP or by calcium-enriched vesicles. The calcium efflux at the serosal side is an active process involving hydrolysis of ATP, sodium-calcium exchange, or vesicular extrusion. Passive calcium absorption, occurring via tight junctions independently of 1,25-$(OH)_2$vitamin D, may play a role at high luminal calcium concentrations.

All segments of the human bowel (jejunum, ileum, colon) can participate in calcium absorption.[32] However, under normal circumstances, the upper small bowel is probably the principal site of calcium absorption, because of the inaccessibility of calcium at distal sites due to enclosure in fecal material.

Calcium Handling in Bone[33]

Bone is composed of matrix (collagen) and mineral (principally calcium phosphate). It is formed when collagen, synthesized by osteoblasts, undergoes mineralization (accretion), with deposition of calcium and phosphate. It is destroyed by osteoclastic resorption, with release of calcium and phosphate. The skeleton in a normal adult man contains about 1000 grams of calcium. Accretion

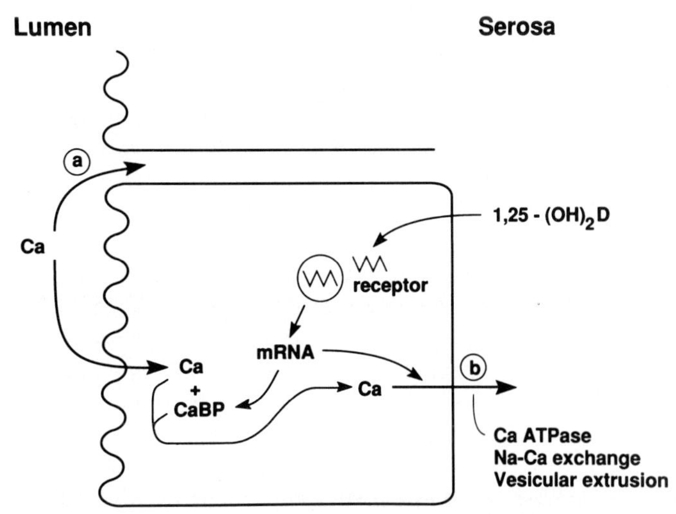

FIGURE 3–4. Scheme for intestinal mucosal calcium transport. Passive transport is indicated by ⓐ and active transport by ⓑ.

and resorption account for a transfer of approximately 0.5 gram of calcium per day each.

The primary stimulus for osteoblastic collagen synthesis is strain on the skeleton. Other stimuli include exogenous material (fluoride) and local growth factors (e.g., somatomedin). Osteoclastic resorption is stimulated by parathyroid hormone (PTH) and 1,25-$(OH)_2$vitamin D and is inhibited by estrogen and calcitonin. Local factors may stimulate it (prostaglandin E_2, interleukin-1) or inhibit it (γ-interferon).

Calcium Homeostatic Mechanism[33]

Calcium homeostasis represents physiologic and hormonal regulation by which the serum concentration of ionized calcium is maintained within a narrow range.

The physiologic regulation constitutes a nonhormonal process by which renal excretion and intestinal secretion of calcium respond to changes in the calcium concentration in serum. In the presence of hypercalcemia, an increased amount of calcium is lost in urine from a rise in the renal filtered load of calcium and from the impaired renal tubular reabsorption of calcium resulting directly from the hypercalcemia. Less certainly, the intestinal secretion of calcium may be increased from an augmented passive diffusion as well. These effects may ameliorate the hypercalcemia. Conversely, hypocalcemia is opposed by a reduced renal excretion of calcium. It is not clearly established whether there is a reduced intestinal secretion of calcium.

The role of the kidney in this physiologic regulation may be appreciated from the following consideration. In a subject with normal renal function, a rise in total serum calcium concentration of 1 mg/dl (which could occur within the normal range) might increase the filtered load and the renal excretion of calcium by 0.8 gram/day. Thus, the input of calcium (from skeletal calcium mobilization and intestinal calcium absorption) into the circulation must generally exceed this amount to cause hypercalcemia.

Hormonal regulation exerts the most important influence on calcium homeostasis. The basis for this regulation is the influence of the serum concentration of calcium (ionized) on the secretion of certain hormones that affect bone and calcium metabolism. Such "calcium-regulatory hormones" include PTH, 1,25-$(OH)_2$vitamin D, calcitonin, and possibly 24,25-$(OH)_2$vitamin D. The classic physiologic response to PTH and to 1,25-$(OH)_2$vitamin D is augmentation of the serum calcium concentration, whereas the net effect of the action of calcitonin and 24,25-$(OH)_2$vitamin D is reduction in the circulating calcium concentration. In hypercalcemia the critical features of calcium homeostasis are the suppression of the secretion or synthesis of PTH and of 1,25-$(OH)_2$vitamin D and the stimulation of the secretion or production of calcitonin. The opposite situation is true in hypocalcemia. When these changes in the secretion of calcium-regulatory hormones are appropriate, marked fluctuations in the circulating concentration of calcium are avoided under ordinary physiologic conditions.

An understanding of the physiologic actions of the calcium-regulatory hormones is critical for the full appreciation of hormonal regulation of calcium homeostasis. Parathyroid hormone promotes bone resorption by increasing the number and activity of osteoclasts. It may do so by binding to the osteoblasts (in which there is a PTH receptor),[34] thereby releasing an unknown factor that then stimulates osteoclasts or precursors. This hormone does not augment intestinal calcium absorption directly but does so indirectly by stimulating the synthesis of 1,25-$(OH)_2$vitamin D in the kidneys[35]; PTH also enhances the renal tubular reabsorption of calcium.[36]

In bone, 1,25-$(OH)_2$vitamin D also stimulates bone resorption,[37] probably by accentuating the activity of osteoclasts. Moreover, it has been suggested that this vitamin D metabolite stimulates osteocytic resorption and causes rapid skeletal mobilization of calcium. In the intestinal tract, 1,25-$(OH)_2$vitamin D probably provides the most potent stimulus to the absorption of calcium.[38] Last, 1,25-$(OH)_2$vitamin D augments the renal tubular reabsorption of calcium.[39] However, this renal action of 1,25-$(OH)_2$vitamin D is less effective than that of PTH, and it probably plays a minor role in calcium homeostasis.

Thus, the hormonal regulation of calcium homeostasis involves appropriate responses in three target organs: intestine, kidney, and bone. This concept may be illustrated by considering the sequelae of ingestion of a high-calcium diet. The ensuing increased absorption of calcium, if unabated, could cause hypercalcemia. However, hypercalcemia is normally averted by compensatory changes that occur as the result of reduced secretion of PTH and impaired PTH-dependent synthesis of 1,25-$(OH)_2$vitamin D. In bone, less calcium is mobilized into the circulation because of reduced resorption. In the intestine a lower fraction of calcium is absorbed because of the decreased availability of 1,25-$(OH)_2$vitamin D. In the kidneys more calcium is excreted following an oral calcium load, since renal tubular reabsorption of calcium is reduced by decreased availability of PTH (and to a lesser extent by a decreased amount of circulating 1,25-$(OH)_2$vitamin D).

This chapter considers the view that the hypercalciuria of nephrolithiasis is composed of several entities of heterogeneous origin. Prevailing major theories of hypercalciuria are incorporated by assigning them a stature as separate entities. This decision was made because no single theory could explain the wide spectrum of characteristics reported in the literature on hypercalciuric nephrolithiasis. It is assumed that the claims in many reports of the existence of a single etiologic scheme might represent a selection bias.

Absorptive Hypercalciuria

The primary abnormality in absorptive hypercalciuria is the intestinal hyperabsorption of calcium, presumed to occur independently of 1,25-$(OH)_2$vitamin D (Fig. 3–5).[6] The consequent increase in the circulating concentration of calcium enhances the renal filtered load and suppresses parathyroid function. Hypercalciuria ensues from the increased filtered load and the reduced tubular reabsorption of calcium consequent to parathyroid suppression. The excessive renal loss of calcium compensates for the high calcium absorption from the intestinal tract and helps to maintain the serum calcium concentration in the normal range. This condition excludes those with a primary renal phosphate leak or an excessive 1,25-$(OH)_2$vitamin D production, which are discussed as separate entities.

The exact cause for the enhancement of intestinal calcium absorption is not known. It may be a primary jejunal disease, since the high calcium absorption has been disclosed only in the jejunum,[40] and the absorption of magnesium and phosphate has been shown to be normal,[32, 41] unlike the action of 1,25-$(OH)_2$vitamin D, which is characterized by a stimulated absorption of calcium in the jejunum, ileum, and colon and of magnesium and phosphate in the jeju-

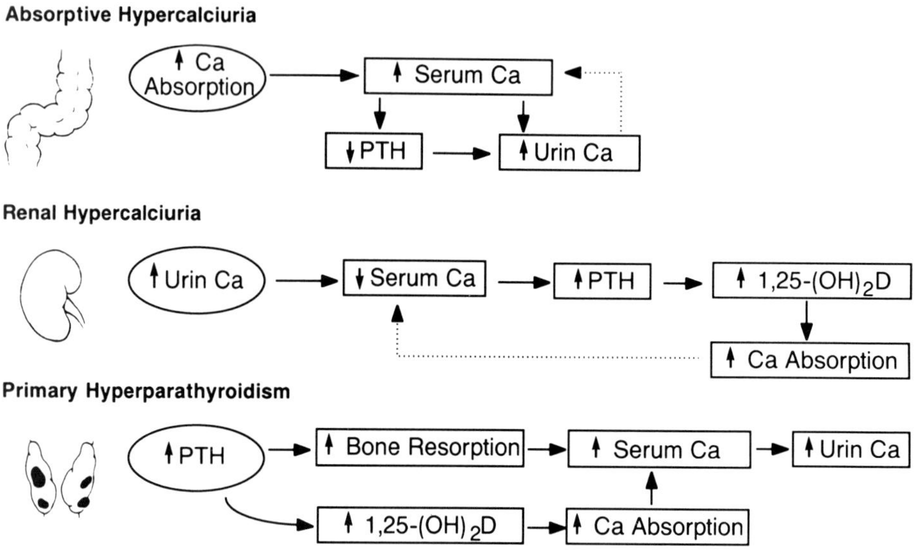

FIGURE 3–5. Schemes for the major forms of hypercalciuria.

num.[32, 41] This conclusion is supported by the finding of a higher uptake of calcium by jejunal (biopsy) tissue from patients with hypercalciuric nephrolithiasis than from control subjects.[42] The calcium uptake was found to be nonsaturable and unaffected by metabolic inhibitors. The results indicated a passive process rather than an active transport, further lending support to the operation of a 1,25-$(OH)_2$vitamin D–independent mechanism.

The primary nature of this disturbance is indicated by the persistence of intestinal hyperabsorption of calcium during treatment with adrenocorticosteroids (which lowers intestinal calcium absorption in sarcoidosis),[43] thiazide (which lowers urinary calcium),[44, 45] and orthophosphate (which reduces the serum concentration of 1,25-$(OH)_2$vitamin D).[46] Although certain dietary aberrations (such as high sodium and animal protein intake)[26] may exaggerate hypercalciuria, the institution of a constant dietary regimen without excesses does not correct the basic abnormality in intestinal calcium absorption.[3] Moreover, this disturbance appears to be inherited as an autosomal dominant trait.[47] Although not all subjects had clinically evident stone disease, the physiologic "marker" of increased calcium absorption was disclosed in the index patient as well as in all cohorts from three generations who were examined. Recently, biochemical and physiologic features of absorptive hypercalciuria were disclosed in inbred hypercalciuric rats, supporting the genetic predisposition for absorptive hypercalciuria.[19] Marked intestinal hyperabsorption of calcium and hypercalciuria were present in the setting of normal values for serum PTH and 1,25-$(OH)_2$vitamin D, indicative of a vitamin D–independent process.

There is no evidence that the skeleton is adversely affected in this condition,[6] consistent with the lack of parathyroid stimulation, hypophosphatemia, or 1,25-$(OH)_2$vitamin D excess. Normal values have been reported for serum osteocalcin, alkaline phosphatase activity, urinary hydroxyproline, and bone density in the radius (shaft) and lumbar vertebrae.[6] No clinically evident bone disease has been attributed to absorptive hypercalciuria. Calcium conservation is intact even when the intestinal calcium absorption is reduced by sodium cellulose phosphate. The absorbed calcium (lumen to blood) exceeds urinary calcium by an amount equivalent to the estimated net secreted calcium.[6]

It has been reported that the majority of patients with hypercalciuric nephrolithiasis excrete calcium in urine that exceeds the intake when challenged by a severe calcium restriction, arguing against the occurrence of primary intestinal hyperabsorption of calcium.[17] However, this study was conducted with an instructed calcium-restricted diet, which could well have overestimated calcium intake. Urinary calcium may exceed calcium intake if calcium restriction is severe enough, even in normal subjects.[48] Moreover, doubts have been raised about the intestinal origin of hypercalciuria because urinary calcium remains higher than in normal subjects despite calcium restriction and because calcium balance has been reported to be negative in many hypercalciuric patients. It should be noted, however, that patients with absorptive hypercalciuria should still absorb a greater fraction of calcium despite a restricted calcium pool and should thus excrete more calcium than normal subjects.[3] During sodium cellulose phosphate therapy (which restricts the intraluminal calcium pool), the actually measured absorbed calcium still exceeded urinary calcium among patients with documented absorptive hypercalciuria.[6] Moreover, calcium balance is a relatively imprecise technique, largely because of inaccuracies in fecal collection and a requirement for long-term stabilization before assessment of balance.

In this classic presentation of absorptive hypercalciuria, evidence for a "primary" renal calcium leak is lacking. Fasting urinary calcium may be secondarily increased in patients with absorptive hypercalciuria from the primary enhancement of intestinal calcium absorption.[49] If the duration of the fast is inadequate and the absorbed calcium is incompletely cleared by the kidneys, the high calcium absorption may cause fasting hypercalciuria by increasing the renal filtered load of calcium and by suppressing parathyroid function, thus impairing the renal tubular reabsorption of calcium. However, fasting hypercalciuria can be eliminated by a prolongation of the fast or by the prior administration of sodium cellulose phosphate (which binds calcium in the intestinal tract and reduces calcium absorption), without provoking hyperparathyroidism.[49] The lack of a generalized disturbance in renal proximal tubular function is shown by a normal calciuric response to carbohydrate load[50] and by a normal natriuretic response to thiazide.[51]

Renal Hypercalciuria

The primary abnormality in renal hypercalciuria is believed to be the impairment of the renal tubular reabsorption of calcium (Fig. 3–5).[15, 52] The consequent reduction in the circulating concentration of calcium stimulates parathyroid function. There may be an excessive mobilization of calcium from bone and an enhanced intestinal absorption of calcium because of the PTH excess and the ensuing stimulation of the renal synthesis of 1,25-$(OH)_2$vitamin D. These effects restore the serum calcium level toward normal. Unlike in primary hyperparathyroidism, the serum calcium level is normal, and the state of hyperparathyroidism is secondary.

Some patients with hypercalciuric nephrolithiasis, albeit a minority in most series, have been shown to have a biochemical presentation supporting operation of the preceding scheme. The occurrence of high serum PTH levels or urinary cyclic adenosine monophosphate (cAMP), as well as elevated serum 1,25-$(OH)_2$vitamin D levels and intestinal calcium absorption, has been shown in such patients in the setting of normal serum calcium values and fasting hypercalciuria (indicative of renal calcium leak).[52]

A high serum osteocalcin level has been reported in renal hypercalciuria, unlike in absorptive hypercalciuria.[53] The correction of renal calcium leak by thiazide restores normal serum 1,25-$(OH)_2$vitamin D levels and fractional calcium absorption, commensurate with the correction of hyperparathyroidism.[45] These findings support the contention that 1,25-$(OH)_2$vitamin D synthesis is enhanced by secondary parathyroid stimulation and that intestinal calcium absorption is high owing to 1,25-$(OH)_2$vitamin D excess.

In some patients with renal hypercalciuria, parathyroid stimulation may not be manifest because of the persistent effect of absorbed calcium.[49] However, secondary hyperparathyroidism may be unmasked by a further dietary calcium restriction or by an inhibition of intestinal calcium absorption with sodium cellulose phosphate. The persistent effect of absorbed calcium also manifests itself in patients with absorptive hypercalciuria by fasting hypercalciuria and normal or suppressed parathyroid function.[49] However, sodium cellulose phosphate restores normal fasting urinary calcium but does not cause secondary hyperparathyroidism. This background is the basis for the improved diagnostic differentiation of renal and absorptive hypercalciurias from the ratio of serum PTH and fractional (intestinal) calcium absorption[54] and from fasting urinary calcium-cAMP discriminant score.[49] Both measures are indices of parathyroid function corrected for the degree of intestinal calcium absorption. Serum PTH and urinary cAMP (measures of parathyroid function), expressed relative to fractional radiocalcium absorption or urinary calcium (reflective of intestinal calcium absorption), were distinctly higher in renal hypercalciuria than in absorptive hypercalciuria.

The occurrence of a primary renal calcium leak is supported by three lines of evidence. First, fasting hypercalciuria is associated with parathyroid stimulation and is inadequately corrected by the inhibition of intestinal calcium absorption (and removing the effect of absorbed calcium) with sodium cellulose phosphate.[49] Second, there is a unique natriuretic response to thiazide. When thiazide is given to block reabsorption of calcium and sodium in the distal (renal) tubule, impaired proximal tubular function would be manifest as an exaggerated renal excretion of these cations. The exaggerated natriuretic and calciuric response to hydrochlorothiazide was encountered only in patients with documented renal hypercalciuria with secondary hyperparathyroidism.[51] Third, an exaggerated calciuric response to 100 grams of glucose was encountered in patients with renal hypercalciuria with secondary hyperparathyroidism, not in those with absorptive hypercalciuria.[50] Ingestion of readily metabolizable carbohydrate (without calcium) normally augments renal calcium excretion, believed to be due to an alteration in renal proximal tubular function.[55]

It has been suggested that renal calcium leak is secondary to an excessive dietary intake of sodium.[56] High urinary sodium is common in the stone-forming population during a random dietary regimen. In normal subjects maintained on a constant dietary regimen, sodium chloride load (240 mEq/day) produces the full biochemical picture of renal hypercalciuria, including increases in urinary calcium, serum PTH, and 1,25-$(OH)_2$vitamin D and in intestinal calcium absorption.[57] Furosemide-induced natriuresis has been shown to cause hypercalciuria, parathyroid stimulation, and enhancement of intestinal calcium absorption.[58] However, renal hypercalciuria has been detected during a customary diet with normal sodium content (100 mEq/day), which does not produce a substantial renal calcium leak.[52] Moreover, in a preliminary study at Dallas, the institution of a very low sodium intake (9 mEq/day) does not eliminate fasting hypercalciuria in most patients with renal hypercalciuria.

Another nutritional cause for renal hypercalciuria is the ingestion of a diet high in animal proteins with sulfur-containing amino acids.[26, 59] The renal calcium leak may be produced by the direct action of an acid load that impairs renal tubular reabsorption of calcium or by poorly reabsorbed sulfate in the renal tubule, which "traps" and retards reabsorption of calcium. However, renal hypercalciuria has been diagnosed in the setting of normal animal protein intake.[52] Thus, this dietary excess, like high sodium intake, probably contributes to, but may not be solely responsible for, the renal hypercalciuria.

That renal calcium leak (and secondary hyperparathyroidism) had been longstanding is shown by changes disclosed in bone density. Although clinical bone disease is rare, bone density, as measured by photon absorptiometry in the distal third of the radius, is reduced in the group with renal hypercalciuria (compared with age- and sex-matched control subjects).[60] These results indicate that secondary hyperparathyroidism exerts deleterious effects on the skeleton. The lack of a more serious involvement is probably due to the compensatory intestinal hyperabsorption of calcium that results from the PTH-induced renal synthesis of 1,25-$(OH)_2$vitamin D. This compensation may be inadequate, since urinary calcium sometimes exceeds absorbed calcium indicative of negative calcium balance.

The danger of an adverse effect on the skeleton is much greater in postmenopausal women with renal hypercalciuria. Because of a disturbed vitamin D metabolism, secondary hyperparathyroidism from renal calcium leak does not stimulate 1,25-$(OH)_2$vitamin D synthesis. Thus, the lack of an increase in intestinal calcium absorption does not compensate for the excessive renal calcium loss, exposing patients to negative calcium balance. Recently, this pathogenetic scheme has been described in a group of postmenopausal women with osteoporosis.[61]

Renal hypercalciuria associated with other metabolic causes (such as distal renal tubular acidosis) is described elsewhere (Chapter 6).

To summarize, there are clearly distinguishing features between absorptive hypercalciuria and renal hypercalciuria in their classic presentations[7] (Table 3–1).

TABLE 3–1. EVIDENCE THAT ABSORPTIVE AND RENAL HYPERCALCIURIAS ARE PHYSIOLOGICALLY DISTINCT

Item	Absorptive Hypercalciuria Type I or Type II	Renal Hypercalciuria
Parathyroid function	Normal or suppressed	Stimulated
Renal calcium leak	Secondary	Primary
Effect of sodium cellulose phosphate	Correctable	Noncorrectable
Natriuretic response to thiazide	Normal	Exaggerated
Intestinal calcium absorption	Primarily increased	Secondarily increased
Jejunal absorption	Increased	Increased
Ileal absorption	Normal	Increased
Intestinal magnesium absorption	Normal	Increased
Serum 1,25-$(OH)_2$vitamin D vs. calcium absorption	No correlation	Correlated
Effect of treatment with:		
thiazide on serum 1,25-$(OH)_2$ vitamin D and calcium absorption	No change	Decreased
sodium cellulose phosphate on		
urinary calcium	Markedly decreased	Less marked
calcium conservation	Intact	Impaired
Skeletal status		
Bone density (radial shaft)	Normal	Decreased
Calcium balance	Normal	Normal or negative

Thus, renal hypercalciuria is characterized by fasting hypercalciuria and secondary hyperparathyroidism. The intestinal calcium absorption is primarily increased in absorptive hypercalciuria, as shown by independence from 1,25-$(OH)_2$vitamin D action, a lack of correction by thiazide diuretic, and the localized involvement of jejunum only. In contrast, the intestinal calcium absorption is secondarily stimulated in renal hypercalciuria, as it is dependent on 1,25-$(OH)_2$vitamin D action and is corrected by thiazide. There may be a more generalized disturbance in renal tubular function in renal hypercalciuria, as shown by an exaggerated natriuretic response to thiazide and an exaggerated calciuric response to carbohydrate load.

Resorptive Hypercalciuria

Resorptive hypercalciuria resulting in kidney stones is generally due to primary hyperparathyroidism. Other causes of excessive bone resorption (such as oncogenic hypercalcemia, thyrotoxicosis, and sarcoidosis) infrequently or less commonly result in stone formation. In primary hyperparathyroidism, the initial event is excessive resorption of bone resulting from hypersecretion of PTH by adenomatous or hyperplastic parathyroid glands (Fig. 3–5). The intestinal absorption of calcium is frequently elevated, because of PTH-dependent stimulation of the renal synthesis of 1,25-$(OH)_2$vitamin D. These effects increase the circulating concentration and the renal filtered load of calcium. The occurrence of hypercalciuria in primary hyperparathyroidism seems paradoxical, since the primary renal effect of PTH is to stimulate tubular reabsorption of calcium. However, hypercalciuria is often encountered in primary hyperparathyroidism because the PTH-dependent augmentation of renal tubular reabsorption of calcium is "overcome" by an increase in the renal filtered load and by a suppressive effect of hypercalcemia on calcium reabsorption.

Stone formation is becoming less commonly encountered in primary hyperparathyroidism, probably reflective of earlier detection. Thus, the physiologic background leading to stone formation in primary hyperparathyroidism requires consideration. The biochemical and clinical features of patients with primary hyperparathyroidism who develop nephrolithiasis may be different from those of patients without stones. Patients with stones are believed to have a longer duration of the disease process, a less severe hypercalcemia, and a smaller amount of abnormal parathyroid tissue than patients who present with bone disease.[62] Hypercalciuria is frequent in stone-forming patients with primary hyperparathyroidism. Hypercalciuria has often been implicated as one of the causes of renal stone formation, since it is also a frequent finding in normocalcemic patients with calcium nephrolithiasis. The hypercalciuria could result from excessive PTH-dependent bone resorption or enhanced intestinal absorption of calcium caused by the PTH-dependent synthesis of 1,25-$(OH)_2$vitamin D or from both. The hypercalciuria of intestinal origin may be more important for the formation of renal stones.[63] Thus, an apparent predilection for nephrolithiasis has been reported in the group of patients with primary hyperparathyroidism who possess a high circulating concentration of 1,25-$(OH)_2$vitamin D and an increased intestinal absorption of calcium. Conversely, patients presenting with bone disease were reported to have a lower glomerular filtration rate and serum 25-hydroxyvitamin D level and higher values for serum PTH, compared with those without bone disease. It has been suggested that reduced renal mass and vitamin

D substrate led to an impaired synthesis of 1,25-$(OH)_2$vitamin D, further exaggerating PTH secretion and causing bone disease.[64]

However, patients with primary hyperparathyroidism who present with renal stones may not be readily distinguished from those without stones on the basis of the biochemical or physicochemical picture.[65] First, there is not a unique histologic picture of parathyroid glands characteristic of stone formation. The prevalence of nephrolithiasis is equivalent in patients with parathyroid hyperplasia and those with parathyroid adenoma. Second, bone density by photon absorptiometry is reduced in both the stone-forming and the non–stone-forming groups.[65] The mean value for the fractional change in bone density is actually lower in the group with stones than in the group without stones, although the difference does not reach statistical significance. It thus seems clear that the stone-forming group also has the skeletal involvement of PTH excess. Third, the biochemical features of patients with stones cannot be distinguished from those of patients without stones, at least in a group with surgically proven primary hyperparathyroidism.[65] Thus, patients with stones have degrees of elevation of serum calcium, PTH, and 1,25-$(OH)_2$vitamin D levels, fractional calcium absorption, and urinary calcium equivalent to those of their non–stone-forming counterparts. Most patients without stones have a high fractional calcium absorption, and some patients with stones have normal absorption. Fourth, no significant difference can be found between patients with primary hyperparathyroidism presenting with nephrolithiasis and those with bone disease with respect to serum calcium level, parathyroid function, urinary calcium, serum 1,25-$(OH)_2$vitamin D concentration, or fractional calcium absorption.[65]

Finally, the urinary environment of patients with stones cannot be distinguished from that of non–stone-forming patients on the basis of usual urinary composition or saturation with stone-forming salts.[65] It is possible that a reduced inhibitor activity in urine contributes to the predilection for stone formation. It has been reported, though not confirmed, that urinary citrate is lower in patients with primary hyperparathyroidism who present with stones than in those without stones, though not different from the amount in normal subjects without stones.[66] A similar reduction in urinary pyrophosphate has been reported in stone-forming patients.[66] It has been suggested that promoter or promoters of stone formation may be present, since the formation product (limit of metastability) of calcium oxalate and brushite in the urine of stone-forming patients with primary hyperparathyroidism has been sometimes shown to be lower than that of synthetic urine devoid of inhibitors.[22, 67] The nature of the promoter or promoters has not been identified.

Although the overall scheme for resorptive hypercalciuria in primary hyperparathyroidism is generally accepted, the mechanisms by which intestinal calcium absorption is controlled need to be elucidated. The high intestinal calcium absorption is customarily ascribed to the enhanced PTH-dependent synthesis of 1,25-$(OH)_2$vitamin D. Thus, the fractional calcium absorption bears a direct relationship to serum 1,25-$(OH)_2$vitamin D.[68] However, in some patients with primary hyperparathyroidism, the intestinal hyperabsorption of calcium persists after parathyroidectomy, despite restoration of normal serum 1,25-$(OH)_2$vitamin D concentration.[69] The results suggest that factors other than 1,25-$(OH)_2$vitamin D contribute to the maintenance of high intestinal calcium absorption in hyperparathyroid patients in the postoperative state.

One possibility, though speculative, is the release from the skeleton of a non–vitamin D factor that stimulates calcium absorption, occurring postoperatively during "bone healing." Another possibility is the co-occurrence of absorptive hypercalciuria and primary hyperparathyroidism as independent but relatively common entities in the same patient.[70] The coexistence of absorptive hypercalciuria should be suspected in patients who continue to have hypercalciuria and suffer from recurrent stone formation despite restoration of normal parathyroid function following parathyroidectomy.

Renal Phosphate Leak

In this condition, hypophosphatemia ensuing from renal phosphate leak has been implicated in the intestinal hyperabsorption of calcium by stimulating the renal synthesis of 1,25-$(OH)_2$vitamin D (Fig. 3–6).[4] This scheme is supported by the following findings:

1. Low tubular threshold concentration of phosphate (TmP) and hypophosphatemia in the setting of hypercalciuria without parathyroid stimulation.
2. Ability of induced hypophosphatemia from limitation of intestinal phosphate absorption to stimulate the renal synthesis of 1,25-$(OH)_2$vitamin D.[71]
3. Significant inverse correlation between serum 1,25-$(OH)_2$vitamin D and serum phosphorus concentration.[72]

Moreover, the presence of hypophosphatemia or a high serum 1,25-$(OH)_2$vitamin D level, or both, provides an explanation (other than PTH excess) for the reported occurrence of fasting hypercalciuria, poor calcium conservation, reduced bone density, and abnormal histomorphometric picture of bone[73, 74] in hypercalciuric patients with normal parathyroid function. Findings on histomorphometric analysis of bone with normal or low osteoclastic resorption, reduced osteoblastic activity with increased osteoid, and a reduction in mineral apposition rate are compatible with a prolonged hypophosphatemic state. By so affecting bone,

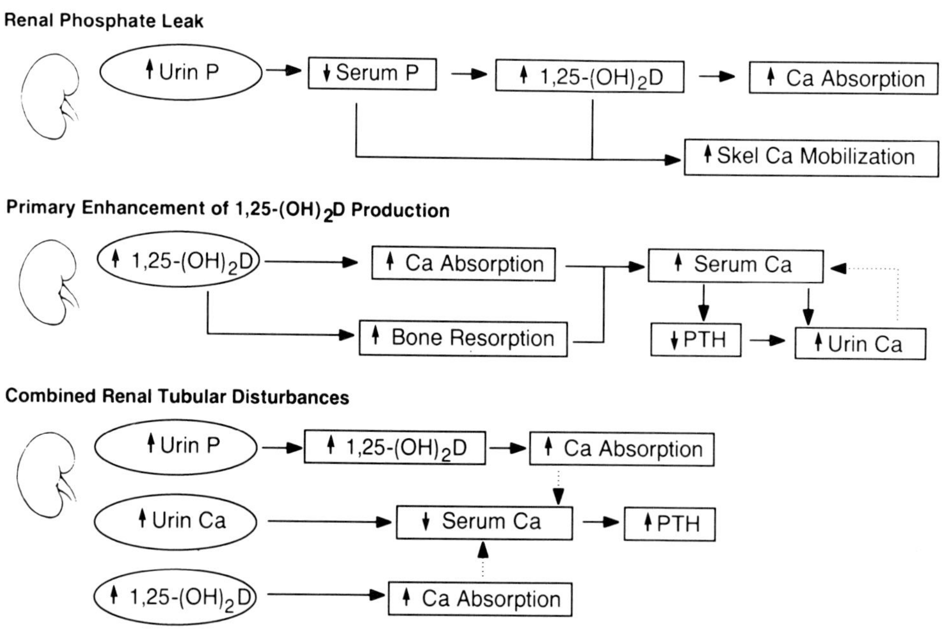

FIGURE 3–6. Schemes for the remaining forms of hypercalciuria.

hypophosphatemia could cause fasting hypercalciuria and negative calcium balance.

In a careful study of patients on a controlled dietary regimen, renal phosphate leak was an uncommon cause of calcium nephrolithiasis.[46] Two patients who satisfied the diagnostic criteria of this entity were shown later to have surgically proven primary hyperparathyroidism. Thus, renal phosphate leak may sometimes represent an early phase of primary hyperparathyroidism. Moreover, orthophosphate treatment failed to restore normal intestinal calcium absorption despite a reduction in serum 1,25-$(OH)_2$vitamin D, arguing against the widespread occurrence of this pathogenetic scheme.[46]

Renal phosphate leak may not be primarily renal in origin but may result from certain dietary or environmental influences. In patients with hypercalciuric nephrolithiasis who presented with a high intestinal calcium absorption and normal serum calcium level, serum phosphorus level and the TmP were low normal while the patients were maintained on a random diet in an outpatient setting.[46] When these patients were evaluated in an inpatient setting while on a constant dietary regimen, serum phosphorus and TmP concentrations rose to the midnormal range.

The exact dietary or environmental factor responsible for this observation is unknown. One possibility is differences in phosphate intake (approximately 1500 mg/day in an outpatient setting and 800 mg/day in an inpatient setting). A high phosphate intake may lead to a stimulated renal excretion of phosphate even in the absence of PTH, by "renal phosphate adaptation."[73] Though unproven, an overly efficient renal adaptive mechanism could explain the fall in serum phosphorus concentration. This speculation is supported by the finding of a fall in serum phosphorus concentration in stone-forming patients treated with orthophosphate in the absence of parathyroid stimulation.[76] Another nutritional cause of renal phosphate leak might be the dietary sodium abuse by the stone-forming population under the random regimen previously alluded to, which leads to a volume-expanded state and impaired proximal tubular reabsorption.

Despite the uncommonness of "true" renal phosphate leak and the possible dietary origin of this disorder, a recent study by Tieder and colleagues suggests that it could occur on a metabolic or genetic basis.[77] They reported a new hereditary syndrome of hypophosphatemic rickets and hypercalciuria in six affected members of one kindred. The afflicted patients presented with low TmP, hypophosphatemia, high serum 1,25-$(OH)_2$vitamin D levels, increased intestinal calcium absorption, and hypercalciuria. Although the full-blown biochemical manifestation of renal phosphate leak was present, the patients suffered from bone disease and not renal stones.

Primary Enhancement of 1,25-$(OH)_2$Vitamin D Production

Many of the biochemical characteristics of absorptive hypercalciuria can be explained by an overproduction of 1,25-$(OH)_2$vitamin D occurring independently (Fig. 3–6). These features include intestinal hyperabsorption of calcium, parathyroid suppression, and hypercalciuria. This conclusion is supported by the biochemical similarity of absorptive hypercalciuria to the state induced in normal subjects by exogenous 1,25-$(OH)_2$vitamin D therapy.[78] Hypercalciuria could also be due to the 1,25-$(OH)_2$vitamin D–dependent stimulation of bone resorption.[79] Exogenous 1,25-$(OH)_2$vitamin D has been shown to augment urinary calcium excretion even when patients are placed on a low-calcium diet, as well as to increase urinary hydroxyproline (a marker of bone resorption) and serum osteocalcin (a marker of bone formation and turnover).[80]

The 1,25-$(OH)_2$vitamin D excess could also cause fasting hypercalciuria. The parathyroid suppression can secondarily produce the high fasting urinary calcium sometimes encountered, because of the loss of PTH-dependent stimulation of the renal tubular reabsorption of calcium.[78] Thus, there is secondary renal calcium leak. The picture of fasting hypercalciuria with suppressed parathyroid function occurs because of a primary increase in 1,25-$(OH)_2$vitamin D synthesis, as a form of an acquired renal calcium leak.

The scheme for excessive 1,25-$(OH)_2$vitamin D production is supported by the finding of high serum 1,25-$(OH)_2$vitamin D levels in some patients with absorptive hypercalciuria and the demonstration of an accelerated in vivo 1,25-$(OH)_2$vitamin D synthesis in patients with absorptive hypercalciuria selected from high extremes of serum 1,25-$(OH)_2$vitamin D levels.[5] This condition probably represents a variable fraction of those presenting with absorptive hypercalciuria and should be distinguished from classic absorptive hypercalciuria (previously described), in which a pathogenetic role of 1,25-$(OH)_2$vitamin D is not implicated.

Prolonged enhanced synthesis of 1,25-$(OH)_2$vitamin D may up-regulate the intestinal receptor for this vitamin D metabolite. Under this circumstance, the serum concentration of 1,25-$(OH)_2$vitamin D may not be clearly increased.[81]

Combined Renal Tubular Disturbances

The occurrence of fasting hypercalciuria with normal parathyroid function could be explained by multiple disturbances in renal proximal tubular function, characterized by varying degrees of calcium leak, a disturbance in phosphate transport, and accelerated 1,25-$(OH)_2$vitamin D synthesis (Fig. 3–6).[17] This unifying scheme could explain the pathogenesis of both renal and absorptive hypercalciurias from the general defect originating in the kidney. The predominance of the renal calcium leak would lead to renal hypercalciuria with secondary hyperparathyroidism. On the other hand, the prominence of 1,25-$(OH)_2$vitamin D synthesis, occurring independently of or secondarily from renal phosphate leak, would produce a picture of absorptive hypercalciuria by enhancing intestinal calcium absorption and masking parathyroid stimulation. The occurrence of both renal calcium leak and renal phosphate leak or increased 1,25-$(OH)_2$vitamin D synthesis may produce a picture of fasting hypercalciuria without parathyroid stimulation. Thus, renal hypercalciuria need not be accompanied by hyperparathyroidism, and absorptive hypercalciuria results secondarily from 1,25-$(OH)_2$vitamin D–dependent stimulation of intestinal calcium absorption.

Other Causes of Hypercalciuria

Hypercalciuria may be due to other causes. Enhanced renal excretion of prostaglandin E_2 has been reported in patients with hypercalciuric nephrolithiasis. The treatment with inhibitors of prostaglandin synthesis reduced urinary calcium in normocalcemic patients with nephrolithiasis,[18,82–84] but not in normal subjects.[85] The reduction in urinary calcium in stone-forming patients occurred with a decline in glomerular filtration rate in one study,[18] but not in another study.[82]

The possibility that prostaglandins may play a causal role in hypercalciuria is intriguing but awaits validation.

Recently, a high interleukin-1 activity was detected in the culture media of peripheral blood monocytes from patients with fasting hypercalciuria and with normal serum PTH and 1,25-$(OH)_2$vitamin D levels.[86] This preliminary study suggests that a stimulated bone resorption by a local growth factor may contribute to hypercalciuria. Even if confirmed, this scheme is unlikely to be a major cause of hypercalciuria because of the infrequent occurrence of clinically evident bone disease.

DIAGNOSTIC CRITERIA

Diagnostic protocols are now available for the differentiation of hypercalciuria[8] (see Chapter 11 for details). The main distinguishing features are summarized in Table 3–2.

Absorptive hypercalciuria Type I is characterized by the following features:

1. Normocalcemia.
2. Normophosphatemia.
3. Normal fasting urinary calcium level (<0.11 mg/dl of glomerular filtrate [GF]).
4. Exaggerated urinary calcium values following an oral calcium load (>0.2 mg per milligram of creatinine).
5. Normal or suppressed parathyroid function (normal serum immunoreactive PTH).
6. Urinary calcium, while the patient is on a restricted diet (400 mg of calcium and 100 mEq of sodium per day), of more than 200 mg/day.[8]

These values reflect increased intestinal calcium absorption, resultant parathyroid suppression, and hypercalciuria. There is a strong male preponderance, with a special predilection for middle-aged white men. A positive family history of stones can be elicited from a majority of patients.

Absorptive hypercalciuria Type II is characterized by the same biochemical features as those of Type I except for normocalciuria (<200 mg/day) while the

TABLE 3–2. DIAGNOSTIC CRITERIA OF DIFFERENT FORMS OF HYPERCALCIURIA

	AH-I	AH-II	RH	PHPT	P Leak	1,25-Excess	Combined
Serum							
Calcium	N	N	N	↑	N	N	N
Phosphorus	N	N	N	↓	↓	N	N, ↓
PTH	N	N	↑	↑	N	N	N
1,25-$(OH)_2D$	N	N	↑	↑	↑	↑	↑
Urinary calcium							
Fasting	N	N	↑	↑	↑	↑	↑
24 hr, restricted	↑	N	↑	↑	↑	↑	↑
Postcalcium load	↑	↑	↑	↑	↑	↑	↑

Abbreviations: AH-I = absorptive hypercalciuria Type I; AH-II = absorptive hypercalciuria Type II; RH = renal hypercalciuria; PHPT = primary hyperparathyroidism; P leak = renal phosphate leak; 1,25-Excess = primary enhancement of 1,25-$(OH)_2$vitamin D production; Combined = combined renal tubular disturbances, PTH = parathyroid hormone; N = normal; ↑ = increase; ↓ = decrease. Restricted urinary calcium refers to 24-hr urinary calcium obtained during maintenance on a diet restricted in calcium (400 mg/day) and sodium (100 mEq/day). Postcalcium load urinary calcium indicates calcium excretion during 4 hr following an oral load of 1 gram of calcium.

patient is on a restricted diet (400 mg of calcium and 100 mEq of sodium per day).[8] If these patients are placed on a diet of 1000 mg of calcium and 100 mEq of sodium per day, urinary calcium exceeds 4 mg/kg/day or 250 mg/day. This condition probably represents a less severe variant of absorptive hypercalciuria Type I.

Renal hypercalciuria has the following features:

1. Normocalcemia.
2. High fasting urinary calcium level (>0.11 mg/dl of GF).
3. Enhanced parathyroid activity (high serum immunoreactive PTH or 24-hour urinary cAMP >5.4 nmol/dl of GF, or both).[8]

These results indicate a renal leak of calcium with compensatory parathyroid stimulation. With the continuing improvement in the PTH assay, the urinary cAMP is being assayed less commonly. Either serum PTH or urinary cAMP, or both, must be elevated to confirm the diagnosis of renal hypercalciuria. In most patients, urinary cAMP or serum PTH, which is high in the fasting state, decreases to the normal range following an oral calcium load, a finding indicative of the suppressibility of parathyroid stimulation. Bone density may be low in patients with renal hypercalciuria, and in some, osteopenia may occur. There is less male preponderance than in absorptive hypercalciuria. A history of urinary tract infection preceding the onset of stone disease may be elicited in many patients.

Primary hyperparathyroidism may be recognized by the presence of hypercalcemia, hypophosphatemia, hypercalciuria, and increased or inappropriately high serum PTH levels. Bone density in the radial diaphysis is often low. Hypercalcemic symptoms, peptic ulcer, or bone disease (osteitis, pathologic fractures, and osteoporosis) may be present. There is a female preponderance, with postmenopausal women being particularly afflicted.

Fasting hypercalciuria with normal parathyroid function is characteristic of normocalcemic hypercalciuric patients with calcium nephrolithiasis in whom the diagnosis of absorptive or renal hypercalciuria cannot be made with certainty. It is typified by normocalcemia, a high fasting urinary calcium (>0.11 mg/dl of GF), and a normal serum PTH level. In many cases, this presentation is accounted for by an incomplete clearance of absorbed calcium in patients with an underlying absorptive or renal hypercalciuria. A more complete elimination of the effect of absorbed calcium by prior treatment with sodium cellulose phosphate may provide further clarification.[49] In patients with persistent fasting hypercalciuria and normal serum PTH levels (despite preparation with sodium cellulose phosphate), one should suspect renal phosphate leak (previously called absorptive hypercalciuria Type III), primary 1,25-$(OH)_2$vitamin D excess, or combined disturbances in renal proximal tubular function. In renal phosphate leak, the serum phosphorus level and renal threshold concentration of phosphorus are less than 2.5 mg/dl and remain low despite examination in an inpatient setting and avoidance of dietary phosphate excess.[46]

MANAGEMENT OF CALCIUM NEPHROLITHIASIS

It is recommended that conservative measures (high fluid intake and avoidance of dietary excesses) be applied in all patients with nephrolithiasis.[87] This conservative treatment program is described in detail in Chapter 12. Briefly, a high fluid intake, as well as restriction of sodium and oxalate, should be applied in all patients with hypercalciuric nephrolithiasis. Calcium restriction is useful in absorptive hypercalciuria, resorptive hypercalciuria, renal phosphate leak, and primary enhancement of 1,25-$(OH)_2$vitamin D synthesis. In renal hypercalciuria, calcium restriction is not indicated, since it could exaggerate secondary hyperparathyroidism, especially if it is applied alone.

When a conservative program fails or is not expected to be completely effective, specific medical treatments should be instituted while still applying conservative measures. This chapter discusses specific medical treatments for the prevention of hypercalciuric nephrolithiasis (Table 3–3).

Absorptive Hypercalciuria Type I

Sodium Cellulose Phosphate. No treatment program is capable of correcting the basic abnormality of absorptive hypercalciuria, although several drugs restore normal calcium excretion. Sodium cellulose phosphate best meets the criteria for optimal therapy.[88, 89] When given orally, this nonabsorbable ion-exchange resin binds calcium and inhibits calcium absorption. However, this inhibition is caused by limiting the amount of intraluminal calcium available for absorption and not by correcting the basic disturbance in calcium transport.

The above-described mode of action accounts for the two potential complications of sodium cellulose phosphate therapy. First, the treatment may cause magnesium depletion by also binding dietary magnesium.[88] Second, sodium cellulose phosphate may produce secondary hyperoxaluria by binding divalent cations in the intestinal tract, reducing divalent cation-oxalate complexation, and making more oxalate available for absorption.[90] These complications may be overcome by oral magnesium supplementation (10 mEq of magnesium citrate twice a day, given separately from sodium cellulose phosphate) and moderate dietary restriction of oxalate (see Chapters 11 and 12). Under such circumstances, sodium cellulose phosphate (10 to 15 grams/day, given with meals) has been shown to lower urinary calcium, reduce urinary saturation of calcium salts, and retard new stone formation, without substantially altering urinary oxalate or magnesium.[91] This drug therapy is contraindicated in other forms of hypercalciuria because it may further stimulate parathyroid function and cause negative calcium

TABLE 3–3. MEDICAL MANAGEMENT OF HYPERCALCIURIC NEPHROLITHIASIS

Condition	Treatment	Typical Dose	Mechanism of Action
AH-I	Sodium cellulose phosphate + magnesium citrate	2.5 grams with meals + 10 mEq bid	Binds dietary calcium Avoid magnesium depletion
	Trichlormethiazide + potassium citrate	4 mg qd + 15 mEq bid	Lower urinary calcium Prevent hypokalemia Increase urinary citrate
AH-II	Dietary calcium restriction	400 mg qd	Lower urinary calcium
RH	Trichlormethiazide + potassium citrate	4 mg qd + 15 mEq bid	Lower urinary calcium Prevent hypokalemia Increase urinary citrate
P leak	Sodium-potassium phosphate (neutral)	0.5 gram phosphorus tid	Prevent hypophosphatemia Lower urinary calcium Increase urinary pyrophosphate and citrate

balance. Because of this potential complication, it may be prudent to restrict the use of sodium cellulose phosphate to severe cases of absorptive hypercalciuria Type I (urinary calcium >350 mg/day) or to thiazide-resistant absorptive hypercalciuria and avoid usage in those with increased risk for bone disease (growing children, elderly persons, and postmenopausal women).

Thiazide. Thiazide is not considered a selective therapy for absorptive hypercalciuria, since it does not decrease intestinal calcium absorption in this condition.[45] However, this drug has been widely used to treat this disorder, because of its hypocalciuric action.[9] This diuretic corrects the hypercalciuria directly by augmenting calcium reabsorption in the distal tubule and indirectly by causing extracellular volume depletion, which then stimulates proximal tubular reabsorption of calcium. Physicochemically, the urinary environment becomes less saturated with respect to calcium oxalate and brushite, largely because of the reduced calcium excretion.[92] Moreover, urinary inhibitor activity, as reflected by an increase in the limit of metastability, occurs during the early period of treatment, probably by transiently stimulating renal excretion of pyrophosphate[93] and zinc.[94]

A recent study indicates that thiazide may have a limited long-term effectiveness in absorptive hypercalciuria Type I.[44] Thiazide is usually effective in reducing urinary calcium during the first 2 years of treatment. Thereafter, however, urinary calcium generally returns to the pretreatment range. In contrast, intestinal calcium absorption remains persistently elevated throughout thiazide treatment. Preliminary studies suggest that thiazide may cause accretion of calcium in bone during the early years of therapy.[21] Bone density, determined in the distal third of the radius by single-photon absorptiometry, increased significantly during thiazide treatment of absorptive hypercalciuria. With continued treatment, however, the rise in bone density stabilized as the hypocalciuric effect of thiazide became attenuated. The results suggest that thiazide treatment may eventually cause a low turnover state of bone, which interferes with a continued calcium accretion in the skeleton. The "rejected" calcium would then be excreted in urine. In contrast, bone density was not significantly altered in renal hypercalciuria in which thiazide was shown to cause a decline in intestinal calcium absorption commensurate with a reduction in urinary calcium.[21]

Thus, thiazide is often ineffective in correcting hypercalciuria in absorptive hypercalciuria after more than 2 years of treatment. Another problem with thiazide is the induction of hypocitraturia (see Chapter 6).[95] Intracellular acidosis resulting from thiazide-induced hypokalemia may augment renal tubular reabsorption of citrate. In this author's experience, thiazide used alone is relatively ineffective in the management of stone disease in patients with absorptive hypercalciuria Type I, probably owing to these changes.

It is recognized that sodium cellulose phosphate does not correct the basic intestinal calcium transport defect in absorptive hypercalciuria Type I and that thiazide treatment may eventually be ineffective in correcting hypercalciuria or is attendant with certain complications. The following guidelines in the use of these two agents are recommended until more selective therapies are found.

Sodium cellulose phosphate might be used in patients with severe absorptive hypercalciuria Type I (urinary calcium >350 mg/day) or those resistant to or intolerant of thiazide therapy. In patients with absorptive hypercalciuria Type I who may be at risk for bone disease (growing children, elderly patients, or postmenopausal women), thiazide might be the first choice. When thiazide becomes ineffective in lowering urinary calcium, this treatment may be temporarily substituted by sodium cellulose phosphate or orthophosphate (for approximately 6 months). Restoration of the hypocalciuric response to thiazide may then ensue, permitting resumption of thiazide therapy.

Complications of thiazide include adverse symptoms of weakness, muscle cramping, fatigability, and impotence, an abnormal biochemical picture of hypokalemia, mild metabolic alkalosis, hyperuricemia, and hepatic dysfunction (rare). Besides hypocitraturia, previously mentioned, urinary uric acid may increase in some stone-forming patients during thiazide therapy, opposing the beneficial hypocalciuric action on stone formation.

In persons weighing more than 60 kg, recommended dosages are hydrochlorothiazide, 50 mg twice a day; trichlormethiazide, 4 mg/day; and chlorthalidone, 50 mg/day. In smaller individuals, one half of these dosages might be used. Potassium citrate (15 to 20 mEq twice a day) should be added to prevent hypokalemia and attendant hypocitraturia. Concurrent use of triamterene, a potassium-sparing agent, should be undertaken with caution because of recent reports of triamterene stone formation.[96] Amiloride may be used with thiazide, since it alone has sometimes been shown to exert a hypocalciuric action, to exaggerate the hypocalciuric action of thiazide and to prevent hypokalemia.[97] However, amiloride itself does not augment citrate excretion.[97] Thus, in patients with hypercalciuric nephrolithiasis presenting with hypocitraturia, in whom the use of potassium citrate is contemplated, it is probably wise to use thiazide alone without a potassium-sparing diuretic. Allopurinol (300 mg/day) may be necessary if hyperuricemia (>8.5 mg/dl) or moderate-to-marked hyperuricosuria (>800 mg/day) develops. Sodium restriction (100 mEq/day) is critical, since a high sodium intake could blunt the hypocalciuric action of thiazide and exaggerate thiazide-induced hypocitraturia.

Absorptive Hypercalciuria Type II

The features of absorptive hypercalciuria Type II are identical with those of absorptive hypercalciuria Type I, except that normocalciuria (<200 mg/day) can be induced by a diet of 400 mg of calcium and 100 mEq of sodium per day.[8] In addition, many patients show disdain for drinking fluids and thus excrete a concentrated urine. A low calcium intake (400 to 600 mg/day) and high fluid intake (sufficient to achieve a minimal urine output of greater than 2 liters/day) would seem ideally indicated, since normocalciuria could be restored by dietary calcium restriction alone[91] and increased urine volume has been shown to reduce the urinary saturation of calcium oxalate, brushite, and monosodium urate and to inhibit spontaneous nucleation of calcium oxalate.[98]

Renal Hypercalciuria

Thiazide is ideally indicated for renal hypercalciuria.[45, 52] By correcting renal calcium leak, thiazide corrects secondary hyperparathyroidism and restores a normal serum 1,25-$(OH)_2$vitamin D level and intestinal calcium absorption. In a recent study, thiazide has been shown to produce a sustained correction of hypercalciuria, commensurate with a restoration of normal serum 1,25-$(OH)_2$vitamin D levels and intestinal calcium absorption (and stability of bone density), during up to 10 years of therapy.[44] Thus, thiazide action in renal hypercalciuria differs from that previously described for absorptive hypercalciuria.

The treatment guidelines for thiazide are the same as those described for absorptive hypercalciuria Type I.

Primary Hyperparathyroidism

SURGICAL TREATMENT. Parathyroidectomy is the optimal treatment for the nephrolithiasis of primary hyperparathyroidism. Following removal of abnormal parathyroid tissue, urinary calcium is restored to normal commensurate with a decline in the serum concentration of calcium and in intestinal calcium absorption. The urinary environment becomes less saturated with respect to calcium oxalate and brushite, and its limit of metastability (formation product ratio) for these calcium salts increases.[67] There is typically a reduced rate of new stone formation, unless urinary tract infection is present. Parathyroidectomy is contraindicated in the secondary hyperparathyroidism of renal hypercalciuria and in absorptive hypercalciuria.

MEDICAL TREATMENT. There is no established medical treatment for the nephrolithiasis of primary hyperparathyroidism. Although orthophosphates (neutral sodium-potassium phosphate, 0.5 gram of phosphorus three to four times a day) have been recommended for disease of mild-to-moderate severity, their safety or efficacy has not yet been proved.[99] They should be used only when parathyroid surgery cannot be undertaken.

Estrogen is a reasonable alternative in postmenopausal women with primary hyperparathyroidism in whom surgery is refused or contraindicated.[100] This treatment (e.g., conjugated estrogen, 0.625 mg/day, 25 days of each month) has been shown to reduce the serum calcium concentration (by inhibiting PTH-induced bone resorption) and thereby decrease urinary calcium.

Thiazide is contraindicated in primary hyperparathyroidism, because of the potential aggravation of hypercalcemia.

Renal Phosphate Leak

ORTHOPHOSPHATE. Orthophosphate (neutral salt of sodium or potassium or both, 0.5 gram of phosphorus three to four times a day) would seem to be the logical treatment because of its potential for the inhibition of 1,25-$(OH)_2$vitamin D synthesis.[46, 101] However, there is currently no convincing evidence that this treatment restores normal intestinal calcium absorption in this condition.[46] Orthophosphate reduces urinary calcium probably by directly enhancing the renal tubular reabsorption of calcium. Urinary phosphorus is markedly increased during therapy, a finding reflecting the absorbability of soluble phosphate. Physicochemically, orthophosphate reduces the urinary saturation of calcium oxalate but increases that of brushite.[102] Moreover, the urinary inhibitor activity is increased, probably owing to the stimulated renal excretion of pyrophosphate and citrate. At the usual recommended dosages, the citraturic effect of orthophosphate is approximately one-third that of potassium citrate (see Chapter 6). Although reports to the contrary have appeared, this treatment program has been observed to cause soft tissue calcification and parathyroid stimulation.[103] A minor but frequent side effect is diarrhea. It is contraindicated in nephrolithiasis complicated by urinary tract infection.

Primary Enhancement of 1,25-$(OH)_2$Vitamin D Synthesis

There is no known treatment that is capable of correcting this disturbance. Adrenocorticosteroids do not reduce serum 1,25-$(OH)_2$vitamin D or calcium absorption in hypercalciuric nephrolithiasis, unlike in sarcoidosis.[43] Although orthophosphate has been shown to reduce serum 1,25-$(OH)_2$vitamin D, it does not correct hyperabsorption of calcium from the intestinal tract.[46]

Since the skeleton may be adversely affected owing to the bone-resorptive capacity of 1,25-$(OH)_2$vitamin D, thiazide may be preferable to sodium cellulose phosphate in controlling hypercalciuria. Eventual attenuation of the hypocalciuric action to thiazide is likely, as in absorptive hypercalciuria Type I.

A potentially useful agent is one that either inhibits the synthesis or facilitates the clearance of 1,25-$(OH)_2$vitamin D, such as ketoconazole[104] or 25,26-$(OH)_2$vitamin D,[105] as preliminary studies from Dallas indicate.

Combined Disturbance in Renal Tubular Function

Since renal calcium leak is presumed to be an invariant feature, coexisting with either phosphate leak or excessive 1,25-$(OH)_2$vitamin D synthesis, thiazide treatment should be attempted first. If this treatment is ineffective in controlling hypercalciuria or should hypercalcemia develop, orthophosphate or sodium cellulose phosphate may be added to the treatment program.

REFERENCES

1. Flocks RH: Calcium and phosphorus excretion in the urine of patients with renal or ureteral calculi. JAMA 113:1466–1471, 1939.
2. Nordin BEC, Peacock M, Wilkinson R: Hypercalciuria and calcium stone disease. *In* McIntyre I (ed): Clinics in Endocrinology and Metabolism. Philadelphia, WB Saunders Company, 1972, pp 169–183.
3. Pak CYC, Ohata M, Lawrence EC, Snyder W: The hypercalciurias: Causes, parathyroid functions and idiopathic criteria. J Clin Invest 54:387–400, 1974.
4. Shen FH, Baylink DJ, Neilsen RL, et al: Increased serum 1,25-dihydroxyvitamin D in idiopathic hypercalciuria. J Lab Clin Med 90:955–962, 1977.
5. Insogna KL, Broadus AE, Dreyer BE, et al: Elevated production rate of 1,25-dihydroxyvitamin D in patients with absorptive hypercalciuria. J Clin Endocrinol Metab 61:490–495, 1985.
6. Pak CYC: Pathogenesis of hypercalciuria. *In* Peck WA (ed): Bone and Mineral Research/4. New York, Elsevier, 1985, pp 303–334.
7. Pak CYC: Medical management of nephrolithiasis in Dallas: Update 1987. J Urol 140:461–467, 1988.
8. Pak CYC, Britton F, Peterson R, et al: Ambulatory evaluation of nephrolithiasis: Classification, clinical presentation and diagnostic criteria. Am J Med 69:19–30, 1980.
9. Yendt ER, Guay GF, Garcia DA: The use of thiazides in the prevention of renal calculi. Can Med Assoc J 102:614–620, 1970.
10. Pak CYC, Delea CS, Bartter FC: Successful treatment of recurrent nephrolithiasis (calcium stones) with cellulose phosphate. N Engl J Med 290:175–180, 1974.
11. Pak CYC: Role of medical prevention. J Urol 141:798–801, 1989.
12. Pak CYC: Medical management of nephrolithiasis. J Urol 128:1157–1164, 1982.
13. Albright F, Henneman P, Benedict PH, Forbes AP: Idiopathic hypercalciuria: A preliminary report. Proc R Soc Med 46:1077–1081, 1953.

14. Henneman PH, Benedict PH, Forbes AP, Dudley HR: Idiopathic hypercalciuria. N Engl J Med 259:802–807, 1958.
15. Coe FL, Canterbury JM, Firpo JJ, Reiss E: Evidence for secondary hyperparathyroidism in idiopathic hypercalciuria. J Clin Invest 52:134–142, 1973.
16. Lemann J, Gray RW, Dominguez JH: 25-OH-vitamin D metabolism in calcium stone formers. *In* Fleisch H, Robertson WG, Smith LH, Vahlensieck W (eds): Urolithiasis Research. New York, Plenum Press, 1976, pp 467–472.
17. Coe FL, Favus MJ, Crockett T, et al: Effects of low-calcium diet on urine calcium excretion, parathyroid function and serum 1,25-$(OH)_2D_3$ levels in patients with idiopathic hypercalciuria and in normal subjects. Am J Med 72:25–32, 1982.
18. Buck AC, Sampson WF, Lote CJ, Blacklock NJ: The influence of renal prostaglandins on glomerular filtration rate (GFR) and calcium excretion in urolithiasis. Br J Urol 53:485, 1981.
19. Bushinsky DA, Johnston RB, Nalbantian CE, Favus MJ: Increased calcium absorption and retention without elevated serum 1,25$(OH)_2D_3$ in genetically hypercalciuric rats. *In* Abstract Program, The American Society of Nephrology, 20th Annual Meeting, December 13–16, 1987, Washington, DC, 55:189A.
20. Coe FL, Parks JH, Bushinsky DA, et al: Chlorthalidone promotes mineral retention in patients with idiopathic hypercalciuria. Kidney Int 33:1140–1146, 1988.
21. Pak CYC, Nicar MJ, Northcutt C: The definition of the mechanism of hypercalciuria is necessary for the treatment of recurrent stone formers. Contrib Nephrol 33:136–151, 1982.
22. Pak CYC, Holt K: Nucleation and growth of brushite and calcium in urine of stone-formers. Metabolism 25:665–673, 1976.
23. Pak CYC, Breslau NA, Harvey JA: Nutrition and metabolic bone disease. Nutr Dis 15:215–240, 1986.
24. Zerwekh JE, Holt K, Pak CYC: Attenuation by the urate salts of the inhibitory effect of naturally occurring urinary macromolecules on calcium oxalate nucleation and crystal growth. Kidney Int 23:838–841, 1983.
25. Harvey JA, Hill KD, Pak CYC: Similarity of urinary risk factors among stone-forming patients in five regions of the United States. J Lithotripsy Stone Disease. (Accepted).
26. Breslau NA, Brinkley L, Hill KD, Pak CYC: Relationship role of animal protein–rich diet to kidney stone formation and calcium metabolism. J Clin Endocrinol Metab 66:140–146, 1988.
27. Wills MR, Gill JR Jr, Bartter FC: The interrelationships of calcium and sodium excretions. Clin Sci (Oxford) 37:621–630, 1969.
28. Preminger GM, Sakhaee K, Skurla C, Pak CYC: Prevention of recurrent calcium stone formation with potassium citrate therapy in patients with distal renal tubular acidosis. J Urol 134:20–23, 1985.
29. Sutton RA: Disorders of renal calcium excretion. Kidney Int 23:665–673, 1983.
30. Pak CYC, Fordtran JS: Disorders of mineral metabolism. *In* Sleisenger MH, Fordtran JS, Ingelfinger FJ (eds): Gastrointestinal Disease. Philadelphia, WB Saunders Company, 1978, pp 251–271.
31. Sheikh MS, Ramirez A, Emmett M, et al: Role of vitamin D–dependent and vitamin D–independent mechanisms in absorption of food calcium. J Clin Invest 81:126–132, 1988.
32. Pak CYC, Nicar MJ, Krejs GJ: Intestinal absorption of calcium, magnesium, phosphate and oxalate: Deviation from normal in idiopathic urolithiasis. *In* Schwille PO, Smith LH, Robertson WG, Vahlensieck W (eds): Urolithiasis and Related Clinical Research. Garmisch-Partenkirchen, Germany, Plenum Publishing, 1985, pp 127–133.
33. Pak CYC: Calcium disorders: Hypercalcemia and hypocalcemia. *In* Kokko JP, Tannen RL (eds): Fluids and Electrolytes. 2nd ed. Philadelphia, WB Saunders Company (in press).
34. Majeska RJ, Rodan SB, Rodan GA: Parathyroid hormone responsive clonal cell lines from rat osteosarcoma. Endocrinology 107:1494–1503, 1980.
35. Garabedian M, Holick MJ, DeLuca HF, Boyle IT: Control of 25-hydroxycholecalciferol metabolism by parathyroid glands. Proc Natl Acad Sci USA 69:1673–1676, 1973.
36. Sutton RAL, Dirks JH: Renal handling of calcium: Overview. In Massry SR, Ritz E (eds): Phosphate Metabolism. New York, Plenum Press, 1976, pp 15–27.
37. Raisz LG, Trummel CL, Holick MF, DeLuca HF: 1,25-Dihydroxycholecalciferol: A potent stimulator of bone resorption in tissue culture. Science 175:768, 1972.
38. Stern PH: A monolog on analogs: In vitro effects of vitamin D metabolites and consideration of the mineralization question. Calcif Tissue Int 33:1–4, 1981.
39. Pushett JB, Fernandez PC, Boyle JT, et al: The acute renal tubular effects of 1,25-dihydroxy-cholecalciferol. Proc Soc Endocrinol Metab 141:379–384, 1972.
40. Brannon PG, Morawski S, Pak CYC, Fordtran J: Selective jejunal hyperabsorption of calcium in absorptive hypercalciuria. Am J Med 66:425–428, 1979.
41. Schmulen C, Lerman M, Pak CYC, et al: Effect of 1,25-$(OH)_2D_3$ therapy on jejunal absorption of magnesium in patients with chronic renal disease. Am J Physiol 238:G349–G352, 1980.
42. Duncombe VM, Watts RWE, Peters TJ: In-vitro calcium uptake by jejunal biopsy specimens from patients with idiopathic hypercalciuria. Lancet 2:1334–1336, 1980.
43. Zerwekh JE, Pak CYC, Kaplan RA, et al: Pathogenetic role of 1,25-dihydroxyvitamin D in sarcoidosis and absorptive hypercalciuria: Different response to prednisolone therapy. J Clin Endocrinol Metab 51:381–386, 1980.

44. Preminger GM, Pak CYC: Eventual attenuation of hypocalciuric response to hydrochlorothiazide in absorptive hypercalciuria. J Urol 137:1104–1108, 1986.
45. Zerwekh JE, Pak CYC: Selective effects of thiazide therapy on serum 1,25-dihydroxyvitamin D and intestinal calcium absorption in renal and absorptive hypercalciurias. Metabolism 29:13–17, 1980.
46. Barilla DE, Zerwekh JE, Pak CYC: A critical evaluation of the role of phosphate in the pathogenesis of absorptive hypercalciuria. Miner Electrolyte Metab 2:302–309, 1979.
47. Pak CYC, McGuire J, Peterson R, et al: Familial absorptive hypercalciuria in a large kindred. J Urol 126:717–719, 1981.
48. Maierhofer WJ, Gray RW, Cheung HS, Lemann J Jr: Bone resorption stimulated by elevated serum 1,25-$(OH)_2$vitamin D concentrations in healthy men. Kidney Int 24:555–560, 1983.
49. Pak CYC, Galosy RA: Fasting urinary calcium and adenosine 3′, 5′-monophosphate: A discriminant analysis for the identification of renal and absorptive hypercalciurias. J Clin Endocrinol Metab 48:260–265, 1979.
50. Barilla DE, Townsend J, Pak CYC: An exaggerated augmentation of renal calcium excretion following oral glucose ingestion in patients with renal hypercalciuria. Invest Urol 15:468–486, 1978.
51. Sakhaee K, Nicar MJ, Brater DC, Pak CYC: Exaggerated natriuretic and calciuric response to hydrochlorothiazide in renal hypercalciuria but not in absorptive hypercalciuria. J Clin Endocrinol Metab 61:825–829, 1985.
52. Pak CYC: Physiological basis for absorptive and renal hypercalciurias. Am J Physiol 237:F415–F423, 1979.
53. Urivetzky M, Anna PS, Smith AD: Plasma osteocalcin levels in stone disease: A potential aid in the differential diagnosis of calcium nephrolithiasis. J Urol 139:12–14, 1988.
54. Pacifici R, Filipponi P, Mannarelli C, et al: Classification of idiopathic hypercalciuric patients by isotopic calcium absorption: A comparison with oral calcium tolerance test. Calcif Tissue Int 37:467–473, 1985.
55. Lemann J, Piering WF, Lennon EJ: Possible role of carbohydrate-induced calciuria in calcium oxalate kidney-stone formation. N Engl J Med 280:232–237, 1969.
56. Muldowney FP, Freaney R, Moloney MF: Importance of dietary sodium in the hypercalciuria syndrome. Kidney Int 22:292–296, 1982.
57. Breslau NA, McGuire JL, Zerwekh JE, Pak CYC: The role of dietary sodium on renal excretion and intestinal absorption of calcium and on vitamin D metabolism. J Clin Endocrinol Metab 55:369–373, 1982.
58. Bushinsky DA, Favus MJ, Langman CB, Coe FL: Mechanism of chronic hypercalciuria with furosemide: Increased calcium absorption. Am J Physiol 251 (Renal Fluid Electrolyte Physiol 20):F17–F24, 1986.
59. Tschope W, Ritz E: Sulfur-containing amino acids are a major determinant of urinary calcium. Miner Electrolyte Metab 11:137–139, 1985.
60. Lawoyin S, Sismilich S, Browne R, Pak CYC: Bone mineral content in patients with primary hyperparathyroidism, osteoporosis, and calcium urolithiasis. Metabolism 28:1250–1254, 1979.
61. Pak CYC: Getting out from under kidney stones. Acute Care Med, June 1985, pp 10–23.
62. Lloyd HM: Primary hyperparathyroidism: An analysis of the role of the parathyroid tumor. Medicine 47:53, 1968.
63. Broadus AE, Horst RL, Lang R, et al: The importance of circulating 1,25-dihydroxyvitamin D in the pathogenesis of hypercalciuria and renal-stone formation in primary hyperparathyroidism. N Engl J Med 302:421–426, 1980.
64. Patron P, Gardin J-P, Paillard M: Renal mass and reserve of vitamin D: Determinants of plasma $1,25(OH)_2D_3$ in primary hyperparathyroidism. Kidney Int 31:1174–1180, 1987.
65. Pak CYC, Nicar MJ, Peterson R, et al: A lack of unique pathophysiologic background for nephrolithiasis of primary hyperparathyroidism. J Clin Endocrinol Metab 53:536–542, 1981.
66. Smith LH, Werness PG, Lee KE, et al: Inhibitors of crystal growth and aggregation in calcium urolithiasis. Clin Res 26:727A, 1979.
67. Pak CYC: Effect of parathyroidectomy on crystallization of calcium salts in urine of patients with primary hyperparathyroidism. Invest Urol 17:146–148, 1979.
68. Kaplan RA, Haussler MR, Deftos LJ, et al: The role of 1α,25-dihydroxyvitamin D in the mediation of intestinal hyperabsorption of calcium in primary hyperparathyroidism and absorptive hypercalciuria. J Clin Invest 59:756–760, 1977.
69. Bone HG III, Zerwekh J, Haussler MR, et al: Effect of parathyroidectomy on serum 1α,25-dihydroxyvitamin D and on intestinal calcium absorption in primary hyperparathyroidism. J Clin Endocrinol Metab 48:877–879, 1979.
70. Breslau NA, Pak CYC: Combined primary hyperparathyroidism and absorptive hypercalciuria: Clinical implications. *In* Sutton RAL, Cameron EC, Walker V (eds): Urolithiasis: VIth International Meeting on Urolithiasis and Related Clinical Research, July 24–29, 1988, Vancouver, British Columbia.
71. Dominguez JH, Gray RW, Lemann J: Dietary phosphate deprivation in women and men: Effects on mineral and acid balances, parathyroid hormone and the metabolism of 25-OH-vitamin D. J Clin Endocrinol Metab 43:1056–1068, 1976.
72. Gray RW, Wilz DR, Caldas AE, Lemann J: The importance of phosphate in regulating plasma

1,25-$(OH)_2$vitamin D levels in humans: Studies in healthy subjects, in calcium-stone formers and in patients with primary hyperparathyroidism. J Clin Endocrinol Metab 45:299–306, 1977.
73. Bordier R, Ryckewart A, Gueris J, Rasmussen HR: On the pathogenesis of so-called idiopathic hypercalciuria. Am J Med 63:398–409, 1977.
74. Malluche HH, Tschoepe W, Ritz E, et al: Abnormal bone histology in idiopathic hypercalciuria. J Clin Endocrinol Metab 50:654–658, 1980.
75. Steele TH, DeLuca HF: Influence of dietary phosphorus on renal phosphate reabsorption in the parathyroidectomized rat. J Clin Invest 57:867–874, 1976.
76. Smith LH, Thomas WC, Arnaud CD: Orthophosphate therapy in calcium renal lithiasis: Urinary calculi. *In* International Symposium on Renal Stone Research, Basel, S Karger, 1973, pp 189–197.
77. Tieder M, Modai D, Samuel R, et al: Hereditary hypophosphatemic rickets with hypercalciuria. N Engl J Med 312:611–617, 1985.
78. Broadus AE, Erickson SB, Gertner JM, et al: An experimental human model of 1,25-dihydroxyvitamin D–mediated hypercalciuria. J Clin Endocrinol Metab 59:202–206, 1984.
79. Reynolds JJ, Holick MF, DeLuca HF: The role of vitamin D metabolites on bone resorption. Calcif Tissue Res 12:295–301, 1973.
80. Zerwekh JE, Sakhaee K, Pak CYC: Short term 1,25-dihydroxyvitamin D_3 administration raises serum osteocalcin in patients with postmenopausal osteoporosis. J Clin Endocrinol Metab 60:615–617, 1985.
81. Lemann J Jr, Gray RW: Hypercalciuric kidney stone formers exhibit enhanced intestinal calcium absorption (Ca_A) despite only slightly elevated serum 1,25-$(OH)_2$-D concentrations. *In* Abstract Program, The American Society of Nephrology, 20th Annual Meeting, December 13–16, 1987, Washington, DC, 139:196A.
82. Buck AC, Lote CJ, Sampson WF: The influence of renal prostaglandins on urinary calcium excretion in idiopathic urolithiasis. J Urol 129:421–426, 1983.
83. Rao PN, Blacklock NJ: A non-steroidal anti-inflammatory drug (flurbiprofen) to control idiopathic hypercalciuria resistant to dietary manipulation. Br J Urol 55:599–602, 1983.
84. Houser M, Zimmerman B, Davidman M, et al: Idiopathic hypercalciuria associated with hyperreninemia and high urinary prostaglandin E. Kidney Int 26:176–182, 1984.
85. Rocco VK, Sakhaee K, Pak CYC, Brater DC: Lack of effect of prostaglandin inhibition on calcium excretion in normal volunteers. J Urol 133:1093–1094, 1985.
86. Pacifici R, Rothstein M, Rifis L: Increased interleukin-1 activity and decreased bone density in patients with fasting hypercalciurias (FN). Urol Res 16:218, 1988.
87. Pak CYC, Smith LH, Resnick MI, Weinerth JL: Dietary management of idiopathic calcium urolithiasis. J Urol 131:850–852, 1984.
88. Pak CYC: Sodium cellulose phosphate: Mechanism of action and effect on mineral metabolism. J Clin Pharmacol 13:15–27, 1973.
89. Pak CYC: A cautious use of sodium cellulose phosphate in the management of calcium nephrolithiasis. Invest Urol 19:187–190, 1981.
90. Hayashi Y, Kaplan RA, Pak CYC: Effect of sodium cellulose phosphate therapy on crystallization of calcium oxalate in urine. Metabolism 24:1273–1278, 1975.
91. Pak CYC, Peters P, Hurt G, et al: Is selective therapy of recurrent nephrolithiasis possible? Am J Med 71:615–622, 1981.
92. Woelfel A, Kaplan RA, Pak CYC: Effect of hydrochlorothiazide therapy on crystallization of calcium oxalate in urine. Metabolism 26:201–205, 1977.
93. Pak CYC: Hydrochlorothiazide therapy in nephrolithiasis: Effect on urinary activity product and formation product of brushite. Clin Pharmacol Ther 14:209–217, 1973.
94. Pak CYC, Ruskin B, Diller E: Enhancement of renal excretion of zinc by hydrochlorothiazide. Clin Chim Acta 39:511–517, 1972.
95. Pak CYC, Peterson R, Sakhaee K, et al: Correction of hypocitraturia and prevention of stone formation by combined thiazide and potassium citrate therapy in thiazide-unresponsive hypercalciuric nephrolithiasis. Am J Med 79:284–288, 1985.
96. Ettinger B, Oldroyd NO, Sorge F: Triamterene nephrolithiasis. JAMA 244:2443–2445, 1980.
97. Leppla D, Browne R, Hill K, et al: Effect of amiloride with or without hydrochlorothiazide on urinary calcium and saturation of calcium salts. J Clin Endocrinol Metab 57:920–924, 1983.
98. Pak CYC, Sakhaee K, Crowther C, Brinkley L: Evidence justifying a high fluid intake in treatment of nephrolithiasis. Ann Intern Med 93:36–39, 1980.
99. Broadus AE, Magee JS, Mallette LE, et al: A detailed evaluation of oral phosphate therapy in selected patients with primary hyperparathyroidism. J Clin Endocrinol Metab 56:953–961, 1983.
100. Selby PL, Peacock M: Ethinyl estradiol and norethindrone in the treatment of primary hyperparathyroidism in postmenopausal women. N Engl J Med 314:1481–1485, 1986.
101. Van Den Berg CJ, Kumar R, Wilson MD, et al: Orthophosphate therapy decreases urinary calcium excretion and serum 1,25-dihydroxyvitamin D concentrations in idiopathic hypercalciuria. 51:998–1001, 1980.
102. Pak CYC, Galosy RA: Propensity for spontaneous nucleation of calcium oxalate: Quantitative assessment by urinary FPR-APR discriminant score. Am J Med 69:681–689, 1980.

103. Dudley FJ, Blackburn CRB: Extraskeletal calcification complicating oral neutral-phosphate therapy. Lancet 2:628–630, 1970.
104. Glass AR, Eil C: Ketoconazole-induced reduction in serum 1,25-dihydroxyvitamin D. J Clin Endocrinol Metab 63:766, 1986.
105. Zerwekh JE, Harvey JA, Pak CYC: Administration of pharmacologic amounts of 25(s), 26-dihydroxyvitamin D_3 reduces serum 1,25-dihydroxyvitamin D_3 levels in rats. Endocrinology 121:1671–1677, 1987.

4

Hyperoxaluric Calcium Nephrolithiasis

Charles Y.C. Pak

Oxalate is a constituent of the most common kidney stone—calcium oxalate stone. Hyperoxaluria is therefore one of the major risk factors for stone formation.

Much is known about the chemistry and biochemistry of oxalate. It has been realized for many centuries that oxalic acid is a constituent of certain foods, particularly dark green vegetables. Oxalic acid has long had industrial applications as a bleaching and cleaning agent and in beer making. Its biosynthetic pathway has been largely clarified, permitting identification of the enzymatic defect in primary hyperoxalurias. Reliable methods are now available for the measurement of oxalate in urine.

However, therapeutic efforts directed toward the reduction of oxalate excretion in urine continue to be disappointing. For most patients with calcium oxalate stones, there is little in the way of lowering oxalate excretion except dietary manipulation. This situation contrasts with that of hypercalciuria, hyperuricosuria, hypocitraturia, and undue urinary acidity, other major urinary risk factors for which effective therapeutic modalities are available. The difficulty in the correction of hyperoxaluria probably accounts for the lack of emphasis and consideration oxalate has received in the discussion on nephrolithiasis.

HISTORICAL CONSIDERATIONS

The bitter and sour taste in sorrel, due to the presence of oxalic acid, was known to the ancient Greeks. In 1668, Duclos isolated potassium oxalate from sorrel juice.[1] In 1784, Scheele, who isolated uric acid in a urinary stone, showed oxalate to exist in rhubarb and other vegetables as the calcium salt.[2] In 1797, Wollaston first noted the presence of calcium oxalate in a urinary stone of mulberry appearance.[3] Calcium oxalate monohydrate was first reported in rocks by Brooke in 1840,[4] and calcium oxalate dihydrate was found in the bottoms of the Weddell Sea in Antarctica by Bannister and Hey in 1936.[5] In 1967, Lloyd H. Smith and colleagues uncovered the enzymatic disturbance in primary hyperoxaluria Type I.[6] In 1968, Williams and Lloyd H. Smith discovered the enzymatic defect in primary hyperoxaluria Type II.[7] In 1970, Lynwood H. Smith and coworkers first noted the association of hyperoxaluria with calcium oxalate nephrolithiasis after a small bowel resection.[8]

PATHOGENETIC ROLE OF HYPEROXALURIA IN CALCIUM STONE FORMATION

Hyperoxaluria contributes to calcium oxalate stone formation by increasing the urinary saturation of calcium oxalate. In the simulated environment of urine, a rise in oxalate concentration is equally effective as a rise in calcium concentration in augmenting the activity product (saturation) of calcium oxalate (see Chapter 3).[9] In patients with recurrent calcium nephrolithiasis and in normal subjects, urinary saturation of calcium oxalate is directly correlated with urinary oxalate concentration (Fig. 4–1). In patients with primary hyperoxaluria, the urinary saturation of calcium oxalate is more than threefold greater than that of control subjects, despite a lack of difference in any of the urinary biochemistry except for higher urinary oxalate.[10] Finally, hyperoxaluria has been identified as an important risk factor for stone formation in the risk factor analysis.[11]

PATHOPHYSIOLOGY OF HYPEROXALURIA

In normal subjects maintained on a customary diet, approximately 35 mg of the oxalate that appears in urine is composed of 2 mg from intestinal absorption, 13 mg from endogenous production of ascorbic acid, and 20 mg from other routes of endogenous synthesis.

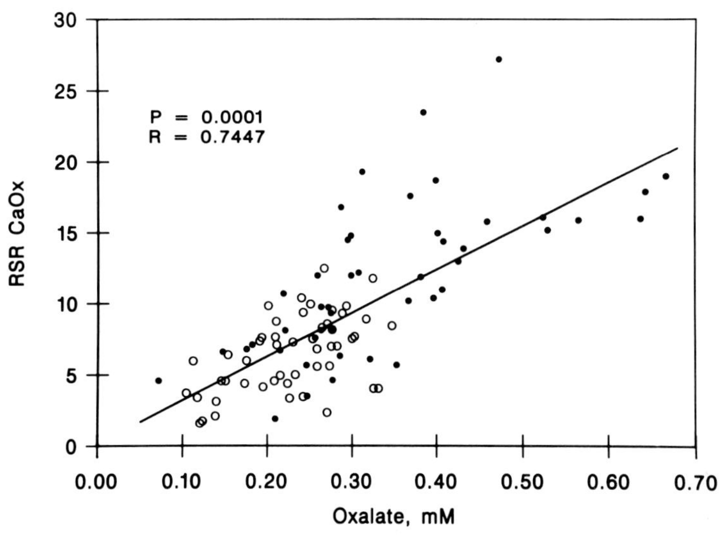

FIGURE 4–1. The dependence of urinary relative saturation ratio (RSR) of calcium oxalate (CaOx) on urinary oxalate concentration. RSR is the degree of saturation with respect to calcium oxalate, where a value of 1 is saturation and above 1 is supersaturation. Open circles represent urine samples collected from normal subjects and closed circles those obtained from patients with stones. The regression line is shown with the correlation coefficient (R) and *P* value.

Intestinal Absorption of Oxalate

Oxalate is absorbed by passive diffusion.[12] There is no evidence for a rate-limiting, active transport process. Although the entire intestinal tract is capable of absorbing oxalate, the distal bowel is believed to be more efficient than the proximal bowel.

Determinants of oxalate absorption are therefore as follows:

1. The concentration of free oxalate in the lumen.
2. Assessibility of the "more efficient" distal bowel.
3. Factors that affect the membrane permeability of oxalate.

The free oxalate pool would be affected by the dietary oxalate intake and by binding to calcium, magnesium, fatty acids, and bile salts.[13] Diseases of the proximal bowel may expose the distal bowel for oxalate absorption.[14] Oxalate permeability may be enhanced by certain substances (bile salts and fatty acids).[15]

Renal Handling of Oxalate

Renal excretion is the only route of oxalate elimination from the body. Oxalate is freely filtered at the glomerulus, with little evidence for substantial protein binding. The normal serum concentration of oxalate is 2 μmol/liter. The oxalate clearance normally ranges from 50 to 200 ml/min. The fractional excretion of oxalate (ratio of oxalate and creatinine clearances) ranges from 0.2 to 1.8, with a mean of approximately 0.5. The high fractional excretion (exceeding 1) sometimes encountered suggests that oxalate is normally secreted in the renal tubule. It is unknown if oxalate is reabsorbed in the renal tubule.

The renal handling of oxalate may be disturbed in patients with nephrolithiasis.[16] In primary hyperoxaluria and enteric hyperoxaluria, the fractional excretion of oxalate averaged 2.74 and 3.73, respectively, suggesting a renal leak of oxalate. In patients with hypercalciuric nephrolithiasis, oxalate clearance has been reported to be normal or slightly increased.

De Novo Synthesis of Oxalate

Like uric acid, oxalate is a useless end product of metabolism (Fig. 4–2). Approximately 50 per cent of oxalate synthesis is normally accounted for by direct metabolic conversion of ascorbic acid and tryptophan. The remaining half is attributable to oxidation of glyoxylate, which serves as a major substrate for oxalate synthesis. Two major pathways for glyoxylate degradation are its transamination to glycine and to alanine. Hydroxyproline serves as a substrate, albeit a minor one, for glyoxylate synthesis. Factors that affect the glyoxylate pool, by inhibiting its degradation or enhancing its synthesis, could influence oxalate synthesis.

Clinical Disorders of Hyperoxaluria

Clinically, hyperoxaluria is due to an enzymatic disturbance in oxalate biosynthesis, to increased availability of substrate, and to intestinal hyperabsorp-

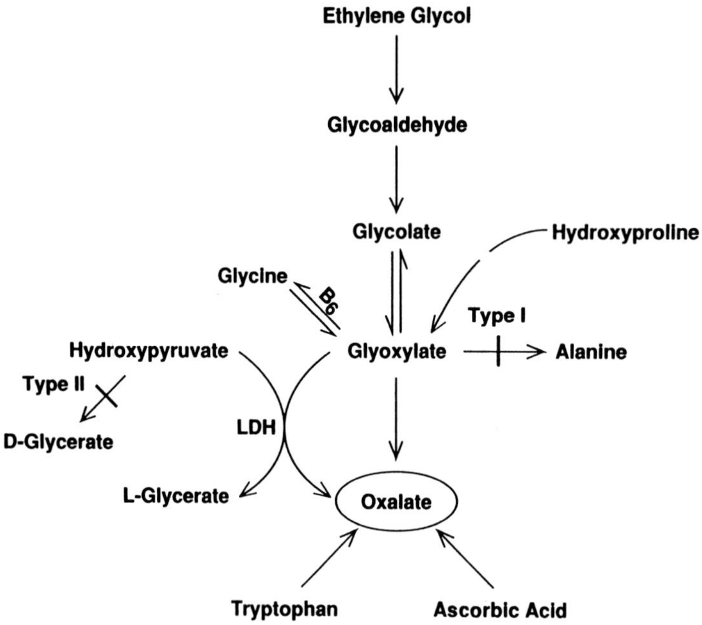

FIGURE 4–2. Biosynthetic pathway for oxalate.

tion of oxalate[10] (Table 4–1). The first category is composed of primary hyperoxaluria and pyridoxine deficiency.

PRIMARY HYPEROXALURIA. Primary hyperoxaluria is composed of two types, representing rare inborn errors of metabolism. Type I (glycolic aciduria) is inherited as an autosomal recessive trait, with the disease being manifest only in the homozygous state.[6] The nature of inheritance for Type II (L-glyceric aciduria) has not been disclosed.[7]

The metabolic defect in primary hyperoxaluria Type I is the inhibition of the conversion of glyoxylate to alanine due to the deficiency of the enzyme alanine glyoxylate aminotransferase (Fig. 4–2). Thus, there is an accumulation of glyoxylate, resulting in enhanced oxalate synthesis and hyperoxaluria. Urinary excretion of glycolate is increased, since this substrate is increased as well; hence the term glycolic aciduria has been applied to distinguish this type from the Type II presentation.

In primary hyperoxaluria Type II, a deficiency of the enzyme D-glyceric dehydrogenase leads to the accumulation of hydroxypyruvate (Fig. 4–2).[7] Hydroxypyruvate excess facilitates its conversion to L-glycerate in the presence of lactic dehydrogenase (LDH), resulting in enhanced renal excretion of L-glyceric acid (hence the term L-glyceric aciduria). The oxidation-reduction of glyoxylate

TABLE 4–1. CAUSES OF HYPEROXALURIA

1. Enhanced oxalate synthesis due to enzymatic disturbances
   a. Primary hyperoxaluria, Type I and Type II
   b. Pyridoxine deficiency
2. Increased availability of substrate
   a. Ascorbic acid
   b. Ethylene glycol and methoxyflurane
3. Intestinal hyperabsorption of oxalate
   a. Enteric hyperoxaluria
   b. High-oxalate diet
   c. Imbalance between intraluminal calcium and oxalate

and hydroxypyruvate is apparently coupled by their common reactivity with lactic dehydrogenase. Thus, the hydroxypyruvate accumulation also stimulates oxalate synthesis from glyoxylate.

Type I can be distinguished from Type II by the concurrent rise in glycolic acid in the former and in L-glyceric acid in the latter. Hyperoxaluria is marked (>60 mg/1.73 meter^2/24 hr). Unless effectively treated, primary hyperoxaluria runs a malignant course, with early death from renal failure and generalized oxalosis.

As previously noted, a renal leak of oxalate may contribute to hyperoxaluria.[16]

Pyridoxine Deficiency.[17] The transamination of glyoxylate to glycine requires pyridoxine (vitamin B_6) as a cofactor (Fig. 4–2). Thus, in pyridoxine deficiency, glyoxylate accumulation leads to enhanced oxalate synthesis and hyperoxaluria. In some patients with primary hyperoxaluria, pharmacologic doses of pyridoxine may reduce the degree of hyperoxaluria. This action is not likely to be prominent in most patients with calcium oxalate nephrolithiasis who do not display a disturbance in oxalate biosynthesis.

There is a recent report that pyridoxine might be useful in controlling hyperoxaluria in an apparent new syndrome called mild metabolic hyperoxaluria.[18] Persons with this condition display a moderate hyperoxaluria (55 to 80 mg/day). Coexisting glycolic aciduria suggests that it may be a mild form of primary hyperoxaluria. However, this conclusion is not supported because of the lack of a family history, an onset at any age, and a clinical course sometimes characterized by spontaneous remission or relapse.

Increased Availability of Substrate. As previously mentioned, ascorbic acid normally accounts for about 40 per cent of oxalate synthesized de novo, by serving as a substrate for oxalate synthesis.[19] In normal subjects, the increment in urinary oxalate has been reported to be 12 mg/day with a vitamin C dosage of 4 grams/day, 45 mg/day with an intake of 8 grams/day, and 60 mg with administration of 9 grams of vitamin C per day.[20] Some patients with calcium oxalate nephrolithiasis may show a significant rise in urinary oxalate even when taking 500 mg of supplemental vitamin C a day.

Ethylene glycol is an antifreeze that is sometimes taken as an alcohol substitute.[21] It is catalyzed to glycoaldehyde, which is then converted to oxalate via glycolate and glyoxylate (Fig. 4–2). Its ingestion may lead to massive hyperoxaluria, oxalosis, renal failure, and death. Methoxyflurane, a general anesthetic, may be converted to oxalate via two pathways that do not involve participation of glyoxylate substrate.[22] Prolonged anesthesia with this agent may cause hyperoxaluria and nephrotoxicity.

It has been suggested that a diet high in animal proteins may augment oxalate excretion by stimulating de novo synthesis of oxalate. The concurrent rise in urinary glycolate supported this hypothesis. However, in a controlled study, urinary oxalate was found to be lower on a diet high in animal protein compared with a diet of vegetable protein.[23]

Intestinal Hyperabsorption of Oxalate. Enteric hyperoxaluria is the hallmark of hyperoxaluria due to intestinal hyperabsorption of oxalate.[24] Gastrointestinal diseases that have been associated with this entity are those characterized by an absence or nonfunction of small bowel (regional enteritis, small bowel resection or bypass) and those causing defective absorption of fat or bile acids (chronic pancreatitis, pancreatectomy, nontropical sprue, biliary cirrhosis, and blind loop syndrome). In the former group of diseases, the involvement of the upper bowel "exposes" the colon to perform an absorptive function. There is malabsorption of fat and bile salts as well.

Common denominators of enteric hyperoxaluria are therefore malabsorption and function of the colon. They are critical factors in causing the intestinal hyperabsorption of oxalate. First, unabsorbed bile acids and fatty acids directly increase the permeability of the colon to oxalate (Fig. 4–3).[15] Second, the intestinal fat malabsorption may leave unabsorbed fatty acids to react with divalent cations (calcium and magnesium). This "soap formation" would limit the amount of free divalent cations to complex oxalate, thereby raising the available oxalate pool.[13, 25] Oxalate absorption is thus increased from an enlargement of the intraluminal pool of oxalate available for absorption. Third, the efficient site of oxalate (colon) is allowed to participate in oxalate absorption because of involvement of the upper bowel. The essentiality of the colon in the production of enteric hyperoxaluria is indicated by the absence of hyperoxaluria in subjects with diseases of the colon and upon ileostomy.[14]

In addition to the disturbance in oxalate metabolism, the intestinal absorption and renal excretion of calcium are often decreased in enteric hyperoxaluria, probably a reflection of the loss of the intestinal site of calcium absorption from disease or resection, of intraluminal binding of calcium by nonabsorbed fatty acids, or of vitamin D deficiency associated with fat malabsorption. Urine output may be substantially reduced consequent to fluid loss from the intestinal tract. Urinary citrate is low because of metabolic acidosis and hypokalemia (see Chapter

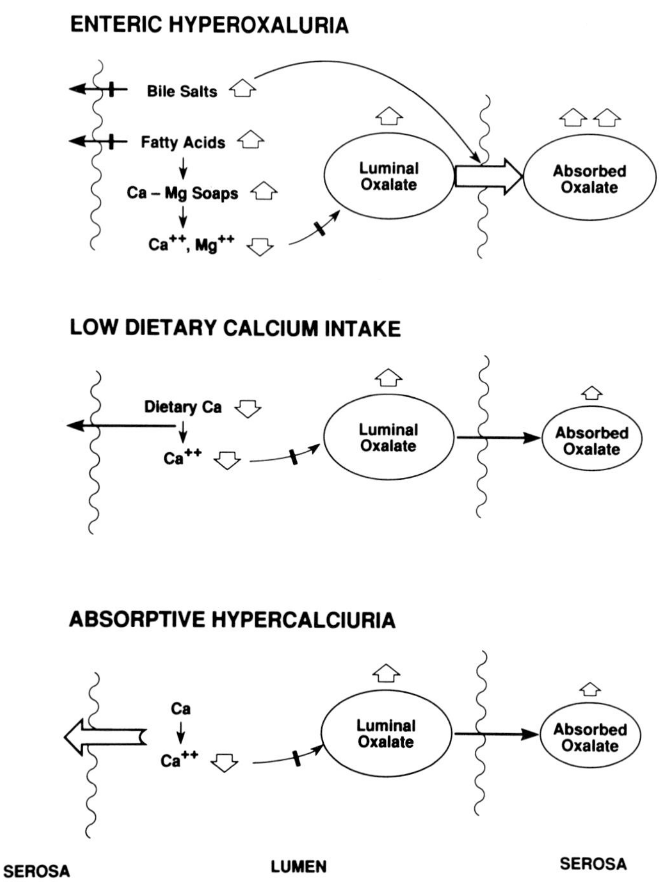

FIGURE 4–3. Schemes for hyperoxaluria due to increased intestinal oxalate absorption.

6).[26] Low urinary magnesium may result from impaired intestinal magnesium absorption.

The cause of the formation of calcium oxalate stones in enteric hyperoxaluria is multifactorial and includes hyperoxaluria as well as some of the other disturbances previously described (Fig. 4–4).[10] Saturation of urine with respect to calcium oxalate may be increased because of high oxalate concentration and low urinary citrate and magnesium (which reduces complexation of calcium and oxalate, respectively), even though urinary calcium may be low. Low urine volume exaggerates urinary supersaturation. Moreover, the inhibitor activity against the crystallization of calcium salts is reduced because of a low renal excretion of citrate. Low urinary pH resulting from intestinal alkali loss increases the amount of undissociated uric acid in urine and predisposes to uric acid lithiasis (see Chapter 7).

Two other causes of intestinal hyperabsorption of oxalate and hyperoxaluria are an excessive dietary oxalate intake and an imbalance between intraluminal calcium and oxalate. Moderate-to-severe hyperoxaluria uncommonly arises solely from an excessive oxalate intake because of a limited absorbability of oxalate from food. Foods of high oxalate content include rhubarb, spinach, beet greens, Swiss chard, sorrel, parsley, turnip greens, dill, nuts, chocolate, cocoa, and tea. However, the content of oxalate of a given food item may vary, depending on the species, areas where grown, age of the plant, and time of the year. The oxalate bioavailability may be restricted because oxalate is often present as an insoluble salt with calcium in food. The oxalate absorption may also depend on whether the oxalate-rich food item is taken on an empty stomach or with food.

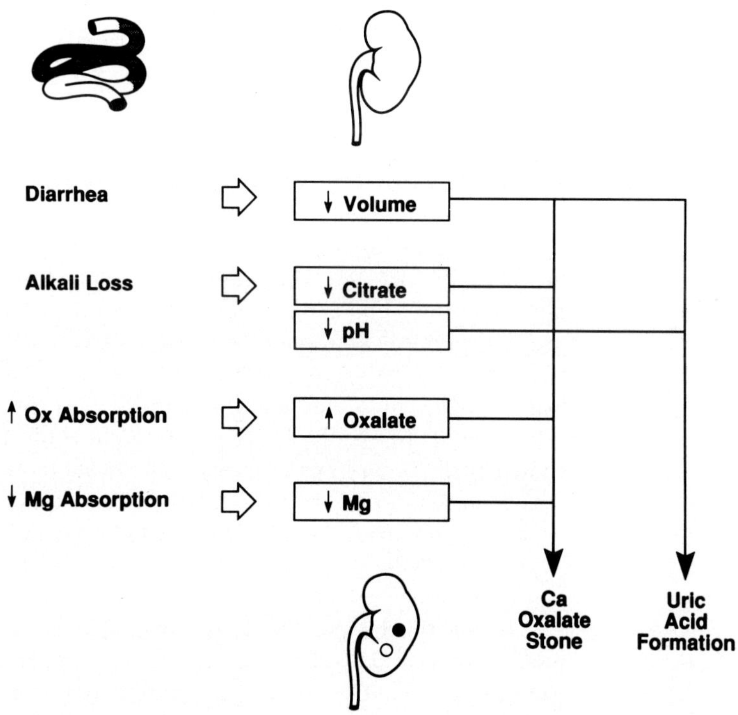

FIGURE 4–4. Multifactorial causes for calcium and uric acid stone formation in enteric hyperoxaluria. In the picture of the kidney below, calcium oxalate stone is indicated by a closed circle and uric acid (stone) formation by an open circle.

These considerations are discussed in Chapter 11. In general, only 2 to 5 per cent of oxalate from food is normally absorbed.[27] However, in patients with an underlying intestinal hyperabsorption of oxalate, an ingestion of oxalate-rich foods can substantially exaggerate hyperoxaluria.

Mild hyperoxaluria may be encountered in patients with intestinal hyperabsorption of calcium, for two reasons (see Fig. 4–3).[28, 29] First, they are often kept on a low-calcium diet to control hypercalciuria. The reduced amount of calcium in the intestinal lumen limits the binding of oxalate by calcium, thus enlarging the pool of oxalate available for absorption.[30] Second, the reduced luminal content of calcium with the same sequelae as described previously results from an enhanced intestinal hyperabsorption of calcium. This problem may be particularly acute in patients with absorptive hypercalciuria who are treated with sodium cellulose phosphate (which binds dietary calcium) while maintained on a calcium-restricted diet (see Chapter 3).[31] Urinary oxalate excretion may approach 100 mg/day.

Oxalate Handling in Absorptive Hypercalciuria. The demonstration of an intestinal hyperabsorption of oxalate in patients with absorptive hypercalciuria does not indicate that they suffer from an intrinsic "absorptive hyperoxaluria" as well. The absorption of oxalate given in a soluble form has been shown to be normal.[32] The high oxalate absorption from food displayed by these patients is therefore secondary to the imbalance in the intraluminal content of calcium and oxalate.

Three intriguing reports have recently appeared regarding oxalate transport in patients with idiopathic calcium oxalate nephrolithiasis, many of whom probably suffered from absorptive hypercalciuria. In one report, these patients were found to have an intestinal malabsorption of ascorbic acid.[33] The conversion of ascorbic acid to oxalic acid in the intestinal lumen and the subsequent absorption of the latter have been implicated in the pathogenesis of mild-to-moderate hyperoxaluria. However, this explanation remains largely a speculation and needs validation. There is no evidence that the vitamin C conversion to oxalate is more efficient in the intestinal lumen than in tissues.

In another report,[34] oxalate exchange across red blood cells was shown to be increased in patients with idiopathic calcium oxalate nephrolithiasis and was demonstrated to be correctable by treatment with thiazide or amiloride or both. This biochemical abnormality was expressed as an autosomal monogenic dominant trait and was associated with an exaggerated oxaluric response to oral oxalate load, suggestive of increased intestinal absorption of oxalate. However, the relevance of the results in stone formation could be questioned, because of the similarity of the 24-hour urinary oxalate of subjects with versus without abnormal oxalate fluxes in erythrocytes, a lack of correlation between oxalate flux rate and urinary oxalate excretion rate, and the failure to demonstrate an intrinsic intestinal hyperabsorption of oxalate (from soluble oxalate) in patients with absorptive hypercalciuria.[32]

In the third report,[16] the serum oxalate level was slightly reduced and the renal fractional excretion of oxalate was slightly increased in patients with "idiopathic" calcium oxalate nephrolithiasis compared with normal subjects. However, this intriguing finding needs confirmation, since only eight patients were studied.

DIAGNOSIS OF HYPEROXALURIA

Hyperoxaluria, defined as a urinary oxalate higher than 44 mg/day, is associated with calcium oxalate stones. If urinary oxalate is more than 80 mg/day, primary or enteric hyperoxaluria is probably present. In primary hyperoxaluria, urinary glycolate (in Type I) or glycerate (in Type II) may be increased in addition to oxalate. Moreover, oxalosis (tissue deposition of calcium oxalate), anemia, and renal failure are common in primary hyperoxaluria. In enteric hyperoxaluria, there is a history of small bowel disease, ileal bypass, small bowel resection, chronic pancreatitis, nontropical sprue, biliary cirrhosis, or blind loop syndrome. Urinary calcium is typically low (<100 mg/day), as is urinary magnesium (<50 mg/day). Serum calcium and magnesium levels may be low or low normal, and parathyroid function may be stimulated. The serum bicarbonate level and urinary citrate may be reduced. Women are more commonly affected than men.

Even in the absence of intestinal disease, a mild-to-moderate hyperoxaluria (urinary oxalate of 44 to 80 mg/day) may occur with vitamin C therapy, overindulgence in oxalate-rich foods (particularly spinach), or severe dietary calcium deprivation. Mild hyperoxaluria may also occur in patients with increased calcium absorption, such as those suffering from absorptive hypercalciuria.

A careful history should be taken for intestinal disease, certain dietary excesses (ingestion of oxalate-rich foods, vitamin C supplementation, and severe calcium restriction), and a family history of stones, oxalosis, and early death from renal failure.

Characteristic features of the three main forms of hyperoxaluria are summarized in Table 4–2.

TREATMENT OF HYPEROXALURIC CALCIUM NEPHROLITHIASIS

Enteric Hyperoxaluria

The cause of stone formation in enteric hyperoxaluria is multifactorial.[10] The treatment should therefore be directed at correcting the various disturbances present, including hyperoxaluria, hypocitraturia and low urinary pH, hypomagnesiuria, and low urine volume (Table 4–3).

TABLE 4–2. DIAGNOSTIC FEATURES OF HYPEROXALURIAS

Feature	Primary Hyperoxaluria	Enteric Hyperoxaluria	Absorptive Hypercalciuria
Serum			
Carbon dioxide	N	↓	N
Potassium	N	↓	N
Urinary			
Calcium	N	↓	↑
Magnesium	N	↓	N
Oxalate	↑ ↑ ↑	↑ ↑ ↑	N or ↑
Citrate	N	↓	N
pH	N	↓	N
Stone composition	Calcium oxalate	Calcium oxalate zUric acid	Calcium oxalate Calcium phosphate
Oxalosis	Common	Seldom	Rare
Renal function	↓ ↓	N or ↓	N
Sex predominance	Equivalent	Female	Male

N = normal; ↑ = increase; ↓ = decrease.

TABLE 4–3. TREATMENT OF HYPEROXALURIAS

Condition	Treatment and Customary Dose	Mechanism of Action
Enteric hyperoxaluria	High fluid intake	Increase urine volume
	Low-oxalate diet	Lower urinary oxalate
	Potassium citrate, 60–120 mEq/day	Increase urinary pH and citrate
	Magnesium citrate, 20–40 mEq/day	Increase urinary pH, magnesium, and citrate
	Calcium citrate, 1.2 grams of calcium per day	Lower urinary oxalate and increase urinary pH and citrate
Primary hyperoxaluria	Orthophosphate, 1.5–2.5 grams of phosphorus per day	Increase urinary citrate and pyrophosphate, lower calcium
	Pyridoxine, 200 mg/day	Lower urinary oxalate

The control of hyperoxaluria requires a rigid dietary oxalate restriction, broadly applied to all known oxalate-rich foods (see Chapter 11). Oxalate bioavailability from food is generally higher in patients with enteric hyperoxaluria than in normal subjects.[32] Thus, certain foods (e.g., chocolate) from which little oxalate is normally absorbed may produce a substantial rise in urinary oxalate among patients with intrinsic increased oxalate absorption.

Oral administration of large amounts of calcium (0.25 to 1.0 gram four times a day) or magnesium has been recommended for the control of hyperoxaluria.[13] Although urinary oxalate may decrease (probably from binding of oxalate by divalent cations), the concurrent rise in urinary calcium may obviate the beneficial effect of this therapy, at least in some patients.[32] Cholestyramine does not cause a sustained reduction in oxalate excretion.[24] A partial replacement of dietary fat with medium-chain fatty acids may be helpful in those patients who also have malabsorption.

The treatment of low urinary citrate and pH with potassium citrate[35] is considered in detail in Chapter 6. A liquid preparation is preferred, to be given at frequent intervals (three to four times a day). A high dose may sometimes be required (up to 120 mEq/day). The use of sodium-potassium citrate should be considered if there is sodium deficiency from diarrheal loss.

Hypomagnesiuria is due to an impaired intestinal absorption of magnesium. It contributes to calcium oxalate stone formation because of a reduced complexation of oxalate by magnesium and a consequent rise in the urinary saturation of calcium oxalate. Oral magnesium supplementation could partially correct hypomagnesiuria, although it may provoke further diarrhea. Magnesium citrate (10 mEq two to four times a day) is better tolerated and absorbed than magnesium oxide or hydroxide.[36] It may also raise urinary citrate and pH and lower urinary oxalate. Magnesium chloride is contraindicated, since it will exaggerate metabolic acidosis.

A high fluid intake is recommended to ensure adequate urine volume. Control of excessive intestinal fluid loss with an antidiarrheal agent may be necessary before a sufficient urine output can be achieved.

Calcium citrate (400 mg of calcium with meals) may theoretically have a role in the management of enteric hyperoxaluria.[37] This treatment may lower urinary oxalate by binding oxalate in the intestinal tract.[32] It may raise urinary citrate and pH by providing an alkali load.[38] Finally, it may correct the malabsorption of calcium and adverse effects on the skeleton by providing an efficiently absorbed calcium. If there is coexistent bone disease, 25-OH vitamin D (50 μg every other day) may be provided along with calcium citrate. If hypercalciuria develops, thiazide (e.g., trichlormethiazide, 2 to 4 mg/day) may be administered to control it.

Treatment of Other Hyperoxaluric States

Primary Hyperoxaluria. In this condition, the established treatment regimen comprises orthophosphate, 1.5 to 2.5 grams of phosphorus per day in three or four divided doses, and pyridoxine, 100 mg twice a day.[10] This treatment has been shown to inhibit further stone formation in most persons and to reduce residual stone mass in some. Orthophosphate reduces urinary calcium and augments urinary pyrophosphate (see Chapter 3). If it is given in a neutral form, it increases citrate excretion by 100 to 200 mg/day. Thus, the urinary saturation of calcium oxalate is reduced (from a reduction in urinary calcium and the citrate complexation of calcium), and the inhibitor activity against calcium oxalate crystallization may be augmented (from the action of pyrophosphate). Pyridoxine may reduce urinary oxalate excretion (by stimulating transamination of glyoxylate to glycine) in some patients, thereby reducing the urinary saturation of calcium oxalate.

Magnesium oxide supplementation has been reported to be useful in the prevention of recurrent calcium oxalate nephrolithiasis in primary hyperoxaluria.[39] Magnesium exerts its action by forming a soluble complex with oxalate, thereby reducing ionic oxalate concentration and the urinary saturation of calcium oxalate. However, magnesium oxide has a limited intestinal absorbability because of its low solubility, except in patients with high gastric acid secretion. Thus, the rise in urinary magnesium, necessary for the physicochemical action, is modest. As discussed before, magnesium citrate (10 mEq three or four times a day) may be preferable because of its greater solubility, magnesiuric action, and citraturic effect.[36]

Vitamin C Supplementation. There is no controlled study showing that ascorbic acid supplementation could cause calcium oxalate stone formation; rather, the evidence is mainly anecdotal. However, there is such a strong physicochemical and physiologic basis for a causal role that it would be prudent to avoid vitamin C supplementation in excess of 500 mg/day in patients with calcium oxalate nephrolithiasis. However, there is no reason to withhold vitamin C–rich foods. An ingestion of 1 quart of fresh orange juice per day provides less than 500 mg of vitamin C.

Vitamin C is sometimes used as an acidifying agent in patients with urinary tract infection.[40] This practice should be abandoned. There is no evidence that it could lower urinary pH.[41] On the other hand, it may cause or exaggerate stone formation by augmenting oxalate excretion.

Dietary Hyperoxaluria. Dietary calcium restriction is not necessary or recommended in patients with normal intestinal calcium absorption or in those with renal hypercalciuria in whom high calcium absorption results from renal leak of calcium. Even in those with a primary increase in intestinal calcium absorption (absorptive hypercalciuria), severe dietary calcium restriction (<400 mg/day) is not indicated. Under these circumstances, calcium restriction could increase renal oxalate excretion as well as exert a deleterious effect on bone.

A moderate dietary restriction of oxalate is justified in all patients with calcium oxalate nephrolithiasis, regardless of etiology. It may comprise avoidance of nuts, brewed and "sun" tea, chocolates, and dark greens (like spinach) (see Chapter 12). Such a restriction should not adversely influence general well-being. If hyperoxaluria is present or persists, a more rigid dietary oxalate restriction may be required by avoiding other oxalate-rich foods (green beans, beets, parsley, sweet potatoes, certain spices [dill, sorrel], cocoa, and pepper).

REFERENCES

1. Duclos SC (1668): Histoire de l'Académie Royale des Sciences Dupuis 1666 Jusqu'à son Renouvellement en 1699. Quoted by Partington, Paris, 1733, i. 57, 1962.
2. Scheele CW: On the constituents of Earth of rhubarb; together with the method to prepare the acid of sorrel. Kongliga Vetenskaps Academiens Nya Handlinger 5:180, 1784.
3. Wollaston WH: On gouty and urinary concretions. Philos Trans Soc Lond 87:386–400, 1797.
4. Brooke HJ: On crystallized native oxalate of lime. Philos Mag 16:449–450, 1840.
5. Bannister FA, Hey MH: Reports on some crystalline components of the Weddell Sea deposits. Discovery Rep 13:60–69, 1936.
6. Koch J, Stokstad ELR, Williams HE, Smith LH: Deficiency of 2-oxoglutarate glyoxylate carboligase activity in primary hyperoxaluria. Proc Natl Acad Sci USA 57:1123–1129, 1967.
7. Williams HE, Smith LH Jr: L-Glyceric aciduria: A new genetic variant of primary hyperoxaluria. N Engl J Med 278:233, 1968.
8. Smith LH, Hofmann AF, McCall JT, Thomas PJ: Secondary hyperoxaluria in patients with ileal resection and oxalate nephrolithiasis (abstract). Clin Res 18:541, 1970.
9. Pak CYC, Nicar MJ, Northcutt C: The definition of the mechanism of hypercalciuria is necessary for the treatment of recurrent stone formers. Contrib Nephrol 33:136–151, 1982.
10. Smith LH: Enteric hyperoxaluria and other hyperoxaluric states. *In* Coe FL, Brenner BM, Stein JH (eds): Contemporary Issues in Nephrology. Vol 5. New York, Churchill Livingstone, 1980, pp 43–71.
11. Robertson WG, Peacock M, Heyburn PJ, et al: Risk factors in calcium stone disease of the urinary tract. Br J Urol 50:449–454, 1978.
12. Hodgkinson A: Oxalate metabolism in animals and man. *In* Oxalic Acid in Biology and Medicine. London, Academic Press, 1977, pp 161–164.
13. Earnest DL, Williams HE, Admirand WH: A physicochemical basis for treatment of enteric hyperoxaluria. Trans Assoc Am Physicians 88:224–234, 1975.
14. Dobbins JW, Binder HJ: Importance of the colon in enteric hyperoxaluria. N Engl J Med 296:298, 1977.
15. Dobbins JW, Binder HJ: Effect of bile salts and fatty acids on the colonic absorption of oxalate. Gastroenterology 70:1096, 1976.
16. Wilson DM, Smith LH, Liedtke RR: Renal handling of oxalate in normals and patients with primary and secondary hyperoxaluria and idiopathic stone disease. Urol Res 16:215(B27), 1988.
17. Gershoff SN, Faragalla FF: Endogenous oxalate synthesis and glycine, serine, deoxypyridoxine interrelationships in vitamin B_6-deficient rats. J Biol Chem 234:2391, 1959.
18. Gill HS, Rose A: Mild metabolic hyperoxaluria and its response to pyridoxine. Urol Int 41:393–396, 1986.
19. Atkins GL, Dean B, Griffin M, et al: Quantitative aspects of ascorbic acid metabolism in man. J Biol Chem 239:2975, 1964.
20. Lamden MP, Chrystowski GA: Urinary oxalate excretion by man following ascorbic acid ingestion. Proc Soc Exp Biol Med 85:190–192, 1954.
21. Berman LB, Schreiner GE, Feys J: The nephrotoxic lesion of ethylene glycol. Ann Intern Med 46:611, 1957.
22. Paddock RB, Parker JW, Guadagni NP: The effects of methoxyflurane on renal function. Anesthesiology 25:707, 1964.
23. Breslau NA, Brinkley L, Hill K, Pak CYC: Relationship role of animal protein–rich diet to kidney stone formation and calcium metabolism. J Clin Endocrinol Metab 66:140–146, 1988.
24. Smith LH, Fromm H, Hofmann AF: Acquired hyperoxaluria, nephrolithiasis, and intestinal disease. N Engl J Med 286:1371–1375, 1972.
25. Earnest DL, Johnson G, Williams HE, Admirand WH: Hyperoxaluria in patients with ileal resection: An abnormality in dietary oxalate absorption. Gastroenterology 66:1114, 1974.
26. Rudman D, Dedonis JL, Fountain MT, et al: Hypocitraturia in patients with gastrointestinal malabsorption. N Engl J Med 303:657–661, 1980.
27. Brinkley L, McGuire J, Gregory J, Pak CYC: Bioavailability of oxalate in foods. Urology 17:534–538, 1981.
28. Zarembski PM, Hodgkinson A: Some factors influencing the urinary excretion of oxalic acid in man. Clin Chim Acta 25:1, 1969.
29. Hodgkinson A: Evidence of increased oxalate absorption in patients with calcium-containing renal stones. Clin Sci Mol Med 54:291–294, 1978.
30. Jaeger P, Portmann L, Jacquet A-F, Burckhardt P: Influence of the calcium content of the diet on the incidence of mild hyperoxaluria in idiopathic renal stone formers. Am J Nephrol 5:40–44, 1985.
31. Hayashi Y, Kaplan RA, Pak CYC: Effect of sodium cellulose phosphate therapy on crystallization of calcium oxalate in urine. Metabolism 24:1273–1278, 1975.
32. Barilla DE, Notz C, Kennedy D, Pak CYC: Renal oxalate excretion following oral oxalate loads in patients with ileal disease and with renal and absorptive hypercalciurias: Effect of calcium and magnesium. Am J Med 64:576–585, 1978.

33. Cowley DM, McWhinney BC, Brown JM, Chalmers AH: Chemical factors important to calcium nephrolithiasis: Evidence for impaired hydroxycarboxylic acid absorption causing hyperoxaluria. Clin Chem 33:243–247, 1987.
34. Baggio B, Gambaro G, Marchini F, et al: An inheritable anomaly of red-cell oxalate transport in "primary" calcium nephrolithiasis correctable with diuretics. N Engl J Med 314:599–604, 1986.
35. Zerwekh JE, Sakhaee K, Pak CYC: Short-term 1,25-dihydroxyvitamin D_3 administration raises serum osteo-calcin in patients with postmenopausal osteoporosis. J Clin Endocrinol Metab 60:615–617, 1985.
36. Lindberg JS, Zobitz MM, Poindexter JR, Pak CYC: Magnesium bioavailability from magnesium citrate and magnesium oxide. Am J Clin Nutr (in press).
37. Pak CYC: The problem of idiopathic stone formers presenting with no metabolic disorders: Pathogenesis and management. *In* Third International Symposium on Recent Advances in Pathogenesis and Treatment of Nephrolithiasis, March 1987, Turin. Contrib Nephrol 58:164–171, 1987.
38. Harvey JA, Zobitz MM, Pak CYC: Calcium citrate: Reduced propensity for the crystallization of calcium oxalate in urine resulting from induced hypercalciuria of calcium supplementation. J Clin Endocrinol Metab 61:1223–1225, 1985.
39. Dent CE, Stamp TCB: Treatment of primary hyperoxaluria. Arch Dis Childhood 45:735, 1970.
40. McDonald DF, Murphy GP: Bacteriostatic and acidifying effects of methionine, hydrolyzed casein and ascorbic acid on the urine. N Engl J Med 261:803–805, 1959.
41. Barton CH, Sterling ML, Thomas R, et al: Ineffectiveness of intravenous ascorbic acid as an acidifying agent in man. Arch Intern Med 141:211–212, 1981.

5

Hyperuricosuric Calcium Nephrolithiasis

Charles Y.C. Pak

Traditionally, hyperuricosuria has been associated with uric acid nephrolithiasis. However, it is now recognized that this biochemical abnormality may lead to the development of calcium stones as well.[1] This condition has received the appellation of hyperuricosuric calcium nephrolithiasis (HUCN). Although calcium stones may develop in patients with gout, HUCN should be distinguished from gout and gouty diathesis, which are discussed in Chapter 7. In HUCN, the classic biochemical features of gout of significant hyperuricemia and unusually acid urine are lacking.

In its pure presentation, HUCN is encountered in about 10 per cent of patients.[2] It coexists with other abnormalities in 40 per cent of patients.

HISTORICAL BACKGROUND

The saga of HUCN began in 1968 with three noteworthy publications. In their report on analysis of stones, Prien and Prien observed that some stones containing or composed of calcium oxalate originated from patients with gout.[3] Gutman and Yu noted that patients with gout not only formed uric acid stones but also frequently developed calcium oxalate stones.[4] That same year, Lonsdale reported that sufficient structural conformity existed among crystals of calcium oxalate, uric acid, and sodium urate to permit epitaxial growth of one phase over another.[5] A short time later in 1969, Vernon Smith and associates, noting a higher serum urate concentration in patients with idiopathic calcium oxalate nephrolithiasis than in normal subjects, suggested the use of allopurinol to control formation of recurrent calcium oxalate stones.[6] Coe and Raisen were the first to note the potential pathogenetic role of hyperuricosuria in calcium oxalate stone formation.[7] In 1973, they reported the inhibition of calcium oxalate stone formation by allopurinol treatment in patients with idiopathic calcium oxalate nephrolithiasis who presented with hyperuricosuria without gouty arthritis or significant hyperuricemia.

In 1975, Coe and colleagues[8] and Pak and coworkers[9] simultaneously showed that seeding with monosodium urate of a solution metastably supersaturated with respect to calcium oxalate in vitro induced heterogeneous nucleation of calcium oxalate, providing experimental verification of HUCN. In 1978, Robertson and associates[10] speculated that colloidal monosodium urate could form in the supersaturated urinary environment of patients and could attenuate the inhibitor activity against calcium oxalate crystallization by binding glycosaminoglycans. In 1980, Pak and colleagues[11] reported that the urinary pH of patients with HUCN was normal (>5.5) and not low (<5.5), as in uric acid lithiasis, and showed that the urinary environment of afflicted patients was supersaturated with respect to monosodium urate. In 1986, Ettinger and associates[12] showed in a placebo-controlled randomized trial that allopurinol inhibits calcium oxalate stone formation.

PATHOGENETIC ROLE OF HYPERURICOSURIA IN CALCIUM STONE FORMATION

The essential biochemical features of HUCN are hyperuricosuria and a urinary pH that is normal (>5.5).[11, 13, 14] It has been proposed that this circumstance leads to calcium stone formation from the operation of the following scheme (Fig. 5–1).[15] The urinary environment may be supersaturated with respect to monosodium urate because of a high urinary content of uric acid and a favorable urinary pH (>pK_a for the first proton of uric acid of 5.47) in which adequate dissociation of uric acid occurs. Either a colloidal or a crystalline monosodium urate could theoretically form in such an environment. The urinary environment of patients with HUCN has been shown to be supersaturated with

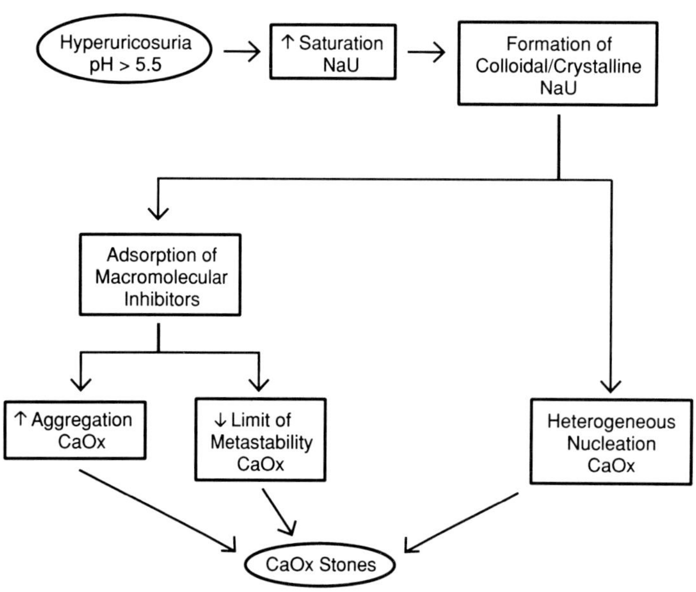

FIGURE 5–1. Scheme for calcium oxalate stone formation from hyperuricosuria. NaU = monosodium urate; CaOx-calcium oxalate.

respect to monosodium urate, unlike normal urine. The possible presence of colloidal urate in the urine of patients with HUCN is indicated by the loss of urate following ultrafiltration of filtered urine.[16]

The monosodium urate so formed can then initiate the crystallization of calcium oxalate by direct induction of heterogeneous nucleation of calcium oxalate or by removing urinary macromolecules through adsorption, thereby attenuating their inhibitor activity.[15,17] In a synthetic solution metastably supersaturated with respect to calcium oxalate, the addition of a small amount of solid crystals of monosodium urate causes precipitation of calcium oxalate.[8, 9] Moreover, monosodium urate (solid) has been shown to bind heparin (a model glycosaminoglycan)[15, 18] and naturally occurring urinary macromolecules (probably glycopeptide),[17] reducing the inhibitor activity of these macromolecules against spontaneous nucleation and crystal growth of calcium oxalate. Recently, increasing the urate concentration of urine in vitro with the addition of uric acid has been shown to facilitate calcium oxalate crystallization. Since the urinary environment was devoid of crystalline urate, the results suggested a "promotive" role of colloidal urate.[19]

The conclusions from the in vitro studies cited in the previous paragraphs are supported by an in vivo study.[16] In patients with HUCN, urinary uric acid was manipulated over a wide range, from low values produced by purine restriction and allopurinol to high values from oral purine loading. During induced hyperuricosuria, the urinary environment was supersaturated with respect to monosodium urate. With increasing urinary supersaturation of monosodium urate, there was a decreasing limit of metastability of calcium oxalate, as reflected in the fall of the formation product ratio (see Chapter 2), indicative of stimulation of calcium oxalate crystallization by monosodium urate.

Unfortunately, crystalline monosodium urate has rarely been found in urine or stones. Although its lack could be explained by the participation of colloidal monosodium urate, the presence of colloidal urate has not been directly demonstrated.

PATHOPHYSIOLOGY OF HYPERURICOSURIA

Normal Uric Acid Metabolism[20, 21]

Uric acid is an end product of purine metabolism, with no useful biochemical function yet recognized. It is formed by irreversible oxidation of purines derived from three sources: de novo synthesis, diet, and tissue catabolism.

In de novo synthesis, "key" nucleotide (inosinic acid) is produced by the incorporation of ribose and phosphate on a "backbone" of glycine (Fig. 5–2). The inosinic acid not only produces adenylic acid and guanylic acid but also gives rise to uric acid. Uric acid is formed from the dephosphorylation of inosinic acid (to form inosine), deribosylation of inosine (to form hypoxanthine), oxidation of hypoxanthine (to form xanthine), and further oxidation of xanthine by xanthine oxidase. An alternate pathway is the conversion of inosinic acid to xanthylic acid, which is dephosphorylated and deribosylated to form xanthine.

Diet contributes to uric acid production by providing purine (ribonucleic acid [RNA] and purine bases, adenine, and guanine) (Fig. 5–2). Tissue catabolism further adds to uric acid synthesis by releasing RNA.

Under normal circumstances, urate synthesized de novo and from tissue

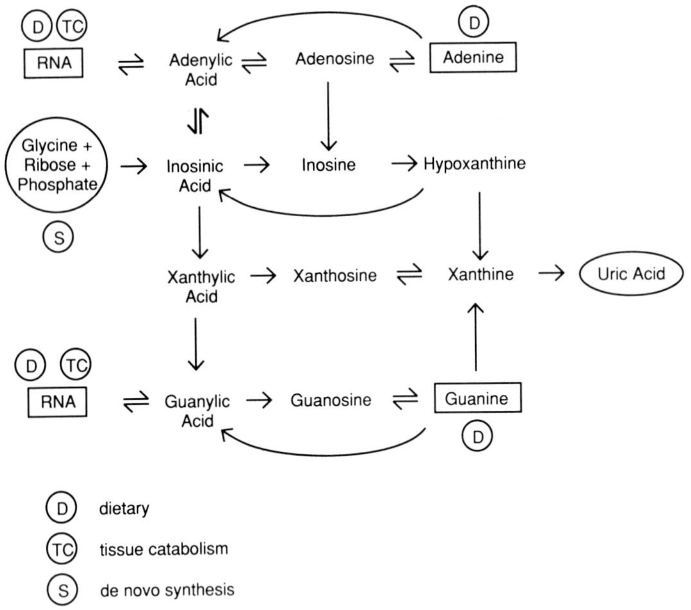

FIGURE 5–2. Normal pathway for de novo synthesis of uric acid.

catabolism is relatively constant, accounting for about 400 mg/day (Fig. 5–3). An additional 400 mg of uric acid is produced from the substrate provided by the diet each day.[22] The synthesized uric acid is eliminated from the body by two main routes. Approximately 25 per cent, or 200 mg/day, is eliminated via the intestinal tract (by "intestinal uricolysis"),[23] where secreted uric acid is degraded to allantoin and allantoic acid by enteric bacteria. The remaining 75 per cent, or 600 mg, of uric acid is eliminated by the kidneys each day.

Normal Renal Handling of Uric Acid[24, 25]

Uric acid is freely filtered at the glomerulus, since there is negligible binding to proteins at physiologic temperature and pH. More than 90 per cent of filtered urate is reabsorbed in the proximal tubule. Urate secretion also takes place probably in the proximal tubule by an amount approximating the filtered load. Subsequent reabsorption of urate (postsecretory absorption), accounting for more

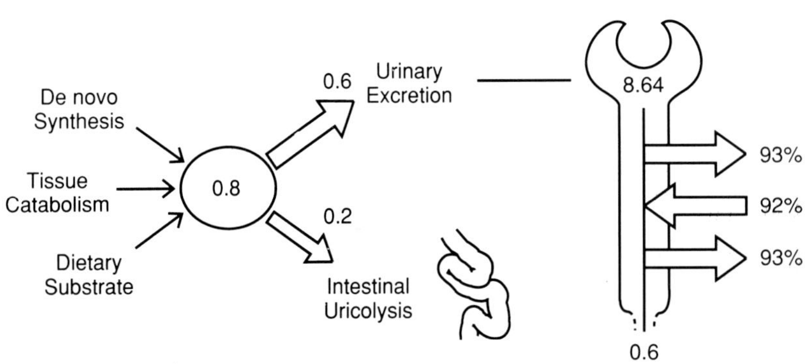

FIGURE 5–3. Sources and fate of synthesized urate. Numbers indicate the amount of uric acid in grams per day.

than 90 per cent of nonreabsorbed filtered and secreted urate, provides the final regulation of urate excretion.

In the example of a normal man given previously, 8.64 grams of uric acid would be filtered each day, assuming a serum uric acid concentration of 6 mg/dl and a glomerular filtration rate of 100 ml/min (Fig. 5–3). After 93 per cent reabsorption, 0.61 gram of uric acid would be left. Secretion of 7.96 grams (equivalent to 92 per cent of the filtered load) would give 8.57 grams, from which 93 per cent postsecretory reabsorption would leave a urinary excretion of 0.6 gram/day.

Control of Urinary Uric Acid Excretion

From the preceding considerations, it is clear that the degree of urinary uric acid excretion would be influenced by alteration in the various steps in its metabolic pathway and in renal excretion (Fig. 5–4). Dietary purine intake could increase urinary uric acid by raising serum concentration and the filtered load of urate. When the individual is placed on a low-purine diet, serum and urinary uric acid values approach 3 mg/dl and 300 mg/dl, respectively.[16, 22] When the individual is placed on a high-protein diet, the serum uric acid level might increase to a high normal range (6 to 7 mg/dl), and urinary uric acid might exceed 1000 mg/day.[16, 22] Accelerated de novo synthesis of urate or exaggerated tissue catabolism might be expected to cause a similar enhancement of urate excretion (see Chapter 7).

Ketone bodies and lactate reduce urate excretion, probably by inhibiting tubular secretion.[26] This observation probably accounts for hyperuricemia, which develops during diabetic ketoacidosis and during fasting. Diuretics, such as thiazide and furosemide, augment tubular reabsorption and inhibit secretion, reducing renal urate excretion and causing hyperuricemia. However, these effects

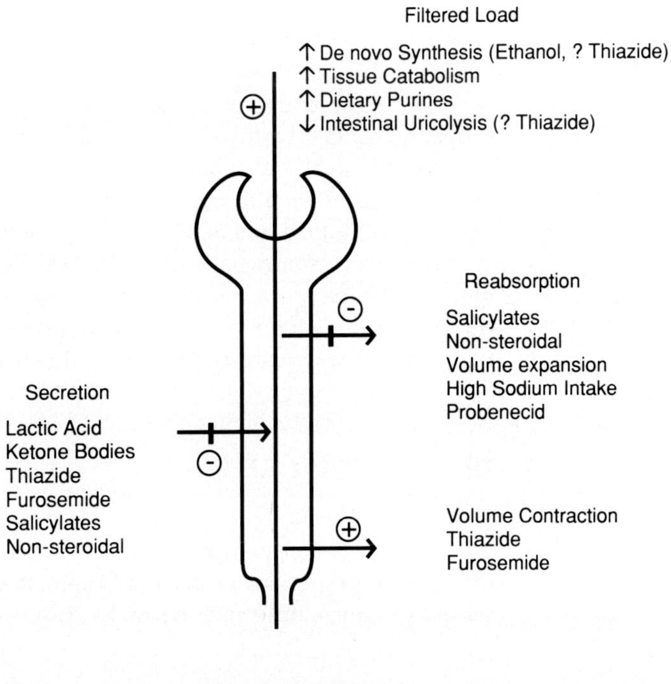

FIGURE 5–4. Factors affecting uric acid excretion. Enhanced uric acid excretion is promoted by factors that increase the filtered load of urate and those that reduce the tubular reabsorption of urate. Diminution of uric acid excretion occurs from the action of factors that reduce the secretion of uric acid and those that augment renal tubular reabsorption of urate. ⊕ = increase; ⊖ = decrease.

are manifested only if there is volume depletion. A finding of relevance to nephrolithiasis is the disclosure that long-term thiazide treatment causes an elevation in urinary and serum uric acid in some patients with calcium nephrolithiasis.[27] Although the precise mechanism is unknown, the results suggest accelerated urate synthesis, reduced extrarenal disposal (intestinal uricolysis) of urate, or both. Salicylates and certain nonsteroidal antiinflammatory agents inhibit both tubular reabsorption and the secretion of urate.[28] At high doses, they are uricosuric because of the prominence of the inhibition of reabsorption. However, they are antiuricosuric at low doses owing to the prominence of secretory inhibition.

Volume expansion (e.g., by high sodium intake) augments urate clearance and lowers serum urate concentration, probably by inhibiting the proximal tubular reabsorption of urate. Although urinary uric acid excretion increases initially during a high sodium intake, it gradually returns to the control level as the sodium load is continued.[29] A new steady-state is reached at a lower level of serum urate concentration. The same remarks apply to probenecid, a drug well known to inhibit tubular urate reabsorption and sometimes used to control hyperuricemia. The enhanced renal excretion of urate and the danger of urate-induced stone formation are present during the early course of treatment, but not late.

Consumption of alcoholic beverages has a variable effect on urate excretion. During ethanol abuse, the hyperlactacidemia achieved may be sufficient to suppress the renal excretion of uric acid by inhibiting secretion.[30] However, this hypouricosuric effect may be opposed by ethanol-induced enhancement of urate synthesis[31] and by provision of exogenous purines (yeast) by certain alcoholic beverages (beer and wine).

Rarely, hyperuricosuria may be present as a genetic defect caused by a defective renal handling of uric acid. In hereditary renal hypouricemia, hyperuricosuria is associated with a high renal urate clearance and low serum urate concentration. Coincidental findings are hypercalciuria and reduced bone density.

Physiologic Derangement in Hyperuricosuric Calcium Nephrolithiasis

The most common cause of hyperuricosuria in patients with HUCN is probably "dietary overindulgence" with purine-rich foods.[1] Such individuals have a history of a liberal intake of meat, poultry, and fish, and estimated purine intake is higher than in the control group. Hyperuricosuria may be produced by an oral purine load and ameliorated by dietary purine deprivation.

However, some patients with HUCN (approximately 30 per cent) have hyperuricosuria as a result of uric acid overproduction.[1, 16] Hyperuricosuria persists despite long-term purine deprivation. No further studies have been performed to elucidate the nature of this apparent urate overproduction.

DIAGNOSTIC CRITERIA

HUCN (in its pure presentation) is characterized by hyperuricosuria (urinary uric acid >600 mg/day on mean of three samples and on at least two of the three samples)[14]; normocalcemia; normal fasting and calcium load response and normal urinary calcium and oxalate (<44 mg/day); and calcium nephrolithiasis. Hyperuricosuria, defined functionally here by the upper normal limit of 600 mg/day, correlates with the urinary supersaturation with respect to monosodium urate and with the propensity for calcium stone formation. (Other laboratories employ a higher upper limit for urinary uric acid, e.g., 750 mg/day for women and 800 mg/day for men.) Urinary pH is typically greater than 5.5, though it is often low normal (5.5 to 6.0). Hyperuricosuria may be the only major abnormal stone risk in patients with calcium stones, or it may coexist with various forms of hypercalciuria. Serum uric acid is usually high normal (6 to 7 mg/dl). Frank hyperuricemia is uncommon; if present, gouty diathesis should be suspected (see Chapter 7). Urinary sulfate and phosphorus may be increased (>30 mEq/day and >1000 mg/day), indicative of a dietary excess of animal protein. Gouty arthritis is not a part of the HUCN syndrome; if present, a search should be made for gouty diathesis (see Chapter 7). HUCN shares the same demographic features as absorptive hypercalciuria in its predilection for middle-aged white men. Many patients give a history of a preference for or overindulgence of animal proteins (meat, poultry, and fish).

MANAGEMENT OF HYPERURICOSURIC CALCIUM NEPHROLITHIASIS (Table 5–1)

Dietary purine restriction might be useful in controlling hyperuricosuria in many patients with HUCN, whose excessive urate synthesis is due to dietary purine excess. A common fallacy is the belief that a substitution of red meat by poultry and fish constitutes purine restriction. Poultry and fish are as rich in purines as red meat. An adequate purine restriction requires limiting all three types of meat and making up the caloric need with vegetables and fruits.

Because purine restriction is often impractical and poorly followed, allopurinol represents the treatment of choice.[12] By inactivating xanthine oxidase, allopurinol inhibits the oxidation of hypoxanthine to xanthine and of xanthine to uric acid. Thus, by inhibiting urate synthesis, allopurinol causes a prompt reduction in serum and urinary uric acid. With this inhibition, increased amounts of precursors, hypoxanthine and xanthine, are produced. In patients with HUCN, allopurinol at a customary dose of 300 mg/day usually produces a sustained restoration of normal urinary uric acid (<600 mg/day) and reduces the serum uric acid level by about 2 mg/dl. Allopurinol has been reported to reduce oxalate excretion.[32] However, such an action might have been an "artifact" of the diet, since it could not be demonstrated under a constant dietary regimen.[16] Allopurinol is surprisingly well tolerated in patients with HUCN, the principal side effects being represented by an uncommon skin rash and rare hepatic enzymatic abnormalities. The appearance of the latter complication mandates cessation of drug treatment.

TABLE 5–1. MANAGEMENT OF HYPERURICOSURIC CALCIUM NEPHROLITHIASIS

Mode of Therapy	Mechanism of Action
Dietary purine restriction	Reduced substrate for uric acid synthesis
Allopurinol, 300 mg/day	Inhibition of uric acid synthesis from xanthine
Potassium citrate, 30–60 mEq/day	Increase urinary citrate and pH Inhibition of calcium oxalate crystallization

Physicochemical changes ensuing from restoration of normal urinary uric acid by allopurinol include an increase in the urinary limit of metastability of calcium oxalate.[16] Thus, the spontaneous nucleation of calcium oxalate is retarded by treatment, probably via inhibition of monosodium urate–induced stimulation of calcium oxalate crystallization. Because of the potential exaggeration of monosodium urate–induced calcium oxalate crystallization from excessive sodium intake, a moderate sodium restriction (<150 mEq/day) is also advisable.

Potassium citrate represents an effective alternative to allopurinol in the treatment of this condition.[33] Citrate added to a synthetic medium metastably supersaturated with respect to calcium oxalate[34] inhibits the heterogeneous nucleation of calcium oxalate by monosodium urate. When potassium citrate (30 to 60 mEq/day in divided doses) is given to patients with hyperuricosuric calcium oxalate nephrolithiasis, urinary citrate rises significantly.[33] The induced hypercitraturia not only reduces the urinary saturation of calcium oxalate (by complexing calcium) but also inhibits urate-induced crystallization of calcium oxalate.

Potassium citrate may be particularly useful in patients with mild-to-moderate hyperuricosuria (600 to 800 mg/day) in whom hypocitraturia is also present. However, allopurinol is probably preferred in patients with more marked hyperuricosuria. Allopurinol is also recommended if significant hyperuricemia (>8.5 mg/dl) coexists and gouty diathesis is suspected.

REFERENCES

1. Coe FL: Hyperuricosuric calcium oxalate nephrolithiasis. Kidney Int 13:418–426, 1978.
2. Pak CYC: Medical management of nephrolithiasis: Update 1987. J Urol 140:461–467, 1988.
3. Prien EL, Prien, EL Jr: Composition and structure of urinary stone. Am J Med 45:654–672, 1968.
4. Gutman AB, Yu TF: Uric acid nephrolithiasis. Am J Med 45:756–779, 1968.
5. Lonsdale K: Epitaxy as a growth factor in urinary calculi and gallstones. Nature 217:56–58, 1968.
6. Smith MJV: Placebo versus allopurinol for renal calculi. J Urol 117:690–692, 1977.
7. Coe FL, Raisen L: Allopurinol treatment of uric-acid disorders in calcium stone formers. Lancet 1:129–131, 1973.
8. Coe FL, Lawton RL, Goldstein RB, Tembe V: Sodium urate accelerates precipitation of calcium oxalate in vitro. Proc Soc Exp Biol Med 149:926–929, 1975.
9. Pak CYC, Arnold LH: Heterogeneous nucleation of calcium oxalate by seeds of monosodium urate. Proc Soc Exp Biol Med 149:930–932, 1975.
10. Robertson WG, Knowles F, Peacock M: Urinary acid mucopolysaccharide inhibitors of calcium oxalate crystallization. *In* Fleisch H, Robertson WG, Smith LH, Vahlensieck W (eds.): Urolithiasis Research. New York, Plenum Publishing, 1978, pp 331–338.
11. Pak CYC, Holt K, Britton F, et al: Assessment of pathogenetic roles in uric acid, monopotassium urate, monoammonium urate and monosodium urate in hyperuricosuric calcium oxalate nephrolithiasis. J Clin Endocrinol Metab 50:593–596, 1980.
12. Ettinger B, Tang A, Citron JT, et al: Randomized trial of allopurinol in the prevention of calcium oxalate calculi. N Engl J Med 315:1386–1389, 1986.
13. Pak CYC, Waters O, Arnold L, et al: Mechanism for calcium nephrolithiasis among patients with hyperuricosuria: Supersaturation of urine with respect to monosodium urate. J Clin Invest 59:426–431, 1977.
14. Pak CYC, Britton F, Peterson R, et al: Ambulatory evaluation of nephrolithiasis: Classification, clinical presentation and diagnostic criteria. Am J Med 69:19–30, 1980.
15. Pak CYC, Holt K, Zerwekh JE: Attenuation by monosodium urate of the inhibitory effect of glycosaminoglycans on calcium oxalate nucleation. Invest Urol 17:138–140, 1979.
16. Pak CYC, Barilla DE, Holt K, et al: Effect of oral purine load and allopurinol on the crystallization of calcium salts in urine of patients with hyperuricosuric calcium urolithiasis. Am J Med 65:593–599, 1978.
17. Zerwekh JE, Holt K, Pak CYC: Natural urinary macromolecular inhibitors: Attenuation of inhibitory activity by urate salts. Kidney Int 23:838–841, 1983.
18. Finlayson B, DuBois L: Adsorption of heparin on sodium acid urate. Clin Chim Acta 84:203–206, 1978.

19. Glover PK, Ryall RL, Marshall VR: The effect of increasing urate concentration on the precipitation of calcium oxalate from human urine. Urol Res 16:181 (A27), 1988.
20. Seegmiller JE, Laster L, Howell R: Biochemistry of uric acid and its relation to gout. N Engl J Med 268:712–716, 764–773, 821–827, 1963.
21. Wyngaarden JB, Kelley WN: Gout. *In* Stanbury JB, Wyngaarden JB, Fredrickson DS (eds.): The Metabolic Basis of Inherited Disease. New York, McGraw-Hill Company, 1972, pp 889–968.
22. Zollner N, Griebsch A: Uric acid lithiasis. *In* Urinary Calculi: International Symposium on Renal Stone Research, Madrid. Basel, S Karger, 1973, pp 84–88.
23. Sorenson LB: Elimination of uric acid in men studied by means of C^{14}-labeled uric acid. Scand J Clin Lab Invest 12(54):1–214, 1960.
24. Gutman AB, Yu TF: A three-component system for regulation of renal excretion of uric acid in man. Trans Assoc Am Physicians 74:353–365, 1961.
25. Steele TH: Control of uric acid excretion. Med Intelligence 284:1193–1196, 1971.
26. Goldfinger S, Klinenberg JR, Seegmiller JE: Renal retention of uric acid induced by infusion of beta-hydroxybutyrate and acetoacetate. N Engl J Med 272:351–355, 1965.
27. Pak CYC, Tolentino R, Stewart A, Galosy RA: Enhancement of renal excretion of uric acid during long-term thiazide therapy. Invest Urol 3:191–193, 1978.
28. Gutman AB: Uricosuric drugs, with special references to probenecid and sulfinpyrazone. Adv Pharmacol Chemother 4:91–142, 1966.
29. Breslau NA, Pak CYC: Lack of effect of salt intake on urinary uric acid excretions. J Urol 129:531–532, 1983.
30. Lieber CS, Davidson CS: Some metabolic effects of ethyl alcohol. Am J Med 33:319–327, 1962.
31. Faller J, Fox IH: Ethanol-induced hyperuricemia: Evidence for increased urate production by activation of adenine nucleotide turnover. N Engl J Med 307:1598–1602, 1982.
32. Scott R, Paterson PJ, Smith M, Mathieson A: Reduction in urinary oxalate values by allopurinol. Urology 12:212–214, 1978.
33. Pak CYC, Peterson R: Successful treatment of hyperuricosuric calcium oxalate nephrolithiasis with potassium citrate. Arch Intern Med 146:863–868, 1986.
34. Nicar MJ, Hill K, Pak CYC: Inhibition by citrate of spontaneous precipitation of calcium oxalate, *in vitro*. J Bone Min Res 2:215–220, 1987.

6

Hypocitraturic Calcium Nephrolithiasis

Charles Y.C. Pak

During the past decade, citrate has received increasing and renewed interest as an important pathogenetic factor in stone formation and as an exciting modality in the prevention of new stone formation.[1] The physicochemical background responsible for the inhibitor activity of citrate is being elucidated. It is now generally recognized that hypocitraturia is a frequent biochemical disturbance among patients with nephrolithiasis. The approval of potassium citrate by the Food and Drug Administration (FDA) in 1985 has introduced a new dimension in the management of a wide variety of stone-forming disorders.

The facility with which urinary citrate can be measured and manipulated undoubtedly has been responsible, in a very large measure, for this development. This situation contrasts with that of other inhibitors, such as glycosaminoglycans and glycoproteins, which have not been accorded similar interest, possibly because of the lack of a reliable assay system and of a therapeutic modality that could alter their urinary excretion.

This chapter reviews the physicochemistry and physiology of citrate and concludes with a discussion of the therapeutic value of potassium citrate. To provide an appropriate perspective, a brief historical background precedes this discussion.

HISTORICAL BACKGROUND

The development of potassium citrate for the treatment of hypocitraturic calcium nephrolithiasis has been commonly attributed to the studies conceived and initiated at Dallas. However, it is clear that the potential therapeutic role of alkali had been appreciated for many years before.

In 1826, Sir Astley Cooper prescribed "liquor potassae, potassium carbonate and sodium carbonate" for nephrolithiasis, presumably for stones of uric acid composition.[2] In 1940, Albright and colleagues described the case of a 13-year-old girl suffering from rickets due to distal renal tubular acidosis.[3] Treatment with a sodium citrate–citric acid mixture corrected the acidosis, improved calcium balance and bone disease, and reestablished growth. One year later, Kissin and Locks observed reduced citrate excretion in patients with calcium nephrolithiasis and suggested that "increasing the citrate concentration of urine, by the administration of citrates . . . may offer a new prophylactic or even therapeutic measure" in nephrolithiasis.[4] In 1954, Howard used a mixture of sodium citrate, potassium citrate, and citric acid as an alkalinizing agent to treat patients with stones composed of uric acid or cystine.[5]

In 1981, Gregory and associates administered to patients with enteric hyperoxaluria sodium bicarbonate at a dosage sufficient to alkalinize the urine.[6] They observed a reduction in urinary calcium, the urinary saturation of calcium oxalate, and crystalluria. That same year, Butz and Dulce reported that a mixture of potassium and sodium citrate could lower urinary calcium and raise urinary citrate in patients with idiopathic calcium oxalate nephrolithiasis.[7] In 1983, Sakhaee and coworkers found a distinction between potassium citrate action and sodium citrate action in uric acid lithiasis.[8] Whereas potassium citrate lowered urinary calcium and calcium oxalate saturation and increased the inhibitor activity against calcium oxalate crystallization, sodium citrate was devoid of hypocalciuric action and did not augment inhibitor activity. This finding provided the explanation for the complication of calcium stones during sodium alkali therapy in patients with uric acid lithiasis reported several years later.[9] In 1985, another unique advantage of potassium citrate was disclosed.[10] This treatment was shown to prevent hypokalemia, augment citrate excretion, and prevent recurrent calcium stone formation in patients with hypercalciuric nephrolithiasis who continued to form stones on thiazide therapy. In 1983, a preliminary report indicated that potassium citrate treatment could cause dissolution of calcium stones in vivo,[11] an occurrence heretofore considered a possibility only for radiolucent stones.

PATHOGENETIC ROLE OF CITRATE IN CALCIUM NEPHROLITHIASIS

Citrate retards the crystallization of stone-forming calcium salts by two broad means (Fig. 6–1). First, it complexes calcium and reduces ionic calcium concentration in urine,[12, 13] thereby reducing the urinary saturation of calcium oxalate and calcium phosphate. Thus, the "driving force" for the crystallization of these salts is reduced. If citrate complexation of calcium is sufficient to produce undersaturation, dissolution of preformed calcium salts could occur.

Second, citrate directly inhibits the crystallization of calcium oxalate and calcium phosphate. Citrate has been shown to inhibit the spontaneous precipitation of calcium oxalate[14] and retard the agglomeration of preformed calcium oxalate crystals.[15] Citrate has a modest inhibitory effect against the crystal growth of calcium oxalate when corrected for the reduction in activity product occurring from ion pair formation.[12] Citrate is believed to be a more potent inhibitor of the crystal growth of calcium phosphate. Finally, citrate has been found to prevent the heterogeneous nucleation of calcium oxalate by monosodium urate.[16] It is therefore expected that in the setting of hypocitraturia, which is frequently

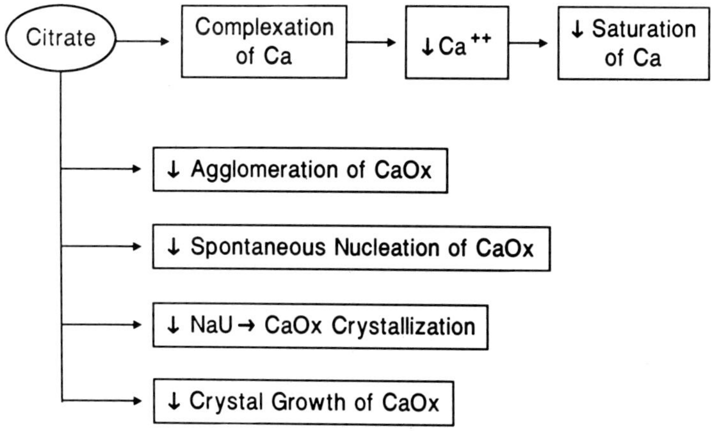

FIGURE 6–1. Scheme for the inhibitor activity of citrate.

encountered in nephrolithiasis, the crystallization of calcium oxalate and calcium phosphate would be facilitated and stone formation exaggerated.

When expressed relative to molecular weight, the inhibitor activity of citrate is much less prominent than that of pyrophosphate, glycosaminoglycan, glycoprotein, or Tamm-Horsfall protein (see Chapter 2). However, the amount of citrate normally present in urine is many times that of other inhibitors. At "physiologic" concentrations in urine, citrate clearly inhibits spontaneous nucleation, crystal growth, and crystal agglomeration of calcium oxalate.[1]

Because of these inhibitor actions of citrate, the urinary environment of patients with hypocitraturic nephrolithiasis is characterized by an increased propensity for the crystallization of calcium salts.

PATHOPHYSIOLOGY OF HYPOCITRATURIA

Physiologic Basis for Hypocitraturia

Normal Physiology. Citrate is a key component of the citric acid cycle. Thus, it is ubiquitous in the body, constituting an important energy source. Of the large amount of citrate that is metabolized by the whole organism, only a very small fraction appears in urine. Dietary citrate is a poor source of citrate, since only about 0.7 per cent of it appears in urine.[17]

In the circulation, citrate is normally present at a concentration of about 0.14 mM, largely as a free trivalent anion. Of the 9 μmol of citrate that are filtered in the kidneys each minute, 75 per cent, or 6.75 μmol, are reabsorbed mostly in the proximal tubule, leaving 25 per cent, or 2.25 μmol, in urine (Fig. 6–2).[18] The proximal tubular cell also extracts citrate from postglomerular blood. An average amount of this peritubular uptake of citrate is 1.5 μmol/min. Thus, total citrate uptake by the proximal tubules from tubular fluid and postglomerular blood is 8.25 μmol/min. The subsequent citrate oxidation to carbon dioxide and water via the citric acid cycle in the mitochondria of the tubular cells provides an important source of energy for the kidney. The tubular uptake of citrate also accounts for the fact that citrate concentration in the renal cortex often exceeds that of peripheral blood.

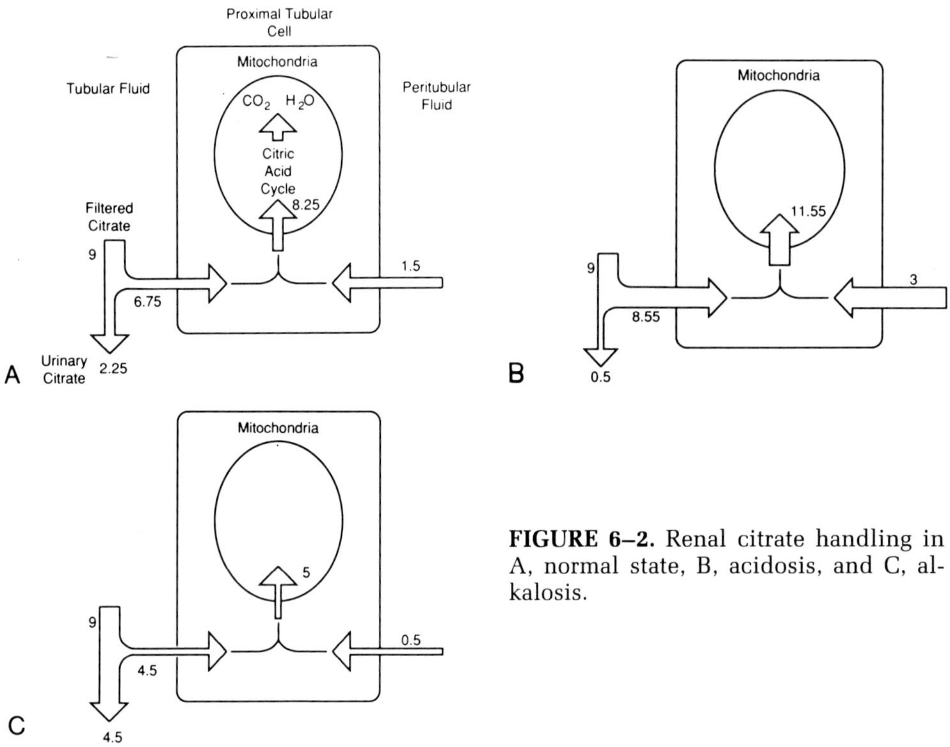

FIGURE 6–2. Renal citrate handling in A, normal state, B, acidosis, and C, alkalosis.

Alteration in Renal Citrate Handling by Changes in Acid-Base Status. An alteration in acid-base status profoundly influences the renal handling of citrate. It is therefore a major determinant of urinary citrate excretion.

Metabolic acidosis facilitates the influx and inhibits the efflux of citrate from renal mitochondria, promoting citrate oxidation (Fig. 6–2). A subsequent fall in cytosolic citrate concentration leads to enhanced citrate uptake by the tubular cell, involving the sodium-citrate cotransporter in the brush border basement membrane.[19] The peritubular uptake of citrate is stimulated as well. The increased tubular reabsorption of citrate reduces urinary citrate excretion, while stimulated mitochondrial citrate oxidation lowers the tissue content of citrate. Thus, reduced citrate clearance parallels the fall in citrate concentration of the renal cortex.

These changes often occur without a substantial alteration in serum citrate concentration. Moreover, negligible citrate is secreted or synthesized during metabolic acidosis. Thus, citrate appearing in urine is that small fraction of citrate that escapes reabsorption. Metabolic acidosis reduces citrate excretion by augmenting citrate reabsorption.

Exactly the opposite sequence prevails in metabolic alkalosis. Mitochondrial uptake of citrate is reduced (Fig. 6–2), retarding citrate oxidation. Cytosolic citrate concentration rises, leading to reduced tubular reabsorption and peritubular uptake of citrate. Urinary citrate increases, since a smaller fraction of filtered citrate is reabsorbed.

Other Determinants of Citrate Excretion. *Hypokalemia* causes an intracellular metabolic acidosis in the renal cortex.[20] Thus, it leads to reduced citrate excretion by the same mechanism as in metabolic acidosis.

Organic acids (such as malate, succinate, and fumarate) stimulate intrarenal citrate synthesis by providing substrate.[21] In addition, they provide an alkali load. These compounds enhance citrate excretion mostly through the effect of alkali on renal citrate handling, previously described, and partly from the escape into the urine of the synthesized citrate. The ingestion of tamarind, a food item rich in tartaric acid, is believed to be useful in preventing stone formation.[22] The ability of tartaric acid to stimulate citrate excretion may explain this action.

Certain hormones may affect renal citrate excretion by a mechanism still poorly defined. Urinary citrate excretion is higher during the latter half of the normal menstrual cycle than the first half (by 100 to 200 mg/day).[23] During pregnancy, urinary citrate increases by 500 to 1000 mg/day. These results have been attributed to the action of *estrogen* or progesterone or both. *Parathyroid hormone* is also believed to augment citrate excretion.[24] This conclusion is supported by the finding of high urinary citrate in patients suffering from primary hyperparathyroidism. It has been suggested that vitamin D and calcitonin augment, while androgens reduce, citrate secretion. These presumed actions, however, have little clinical relevance.

Frequency of Hypocitraturia in Calcium Nephrolithiasis

Hypocitraturia has been reported in 19 to 63 per cent of patients with nephrolithiasis in various reports.[1] This wide variation probably reflects different normal ranges for urinary citrate established by different laboratories. Moreover, attempts have been made to define hypocitraturia separately for men and women and according to age. This convention was suggested because urinary citrate is normally greater in women than in men and in premenopausal rather than in postmenopausal women. When so analyzed, hypocitraturia is believed to be more common in stone-forming women than in men.

In the laboratory at Dallas, the low normal limit for citrate has been established at 320 mg/day for both men and women and, irrespective of age (>18 years), for the following reasons.[25] This value of 320 mg/day is one actually derived from a large number of normal subjects in this laboratory. Among stone-forming patients, no significant difference in urinary citrate was found between men and women. When urinary citrate for the same sex was compared between control subjects and stone-forming patients, a significant reduction in urinary citrate was encountered among patients with stones in both sexes.[25] In distal renal tubular acidosis (complete as well as incomplete), urinary citrate is invariably below 320 mg/day.[26] Finally, this limit provides a good empirical definition of hypocitraturia, since patients with urinary citrate below this level often show a clinical response to potassium citrate therapy superior to those whose citrate exceeds 320 mg/day.[27]

Using the preceding definition, hypocitraturia occurred alone in 5 per cent and coexisted with other abnormalities in 50 per cent of patients.[25]

Clinical Conditions Associated with Hypocitraturic Calcium Nephrolithiasis (Table 6–1)

Among various factors that could cause hypocitraturia, which were previously discussed, acidosis probably plays the most important role in producing hypocitraturia among patients with calcium nephrolithiasis. It accounts for the occurrence of hypocitraturia in distal renal tubular acidosis (complete and incomplete),

TABLE 6–1. CAUSES OF HYPOCITRATURIC CALCIUM NEPHROLITHIASIS

1. Distal renal tubular acidosis
   a. Complete
   b. Incomplete
2. Chronic diarrheal syndrome
3. Thiazide-induced hypocitraturia
4. Idiopathic
   a. Diet high in animal protein
   b. Strenuous physical exercise
   c. High sodium intake
   d. Active urinary tract infection
   e. Intestinal malabsorption of citrate

chronic diarrheal state, and thiazide therapy. The urinary citrate may also be low following a diet high in animal protein,[28] strenuous physical exercise (from acquired acidosis),[29] and high sodium intake (probably from sodium-induced mild metabolic acidosis).

Distal Renal Tubular Acidosis.[26, 30] Distal acidification defect (type I) is the only form of renal tubular acidosis that is associated with nephrolithiasis. Among the stone-forming population, the incomplete form is more common than the complete form. Nephrolithiasis and nephrocalcinosis are both present, usually in the complete form, whereas calcium-containing stones may be present without nephrocalcinosis in the incomplete form. There is systemic metabolic acidosis on presentation in the complete form. In the incomplete form, systemic acidosis may be lacking initially; however, defective acidification is disclosed upon exogenous challenge with an acid load (ammonium chloride).

In the complete form, the defective excretion of hydrogen ions in the distal tubule causes high urinary pH, and systemic acidosis causes skeletal loss of calcium, impaired renal tubular absorption of calcium, and hypocitraturia. Calcium phosphate crystallization is promoted because of increased urinary saturation (from increased dissociation of phosphate and hypercalciuria) and reduced inhibitor activity (from hypocitraturia). The crystallization of calcium oxalate may be enhanced as well owing to increased saturation (from hypercalciuria and reduced citrate complexation of calcium) and impaired inhibitor activity (from hypocitraturia). Thus, the predominant stone constituent is calcium phosphate (hydroxyapatite). Calcium oxalate is also present in the stone typically, albeit as a minor constituent. In an incomplete form, hypocitraturia is invariably present, though usually not as severe as in the complete form. Urinary calcium may be moderately increased, and urinary pH is usually high normal.

In longstanding distal tubular acidosis, the skeleton may be adversely affected. In a severe form of complete distal renal tubular acidosis, osteomalacia or rickets may occur. In the more commonly encountered incomplete form seen among the stone-forming population, clinical bone disease is uncommon. However, subjects may be at increased risk for osteoporosis, since they are often in negative calcium balance.[31] Hypercalciuria of resorptive and renal forms may be present because acidosis causes excessive skeletal resorption and impaired renal tubular resorption of calcium. However, intestinal calcium absorption may be low (via a vitamin D–independent mechanism). A picture of distal renal tubular acidosis with stones may develop following long-term treatment with acetazolamide (a carbonic anhydrase inhibitor).[32]

There is no evidence that nephrolithiasis is associated with proximal renal tubular acidosis (Type II) or with hyporeninemic hypoaldosteronism (Type IV). Urinary citrate may be low because of acidosis. However, urinary calcium is often low owing to bicarbonaturia in Type II and renal insufficiency in Type IV. Moreover, urinary pH is normal in Type IV.

Chronic Diarrheal Syndrome.[33, 34] Underlying gastrointestinal disorders producing this syndrome include postgastrectomy state, inflammatory disease of the small bowel, bowel resection or bypass, and colitis. The cause of the hypocitraturia is metabolic acidosis resulting from intestinal alkali loss from frequent diarrhea. Hypomagnesemia and hypomagnesiuria may result from intestinal malabsorption of magnesium, and hypokalemia may result from intestinal potassium loss. These factors may contribute to the development of hypocitraturia. Hypocitraturia may be very severe and correlates with the degree of diarrhea. If the intestinal disease is associated with malabsorption of fat, hyperoxaluria may be present as well (see Chapter 4). Unlike in distal renal tubular acidosis, urinary pH is reduced. Urine volume is low because of intestinal fluid loss.

Stone formation is multifactorial (see Chapter 4). Calcium stone formation is due to hypocitraturia (reduced inhibitor activity), low urine volume (increased concentration of stone-forming constituents), hypomagnesiuria (reduced complexation of oxalate), and hyperoxaluria. It may occur even in the absence of hyperoxaluria, though it is usually less severe than if hypoxaluria is also present. Low urinary calcium (from intestinal malabsorption) protects against stone formation. Uric acid stones may develop from low urinary pH, which impairs the dissociation of uric acid and increases the amount of undissociated uric acid (see Chapter 7).

Thiazide-Induced Hypocitraturia. Thiazides are widely used for the control of hypercalciuric calcium nephrolithiasis (see Chapter 3).[35] This diuretic has been shown to reduce the urinary saturation of stone-forming calcium salts, principally by reducing calcium excretion. However, thiazides may reduce citrate excretion, probably by causing hypokalemia and intracellular acidosis.[10, 35, 36] Yendt and Cohanim were the first to report this complication.[35] The induced hypocitraturia, if unchecked, may oppose the beneficial effect of the fall in calcium excretion and may cause relapse in the patient receiving thiazide treatment.

Idiopathic Hypocitraturic Calcium Nephrolithiasis. In some patients, the exact cause for the hypocitraturia is not known.[1, 37] It could be related to consumption of a diet rich in animal proteins consisting of sulfur-containing amino acids (producing an acid load) (see Chapter 11),[28] strenuous physical exercise,[29] and high sodium intake in the setting of low potassium intake. Active urinary tract infection could also reduce urinary citrate, probably from bacterial enzymatic degradation of citrate.

There is preliminary evidence that the intestinal absorption of citrate may be impaired in some patients with calcium nephrolithiasis, accounting for their hypocitraturia.[38] This intriguing report awaits verification.

DIAGNOSTIC CRITERIA

The diagnosis of hypocitraturic calcium nephrolithiasis may be made from an ambulatory evaluation,[25, 39] the protocol of which is described in Chapter 11.

Diagnostic criteria for the main forms of hypocitraturia are summarized in Table 6–2.

Hypocitraturic calcium nephrolithiasis in the pure presentation refers to the condition in which hypocitraturia (urinary citrate <320 mg/day) is present alone without other physiologic derangements (such as hypercalciuria or hyperuricosuria).[25] However, hypocitraturia often coexists with other abnormalities.

Complete distal renal tubular acidosis is characterized by hyperchloremic metabolic acidosis (high serum chloride levels and low serum potassium and carbon dioxide levels) and high urinary pH (>6.8) in the absence of infection of the urinary tract. In incomplete distal renal tubular acidosis,[26] serum electrolytes are normal, but there is an impaired ability to acidify the urine following an ammonium chloride load. After an oral administration of ammonium chloride (100 mg/kg), urinary pH does not decline below 5.3. The distal renal tubular acidosis is excluded if the fasting urinary pH is lower than 5.3 in the setting of normal serum electrolytes. Both complete and incomplete forms may be associated with hypercalciuria, hypocitraturia, calcium nephrolithiasis, and nephrocalcinosis. A typical stone analysis shows a preponderance of hydroxyapatite, with calcium oxalate as a minor constituent. As noted before, the degrees of hypercalciuria and hypocitraturia are more severe, and nephrocalcinosis and bone disease are more common in the complete than in the incomplete form.

Chronic diarrheal syndrome[1, 34] capable of producing hypocitraturia and calcium nephrolithiasis includes ileal disease or resection, gastrectomy, ulcerative colitis, and colectomy. The degrees of hypocitraturia are generally proportional to the severity of intestinal fluid loss. In severe diarrheal states, urinary citrate may be very low (<50 mg/day). Besides hypocitraturia, there may be hypokalemia, hypomagnesemia, and low urine volume and pH (<5.5). Urinary calcium and magnesium may be low (<100 and <50 mg/day, respectively). Some patients, particularly those with ileal disease, may have hyperoxaluria.

In thiazide-induced hypocitraturia,[10] the serum potassium level is low or low normal, and urinary citrate is low (<320 mg/day). The serum carbon dioxide level may be high, the serum chloride level low, and urinary calcium normal, owing to the action of thiazide.

A careful history should be taken for excessive ingestion of animal proteins, strenuous physical exercise, salt abuse, urinary tract infection, laxative abuse, and acetazolamide therapy, as well as for intestinal disease and diuretic therapy. A biochemical picture simulating distal renal tubular acidosis and calcium nephrolithiasis could develop during treatment with an inhibitor of carbonic anhydrase.

TABLE 6–2. DIAGNOSTIC CRITERIA FOR HYPOCITRATURIC CALCIUM NEPHROLITHIASIS

	Complete Renal Tubular Acidosis	Incomplete Renal Tubular Acidosis	Chronic Diarrheal Syndrome	Thiazide Induced Hypocitraturia
Serum				
Potassium	↓	N	↓	↓
Chloride	↑	N	N, ↑	↓
Carbon dioxide	↓	N	N, ↓	↑
Urinary				
pH	↑	↑, N	↓	N
Calcium	↑	↑, N	↓	↓
Citrate	↓↓	↓	↓↓	↓

N = normal; ↑ = increase; ↓ = decrease.

MEDICAL MANAGEMENT

In the preceding discussion, it was shown that citrate is an important inhibitor of the crystallization of stone-forming salts and that hypocitraturia is common among patients with calcium nephrolithiasis. Thus, it is apparent that maneuvers that maintain urinary pH between 6 and 7 and that raise urinary citrate to normal levels would be desirable in preventing the formation of calcium oxalate stones. There is ample evidence showing that potassium citrate treatment optimally meets this purpose.

Physiologic Action of Potassium Citrate

Under normal circumstances, most of the potassium citrate that is taken orally is probably absorbed (Fig. 6–3). The absorbed citrate is largely oxidized in vivo, whereas the potassium ion remains, thus leaving an alkali load. The alkali load raises urinary citrate by the mechanism previously outlined and increases urinary pH. There is recent evidence that a small amount of absorbed citrate escapes oxidation and appears in urine, contributing in a minor way to the citraturic action of potassium citrate.[40] In the presence of hypokalemia, the potassium ion itself may augment citrate excretion by correcting intracellular acidosis.

During long-term treatment, potassium citrate has been shown to cause a sustained rise in urinary citrate and pH.[1] In patients with mild-to-moderate hypocitraturia (100 to 320 mg/day), potassium citrate (60 mEq/day) increases urinary citrate by about 400 mg/day. The urinary pH rises by about 0.5 unit and can be maintained at about 6.5. The citraturic action is less prominent in those with severe hypocitraturia (e.g., complete renal tubular acidosis and severe chronic diarrheal syndrome). The total rise in urinary pH is less marked in renal tubular acidosis in which urinary pH is high to begin with.

There is a sustained reduction in urinary calcium during long-term treatment of patients with distal renal tubular acidosis.[31] However, in others, the hypocalciuric action tends to be transient.[41]

Physicochemical Action of Potassium Citrate

The physicochemical effects of potassium citrate therapy may be ascribed to its citraturic and alkalinizing action (Fig. 6–4).[1] There is an inhibition of the crystallization of calcium salts in urine because of the rise in urinary citrate[1, 42]

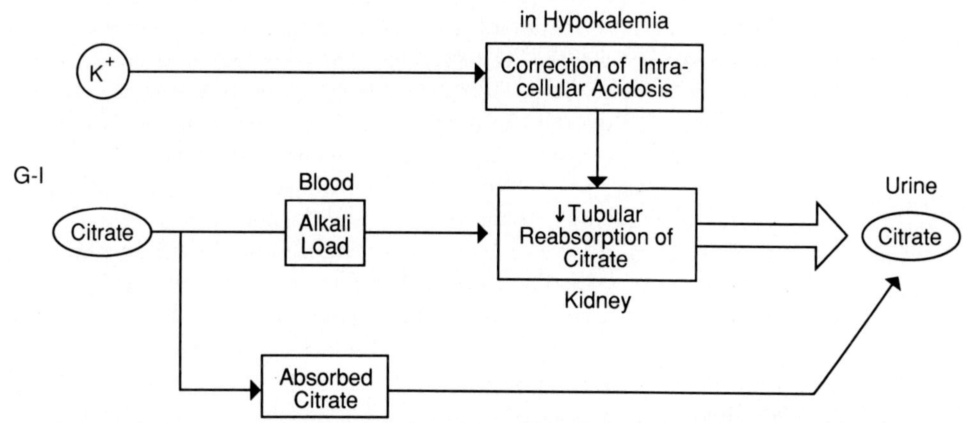

FIGURE 6–3. Scheme for the citraturic action of potassium citrate.

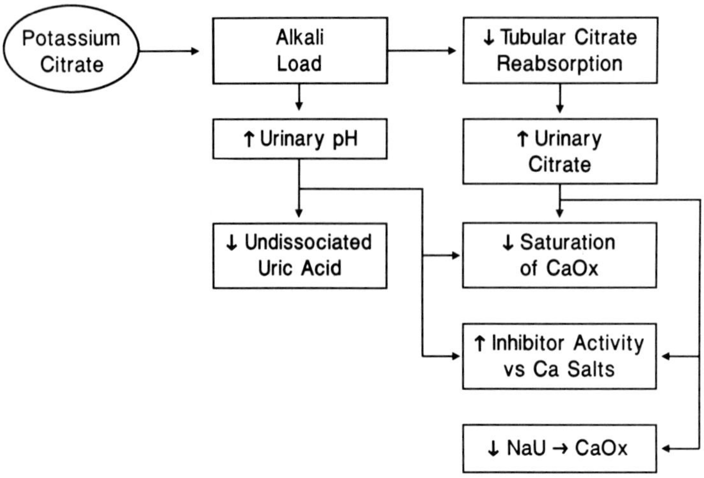

FIGURE 6–4. Physicochemical action of potassium citrate.

by mechanisms previously described. Moreover, the rise in urinary pH contributes to the retardation of the crystallization of calcium salts and inhibits uric acid crystallization. At a higher pH, more phosphate and citrate ions become dissociated, augmenting the complexation of calcium. The resulting reduction in ionized calcium concentration lowers the urinary saturation of stone-forming calcium salts. The further dissociation of citrate, pyrophosphate, and certain macromolecules may accentuate their inhibitor activity against crystallization of calcium salts. Finally, the rise in urinary pH increases the dissociation of uric acid, reducing the concentration of undissociated uric acid and the propensity for uric acid lithiasis (see Chapter 7).[9]

Thus, potassium citrate therapy has the capacity for reducing the propensity for the crystallization of calcium salts. During long-term treatment with potassium citrate, a sustained reduction in the urinary saturation of calcium oxalate has been shown.[1] Moreover, the inhibitor activity measured in whole urine (formation product ratio or limit of metastability of calcium oxalate; see Chapter 2) significantly increases during potassium citrate treatment.[1, 34]

Treatment of Hypocitraturic Calcium Nephrolithiasis

Renal Tubular Acidosis (Distal).[26] Potassium citrate therapy is capable of correcting both metabolic acidosis and hypokalemia. Moreover, it may restore normal urinary citrate, although large doses (up to 120 mEq/day) may be required in severe acidotic states. Urinary calcium typically declines with the correction of acidosis. The overall rise in urinary pH is generally below 7.5 during treatment unless there is a complication by a urinary tract infection.

Thus, potassium citrate treatment produces a sustained decline in the urinary saturation of calcium oxalate (from reduction in urinary calcium and in citrate complexation of calcium). The urinary saturation of calcium phosphate does not increase because the rise in phosphate dissociation is relatively small (owing to a modest rise in pH) and is adequately compensated for by a decline in ionic calcium concentration. Moreover, inhibitor activity against the crystallization of calcium oxalate and calcium phosphate is augmented because of the direct action of citrate.

If there is substantial renal sodium leak, alkali might be provided as a mixed sodium-potassium salt. However, renal sodium wasting is not prominent in most patients with renal tubular acidosis who present with stones. Potassium citrate is contraindicated in patients with moderate-to-severe renal disease (endogenous creatinine clearance of <40 ml/min). If it were to be used in those with moderate renal disease, it should be begun at a lower dose and the serum potassium concentration should be carefully monitored.

CHRONIC DIARRHEAL SYNDROME.[1, 34] In patients with mild-to-moderate severity of intestinal fluid loss in whom hypocitraturia is not severe (urinary citrate being in the range of 100 to 320 mg/day), potassium citrate (40 to 60 mEq in three to four divided doses in a liquid form) is generally effective in restoring normal urinary citrate and pH. Urinary calcium generally remains low. In those with severe hypocitraturia (with urinary citrate <100 mg/day), even excessive doses of potassium citrate (up to 120 mEq/day) may be ineffective in restoring normal urinary citrate.

It is recommended that a liquid preparation of potassium citrate be used rather than a slow-release tablet preparation in these states, because some of these patients may have intestinal adhesions and may be more prone to obstruction from a tablet preparation. Furthermore, a slow-release medication may be poorly absorbed owing to rapid intestinal transit.

A frequent dose schedule (three or four times a day is advisable) for the liquid preparation because of the relatively short duration of biologic action. In other hypocitraturic conditions, the solid slow-release preparation is preferable or is better tolerated. A less frequent dose schedule (twice a day) is acceptable for the solid preparation because of its slow-release characteristic.

Other drugs may be necessary for the treatment of additional disturbances. If hypomagnesiuria is present, magnesium citrate, 10 mEq two to four times a day, may raise urinary magnesium, as well as increase urinary citrate and pH, without substantially aggravating diarrhea. When hyperoxaluria coexists, dietary oxalate restriction is critical (see Chapter 12). In patients in whom hyperoxaluria and hypocalciuria exist, calcium citrate might be useful. This drug might lower renal excretion of oxalate by binding it in the intestinal tract, raise urinary citrate, correct malabsorption of calcium, and avert potential development of bone disease (see Chapter 4). A high fluid intake is critical.

THIAZIDE-INDUCED HYPOCITRATURIA.[10] Hypokalemia resulting from thiazide may cause hypocitraturia, probably by producing intracellular acidosis, and may thereby attenuate the beneficial hypocalciuric effect of therapy on renal stone formation.

It has been suggested that potassium citrate may be less effective than potassium chloride in correcting the thiazide-induced hypokalemia, because of the poor reabsorbability of citrate from the renal tubules. However, severe chloride depletion is uncommon in patients with thiazide-induced hypocitraturia. Thus, potassium citrate has been shown to be equally effective as potassium chloride in correcting thiazide-induced hypokalemia.[36] Moreover, the addition of potassium citrate to thiazide therapy raises urinary pH and citrate. Potassium citrate has been shown to inhibit stone formation in patients who continue to form stones while taking thiazide alone.

It is recommended that potassium citrate (15 to 20 mEq twice a day) be given to all patients being treated with thiazide for hypercalciuric nephrolithiasis (see Chapter 3).

Idiopathic Hypocitraturic Calcium Nephrolithiasis.[37] This entity, idiopathic hypocitraturic calcium oxalate nephrolithiasis, includes hypocitraturia occurring alone with calcium stones and hypocitraturia occurring in conjunction with absorptive and renal hypercalciurias and hyperuricosuric calcium oxalate nephrolithiasis. Stones formed are predominantly composed of calcium oxalate.

Potassium citrate treatment (15 to 30 mEq twice a day) has been shown to produce a sustained increase in urinary citrate excretion. Urinary pH can be maintained at 6.5 to 7.0. Along with these changes, the urinary saturation of calcium oxalate declines to normal limits.

Update on Long-Term Clinical Trial with Potassium Citrate at Dallas[41]

Since 1979, 91 patients with nephrolithiasis have been followed on long-term potassium citrate therapy (for a mean duration of 3.5 years) at Dallas. The group comprised 16 patients with distal renal tubular acidosis, 15 with chronic diarrheal syndrome, 10 with thiazide-induced hypocitraturia, and 50 with idiopathic hypocitraturia.

In all four conditions, potassium citrate therapy has been shown to be clinically efficacious. The group stone formation rate decreased from 1.83 to 6.04 per patient-year before treatment to 0.15 to 0.60 per patient-year during treatment. The individual stone formation rate fell in 90 to 100 per cent of patients during treatment, and remission was encountered in 67.7 to 82.6 per cent of patients. Moreover, none of the patients required surgery for newly formed stones, and approximately 40 per cent of patients with preexisting stones exhibited reduced stone mass after treatment.

Uniqueness of Potassium Citrate Compared with Other Alkali

The action of potassium citrate differs from that of potassium bicarbonate and sodium citrate (Table 6–3).

Compared with potassium bicarbonate, potassium citrate exerts a more prolonged rise in urinary citrate and pH. Moreover, the increment in urinary citrate is more pronounced with potassium citrate, probably owing to the renal excretion of a small amount of absorbed citrate that has escaped oxidation.

Under a constant metabolic dietary regimen, potassium citrate has been shown to reduce calcium excretion, probably by augmenting the renal tubular reabsorption of calcium.[8, 31] Sodium citrate does not. This unique hypocalciuric action of potassium alkali has now been confirmed using bicarbonate salts of

TABLE 6–3. COMPARISON OF POTASSIUM CITRATE ACTION WITH THAT OF SODIUM CITRATE

	Potassium Citrate	Sodium Citrate
Urinary calcium	↓	=, ↑
Urinary citrate	↑ ↑ ↑	↑ ↑
Inhibitor activity, calcium oxalate	↑	=, ↓
Prevention of calcium stones	+ + +	+ +
Urinary pH	↑	↑
Prevention of uric acid stones	+ +	+ +

potassium and sodium in normal subjects (J. Lemann, personal communication). In patients with hypokalemia, potassium citrate causes a more pronounced rise in citrate excretion than does sodium citrate.[43] Urinary sodium remains unaltered with potassium citrate therapy but increases during sodium citrate therapy.

Physicochemically, the urinary saturation of calcium oxalate declines more prominently with potassium citrate than with sodium citrate.[8, 43] The limit of metastability of calcium oxalate (a measure of inhibitor activity; see Chapter 2) may increase during potassium citrate therapy, but not so during sodium citrate therapy. During the latter therapy, the inhibitor action of citrate may be blunted by the sodium urate–induced crystallization of calcium oxalate. These effects probably account for the complication of calcium stones encountered during the sodium alkali therapy of patients with uric acid lithiasis.[9] However, potassium and sodium citrates cause an equivalent rise in urinary pH and an equivalent reduction in the urinary content of undissociated uric acid. Thus, both alkali should be useful in the prevention of uric acid lithiasis.

Side Effects of Potassium Citrate Therapy

Two formulations of potassium citrate approved by the FDA in the United States for use in the prevention of hypocitraturic calcium nephrolithiasis are a tablet preparation (wax matrix) and a liquid preparation.[34]

Minor gastrointestinal complaints are more common with the liquid preparation than with the tablet preparation.[34] Gastric erosions and intestinal obstruction are possible with the tablet preparation (though not reported). Most patients find the tablet preparation to be more convenient to take than the liquid preparation. However, the low citrate content (5 mEq per tablet) requires multitablet dosing. The tablet preparation confers a more prolonged half-life because of its slow release from the wax matrix. Thus, it could be given on a twice-daily schedule, whereas a more frequent dosing is desired for the liquid preparation. These properties provide the rationale for the use of the liquid preparation in chronic diarrheal states and of the tablet preparation in other hypocitraturic states, as recommended previously.

Extrarenal Effects of Potassium Citrate Therapy

In patients with distal renal tubular acidosis, potassium citrate reduces calcium excretion and augments intestinal calcium absorption without a change in the serum 1,25-$(OH)_2$vitamin D level.[31] In so doing, this alkali therapy corrects negative calcium balance and produces a more positive calcium balance. Thus, this treatment not only prevents stone formation but also averts an extrarenal manifestation (bone disease) of distal renal tubular acidosis.

In stone-forming patients without acidosis, a short-term treatment with potassium alkali induces a more positive calcium balance, principally by reducing calcium excretion. However, during long-term treatment, urinary calcium returns to the pretreatment range. The effect on intestinal calcium absorption has not been rigorously examined. During long-term treatment of stone-forming women with potassium citrate at Dallas, the density of the radial shaft showed a small but significant increase.[41] The results suggest that potassium citrate may have bone-sparing action even in the absence of apparent metabolic acidosis.

Overall Comments on Potassium Citrate Therapy

From the preceding discussion, it is clear that potassium citrate not only inhibits new stone formation but also reduces the requirement for surgical removal of stones (by conventional and newer methods), causes dissolution of existing stones in some, and corrects nonrenal manifestations of the disease process (e.g., bone disease of distal renal tubular acidosis). This treatment therefore fulfills the criteria for optimal medical treatment, to be discussed in Chapter 12.

Potassium citrate is also useful in the management of hyperuricosuric calcium nephrolithiasis and uric acid lithiasis. These topics are reviewed in Chapters 5 and 7, respectively.

REFERENCES

1. Pak CYC: Citrate and renal calculi. Miner Electrolyte Metab 13:257–266, 1987.
2. Atsmon A, De Vries A, Frank M: Uric Acid Lithiasis. New York, Elsevier Publishing Company, 1963.
3. Albright F, Consolazio WV, Coombs FS, et al: Metabolic studies and therapy in a case of nephrocalcinosis with rickets and dwarfism. Bull Johns Hopkins Hosp 66:7, 1940.
4. Kissin B, Locks MO: Urinary citrates in calcium urolithiasis. Proc Soc Exp Biol Med 46:216–218, 1941.
5. Howard JE: Clinical and laboratory research concerning mechanisms of formation and control of calculous disease of the kidney. J Urol 72:999, 1954.
6. Gregory JG, Park KY, Wilt R, Feigl A: Therapy for enteric hyperoxaluria: A comparison of calcium supplementation and urinary alkalinization. *In* Smith LH, Robertson WG, Finlayson B (eds.): Urolithiasis: Clinical and Basic Research. New York, Plenum Press, 1981, pp 179–190.
7. Butz M, Dulce HJ: Enhancement of urinary citrate in oxalate stone formers by the intake of alkaline salts. *In* Smith L, Robertson WG, Finlayson B (eds.): Urolithiasis: Clinical and Basic Research. New York, Plenum Press, 1981, pp 881–884.
8. Sakhaee K, Nicar M, Hill K, Pak CYC: Contrasting effects of potassium citrate and sodium citrate therapies on urinary chemistries and crystallization of stone-forming salts. Kidney Int 24:348–352, 1983.
9. Pak CYC, Sakhaee K, Fuller C: Successful management of uric acid nephrolithiasis with potassium citrate. Kidney Int 30:422–428, 1986.
10. Pak CYC, Peterson R, Sakhaee K, et al: Correction of hypocitraturia and prevention of stone formation by combined thiazide and potassium citrate therapy in thiazide-unresponsive hypercalciuric nephrolithiasis. Am J Med 79:284–288, 1985.
11. Pak CYC, Sakhaee K, Fuller CJ: Physiological and physicochemical prevention of calcium-stone formation by potassium citrate therapy. Trans Assoc Am Physicians 96:294–305, 1983.
12. Meyer JL, Smith LH: Growth of calcium oxalate crystals. Invest Urol 13:36–39, 1975.
13. Pak CYC, Nicar MJ, Northcutt C: The definition of the mechanism of hypercalciuria is necessary for the treatment of recurrent stone formers. Contrib Nephrol 33:136–151, 1982.
14. Nicar MJ, Hill K, Pak CYC: Inhibition by citrate of spontaneous precipitation of calcium oxalate, *in vitro*. J Bone Min Res 2:215–220, 1987.
15. Kok DJ, Papapoulos SE, Bijvoet OLM: Excessive crystal agglomeration with low citrate excretion in recurrent stone-formers. Lancet 10:1056–1058, 1986.
16. Pak CYC, Peterson R: Successful treatment of hyperuricosuric calcium oxalate nephrolithiasis with potassium citrate. Arch Intern Med 146:863–868, 1986.
17. Sherman CC, Mendel LB, Smith AH: The metabolism of orally administered citric acid. J Biol Chem 113:265–271, 1936.
18. Simpson DP: Citrate excretion: A window on renal metabolism. Am J Physiol 244 (Renal Fluid Electrolyte Physiol 13):F223–F234, 1983.
19. Jenkins AD, Dousa TP, Smith LH: Transport of citrate across renal brush border membrane: Effects of dietary acid and alkali loading. Am J Physiol 249 (Renal Fluid Electrolyte Physiol 18):F590–F595, 1985.
20. Fourman P, Robinson JR: Diminished urinary excretion of citrate during deficiencies of potassium in man. Lancet 2:656–657, 1953.
21. Baruch SB, Burich RL, Eun CK, King VF: Renal metabolism of citrate. Med Clin North Am 59:569–582, 1975.

22. Down WH, Sacharin RN, Shasseaud LF, et al: Renal and bone uptake of tartaric acid in rats: Comparison of L(+) and DL− forms. Toxicology 8:333–346, 1977.
23. Shorr E, Bernheim AR, Taussky H: The relation of urinary citric acid excretion to the menstrual cycle and the steroidal reproductive hormones. Science 95:606–607, 1942.
24. Costello LC, Stacey R, Franklin R: Parathyroid hormone effects on soft tissue citrate levels. Horm Metab Res 2:242–245, 1970.
25. Nicar MJ, Skurla C, Sakhaee K, Pak CYC: Low urinary citrate excretion in nephrolithiasis. Urology 21:8–14, 1983.
26. Preminger GM, Sakhaee K, Skurla C, Pak CYC: Prevention of recurrent calcium stone formation with potassium citrate therapy in patients with distal renal tubular acidosis. J Urol 134:20–23, 1985.
27. Pak CYC: Role of medical prevention. J Urol 141:798–801, 1989.
28. Breslau NA, Brinkley L, Hill KD, Pak CYC: Relationship role of animal protein–rich diet to kidney stone formation and calcium metabolism. J Clin Endocrinol Metab 66:140–146, 1988.
29. Sakhaee K, Nigam S, Snell P, et al: Assessment of the pathogenetic role of physical exercise in renal stone formation. J Clin Endocrinol Metab 65:974–979, 1987.
30. Morris RC Jr: Relation of stone formation to renal tubular acidosis. Presented at the VIth International Symposium on Urolithiasis, July 24–28, 1988, Vancouver, Canada.
31. Preminger GM, Sakhaee K, Pak CYC: Hypercalciuria and altered intestinal calcium absorption occurring independently of vitamin D in distal renal tubular acidosis. Metabolism 36:176–179, 1987.
32. Parfitt AM: Acetazolamide and sodium bicarbonate induced nephrocalcinosis and nephrolithiasis. Arch Intern Med 124:736–740, 1969.
33. Rudman D, Dedonis JL, Fountain MT, et al: Hypocitraturia in patients with gastrointestinal malabsorption. N Engl J Med 303:657–661, 1980.
34. Pak CYC, Fuller C, Sakhaee K, et al: Long term treatment of calcium nephrolithiasis with potassium citrate. J Urol 134:11–19, 1985.
35. Yendt ER, Cohanim M: Prevention of calcium stones with thiazide. Kidney Int 13:397–409, 1978.
36. Nicar MJ, Peterson R, Pak CYC: Use of potassium citrate as potassium supplement during thiazide therapy of calcium nephrolithiasis. J Urol 131:430–433, 1984.
37. Pak CYC, Fuller C: Idiopathic hypocitraturic calcium oxalate nephrolithiasis successfully treated with potassium citrate. Ann Intern Med 104:33–37, 1986.
38. Cowley DM, McWhinney BC, Brown JM, Chalmers AH: Chemical factors important to calcium nephrolithiasis: Evidence for impaired hydroxycarboxylic acid absorption causing hyperoxaluria. Clin Chem 33:243–247, 1987.
39. Pak CYC, Britton F, Peterson R, et al: Ambulatory evaluation of nephrolithiasis: Classification, clinical presentation and diagnostic criteria. Am J Med 69:19–30, 1980.
40. Sakhaee K, Pak CYC: Contrasting effects of various potassium salts on acid-base status, urinary citrate excretion, and renal citrate clearance. Abstract from Urologic Research: VIth International Symposium on Urolithiasis and Related Clinical Research, July 24–29, 1988, Vancouver, British Columbia, p 197.
41. Pak CYC: Physicochemical action and extrarenal manifestations of alkali therapy. Presented at Urologic Research: VIth International Meeting on Urolithiasis and Related Clinical Research, Vancouver, British Columbia, July 24–29, 1988.
42. Pak CYC: Medical management of nephrolithiasis: Update 1987. J Urol 140:461–467, 1988.
43. Preminger GM, Sakhaee K, Pak CYC: Alkali action on the urinary crystallization of calcium salts: Contrasting responses to sodium citrate and potassium citrate. J Urol 139:240–242, 1988.

7

Uric Acid Nephrolithiasis

Charles Y.C. Pak

Uric acid lithiasis has long been associated with gout, hyperuricemia, and radiolucency.[1] It is clear, however, that uric acid stones could form in the absence of gouty arthritis, hyperuricemia, or hyperuricosuria[2] and that gouty patients could develop radiopaque calcium-containing stones as well.[1, 3]

It is the object of this chapter to resolve the apparent paradox described above. In this chapter, uric acid lithiasis and associated disorders are distinguished pathogenetically and clinically from hyperuricosuric calcium nephrolithiasis, a separate entity described in Chapter 5.

HISTORICAL ASPECTS OF URIC ACID LITHIASIS

Gout has plagued humans since antiquity.[4] In 1500 BC, Papyrus described a drug that was probably colchicine. In the fifth century BC, Hippocrates provided the first description of gout. In 1683, Sydenham, who himself suffered from renal stones, gave an authoritative clinical description of gout, clearly differentiating it from other joint diseases.[5] In 1776, Scheele isolated uric acid from a renal stone formed by a gouty patient.[6] Wollaston in 1797 and Pearson in 1798 found uric acid in the gouty tophi.[7, 8] In 1863, Garrod suggested that the uric acid concentration in blood is increased in gouty patients.[9]

It is possible that some of the treatment measures recommended by early physicians for stone prevention may have been directed at uric acid lithiasis. The value of high fluid intake was noted by a famous lithotomist, Cyprian, who alleged that he "never had operated on a beer drinker."[4] The utility of alkali was suggested by Whytt in the mid-nineteenth century when he ascribed to a solution made from egg and oyster shells and to lime water an "extraordinary power to dissolve stones."[10] In 1826, Cooper prescribed "liquor potassae," potassium carbonate, and sodium carbonate.[11]

In Western industrialized countries today, uric acid lithiasis accounts for 5 to 8 per cent of stones. Its occurrence rate is higher in Israel and in the Middle East, probably reflective of ethnic origin and hot climate.

PHYSICOCHEMICAL BASIS FOR URIC ACID STONE FORMATION

The principal determinant of uric acid crystallization is the supersaturation of urine with respect to undissociated uric acid.[12, 13] There is no known inhibitor of uric acid crystallization. Thus, precipitation of uric acid is the general rule if the urinary environment is supersaturated with respect to undissociated uric acid.

The urinary saturation of undissociated uric acid is dictated by two factors: pH and uric acid concentration. The first proton of uric acid has a pKa of approximately 5.5.[12] Thus, the solubility of uric acid is pH dependent (Fig. 7–1). Below a pH of 5.5, most of the uric acid remains in an undissociated form, possessing low aqueous solubility of less than 100 mg/liter. This unusually acid environment is therefore conducive to uric acid crystallization. With a rise in pH, more uric acid becomes dissociated into an anionic form, approaching 100 per cent at pH 6.5. In such an environment, the propensity for uric acid crystallization is low because of a low amount of undissociated uric acid. However, the dissociated urate reacts with various cations in urine to form urate salts of varying solubility.[13] Monosodium urate has a much lower solubility than monopotassium urate.[13] Thus, the solubility of dissociated urate depends on the type and concentration of cation present in urine. Increasing sodium concentration decreases soluble urate concentration. An equivalent concentration of potassium produces a much higher concentration of soluble urate.

The second factor that dictates the amount of undissociated uric acid is the urinary uric acid concentration. The urinary saturation of uric acid may be represented by the ratio of total uric acid concentration and the solubility of uric acid at the specified pH. Since the solubility of uric acid is constant at the same

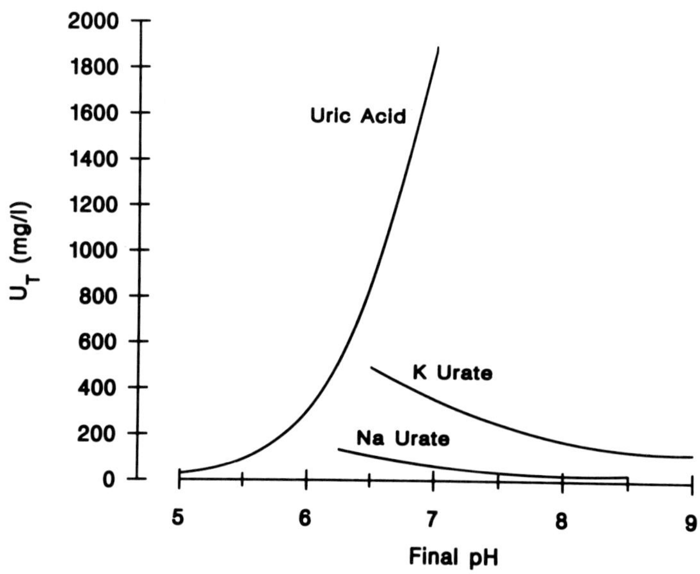

FIGURE 7–1. Uric acid solubility and transformation to urate salts.

pH, the urinary saturation of uric acid increases proportionately with the rise in total uric acid concentration.

The interplay of pH and the solubility characteristics of uric acid and urate salts determines whether uric acid stones or calcium stones are likely to form (Fig. 7–2). At a low urinary pH (<5.5), the low solubility of uric acid leaves an excess of undissociated uric acid to cause uric acid lithiasis. At a higher pH (>5.5), monosodium urate is particularly prone to form because of its low solubility and the normally plentiful sodium content of urine.[13] Potassium urate is much less likely to develop, owing to its higher solubility and to the lower potassium content in urine. This background probably accounts for the implication of monosodium urate, but not monopotassium urate, in calcium oxalate nephrolithiasis via heterogeneous nucleation or binding of inhibitors[14] (see Chapter 5). Moreover, the varying physicochemical properties of urates might explain the complication of calcium stone formation during sodium alkali therapy, but not during potassium alkali treatment, in patients with uric acid lithiasis (to be described).[2]

There is some evidence that uric acid may lead to calcium stones by a similar mechanism as described for monosodium urate. Although uric acid is less efficient than monosodium urate in inducing heterogeneous nucleation of calcium oxalate (on a weight basis),[15, 16] its crystalline dimensions are more compatible with epitaxy.[17] Moreover, uric acid has been shown to remove naturally occurring urinary macromolecular inhibitors, thereby attenuating their activity.[18]

The findings just described could explain the association of calcium stones

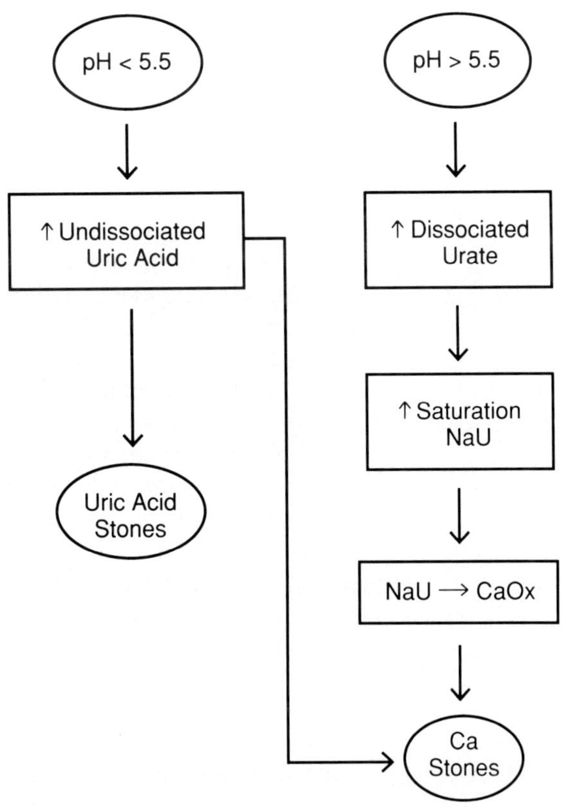

FIGURE 7–2. Interplay of pH and uric acid in the formation of uric acid or calcium stones.

with primary gout and the formation of calcium stones in some patients with uric acid nephrolithiasis.

PATHOPHYSIOLOGY OF URIC ACID LITHIASIS

As might be appreciated from the preceding section, three physiologic or environmental derangements are critical in uric acid lithiasis: undue acidity of urine, hyperuricosuria, and concentrated urine. These urinary risk factors, singly or in combination, are displayed by patients with uric acid lithiasis. Low urinary pH is encountered in patients with primary gout, chronic diarrheal states, and dehydration. Hyperuricosuria is found in primary gout and urate overproduction due to inborn errors of metabolism. Concentrated urine is an invariant feature of chronic diarrheal states and dehydration.

Primary Gout[19, 20]

Primary gout is an inherited disorder transmitted probably as an autosomal dominant trait with variable penetrance. It has a familial incidence of 10 to 30 per cent; men are more commonly affected.

Uric acid lithiasis is encountered in approximately 20 per cent of patients with primary gout. There is a strong correlation between the degree of uric acid excretion and the frequency of uric acid lithiasis.[21] Thus, uric acid stones are formed by more than 50 per cent of patients with marked hyperuricosuria ($>$1000 mg/day).

Three metabolic defects have been disclosed in primary gout: undue acidity of urine, overproduction of uric acid, and impaired renal uric acid clearance.[19, 20] The exact cause for the urate overproduction in primary gout is unknown. It is not due to a specific enzymatic disturbance in the uric acid biosynthetic pathway. In primary gout, the newly synthesized purines from a glycine backbone are not incorporated into tissue nucleic acids and instead are "shunted" toward the synthesis of uric acid.[22] The operation of this shunt pathway has been implicated in urate overproduction.

The metabolic basis for the unusually acid urine is also unclear. Available data indicate that patients with primary gout excrete relatively less ammonium and relatively more titratable acid than do normal subjects.[23] Twenty-four-hour urinary pH is invariably less than 5.5, and there is loss of normal alkaline tide.

Finally, there is an unexplained relative diminution of urate clearance. Thus, the ratio of urate and insulin clearance tends to be lower in gouty subjects than in normal subjects at any specified serum urate concentration.[20] However, hyperuricosuria is generally encountered in gouty patients who are overproducers of uric acid, because of high serum uric acid levels and filtered load of urate.

The defects that have just been described are expressed variably in individual patients with primary gout. Most patients, but not all, express urate overproduction with hyperuricemia and hyperuricosuria. The acidification defect is present in the entire population of patients with primary gout, adding risk for stone formation in overproducers and representing the sole risk in normouricosuric patients. Diminished renal citrate clearance in varying degrees is probably characteristic of all patients with primary gout.

Primary gout may therefore be classified on the basis of varying expression of the three metabolic defects (Table 7–1). *Urate overproduction,* the most common form, is characterized by hyperuricemia, hyperuricosuria, and undue acidity of urine. *Diminished urate clearance* denotes hyperuricemia, normouricosuria, and unusually acid urine. *Latent gout* refers to undue acidity without hyperuricemia or hyperuricosuria. Clinically, gouty arthritis would be manifest in the first two groups with hyperuricemia, but not in the third group without elevation in serum uric acid concentration. All three groups would be at risk for uric acid lithiasis resulting from undue acidity of urine. The overproducers would be particularly at risk because of coexistent hyperuricosuria.

Latent gout may represent an early phase of classic primary gout without articular manifestations.[2] The only biochemical manifestation is undue acidity of urine, and the only clinical problem is uric acid lithiasis often complicated by calcium stones. Some patients give a family history of hyperuricemia or gouty arthritis. No obvious cause for unusually low pH is apparent, since patients deny a history of diarrheal syndrome, strenuous physical exercise, dehydration, or consumption of a diet rich in animal proteins. Although these patients all have renal stones, the stone composition may vary—uric acid alone, calcium oxalate–calcium phosphate alone, or a combination of the two. It is presumed that urate-induced or uric acid–induced crystallization of calcium salts accounts for calcium nephrolithiasis.

It is implied by the use of the term latent gout that these patients suffer from an underlying disturbance of primary gout and that they may ultimately develop the full manifestation of primary gout with hyperuricemia and gouty arthritis. This conclusion is supported by the observation that stone symptoms may precede articular symptoms in 40 per cent of patients with (primary) gouty arthritis, occasionally by more than 10 years.[21] Latent gout resembles the disorder previously termed idiopathic uric acid lithiasis.[1]

The diagnostic criteria of latent gout are far from secure, and the suggestion that it is a forme fruste of primary gout remains largely a speculation. Gastrointestinal and dietary causes of excessive urinary acidification have not been rigorously excluded. However, the designation of latent gout as a special entity is justified because of its positive clinical response to potassium alkali therapy.

The term gouty diathesis was previously used to suggest latent gout. It is now preferred that *gouty diathesis* denote the overall entity of nephrolithiasis associated with primary gout. Thus, it describes uric acid stone formation in all three forms of primary gout, from fully manifest overproducers with gouty arthritis to gouty patients with diminished urate clearance to those with latent gout but without gouty arthritis.

Other Clinical Disorders of Uric Acid Lithiasis

Other causes of uric acid nephrolithiasis (Table 7–2) include certain inborn errors of uric acid metabolism, secondary causes of urate overproduction (exces-

TABLE 7–1. VARIANTS OF GOUTY DIATHESIS (URIC ACID LITHIASIS IN PRIMARY GOUT)

	Urate Overproduction	Diminished Urate Clearance	Latent Gout
Serum uric acid	↑	↑	N
Urinary uric acid	↑	N	N
Urinary pH	↓	↓	↓
Uric acid stones	+	+	+
Gouty arthritis	+	+	0

N = normal; ↑ = increase; ↓ = decrease; + = present; 0 = absent.

TABLE 7–2. CLASSIFICATION OF URIC ACID LITHIASIS

1. Gouty diathesis (primary gout)
   a. Urate overproduction
   b. Diminished urate clearance
   c. Latent gout
2. Urate overproduction with normal urinary pH
   a. Inborn errors of metabolism
   b. Tissue catabolism (myeloproliferative disorders)
3. Passage of concentrated and unduly acid urine
   a. Chronic diarrheal states
   b. Physical exercise
4. Hyperuricosuria without hyperuricemia
   a. Uricosuric drugs
   b. Overindulgence in animal proteins

sive tissue catabolism), chronic diarrheal states, and use of uricosuric agents. Three well-studied but rare enzymatic disorders of uric acid metabolism are hypoxanthineguanine phosphoribosyl transferase deficiency (Lesch-Nyhan syndrome), phosphoribosyl pyrophosphate synthetase overactivity, and glucose-6-phosphatase deficiency (Type I glycogen storage disease).[19, 20] Affected patients have extreme rates of uric acid overproduction. In myeloproliferative disorders, leukemia, neoplasia, or hemolytic anemia, hyperuricemia and hyperuricosuria occur because of an increased rate of nucleoprotein turnover. As many as 50 per cent of patients with myeloproliferative disorders may form uric acid stones, which often is the initial clinical manifestation.

Several gastrointestinal disorders have been associated with a high incidence of uric acid lithiasis.[24] The three most common conditions are ulcerative colitis, regional enteritis, and the presence of ileostomy. The pathogenesis of uric acid stones in these disorders is related to variable degrees of dehydration and bicarbonate loss, resulting in an unusually acid and concentrated urine. The excretion rate of uric acid is usually normal in these patients. A strenuous physical exercise may also cause uric acid lithiasis by reducing urine output (from sweat loss) and lowering pH (from lactic acidosis).[25]

Certain drugs, such as probenecid and high doses of salicylates, as well as radiographic contrast agents, may produce an acute uricosuria.[26] The chronic administration of these agents, however, results in a new steady state, in which the rate of uric acid excretion should be no greater than the pretreatment rate. Thus, the risk of stone formation occurs early and not late, except in the setting of urate overproduction. An overindulgence in animal proteins[27] may cause hyperuricosuria without causing frank hyperuricemia. Despite the associated high acid ash load (from sulfur-containing amino acids), urinary pH typically exceeds 5.5. Thus, calcium nephrolithiasis rather than uric acid lithiasis is characteristically encountered (see Chapter 5).

DIAGNOSIS OF URIC ACID LITHIASIS

Gouty Diathesis

Gouty diathesis, which describes uric acid lithiasis arising from the whole spectrum of primary gout, is characterized by the persistent passage of unusually acid urine (pH <5.5 in 24-hour specimens).[2] The cause for low urinary pH cannot be readily ascertained. Some patients may give a positive personal or family history of gouty arthritis. There is male preponderance. Some patients may present with hyperuricemia, hyperuricosuria, or hypertriglyceridemia. Stones formed may be uric acid alone, calcium oxalate-phosphate alone, or a mixture of the two. Some patients may form uric acid on one occasion and calcium stones on another occasion. Uric acid stones are radiolucent.

TREATMENT OF URIC ACID LITHIASIS

Gouty Diathesis

Potassium citrate is the treatment of choice for this condition.[2] In the study at Dallas, this treatment at a dosage of 30 to 60 mEq/day in divided doses significantly increased urinary pH from the low mean value of 5.30 to above 6.19, but less than 7. There is no need to overtreat to a pH exceeding 7. Owing to the resulting enhanced dissociation of uric acid, the amount of undissociated uric acid significantly decreased to the range encountered in normal subjects without stones (<150 mg/day). Thus, potassium citrate therapy markedly increased the solubility of uric acid, preventing uric acid stone formation. Moreover, potassium citrate therapy inhibited the complication of calcium stones by reducing the urinary saturation of calcium oxalate and retarding the crystallization of calcium oxalate.

It is acknowledged that sodium alkali therapy would be equally effective as potassium citrate in preventing uric acid nephrolithiasis, since it possesses a similar capacity for raising urinary pH and thus lowering the amount of undissociated uric acid. However, the complication of calcium stones, albeit rare, may occur with sodium alkali therapy.[2] Sodium alkali has been shown to be devoid of hypocalciuric action and to promote urate-induced crystallization of calcium oxalate.[28]

In patients who present with hyperuricemia or marked hyperuricosuria (>800 mg/day), allopurinol (e.g., 300 mg/day) is recommended.

REFERENCES

1. Gutman AB, Yu TF: Uric acid nephrolithiasis. Am J Med 45:756–779, 1968.
2. Pak CYC, Sakhaee K, Fuller C: Successful management of uric acid nephrolithiasis with potassium citrate. Kidney Int 30:422–428, 1986.
3. Prien EL, Prien E Jr: Composition and structure of urinary stone. Am J Med 45:654–672, 1968.
4. Atsmon A, deVries A, Frank M: Historical notes. *In* Uric Acid Lithiasis. New York, Elsevier Publishing Company, 1963, pp 1–13.
5. Sydenham T: The Works of Thomas Sydenham, translated by RG Latham. London, Sydenham Society, 1850, Vol II, p 214.
6. Scheele KW: Examen chemicum calculi urinarii. Opuscula 2:73, 1776.
7. Wollaston WH: On gouty and urinary concretions. Philos Trans Lond 87:386, 1797.
8. Pearson G: Experiments and observations, tending to show the composition and properties of urinary concretions. Philos Trans Lond 88:15, 1798.
9. Garrod AB: The Nature and Treatment of Gout and Rheumatic Gout. London, Walton and Maberly, 1863, p 251.
10. Comrie JD: History of Scottish Medicine. Vol I. 2nd ed. London, Balliere, Tindall & Cox, 1932.
11. Wesson MB: Renal calculi: Etiology and prophylaxis. J Urol 34:289, 1935.
12. Finlayson B, Smith A: Stability of first dissociable proton of uric acid. J Chem Eng Data 19:94–97, 1974.
13. Pak CYC, Waters O, Arnold L, et al: Mechanism for calcium nephrolithiasis among patients

with hyperuricosuria: Supersaturation of urine with respect to monosodium urate. J Clin Invest 59:426–431, 1977.
14. Pak CYC, Holt K, Zerwekh JE: Attenuation by monosodium urate of the inhibitory effect of glycosaminoglycans on calcium oxalate nucleation. Invest Urol 17:138–140, 1979.
15. Pak CYC, Arnold LH: Heterogeneous nucleation of calcium oxalate by seeds of monosodium urate. Proc Soc Exp Biol Med 149:930–932, 1975.
16. Coe FL, Lawton RL, Goldstein RB, Tembe V: Sodium urate accelerates precipitation of calcium oxalate in vitro. Proc Soc Exp Biol Med 149:926–929, 1975.
17. Lonsdale K: Epitaxy as a growth factor in urinary calculi and gallstones. Nature 217:56–58, 1968.
18. Zerwekh JE, Holt K, Pak CYC: Natural urinary macromolecular inhibitors: Attenuation of inhibitory activity by urate salts. Kidney Int 23:838–841, 1983.
19. Seegmiller JE, Laster L, Howell RR: Biochemistry of uric acid and its relation to gout. N Engl J Med 268:712–716, 764–773, 821–827, 1963.
20. Wyngaarden JB, Kelley WN: Gout. *In* Stanbury JB, Wyngaarden JB, Fredrickson DS (eds.): The Metabolic Basis of Inherited Disease. New York, McGraw-Hill Book Company, 1972, pp 889–968.
21. Yu TF: Uric acid nephrolithiasis. *In* Kelley WN, Weiner IM (eds.): Handbook of Experimental Pharmacology. Vol 51. New York, Springer-Verlag, 1978, pp 397–442.
22. Benedict JD, Roche M, Yu TF, et al: Incorporation of glycine nitrogen into uric acid in normal and gouty man. Metabolism 1:3–12, 1952.
23. Gutman AB, Yu TF: A three-component system for regulation of renal excretion of uric acid in man. Trans Assoc Am Physicians 74:353–363, 1961.
24. Deren JJ, Porush JG, Levitt MF, Khilnani MT: Nephrolithiasis as a complication of ulcerative colitis and regional enteritis. Ann Intern Med 56:843, 1962.
25. Sakhaee K, Nigam S, Snell P, et al: Assessment of the pathogenetic role of physical exercise in renal stone formation. J Clin Endocrinol Metab 65:974–979, 1987.
26. Steele TH: Control of uric acid excretion. Med Intelligence 284:1193–1196, 1971.
27. Breslau NA, Brinkley L, Hill KD, Pak CYC: Relationship role of animal protein–rich diet to kidney stone formation and calcium metabolism. J Clin Endocrinol Metab 66:140–146, 1988.
28. Sakhaee K, Nicar M, Hill K, Pak CYC: Contrasting effect of potassium citrate and sodium citrate therapies on urinary chemistries and crystallization of stone-forming salt. Kidney Int 24:348–352, 1983.

8

Infection Stones

Malachy J. Gleeson
Donald P. Griffith

Archeologic studies have shown that urolithiasis has affected humans for thousands of years. Excavations at El Amrah, Egypt, by G. Elliot Smith in 1901 uncovered one case of vesical calculi and two cases of renal calculi, which dated to 4800 BC.[1] In 1905, Shattock reported that an Egyptian renal calculus dated 4200 BC was composed of calcium carbonate, calcium phosphate, and calcium oxalate.[2] A struvite and calcium oxalate renal calculus has been found in a late Bronze Age burial mound in Hungary.[3] In the early part of the nineteenth century, the mineral $MgNH_4PO_4 \cdot 6H_2O$ was identified in bat guano by Ulex, a Swedish geologist. He named it "struvite" in honor of his mentor, Baron H.C.G. von Struve, a Russian diplomat and naturalist (1772–1851).[4] Struvite calculi are composed of magnesium ammonium phosphate ($MgNH_4PO_4 \cdot 6H_2O$) and carbonate apatite ($Ca_{10}(PO_4)_6 \cdot CO_3$). Throughout the world literature, struvite calculi have also been referred to as "infection," "infection-induced," "urease," "phosphatic," and "triple-phosphate" stones. The term "triple-phosphate" arises from early chemical analyses of stones wherein three cations (Ca^{2+}, Mg^{2+}, and NH_4^{+}) were found in association with one anion (PO_4^{3-}).[5] Although progress has been made in understanding the underlying pathogenesis of this disease, the treatment is frustrating because of high stone recurrence rates and persistent urinary tract infections. However, many advances in both the medical and the surgical treatment options have been made in the past two decades, which, it is hoped, will lead to further advances and a cure for these patients.

STOICHIOMETRY

Salt crystallization occurs when the solubility product of the component solutes is exceeded. Human urine is replete with the substrates calcium, phosphate, magnesium, and urea. Only in the presence of accelerated ureolysis are urine alkalinity and the concentrations of ammonia, bicarbonate, and carbonate sufficient for crystallization of struvite and carbonate apatite. Struvite will not crystallize if the urine pH is less than 7.19 or if urine alkalinity is not also associated with ammoniuria.[6, 7] Urease-producing bacteria cause hydrolysis of urea:

$$NH_2-CO-NH_2+H_2O \overset{urease}{\rightleftharpoons} 2NH_3 + CO_2$$

Further hydrolysis converts ammonia to ammonium:

$$NH_3+H_2O \rightleftharpoons NH_4^{+}+OH^{-}$$

The carbonate found in carbonate apatite crystals arises from further hydrolysis:

$$CO_2+H_2O \rightleftharpoons H_2CO_3 \rightleftharpoons H^{+}+HCO_3^{-} \rightleftharpoons 2H^{+}+CO_3^{2-}$$

$$pK(NH_3)=9.03;\ pK\ (HCO_3^{-})=6.33;\ pK(CO_3^{2-})=10.1$$

The biochemical changes occurring during a 2-hour period after the addition of urease to normal human urine are shown in Figure 8–1.[8] The factor determining the relative proportions of struvite and carbonate apatite in infection stones is uncertain, but it may be partially due to differing rates of crystallization for either salt with varying urinary pH.

The cause and effect relationship between urea-splitting bacteria and infection stones is now well recognized. In 387 BC, Hippocrates documented renal calculi that were associated with putrefaction and loin abscess.[5] In 1817, Marcet noted the association of putrefaction, ammoniacal urine, alkalinity, and the production of phosphate calculi.[5]

In 1901, Brown proposed the theory that the splitting of urea by bacteria resulted in ammoniacal urine, alkalinity, and stone formation.[9] Urine cultures in

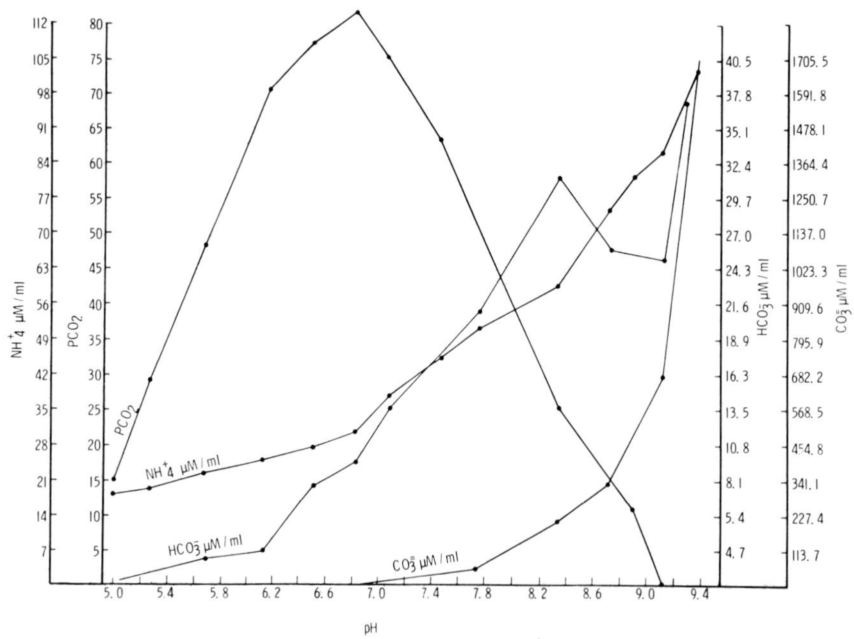

FIGURE 8–1. The biochemical changes occurring during a 2-hour period following the addition of urease to normal human urine. (From Griffith DP: Struvite stones. Kidney Int 13:374, 1978; with permission.)

his six patients revealed *Proteus vulgaris* and staphylococci. *Proteus vulgaris* was also grown from the center of one calculus. In all cases, stone analysis showed "phosphates and carbonates of calcium and magnesium." Hagar and Magath suggested in 1925 that a bacterial protein called urease was responsible for the hydrolysis of urea.[10] In the following year, Sumner reported that he had isolated a new protein from the jack bean *Canavalia ensiformis*.[11] This enzyme (urease) hydrolyzed urea and was in the form of colorless octahedra crystals. He was later awarded the Nobel prize for this work in isolating the first known enzyme.

BACTERIOLOGY

Urinary infection with urease-synthesizing bacteria is an essential prerequisite for infection stone formation. The most widely used method of identifying urease-producing bacteria was described by Christensen in 1946.[12] This technique identifies color changes in urea agar that are caused by the pH change as urea is hydrolyzed. Recently, the "spot test" has been developed for more rapid detection of bacterial urease activity.[13] The most commonly encountered urease-producing bacteria are gram-negative organisms, as shown in Table 8–1. Silverman and Stamey reported that 87 percent of their 46 infection-induced calculi were caused by *Proteus mirabilis* infections.[14] This varies considerably from reports in the first half of this century, when staphylococcal species were the most common causative organisms.[15] Recently, *Ureaplasma urealyticum* has been cited as a causative organism, the detection of which requires specialized culturing techniques.[16] Its calculogenic activity has also been demonstrated in vitro.[17]

Glycosaminoglycans (GAGs) are highly charged macromolecules that are

TABLE 8–1. ORGANISMS THAT MAY PRODUCE UREASE

Organisms	Usually (> 90% of Isolates)	Occasionally (5–30% of Isolates)
Bacteria		
Gram-negative	*Proteus rettgeri* *Proteus vulgaris* *Proteus mirabilis* *Proteus morgani* *Providencia stuartii* *Hemophilus influenzae* *Bordetella pertussis* *Bacteroides corrodens* *Yersinia enterocolitica* *Brucella* spp. *Flavobacterium* spp.	*Klebsiella pneumoniae* *Klebsiella oxytoca* *Serratia marcescens* *Hemophilus parainfluenzae* *Bordetella bronchiseptica* *Aeromonas hydrophila* *Pseudomonas aeruginosa* *Pasteurella* spp.
Gram-positive	*Staphylococcus aureus* *Micrococcus varions* *Corynebacterium ulcerans* *Corynebacterium renale* *Corynebacterium ovis* *Corynebacterium hofmannii*	*Staphylococcus epidermidis* *Bacillus* spp. *Corynebacterium murium* *Corynebacterium equi* *Peptococcus asaccharolyticus* *Clostridium tetani* *Mycobacterium rhodochrous group*
Mycoplasma	T-strain *Mycoplasma* *Ureaplasma urealyticum*	
Yeasts	*Cryptococcus* *Rhodotorula* *Sporobolmyces* *Candida humicola* *Trichosporon cutaneum*	

present in normal urine. Normal bladder mucosa is covered by a layer of GAGs, which acts as a defense against bacterial adherence and infection.[18] Using the rabbit model, Parsons and colleagues showed that ammonium interfered with the GAGs layer and thus increased the ability of bacteria to adhere to the bladder mucosal surface. The mechanism of action is thought to be that ammonium combines with the sulfate group of the GAGs and thus impairs its hydrophilic activity.[19] Recently, it has been demonstrated that the removal of the GAGs layer from rat bladders increases the adherence of struvite and calcium phosphate crystals five to six times compared with that of intact rat bladders.[20]

These studies seem to confirm Griffith's theory of intrarenal struvite calculogenesis (Fig. 8–2).[5] He proposed that the end products of ureolysis in urinary tract infections damage the urothelial GAGs layer and facilitate bacterial adherence, with resultant encrustation. However, the exact role of matrix in the pathogenesis of infection stones is unclear. Boyce and associates showed that the bulk of matrix is made up of a low molecular weight mucoprotein that they called matrix substance A.[21] Matrix stones are characterized by the presence of poorly mineralized, gelatinous, organic stone material in kidneys with advanced parenchymal damage. Nickel and coworkers have studied the ultrastructure of infection stones and have demonstrated bacterial cells growing as microcolonies together with bacterial biofilms within extensive fibrous organic matrices.[22] The biofilm, or glycocalyx, is thought to be secreted by the bacteria themselves and has also been described in relation to infected prostheses, such as cardiac pacemakers, peritoneal dialysis catheters, and hip joints. Its action may be that it protects the bacteria from the appropriate antibiotic therapy.

Thus, the source of some of the matrix may be the bacteria themselves. Khan and colleagues have also demonstrated that urinary macromolecules are absorbed onto crystal surfaces, which may explain a further passive mechanism of matrix formation.[23]

CLINICAL MANIFESTATIONS

Struvite calculi account for between 7 and 31 percent of all renal tract calculi in the Western world.[24] Although calcium oxalate calculi have been reported to be the most common type in the United States, Sarmina and associates have recently reported that struvite-carbonate apatite calculi were the most common type in black patients in Ohio.[25]

Women are more commonly affected than men, in a ratio of 2:1, presumably because of their increased susceptibility to urinary tract infections.[26] Comarr and associates have reported that 8 per cent of patients with spinal cord injury will develop infection stones.[27] The incidence is highest in complete and upper motor neuron lesions.[28] Infection stones are prone to occur in patients with neurogenic bladders, urinary diversions, indwelling Foley catheters, and lower tract voiding dysfunction with abnormal cystometry.[29] Correcting the cystometric abnormalities should eliminate the risk of calculus formation. The correlation between vesicoureteral reflux and the formation of staghorn calculi remains controversial.[30, 31]

The clinical presentation is variable but may include pyrexia, loin pain, dysuria, frequency, and hematuria. Acute pyelonephritis and hydronephrosis may progress to form acute pyonephrosis and renal or perirenal abscesses. Occasionally, xanthogranulomatous pyelonephritis may occur and is characterized by the replacement of renal parenchyma with granulomatous tissue containing

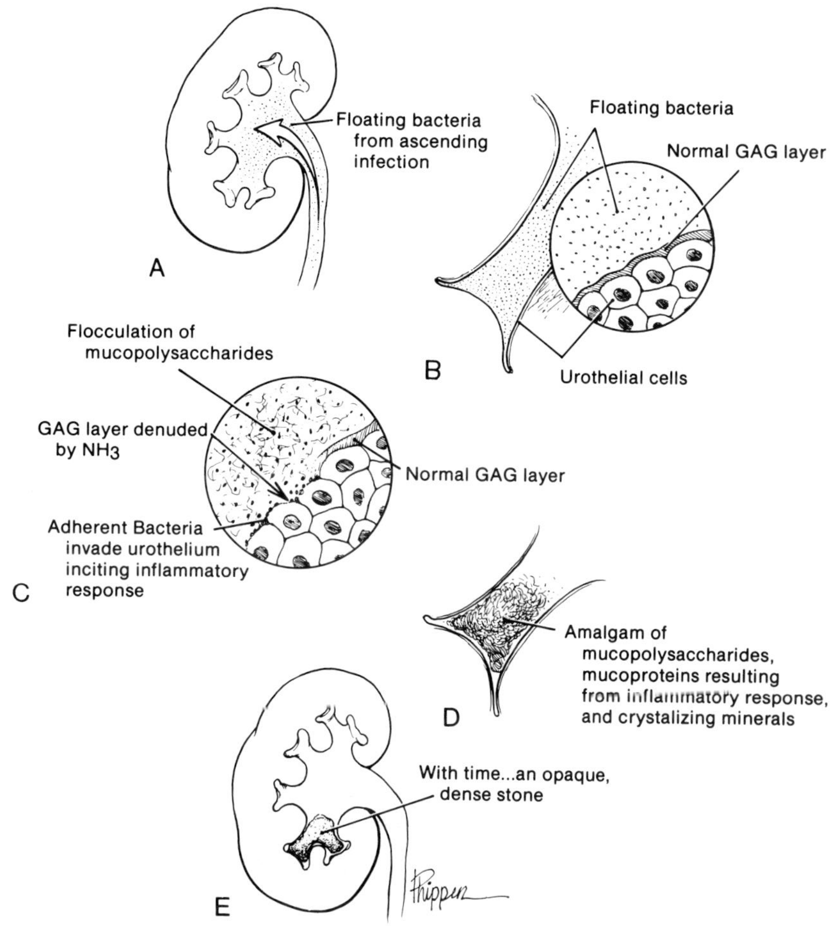

FIGURE 8–2. Glycosaminoglycans and struvite calculogenesis. *A*, Renal infection originates from bacteriuria introduced into the lower urinary tract and ascending to the kidney. *B*, A glycosaminoglycan (GAG) layer normally protects urothelium from bacterial adherence. *C*, End products of urealysis damage the urothelial GAG layer and thereby facilitate (1) bacterial adherence to cells and (2) tissue invasion by bacteria. Urealysis-induced hyperosmolality probably contributes to flocculation of organic compounds. Tissue inflammation brought on by local irritation (mostly ammonia) and bacterial invasion increase the quantity of these organic compounds. *D*, Matrix concretions composed of poorly soluble organic compounds, struvite and carbonate apatite crystals, inflammatory cells, and bacteria form rapidly into immature stone. *E*, With time, the immature stone becomes progressively mineralized owing to continued urealysis by bacteria trapped within the concretion, and the concretion matures into a dense, hard stone.

macrophages. Up to 25 percent of cases may be completely asymptomatic and detected during investigations for unrelated problems.[32] Radiographically, infection stones are usually branched and may grow rapidly to form a cast of the renal collecting system, the so-called staghorn calculus. Approximately 75 percent of staghorn calculi are composed of struvite, carbonate apatite, and matrix, with the remaining 25 percent being composed of calcium oxalate, calcium phosphate, or cystine. Most infection stones are radiopaque, but poorly mineralized matrix stones are faintly radiopaque or radiolucent. Most infection stones are renal in site but occasionally may be found in the bladder, especially in patients with long-term indwelling catheters. Ureteric calculi are rare.

In patients with dual pathology, such as renal calculi and chronic prostatitis, it may be helpful to try to localize the site of infection accurately by taking consecutive selective ureteral urine samples.[33] In the era of open surgical therapy, culture of pelvic urine aspirate and stone washings, both before and after crushing, aided bacterial documentation and treatment.[34]

TREATMENT

The nonoperative management of staghorn calculi was reported in 1976 to result in a 28 percent mortality during 20 years of follow-up, with all survivors having persistent pain and urinary tract infections.[35] Vargas and associates later confirmed the rarity of the "silent staghorn calculus," with only 1 (4.5 percent) of 22 staghorn calculi managed nonsurgically remaining asymptomatic and 17 (77 percent) resulting in significant complications, 2 of which resulted in death after a follow-up period of 1 to 6 years.[36] Treatment rests with initial surgery to render the patient stone free, followed by the various medical options to prevent recurrent infection and subsequent stone formation.

Open Surgical Procedures

Surgical removal has been the cornerstone of treatment for infection stones. The first successful nephrectomy for stone disease was performed by Gustav Simon in 1871.[4] Attempted stone removal from pyonephritic kidneys in both 1872 and 1874 resulted in the deaths of patients. In 1879, Heinecke performed the first successful pyelolithotomy, which was followed in the following year by a successful nephrolithotomy performed by Morris.[5, 37] The open operative alternatives include nephrectomy, partial nephrectomy, pyelolithotomy, extended pyelolithotomy (Gil-Vernet),[38] dismembered pyelolithotomy (Ohshima and coworkers),[39] anatrophic nephrolithotomy (Smith and Boyce),[40] radial nephrolithotomy (Wickham and associates),[41] and bench surgery with autotransplantation (Turini and colleagues).[42] These techniques may be used in conjunction with operative nephroscopy, coagulum pyelolithotomy and hypothermia, and either regional or systemic inosine to minimize ischemic renal damage. In Britain in 1976, intravenous, intraarterial, or intraperitoneal administration of inosine was shown to preserve renal function for up to 1 hour of warm ischemia, enabling safer transparenchymal surgery to be performed.[43] Its use has not been approved by the Food and Drug Administration (FDA) in the United States. Controversy still exists over which procedures cause the least parenchymal damage. Fitzpatrick and colleagues studied renal function and morphology in dogs 48 hours after surgery, using creatinine, inulin, and para-aminohippurate (PAH) clearance.[44] They found no functional or parenchymal loss after the extended sinus approach (Gil-Vernet), 30 percent functional loss and significant parenchymal loss with the anatrophic intersegmental approach, and 50 percent functional loss with considerable parenchymal loss after bivalving the kidney. The following year, Stage and Lewis reported no difference in postoperative functional loss between pyelolithotomy and anatrophic nephrolithotomy in patients who had differential quantitative renal scans using 99-technetium diethylene triaminepentaacetic acid

(DTPA) or ^{131}I Hippuran.[45] It must be remembered that all procedures performed may improve renal function by relieving intrarenal obstruction. The overall residual stone rate after open surgery is approximately 15 percent, with a 30 per cent stone recurrence rate over 6 years and a 40 percent risk of recurrent urinary tract infection.[46]

Percutaneous Nephrolithotomy (PCNL) Monotherapy

Percutaneous nephrolithotomy (PCNL) was described in 1976 by Fernstrom and Johannson.[47] Initially, only small calculi were removed percutaneously, but with the aid of electrohydraulic and ultrasonic lithotripsy, the procedure has been extended to include staghorn calculi.[48, 49] PCNL has been used to treat staghorn calculi with stone-free results in 60 to 90 percent of kidneys (Table 8–2). Adams and associates defined staghorn calculi as those conforming to the branched configuration of two or more calyces but did not refer to stone burden.[50] With an average hospitalization time of 18 days, they rendered 7 of 11 kidneys (63 percent) stone free with PCNL monotherapy. Kerlan and associates reported 90 percent (18 of 20 kidneys) stone free with calculi that "filled the caliceal collecting structures and renal pelvis."[48]

Using a definition of staghorn as a branched calculus more than 5 cm in its greatest diameter, Young and colleagues rendered 68 percent of their 25 kidneys stone free.[51] Sixteen of these calculi were less than 8 cm, and 9 were 8 cm or more in the longest dimension.

Snyder and Smith, using a more standard definition of staghorn as a calculus that fills the renal pelvis and at least two major calyces, rendered 64 of 75 kidneys (85 percent) stone free with PCNL and had an average hospitalization time of 13.3 days.[52] This series was updated more recently by Lee and associates, who reported a similar stone-free rate (85 percent) at time of discharge on 124 kidneys treated.[53] After 6 months of follow-up, the spontaneous passage of residual calculi less than 5 mm increased the stone-free rate to 92 percent.

Eisenberger and colleagues reported their updated series on 151 partial or complete staghorn calculi in 1987.[54] All calculi filled the renal pelvis and at least two branched calyces, and the mean follow-up was 18 months. The stone-free rate at the time of discharge was 69 percent on 42 kidneys treated with PCNL monotherapy, and this increased to 77 percent on follow-up, with a 4 percent stone recurrence rate. However, all long-term results were based on only 89 kidneys (59 percent) of their total series with adequate follow-up. Our own experience has resulted in 18 of 30 kidneys (60 percent) being stone free 3 months postoperatively (MJ Gleeson and DP Griffith, unpublished data).

Experimental studies in dogs have shown that PCNL does not cause any loss of renal function, but these studies referred to a single percutaneous tract

TABLE 8–2. STAGHORN CALCULI TREATED WITH PCNL MONOTHERAPY

Author	Kidneys	Treatments per Kidney	Stone Free at 3 mo (%)
Adams et al[50]	11	2.2	63
Kerlan et al[48]	20	1.8	90
Young et al[51]	25	2.9	68
Snyder and Smith[52]	75	1.24	85
Lee et al[53]	124	1.3	85
Eisenberger et al[54]	42	1.3	69
Gleeson and Griffith (unpublished data)	30	1.43	60

rather than multiple tracts, as are commonly required for removal of staghorn calculi.[55] Comparative studies of PCNL and anatrophic nephrolithotomy show that PCNL is less expensive, is associated with a smaller need for blood transfusion, requires a shorter hospital stay, and allows a more rapid return to work.[52, 56, 57]

Extracorporeal Shock Wave Lithotripsy (ESWL) Monotherapy

Extracorporeal shock wave lithotripsy (ESWL) was introduced clinically in 1980.[58] Its use initially was for small pelvic calculi, but considerable success has resulted in its application to calculi in all parts of the collecting system.[59–61]

ESWL monotherapy has generally resulted in stone-free results ranging from 30 to 66 percent (Table 8–3). Eisenberger and colleagues treated 26 partial and 5 complete staghorn calculi with ESWL monotherapy.[54] Although only 6 (19 percent) kidneys were stone free at the time of discharge, 8 of 16 kidneys (50 percent) followed for 18 months became stone free. Rocco and associates reported that 53 of 84 kidneys (63 percent) were rendered stone free with the added use of in situ irrigation in 20 cases.[62]

A large series of 140 partial staghorn calculi (mean burden = 30 ± 10 mm) and 34 complete staghorn calculi (mean burden = 62 ± 16 mm) treated by Wirth and Frohmuller had a 54 percent stone-free rate at 3 months, which increased to 61 percent at 1 year.[63] However, the results were based on a follow-up rate of 65 percent. Although the total number of procedures per kidney was not reported, 29 percent of partial staghorn calculi and 48 percent of complete staghorn calculi required more than one treatment.

Harada and colleagues rendered 9 of 19 kidneys with complete staghorn calculi (45 percent) and 15 of 28 kidneys with partial staghorn calculi (54 percent) stone free, resulting in an overall stone-free rate of 51 percent.[64] Pode and associates have recently reported a 44 percent stone-free rate with 41 complete staghorn calculi.[65] Complete staghorn calculi were defined as filling the renal pelvis and at least two calyces.

As part of a multicenter prospective randomized study comparing ESWL monotherapy with PCNL-ESWL combination therapy, Sohn and coworkers have reported that 20 of 33 patients were treated with ESWL monotherapy and only 6 of these (30 percent) have become stone free.[66] This compares with 7 of 13 patients with staghorn calculi (54 percent) rendered stone free in the combination PCNL-ESWL group.

In our department, 12 of 18 kidneys (66 percent) have been rendered stone

TABLE 8–3. STAGHORN CALCULI TREATED WTH ESWL MONOTHERAPY

Author	Kidneys	Stone Free at 3 mo (%)
Eisenberger et al[54]	31	50*
Rocco et al[62]	84	63†
Wirth and Frohmuller[63]	174	54
Harada et al[64]	47	51
Sohn et al[66]	20	30
Pode et al[65]	41	44
Gleeson and Griffith (unpublished data)	18	66

*Stone-free rate after 18 months.
†Rocco EXL catheter used in 20 cases.

free with a mean number of treatments of 1.4 per kidney (MJ Gleeson and DP Griffith, unpublished data). Our criteria for this treatment selection included calculi that were less radiopaque than the adjacent ribs and absence of obstruction or hydronephrosis on the preoperative intravenous urogram.

PCNL-ESWL Combination Treatment

The large stone burden of staghorn calculi has resulted in many reports advocating combination PCNL and ESWL, with ESWL being used to treat residual stones after primary debulking with PCNL.[54, 67, 68]

Combination PCNL and ESWL has reportedly resulted in stone-free rates of between 23 and 92 percent (Table 8–4). Although only 23 percent of 78 kidneys with staghorn calculi treated with a combination of PCNL and ESWL by Eisenberger and coworkers were stone free at the time of discharge, this increased to 60 percent after 18 months.[54]

Kahnoski and colleagues treated 52 staghorn calculi, of which 36 had combination PCNL-ESWL therapy.[69] The stone-free outcome for combination therapy was 85 percent, with a mean hospital stay of 12.6 days. A recent update on this series from Indianapolis has reported that 92 percent of kidneys with partial staghorn calculi and 91 percent with complete staghorn calculi became stone free following three-stage procedures consisting of PCNL, ESWL, and flexible PCNL with lavage of residual debris.[70]

A particularly low stone-free rate with struvite staghorn calculi from the Mayo Clinic was attributed to a less aggressive effort at initial PCNL; these authors now favor an aggressive PCNL approach to staghorn calculi.[71] The "sandwich" technique of muliple procedures in a relatively short time was introduced by Streem and is now being used with good effect in Indianapolis.[70, 72] However, Schulze and coworkers treated 77 partial and complete staghorn calculi with combination therapy and had only a 58 percent stone-free rate at 3 months despite a mean hospital stay of 19 days.[68] Our treatment outcome, with 12 of 22 kidneys (55 percent) being stone free, is similar, with a much shorter hospital stay of 10.3 days (MJ Gleeson and DP Griffith, unpublished data).

Urinary Acidification

Alkaline urine, which occurs in patients with urease-producing urinary tract infections, is necessary for urine to become supersaturated with struvite and carbonate apatite. Urinary acidification should therefore be of benefit to increase

TABLE 8–4. STAGHORN CALCULI TREATED WITH PCNL-ESWL COMBINATION

AUTHOR	KIDNEYS	STONE FREE AT 3 MO (%)
Eisenberger et al[54]	78	60
Kahnoski et al[69]	36	85*
Segura et al[71]	16	23†
Lingeman[70]	313	91–92
Schulze et al[68]	87‡	58
Gleeson and Griffith (unpublished data)	22	55

*Includes cases treated with ESWL and PCNL monotherapy.
†Six months follow-up.
‡Seventy-seven calculi were partial or complete staghorns.

the solubility of struvite and carbonate apatite. Ascorbic acid has generally been unsuccessful in acidifying urine, although Murphy and associates have reported acidification with the concomitant use of antimicrobial therapy in the presence of urease-producing bacteria.[73–75] Vermeulen and coworkers used ammonium chloride to acidify urine in rats and thus promoted stone dissolution and prevented stone formation.[76] This work was successfully applied to the ranch mink industry, which was previously plagued by deaths secondary to struvite urolithiasis.[77] Although short-term acidification has been achieved in humans, no long-term studies have been documented.[78] It has been reported that urinary ammonium increases after 6 days, thus counteracting earlier acidification.[79]

In 1978, Froeling used ammonium nitrate (NH_4NO_3) to acidify urine in humans, but no long-term studies were performed.[80] In 1987, Pizzarelli and Peacock reported their experience of long-term urinary acidification with ammonium sulfate ($[NH_4]_2SO_4$).[81] All patients were treated for a minimum of 2 years. Acidic urine and persistent reduction in the relative saturation for calcium phosphate and the stone formation rate were reported. They also noted that metabolic acidosis did not occur in the presence of normal renal function. This is of vital importance, as urinary calcium and phosphate excretion increase during acute or chronic metabolic acidosis.[82, 83] Coe and colleagues have, however, shown that hypercalciuria can be prevented in chronic metabolic acidosis by a low-sodium diet.[84]

Lavage Chemolysis

In 1938, Hellstrom reported his experience with lavage chemolysis for struvite calculi.[15] He used varying combinations of urinary antiseptics and acidifying agents. Albright and coworkers reported their in vitro and in vivo experience with acidic solutions in 1939.[85] They selected citric acid as the most likely effective substance. The resulting equation demonstrates the reaction that occurs:

$$3Ca^{2+} + 2Cit^{2-} \rightarrow Ca_3Cit_2 \rightarrow Ca^{2+} + 2(CaCit)^-$$

The addition of citrate ions to a solution containing calcium ions results in a two-thirds reduction of free calcium ions. The tertiary citrate (Ca_3Cit_2) is produced only in an alkaline pH. At acidic pH levels, primary ($Ca[H_2Cit]_2$) and secondary (Ca H Cit) citrates are formed, and as these are weakly dissociated, there is a marked similar reduction in free calcium ions.

Albright noted that solutions with a pH of 4 caused little tissue irritation. In vitro dissolution of calcium phosphate–calcium carbonate calculi was achieved with a sodium citrate–citric acid mixture of 154 mm/liter (isotonic) at a pH of 4. In vivo experiments were performed in four patients, but successful dissolution occurred in only one patient who had multiple bladder calculi.

In 1943, Suby and Albright reported the development of solution G and their experience with its use.[86] In the original research, citric acid was found to cause marked irritation of rabbit bladder mucosa. This irritation was reduced by the addition of magnesium ions and was thus applied clinically. Solution G was used in six patients and in all cases resulted in partial or complete dissolution of calculi. The irrigant was introduced via nephrostomy tubes in four patients and via ureteral catheters in two patients.

Mulvaney later reported in vitro dissolution of struvite calculi with a similar solution (10 percent hemiacidrin).[87] He also dissolved one patient's renal pelvic calculi by irrigation with 7 percent hemiacidrin through a nephrostomy tube. The main differences between Suby's solution G and 10 per cent hemiacidrin are that Suby's G contains the carbonic acid in the sodium salt rather than in the calcium salt, and hemiacidrin contains additional magnesium salt and D-gluconic acid (Table 8–5). Both are equally effective in dissolving calculi in vitro.[33] The theoretical mode of action is that a calcium ion in the stone is exchanged for a magnesium ion to form the equivalent magnesium salt, which is soluble in the gluconocitrate solution.[34] The FDA later banned renal pelvic irrigation with renacidin (10 percent hemiacidrin) after four deaths were reported.[33] Nemoy and Stamey emphasized that the deaths may have been the result of urosepsis rather than the irrigant solution used.[34] They outlined the precautions necessary when using irrigant chemolysis, which include the following:

1. Maintenance of sterile urine.
2. Unobstructed inflow and outflow.
3. Intrapelvic pressure maintenance less than 30 cm H_2O.
4. Absence of extravasation.
5. Careful monitoring of magnesemia.

Hypermagnesemia is more likely to occur in patients with compromised renal function.[88] Using the aforementioned irrigation precautions, Nemoy and Stamey successfully dissolved renal calculi in eight patients.[34] There have also been reports of successful staghorn stone dissolution through percutaneous nephrostomy tubes and ileal conduit urinary diversions.[89, 90] Recently, outpatient irrigation with 10 percent hemiacidrin has been advocated under carefully controlled conditions. Palmer and coworkers treated 13 patients in this way, with stone dissolution in 78 percent and a 17 percent rehospitalization requirement.[91] Chemolytic irrigation may decrease the incidence of stone recurrences. Silverman and Stamey irrigated 46 kidneys after open surgery and dissolved calculi in 10 of 11 kidneys with residual stones.[14] After a mean follow-up of 7 years, the only stone recurrence was in the kidney with a residual calculus after irrigation.

Dietary Supplementation

In the 1930s, hypovitaminosis A was implicated as a cause of struvite calculogenesis, but dietary supplementation is of doubtful value.[92–94]

TABLE 8–5. COMPARISON OF SUBY'S SOLUTION G AND 10 PER CENT HEMIACIDRIN (RENACIDIN)

COMPONENT	SUBY'S G	10% HEMIACIDRIN
pH	~4.0	3.9
Citric acid	32.25 gram hydrous	28.2 grams
Magnesium oxide	3.84 grams anhydrous	0
Sodium carbonate	4.37 grams anhydrous	0
Calcium carbonate	0	1 gram
D-gluconic acid	0	5 grams
Magnesium hydrocarbonate	0	14.5 grams
Magnesium acid citrate	0	2.5 grams
H_2O	1000 ml	1000 ml

Substrate Depletion

In 1945, Shorr proposed the theoretical advantages of using estrogens and aluminum hydroxide gels in patients with struvite calculi.[95] Citric acid was known to enhance calcium solubility, but when administered orally, it was thought to be mostly metabolized, with little excreted in the urine. The use of estrogens was suggested, as they increase urinary citric acid and decrease calciuria. The mechanism of action of aluminum hydroxide gel is that it binds with phosphate in the gastrointestinal tract to form insoluble aluminum phosphate. Thus, less phosphate absorption occurs, and urinary phosphate is decreased. It was hoped that this combination, coupled with a low-phosphorus diet, would provide protection against calcium phosphate precipitation, even in alkaline urine. Five years later, Shorr and Carter reported their experience with low-calcium, low-phosphorus diets together with aluminum gels in 22 patients.[96] Patients were treated for 2 to 7 years. Basic aluminum carbonate gel (Basaljel) was found to be the most effective in reducing urinary phosphorus excretion. This combination treatment enhanced stone dissolution in 23 percent of stones and prevented stone growth in a further 67 percent. Lavengood and Marshall have reported their experience using the Shorr regimen.[97] They recorded dramatic urinary phosphorus reductions in their patients who were taking 40 ml of basic aluminum gel (Basaljel) after meals and at bedtime, 3 liters of fluid, and a daily diet containing less than 1300 mg of phosphorus. Stones recurred in 9.8 percent of infected patients on the regimen for 3.5 years compared with 30 percent of infected patients not on the regimen. Recurrences in uninfected patients were 0 percent in patients on the regimen compared with 22 percent of those not on the regimen. Dietary compliance was difficult, and many patients developed constipation. The use of aluminum hydroxide must be carefully monitored, as it may cause anorexia, malaise, lethargy, bone pain, and hypercalciuria.[98]

Antimicrobial Agents

The aim of antimicrobial therapy is to sterilize the urine and thus render it undersaturated with respect to struvite. In vitro and in vivo studies have shown that struvite calculi may partially dissolve in the presence of sterile urine.[99, 100] The long-term treatment with suppressive agents such as sulfa, methenamine, and nitrofurantoin has generally resulted in poor suppression of infection. Methenamine is particularly unsuitable, as rapid passage through the upper renal tracts does not allow time for the conversion of methenamine to formaldehyde.[101, 102] Long-term culture-specific antimicrobials may reduce the magnitude of the urinary infection even if sterility does not result. A reduction of the colony count from 10^7 to 10^5 per milliliter reduces the urease production by 99 per cent.[5] In many cases, sterile urine will not be achieved because bacteria are situated within the interstices of the stones and are thus not exposed to the antimicrobial therapy.[34] The majority of urease-producing infections are caused by *Proteus mirabilis*. More than 90 per cent of these are sensitive to penicillin or ampicillin at a concentration of 20 μg/ml of urine.[103] Standard doses of oral penicillin (500 mg every 6 hours) or ampicillin (250 mg every 6 hours) will produce urinary levels of 150 to 300 μg/ml of urine, respectively.[99] Feit and Fair maintained sterile urine in 16 of their 20 patients with long-term oral penicillin.

Tetracyclines are of similar value in patients with *Pseudomonas* or *Ureaplasma urealyticum* urinary tract infections.[16, 104] *Ureaplasma urealyticum* lacks a rigid cell wall and does not synthesize folic acid. It is therefore resistant to antimicrobials that act by interfering with cell wall formation or folic acid synthesis, such as penicillins, cephalosporins, and sulfonamides.[16] Recently, fluorquinolones, such as ciprofloxacin and norfloxacin, have been reported to offer improved coverage against *Pseudomonas*, but they are more expensive than tetracyclines.[105, 106] Griffith and associates reported their ability to maintain sterile urine in nine patients with struvite calculi who were treated with long-term culture-specific antibiotics, including ampicillin, cephalosporin, nalidixic acid, nitrofurantoin, penicillin, sulfisoxazole-trimethoprim, and tetracycline.[100] Five patients had significant stone dissolution, three had no change in stone size, and one had considerable stone growth requiring surgery. They also treated 17 patients (25 stone-containing kidneys) with recalcitrant urinary tract infections with intermittent or continuous antibiotics for up to 4 years. Stone growth occurred in 21 kidneys, slight stone dissolution occurred in 2 kidneys, and no change occurred in 2 kidneys. The long-term use of antibiotics, while possibly preventing stone growth and recurrence, will subject the patient to the risk of developing resistant organisms and the alteration of native bacterial flora. We recommend long-term, low-dose, culture-specific antimicrobials if surgery is contraindicated or if stone clearance is not complete at the time of surgery. The realistic expectation of such therapy is to inhibit stone growth rather than cause stone dissolution.

Preoperative and perioperative antibiotics are vital to prevent urosepsis and to sterilize the renal parenchyma and urine during open surgery, PCNL, ESWL, and lavage chemolysis.

Methylene Blue

In the 1950s, methylene blue was theorized to inhibit struvite stone growth and cause stone dissolution by the exchange of ions of dye for ions of crystal.[107–109] The questionable benefits of cationic dye therapy has resulted in its infrequent use in patients with urolithiasis.

Urease Inhibitors

In 1962, Kobashi and colleagues noted that hydroxamic acids had a molecular structure similar to that of urea (Fig. 8–3) and caused specific inhibition of urease.[110] The site of urease inhibition is the R-CONHOH group, which characterizes the hydroxamate family.[111] Fishbein and Carbone, while studying the actions of hydroxylurea, which is a substrate for urease, noted that acetohydroxamic acid (AHA) was a potent and irreversible inhibitor of urease.[112] Although the mechanism of action has not been established, the ability of urease inhibitors to bind urease is probably related to the nickel atoms in the enzyme.[113]

AHA is the most widely investigated urease inhibitor. In 1973, Griffith and Musher showed that urease was the principal cause of struvite calculogenesis and that AHA prevented the crystallization of struvite and carbonate apatite in vitro and in the rat model.[114] AHA is rapidly absorbed from the gastrointestinal tract when administered orally and reaches peak plasma levels after about 1 hour.[115] The two major metabolites in humans are acetamide and carbon dioxide. Carbon dioxide is eliminated in the breath and accounts for 20 to 45 per cent of the administered dose. Acetamide is excreted in the urine and accounts for 9 to

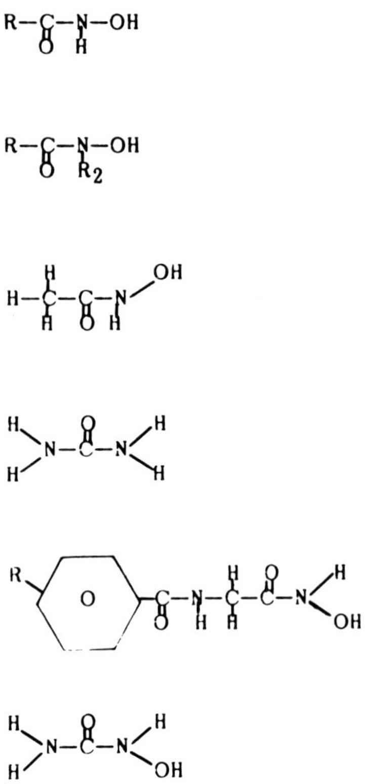

Primary hydroxamic acid

Secondary hydroxamic acid

Acetohydroxamic acid

Urea

Hippurohydroxamic acid

Hydroxyurea

FIGURE 8–3. Molecular structure of urea and examples of urease inhibitors.

14 per cent of the administered dose. The remaining dose (19 to 48 per cent) is excreted as intact AHA in the urine. AHA metabolism in the rat is different, as acetamide is the major metabolite.[116] There is a positive linear relationship between the AHA half-life and creatinine clearance in humans.[65] The half-life is 3.5 to 10 hours in normal subjects, 9 to 13 hours in patients with complicated liver cirrhosis, and 15.3 to 23.7 hours in patients with diminished renal function.[117, 118]

The effectiveness of AHA depends on its concentration in the urine. At the recommended dose of 250 mg every 8 hours, urinary concentrations of 15 to 30 mg/dl are usually achieved in patients with normal renal function.[119] When the serum creatinine level exceeds 2 mg/dl, full therapeutic concentrations of AHA are unachievable. Larger doses of AHA will then increase urinary acetamide and expose the patient to the potential risk of carcinogenesis. AHA has been shown to be teratogenic when administered to female beagle dogs.[120] Pups born to bitches receiving AHA had significantly lower birth weights, higher perinatal mortality, and congenital cardiac and coccygeal anomalies. Hernias also occurred more frequently. Early clinical trials using AHA in patients with staghorn calculi and urease-producing infections showed a reduction in ammoniuria and urine alkalinity in all patients.[46] This was confirmed in a later study from Britain, but Barr and Nuseibeh also reported increased urinary excretion of magnesium and phosphate in their 10 patients.[121] Table 8–6 outlines the results of three double-blind, placebo-controlled clinical trials of AHA in patients with infection-induced renal calculi. In each study, treatment with 250 to 1000 mg of AHA daily was compared with a mannitol placebo. Antimicrobial agents were given concurrently

TABLE 8–6. THE USE OF ACETOHYDROXAMIC ACID FOR INFECTION CALCULI*

	CORNELL[122]	VA[123]	BAYLOR
Patients	37	210	94
Patient population	N + SCI	SCI	N + SCI
Stone growth or recurrence			
Placebo (%)	58 (19 months)	60 (12 months) 60 (24 months)	46 (18 months)
AHA (%)	22 (16 months)	33 (12 months) 42 (24 months)	17 (18 months)
Side effects (%)	45	68	22

*Double-blind, placebo-controlled clinical trials from Cornell University College of Medicine,[122] Baylor College of Medicine (DP Griffith and colleagues, unpublished data), and the Veteran Administration (VA) Cooperative Study Group.[123]

N = normal; SCI = spinal cord injury.

in the Cornell study and were given intermittently in the Veterans Administration and Baylor studies. Sterile urine was not achieved in any group of patients. Similar symptomatic side effects occurred in all three trials. In the Cornell study, these included deep venous thrombosis, tremulousness, and intolerable headache. In the Veterans Administration cooperative study, they included palpitations, edema, nausea, vomiting, diarrhea, headache, tremulousness, loss of taste, hallucinations, rash, alopecia, abdominal pain, anemia, hematocrit decrease, and reticulocyte increase. In the Baylor study, 22 per cent of patients withdrew because of similar side effects. All side effects reversed upon cessation of AHA, and no attributable deaths were recorded.[119] We recommend that AHA be used palliatively in conjunction with antibiotic therapy in patients with infection-induced stones in whom surgical intervention is contraindicated, in the hope of retarding stone growth.

Many other urease inhibitors have been investigated less extensively. In 1981, Martelli and associates compared the effects of AHA and hydroxyurea in 41 patients.[124] They concluded that both drugs, when administered together with antimicrobial agents, facilitated urine sterilization, decreased urinary alkalinity and ammonia, and decreased the incidence of stone recurrence. AHA was the more effective and the less toxic drug. The mutagenic and antibacterial actions of hydroxamic acids are thought to be due to their interaction with cellular deoxyribonucleic acid (DNA).[125]

Propionohydroxamic acid, in combination with antimicrobial agents, reduces urinary ammonia and pH in humans with low dosage (60 mg/day).[126] Few side effects have been reported.

Benurestat [2-(para-chlorobenzamido) acetohydroxamic acid] potentiates the antibiotic inhibition of struvite stone formation and promotes stone dissolution in rats.[127] The theoretical explanation of this potentiation is that antibiotics are unable to act against bacteria that migrate intracellularly to avoid the high pH and ammonia level of the extracellular fluid. When *Proteus ureolysis* is inhibited by Benurestat, infecting *Proteus* organisms may be forced into the extracellular space, where they are accessible to antibiotics.

Biosuppressin (hydroxycarbamide), an antineoplastic agent, has been shown to decrease urinary ammonia and pH in in vitro studies.[128] Its use for this purpose has not been applied clinically because of its leukopenic action.

Nicotinohydroxamic acid prevents stone formation in rats with urinary tract infections, but only 1 percent of the total dose is excreted unchanged in the urine after 24 hours.[129]

Takebe and coworkers reported that struvite stone formation secondary to

Ureaplasma urealyticum infections in human urine was prevented in vitro by *N*-benzoylphosphotriamide, *N*-isopentenoylphosphotriamide, and caprylohydroxamic acid.[17] The mode of action is thought to be a decrease in the adenosine triphosphate (ATP) synthesis in the *Ureaplasma* cells, thus causing their death.

A new hydroxamic acid derivative of hippuric acid, meta-methoxyhippurohydroxamic acid (UCD 11), has been shown to inhibit urine alkalinization caused by *Proteus mirabilis* in vitro and in rats.[130] Although its urinary excretion is less than that of acetohydroxamic acid, its effective index is higher.

Flurofamide, a nonhydroxamate phosphotriamide, is 1000 times more potent than AHA and is effective in retarding stone formation in rats infected with *Proteus mirabilis*.[131] Its use in humans has not been reported.

The search for an ideal urease inhibitor continues. The ideal qualities are as follows:

1. Specific urease inhibition
2. Antibacterial action
3. Potentiation of antimicrobial drugs.

It should also achieve high urinary concentrations, which are nontoxic, nonteratogenic, and nonmutagenic.[132]

In conclusion, although the epidemiology and pathogenesis of infection stones are well documented, effective curative treatment remains problematic. Conservative treatment leads to progressive renal damage, and so treatment rests with attempted complete surgical clearance of the stones, followed by elimination of the urinary tract infection. Although the long-term effects of PCNL and ESWL are not well documented, a combination of PCNL and ESWL appears to offer the patient a less morbid surgical alternative than standard open surgery. Adjunctive medical therapy, such as culture-specific antibiotics, urease inhibitors, and urine acidification, is worthwhile to reduce the morbidity associated with persistent urinary tract infections and further stone recurrences.

REFERENCES

1. Wershub LP: *In* Urology: From Antiquity to the 20th Century. MO, Warren H. Green, 1970, pp 35–36.
2. Shattock SG: A prehistoric or predynastic Egyptian calculus. Trans Pathol Soc Lond 61:275–290, 1905.
3. Schneider HJ: Epidemiology of urolithiasis. *In* Schneider HJ (ed): Urolithiasis: Etiology and Diagnosis. Berlin, Springer-Verlag, 1985, pp 137–184.
4. Dana ES: *In* Descriptive Minerology. New York, John Wiley and Sons, 1920, p 806.
5. Griffith DP, Osborne CA: Infection (urease) stones. Miner Electrolyte Metab 13:278–285, 1987.
6. Elliot JS, Sharp RF, Lewis L: The solubility of struvite in urine. J Urol 81:366–368, 1959.
7. Pitts RF: Production and excretion of ammonia in relation to acid-base regulation. *In* Orloff J, Berlinger RW (eds): Renal Physiology. Washington, DC, American Physiological Society, 1973, p 455.
8. Griffith DP: Struvite stones. Kidney Int 13:372–382, 1978.
9. Brown TR: On the relation between the variety of microorganisms and the composition of stone in calculous pyelonephritis. JAMA 36:1395–1397, 1901.
10. Hagar BH, Magath TB: The etiology of incrusted cystitis with alkaline urine. JAMA 85:1352–1355, 1925.
11. Sumner JB: The isolation and crystallization of the enzyme urease. J Biol Chem 69:435–441, 1926.
12. Christensen WB: Urea decomposition as a means of differentiating proteus and paracolon cultures from each other and from salmonella and shigella types. J Bacteriol 52:461–466, 1946.
13. Qadri SMG, Zubairi S, Hawley HP, Ramirez EG: Simple spot test for rapid detection of urease activity. J Clin Microbiol 20:1198–1199, 1984.

14. Silverman DE, Stamey TA: Management of infection stones: The Stanford experience. Medicine 62:44–51, 1983.
15. Hellstrom J: The significance of staphylococci in the development and treatment of renal and ureteric stones. Br J Urol 10:348–378, 1938.
16. Hedelin H, Brorson JE, Grenabo L, Pettersson S: Ureaplasma urealyticum and upper urinary tract stones. Br J Urol 56:244–249, 1984.
17. Takebe S, Numata A, Kobashi K: Stone formation by Ureaplasma urealyticum in human urine and its prevention by urease inhibitors. J Clin Microbiol 20:869–873, 1984.
18. Parsons CL, Greenspan C, Moore SW, Mulholland SG: Role of surface mucin in primary antibacterial defense of bladder. Urology 9:48–52, 1977.
19. Parsons CL, Stauffer C, Mulholland SG, Griffith DP: The effect of ammonium on bacterial adherence to bladder transitional epithelium. J Urol 132:365–366, 1984.
20. Grenabo L, Hedelin H, Pettersson S: Adherence of urease-induced crystals to rat bladder epithelium. Urol Res 16:49–52, 1988.
21. Boyce WH, King JS Jr, Fielden ML: Total nondialyzable solids (TNDS) in human urine. XIII. Immunological detection of a component peculiar to renal calculous matrix and to urine of calculous patients. J Clin Invest 41:1180–1189, 1962.
22. Nickel JC, Eintage J, Costerton JW: Ultrastructural microbial ecology of infection-induced urinary stones. J Urol 133:622–627, 1985.
23. Khan SR, Finlayson B, Hackett RL: Stone matrix as proteins absorbed on crystal surfaces: A microscopic study. Scan Electron Microsc 1:379–381, 1983.
24. Peacock M, Robertson WC: The biochemical aetiology of renal lithiasis. *In* Wickham JEA (ed): Urinary Calculous Disease. Edinburgh, Churchill Livingstone, 1979, pp 69–95.
25. Sarmina I, Spirnak JP, Resnick MI: Urinary lithiasis in the black population: An epidemiological study and review of the literature. J Urol 138:14–17, 1987.
26. Resnick MI: Evaluation and management of infection stones. Urol Clin North Am 8:265–276, 1981.
27. Comarr AE, Kawaichi GK, Bors E: Renal calculosis in patients with traumatic cord lesions. J Urol 85:647–656, 1962.
28. Bors E: Neurogenic bladder. Urol Survey 7:177–250, 1957.
29. Koff SA, Lapides J: Altered bladder function in staghorn calculus disease. J Urol 117:577–580, 1977.
30. Amar AD, Hutch JA, Katz I: Coexistence of urinary calculi and vesicoureteral reflux. JAMA 206:2312–2313, 1968.
31. Lue TF, Macchia RJ, Pastore L, Waterhouse K: Vesicoureteral reflux and staghorn calculi. J Urol 127:247–248, 1982.
32. Rous SN, Turner WR: Retrospective study of 95 patients with staghorn calculus disease. J Urol 118:902–904, 1977.
33. Shortliffe LMD, Spigelmann SL: Infection stones: Evaluation and management. Urol Clin North Am 13:717–726, 1986.
34. Nemoy NJ, Stamey TA: Surgical, bacteriological, and biochemical management of "infection stones." JAMA 215:1470–1476, 1971.
35. Blandy JP, Singh M: The case for a more aggressive approach to staghorn stones. J Urol 115:505–506, 1976.
36. Vargas AD, Bragin SD, Mendez R: Staghorn calculus: Its clinical presentation, complications and management. J Urol 127:860–862, 1982.
37. Murphy LJT: *In* Part II by L.J.T. Murphy: The History of Urology. Springfield, IL, Charles C Thomas, 1972, pp 191–271.
38. Gil-Vernet J: New concepts in removing renal calculi. Urol Int 20:255–288, 1965.
39. Ohshima S, Ono Y, Mitsuya H: Dismembered pyelolithotomy: New rocedure for removal of renal calculi. Urology 17:22–25, 1981.
40. Smith MJV, Boyce WH: Anatrophic nephrotomy and plastic calycoraphy. J Urol 119:521–527, 1968.
41. Wickham JEA, Coe N, Ward JP: One hundred cases of nephrolithotomy under hypothermia. J Urol 112:702–705, 1974.
42. Turini D, Nicita G, Fiorelli C, et al: Staghorn renal stones: Value of bench surgery and autotransplantation. J Urol 118:905–907, 1977.
43. Fernando AR, Armstrong DMG, Griffiths JR, et al: Enhanced preservation of the ischemic kidney with inosine. Lancet 1:555–557, 1976.
44. Fitzpatrick JM, Sleight MW, Braack A, et al: Intrarenal access: Effects on renal function and morphology. Br J Urol 52:409–414, 1980.
45. Stage KH, Lewis S: Pre- and postoperative evaluation of renal function in patients with staghorn calculi utilizing quantitative renal scanning. Urology 17:29–32, 1981.
46. Griffith DP, Gibson JR, Clinton CW, Musher DM: Acetohydroxamic acid: Clinical studies of a urease inhibitor in patients with staghorn renal calculi. J Urol 119:9–15, 1978.
47. Fernstrom I, Johannson B: Percutaneous pyelolithotomy: A new extraction technique. Scand J Urol Nephrol 10:257–259, 1976.
48. Kerlan RK, Kahn RK, Laberge JM, et al: Percutaneous removal of renal staghorn calculi. AJR 145:797–801, 1985.

49. Clayman RV, Surya V, Miller RP, et al: Percutaneous nephrolithotomy: An approach to branched and staghorn renal calculi. JAMA 250:73–75, 1983.
50. Adams GW, Oke EJ, Dunnick NR, Carson CC: Percutaneous lithotripsy of staghorn calculi. AJR 145:1265–1269, 1985.
52. Snyder JA, Smith AD: Staghorn calculi: Percutaneous extraction versus anatrophic nephrolithotomy. J Urol 136:351–354, 1986.
53. Lee WJ, Smith AD, Cubelli V, Vernace FM: Percutaneous nephrolithotomy: Analysis of 500 consecutive cases. Urol Radiol 8:61–66, 1986.
54. Eisenberger F, Rassweiler J, Bub P, et al: Differentiated approach to staghorn calculi using extracorporeal shock-wave lithotripsy and percutaneous nephrolithotomy: An analysis of 151 consecutive cases. World J Urol 5:248–254, 1987.
55. Webb DR, Fitzpatrick JM: Percutaneous nephrolithotripsy: A functional and morphological study. J Urol 134:587–591, 1985.
56. Charig CR, Webb DR, Payne SR, Wickham JEA: Comparison of treatment of renal calculi by open surgery, percutaneous nephrolithotomy and extracorporeal shock-wave lithotripsy. Br Med J 292:879–882, 1986.
57. Lingeman JE, Saywell RM Jr, Woods JR, Newman DM: Cost analysis of extracorporeal shock-wave lithotripsy relative to other surgical and nonsurgical treatment alternatives for urolithiasis. Med Care 24:1151–1160, 1986.
58. Chaussy C, Brendel W, Schmiedt E: Extracorporally induced destruction of kidney stones by shock waves. Lancet 2:1265–1268, 1980.
59. Gleeson MJ, Shabsigh R, Griffith DP: Outcome of ESWL in patients with multiple renal calculi based on stone burden and location. J Endourol 2:145–149, 1988.
60. Miller K, Hautmann R: Treatment of distal ureteral calculi with ESWL: Experience with more than 100 consecutive cases. World J Urol 5:259–261, 1987.
61. Salvini A, Faustini S, Pizzi P, Quadraccia A: Treatment of urinary bladder stone by ESWL. Presented at 4th Symposium on Shock-Wave Lithotripsy: State-of-the-Art, March 5–6, 1988, Indianapolis.
62. Rocco F, Larcher P, Caimi D, Decobelli O, et al: Treatment of renal staghorn calculi with ESWL monotherapy using the Rocco EXL catheter. Presented at 4th Symposium on Shock-Wave Lithotripsy: State-of-the-Art, March 5–6, 1988, Indianapolis.
63. Wirth MP, Frohmuller HGW: Results of primary treatment of staghorn calculi with extracorporeal shock-wave lithotripsy. Presented at 4th Symposium on Shock-Wave Lithotripsy: State-of-the-Art, March 5–6, 1988, Indianapolis.
64. Harada M, Okuda Y, Maeda H, et al: ESWL treatment of staghorn calculi and large stones. Presented at 4th Symposium on Shock-Wave Lithotripsy: State-of-the-Art, March 5–6, 1988, Indianapolis.
65. Pode D, Verstandig A, Shapiro A, et al: Treatment of complete staghorn calculi by extracorporeal shock-wave lithotripsy monotherapy with special reference to internal stenting. J Urol 140:260–265, 1988.
66. Sohn M, Deutz FJ, Rohrmann D, et al: Anesthesia-free ESWL monotherapy with double J stents versus PCNL/ESWL combined approach in staghorn disease: A prospective randomized study. Presented at 4th Symposium on Shock-Wave Lithotripsy: State-of-the-Art, March 5–6, 1988, Indianapolis.
67. Gilhuis R, Carpentier PJ: Treatment of staghorn calculus by percutaneous lithotripsy followed by ESWL. J Urol 137:279A, 1987.
68. Schulze H, Hertle L, Graff J, et al: Combined treatment of branched calculi by percutaneous nephrolithotomy and extracorporeal shock-wave lithotripsy. J Urol 135:1138–1141, 1986.
69. Kahnoski RJ, Lingeman JE, Coury TA, et al: Combined percutaneous and extracorporeal shock-wave lithotripsy for staghorn calculi: An alternative to anatrophic nephrolithotomy. J Urol 135:679–681, 1986.
70. Lingeman JE: Results of 313 staghorn treatments. Presented at the 4th Symposium on Shock-Wave Lithotripsy: State-of-the-Art, March 5–6, 1988, Indianapolis.
71. Segura JW, Patterson DE, LeRoy AJ: Combined percutaneous ultrasonic lithotripsy and extracorporeal shock-wave lithotripsy for struvite staghorn calculi. World J Urol 5:245–247, 1987.
72. Streem SB, Zelch MG, Risius B, Geisinger MA: Planned endourologic "sandwich" therapy for extensive staghorn calculi. J Urol 137:705A, 1987.
73. McLeod DC, Nabata MC: Inefficacy of ascorbic acid as a urinary acidifier. N Engl J Med 296:1413, 1977.
74. Hetey SK, Kleinberg ML, Parker WC, Johnson EW: Effect of ascorbic acid on urine pH in patients with injured spinal cords. Am J Hosp Pharmacol 37:235–237, 1980.
75. Murphy FJ, Zehman S, Mau W: Ascorbic acid as a urinary acidifying agent: 2. Its adjunctive role in chronic urinary infection. J Urol 94:300–303, 1965.
76. Vermeulen CW, Ragins HD, Grove WJ, Goetz R: Experimental urolithiasis. III. Prevention and dissolution of calculi by alteration of urinary pH. J Urol 66:1–5, 1951.
77. Nielsen IM: Urolithiasis in mink: Pathology, bacteriology and experimental production. J Urol 75:602–614, 1956.

78. Cintron-Nadad E, Lespier LE, Roman-Mircuda A, Martinez-Maldonado M: Renal acidifying ability in subjects with recurrent stone formation. J Urol 118:704–706, 1977.
79. Rector FC Jr, Seldin DW, Copenhaver JH: The mechanism of ammonia excretion during ammonium chloride acidosis. J Clin Invest 34:20–26, 1955.
80. Froeling PGAM: Akute zuurbelastingen. *In* De Zuuruitscheiding bis de Behandeling von Mensen met Nierstenen. 1978, pp 93–106.
81. Pizzarelli F, Peacock M: Effect of chronic administration of ammonium sulfate on phosphatic stone recurrence. Nephron 46:247–252, 1987.
82. Leman J Jr, Litzow JR, Lennon EJ: Studies of the mechanism by which chronic metabolic acidosis augments urinary calcium excretion in man. J Clin Invest 46:1318–1328, 1967.
83. Mahnensmith R, Thier SO, Cooke CR, et al: Effect of acute metabolic acidemia on renal electrolyte transport in man. Metabolism 28:831–842, 1979.
84. Coe FL, Firpo JJ, Hollandsworth DL, et al: Effect of acute and chronic metabolic acidosis on serum immunoreactive parathyroid hormone in man. Kidney Int 8:262–273, 1975.
85. Albright F, Sulkowitch HW, Chute R: Nonsurgical aspects of the kidney stone problem. JAMA 113:2049–2053, 1939.
86. Suby HI, Albright F: Dissolution of phosphatic urinary calculi by the retrograde introduction of a citrate solution containing magnesium. N Engl J Med 228:81–91, 1943.
87. Mulvaney WP: A new solvent for certain urinary calculi: A preliminary report. J Urol 82:546–548, 1959.
88. Cato AR, Tulloch AGS: Hypermagnesemia in a uremic patient during renal pelvis irrigation with renacidin. J Urol 111:313–314, 1974.
89. Brock WA, Nachtseim DA, Parsons CL: Hemiacidrin irrigation of renal pelvic calculi in patients with ileal conduit urinary diversion. J Urol 123:345–347, 1980.
90. Dretler SP, Pfister RC, Newhouse JH: Renal stone dissolution via percutaneous nephrostomy. N Engl J Med 300:341–343, 1979.
91. Palmer JM, Bishai MB, Mallon DS: Outpatient irrigation of the renal collecting system with 10 per cent hemiacidrin: Cumulative experience of 365 days in 13 patients. J Urol 138:262–265, 1987.
92. Higgins CC: Urinary lithiasis: Experimental production and solution with clinical application and end results. J Urol 36:168–177, 1936.
93. McCarrison R: Causation of stone in India. Br Med J 1:1009–1015, 1931.
94. Racic J: Calculus of bladder in Dalmatia. Urol Cutan Rev 39:158–163, 1935.
95. Shorr E: The possible usefulness of estrogens and aluminum hydroxide gels in the management of renal stone. J Urol 53:507–520, 1945.
96. Shorr E, Carter AC: Aluminum gels in the management of renal phosphatic calculi. JAMA 144:1549–1556, 1950.
97. Lavengood RW Jr, Marshall VF: The prevention of renal phosphatic calculi in the presence of infection by the Shorr regimen. J Urol 108:368–371, 1972.
98. Lotz M, Zisman E, Bartter FC: Evidence for a phosphorus depletion syndrome in man. N Engl J Med 278:409–415, 1968.
99. Stamey TA: Infection Stones in Urinary Infections. Baltimore, The Williams and Wilkins Company, 1972, p 213.
100. Griffith DP, Moskowitz PA, Carlton CE Jr: Adjunctive chemotherapy of infection-induced staghorn calculi. J Urol 121:711–715, 1979.
101. Hamilton-Miller JMT, Brumfitt W: Methenamine and its salts as urinary tract antiseptics: Variables affecting the antibacterial activity of formaldehyde, mandelic acid and hippuric acid in vitro. Invest Urol 14:287–291, 1977.
102. Heathcote RSA: Hexamine as a urinary antiseptic. I. Its rate of hydrolysis at different hydrogen ion concentrations. II. Its antiseptic power against various bacteria in urine. Br J Urol 7:9–32, 1935.
103. Feit RM, Fair WR: The treatment of infection stones with penicillin. J Urol 122:592–594, 1979.
104. Musher D, Minuth J, Thorsteinsson SB, Holmes T: Effectiveness of achievable urinary concentrations of tetracyclines against "tetracycline-resistant" pathogenic bacteria. J Infect Dis [Suppl]131:40–44, 1975.
105. Cox CE, McCabe RE, Grad C: Oral norfloxacin versus parenteral treatment of nosocomial urinary tract infections. Am J Med 82 [Suppl 6B]:59–64, 1987.
106. Scully BE, Neu HC, Parry MF, Mandell W: Oral ciprofloxacin therapy of infections due to *Pseudomonas aeruginosa*. Lancet 1:819–822, 1986.
107. Boyce WH, McKinney WM, Long TT, Drach GW: Oral administration of methylene blue to patients with renal calculi. J Urol 97:783–789, 1967.
108. Sobel AE, Burger M: Calcification: Investigation of role of chondroitin sulfate in calcifying mechanism. Proc Soc Exp Biol Med 87:7–13, 1954.
109. Van't Riet B, McKinney WM, Brandt EA, et al: Dye effects on inhibition and dissolution of urinary calculi. Invest Urol 1:446–456, 1964.
110. Kobashi K, Hase J, Uehara K: Specific inhibition of urease by hydroxamic acid. Biochim Biophys Acta 65:380–383, 1962.
111. Kobashi K, Kumaki K, Hase J: Effect of acyl residues of hydroxamic acids on urease inhibition. Biochim Biophys Acta 227:429–441, 1971.

112. Fishbein WN, Carbone PO: Urease catalysis. II. Inhibition of the enzyme by hydroxylurea, hydroxylamine and acetohydroxamic acid. J Biol Chem 240:2407–2414, 1965.
113. Nagarajan K, Fishbein WN: Interaction of urease nickel atoms with thiols and the specific inhibitor, acetodroxamate: A circular dichroism study. Fed Proc 36:700–704, 1977.
114. Griffith DP, Musher DM: Prevention of infected urinary stones by urease inhibition. Invest Urol 11:228–233, 1973.
115. Putcha L, Griffith DP, Feldman S: Pharmacokinetics of acetohydroxamic acid in patients with staghorn renal calculi. Eur J Clin Pharmacol 28:439–445, 1985.
116. Putcha L, Griffith DP, Feldman S: Disposition of ^{14}C-acetohydroxamic acid and ^{14}C-acetamide in the rat. Drug Metab Dispos 12:438–443, 1984.
117. Feldman S, Putcha L, Griffith DP: Pharmacokinetics of acetohydroxamic acid: Preliminary investigations. Invest Urol 15:498–501, 1978.
118. Summerskill WHJ, Thorsell F, Feinberg HJ, Aldrete JS: Effects of urease inhibition in hyperammonemia: Clinical and experimental studies with acetohydroxamic acid. Gastroenterology 54:20–26, 1967.
119. Griffith DP, Khonsari F, Skurnick JH, et al: Experimental and clinical trials of lithostat (acetohydroxamic acid—AHA). *In* Martelli A, Buli P, Marchesini B (eds): Inhibitors of crystallization in Renal Lithiasis and Their Clinical Application. Bologna, Italy, Acta Medica, 1988, pp 229–235.
120. Bailie NC, Osborne CA, Leininger JR, et al: Teratogenic effect of acetohydroxamic acid in clinically normal Beagles. Am J Vet Res 471:2604–2611, 1986.
121. Burr RG, Nureibeh I: The effect of oral acetohydroxamic acid on urinary saturation in stone-forming spinal cord patients. Br J Urol 55:162–165, 1983.
122. Williams JJ, Rodman JS, Peterson CM: A randomized double-blind study of acetohydroxamic acid in struvite nephrolithiasis. N Engl J Med 311:760–764, 1984.
123. Griffith DP, Khonsari F, Skurnick JH, James KE: V.A. Cooperative Study Group: A randomized trial of acetohydroxamic acid for the treatment and prevention of infection induced urinary stones in spinal cord injury patients. J Urol 140:318–324, 1988.
124. Martelli A, Buli P, Cartecchia V: Urease inhibitor therapy in infected renal stones. Eur Urol 7:291–293, 1981.
125. Wang CY, Lee LH: Mutagenicity and antibacterial activity of hydroxamic acids. Antimicrob Agents Chemother 11:753–755, 1977.
126. Martelli A, Buli P, Spatafora S: Clinical experience with low dosage of propionohydroxamic acid (PHA) in infected renal stones. Urology 28:373–375, 1986.
127. Anderson JA: Benurestat, a urease inhibitor for the therapy of infected ureolysis. Invest Urol 12:381–386, 1975.
128. Javor A, Frang D, Nagy Z: Applicability of Biosuppressin as a urease-inhibitor. Int Urol Nephrol 16:191–194, 1984.
129. Takeuchi H, Yoshida O, Kobashi K, et al: Prevention of infected urinary stones by urease inhibitor. II. Urinary excretion of hydroxamic acid and prevention of infected bladder stones in rats. Acta Urol Jpn 23:113–118, 1973.
130. Takeuchi H, Kobashi K, Yoshida O: Prevention of infected urinary stones in rats by urease inhibitor: A new hydroxamic acid derivative. Invest Urol 18:102–105, 1980.
131. Millner OE Jr, Andersen JA, Appler ME, et al: Flurofamide: A potent inhibitor of bacterial urease with potential clinical utility in the treatment of infection induced urinary stones. J Urol 127:346–350, 1982.
132. Rosenstein I: Therapeutic applications of urease inhibitors. J Antimicrob Chemother 10:159–161, 1982.

Cystine Lithiasis

9

Charles Y.C. Pak

Cystinuria is a complex autosomal recessive inherited disorder of amino acid transport involving cystine as well as other dibasic amino acids—ornithine, lysine, and arginine.[1] The transport defect is expressed as an excessive renal excretion and impaired intestinal absorption of these amino acids. This disorder represents an inborn error of membrane transport. The gene responsible has not been mapped to a specific chromosomal locus. Heterozygous cystinuria occurs at a frequency of 1 per 200 individuals, whereas the prevalence of homozygous cystinuria has been estimated at 1 per 20,000 persons in the United States.

The only recognized clinical manifestation is cystine lithiasis, which may develop anytime during life, with peak times for expression during the second and third decades. The stone formation is due to excessive cystine excretion and low solubility of cystine in urine. At very high risk are subjects with homozygous cystinuria, not those with the heterozygous trait. In patients with homozygous cystinuria, urinary cystine exceeds 250 mg/gram of urinary creatinine (or 250 mg/day for a 50-kg person); thus, their urinary environment is often supersaturated with respect to cystine. The heterozygotes are not at risk for stone formation because their cystine excretion, though often higher than in normal subjects, is well below that required to produce supersaturation. The excessive excretion of ornithine, lysine, and arginine does not pose a clinical problem, because of the higher aqueous solubility of these amino acids.

HISTORICAL CONSIDERATIONS

In 1810, Wollaston noted a distinct chemical nature of two bladder stones and called them "cystic oxide" stones, recalling their site of origin.[2] In 1824, Stromeyer provided the classic microscopic description of hexagonal platelike crystals.[3] In 1933, Berzelius, noting the absence of oxide, renamed the compound cystine.[4]

In 1902, Friedman provided the chemical structure of cystine.[5] In 1908, Garrod suggested that an inborn error of metabolism was responsible for cystinuria.[6] In 1963, Crawhall and colleagues introduced D-penicillamine as an effective means of reducing cystine excretion.[7] In 1988, α-mercaptopropionylglycine, a hypocystinuric agent with a lower toxicity profile than D-penicillamine,[8] was approved by the Food and Drug Administration (FDA) for the treatment of cystine lithiasis in the United States.

PATHOGENETIC ROLE OF CYSTINURIA IN CYSTINE LITHIASIS

Cystine stone formation has been ascribed to the low solubility of cystine in the aqueous environment of urine. In the setting of an excessive urinary concentration of cystine (as in homozygous cystinuria), the solubility limit for cystine is often exceeded, creating a supersaturated environment conducive to cystine crystallization.

Factors Affecting Cystine Solubility

It has long been known that cystine solubility is pH dependent, with the lowest solubility at the low range of urinary pH, gradually increased solubility with rising pH to 7.5, and rapid increase in solubility above a pH of 7.5.[9]

Dent and Senior[9] showed that the solubility curve of cystine was the same whether it was obtained in urine from normal subjects or from cystinuric patients and that it was unaffected by the presence of urea or sodium chloride. Studies by Ettinger and Kolb[10] indicated that cystine solubility was greater in urine samples with a specific gravity exceeding 1.01 than in samples with a specific gravity of less than this value. The results suggested that some components of urine might influence cystine solubility. Studies at Dallas have disclosed that the enhanced solubility of cystine in urine is accounted for by mineral electrolytes and macromolecules.[11]

Because of the solvent action of electrolytes and macromolecules,[11] the maximal solubility of cystine determined in *urine* is considerably greater than that derived in a simple synthetic solution (5 mM of sodium), but less than that derived in urine by Dent and Senior (Fig. 9–1). Thus, the saturation of cystine in individual urine samples cannot be estimated by comparing the original cystine concentration with a defined cystine solubility curve. The comparison of urinary cystine value in a given specimen with the curve of Dent and Senior would underestimate urinary cystine saturation, whereas comparison with the cystine solubility curve in a 5 mM sodium solution would overestimate it. It may be more accurately measured as the ratio of original cystine concentration and the directly determined cystine solubility in urine.

Determinants of Cystine Crystallization

The main determinant of cystine crystallization is urinary supersaturation. There is no known inhibitor of cystine crystallization. If the urine sample is supersaturated with respect to cystine, precipitation of cystine invariably occurs. It is virtually impossible to maintain a metastably supersaturated solution. Thus, there is a strong cause and effect relationship between excessive cystine excretion

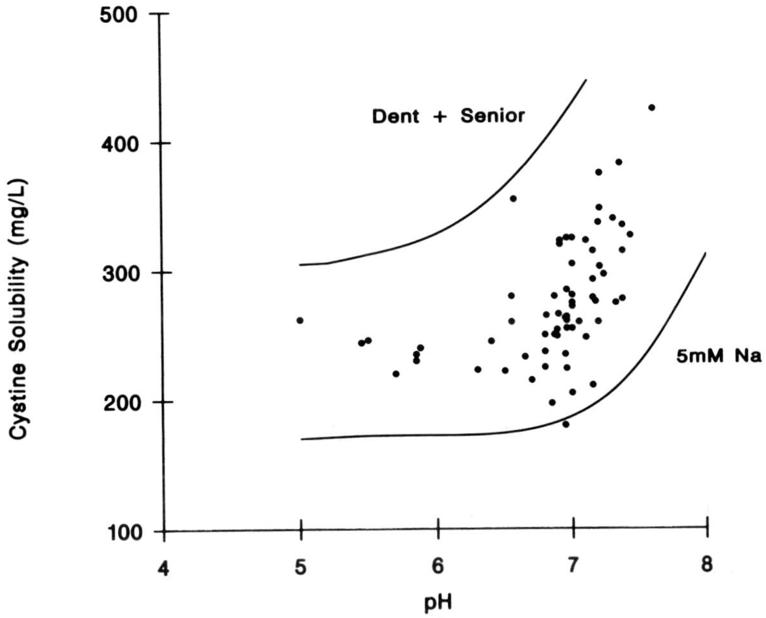

FIGURE 9–1. Solubility of cystine in actual urine specimens, compared with the solubility curve of Dent and Senior and that obtained in a synthetic solution containing 5 mmol of sodium per liter. Solubility in a separate urine sample is indicated by a solid circle.

and cystine stone formation, more so than for any other form of stone disease (e.g., between hypercalciuria and calcium nephrolithiasis).

Although cystine stones often coexist with calcium stones (approximately 30 per cent),[12] no epitaxy or heterogeneous nucleation has been disclosed between cystine and calcium salts.[11]

PATHOPHYSIOLOGY OF CYSTINURIA

Renal Transport Defect

Normally, cystine is filtered and almost completely reabsorbed in the proximal nephron, leaving less than 20 mg in urine each day. In cystinuria, the serum concentration of cystine and hence the renal filtered load of cystine are reduced. Exaggerated cystine excretion under this circumstance suggests a disturbance in the renal handling of cystine.

Normally, specific amino acid transport systems are present in the renal tubule, each mediating the transport of a group of structurally related amino acids, leading to an almost complete reabsorption of these amino acids. The mutant gene in cystinuria codes for an abnormal transport system involving cystinine, ornithine, lysine, and arginine, and not other amino acids.

The probable defect in the renal handling of cystine in cystinuria is illustrated in Figure 9–2.[13] The cystine uptake by the proximal tubular cell from peritubular blood at the basolateral membrane is unaffected. Moreover, the secretion and paracellular leakage of cystine are apparently normal in cystinuria. However, the basic defect in cystinuria is the impaired reabsorption of cystine at the basolateral

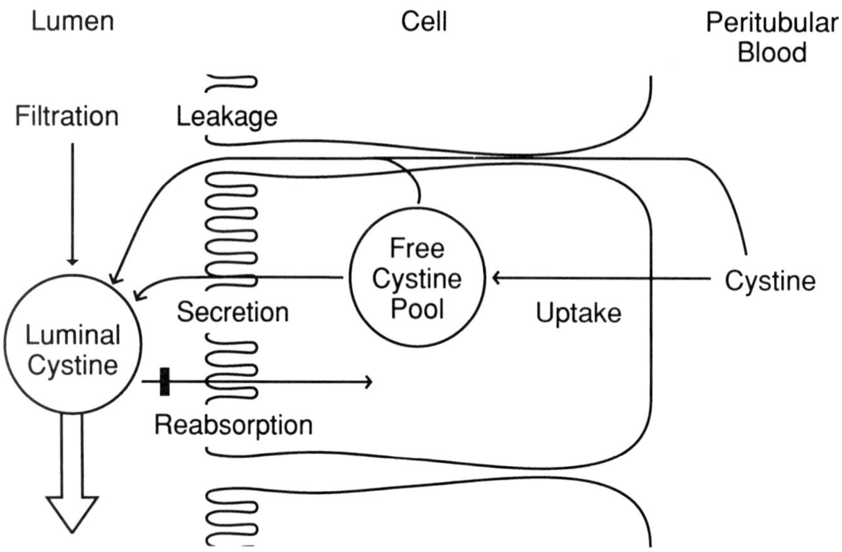

FIGURE 9–2. Renal transport defect in cystinuria.

membrane. Thus, the incomplete reabsorption of cystine (appearing in the proximal tubule by secretion, leakage, and filtration) leads to excessive cystine excretion.

The prevailing evidence suggests that there is impairment in the proximal tubular reabsorption of cystine at the brush border membrane. This characteristic is shared by other dibasic amino acids. However, the peritubular uptake of cystine is apparently independent of that for ornithine, lysine, and arginine.

Recently, it was reported that the urinary excretion of cystine could be reduced by glutamine administration in cystinuria.[14] This finding could not be confirmed.[15] It was later shown that the hypocystinuric action of glutamine occurred only during a high sodium intake and not during a low sodium intake.[16] Since sodium load augments cystine excretion to a modest degree, the effect of glutamine in lowering urinary cystine was equivalent to that produced by dietary sodium restriction.

Intestinal Transport Defect

There is also a defect in the intestinal transport of dibasic amino acids in cystinuria. Cystinuria has been classified into three types based on varying intestinal transport disturbances for these amino acids.[17] The intestinal transport has been assessed from the in vitro uptake of radiolabeled amino acid by specimens of jejunal mucosa obtained by peroral biopsy and from elevation of plasma cystine levels following an oral cystine load. In Type I cystinuria, there is no uptake of cystine, lysine, or arginine by jejunal mucosa, and there is no plasma cystine elevation following an oral cystine load. Thus, there is total abrogation of intestinal transport for these dibasic amino acids. In Types II and III, the intestinal transport of dibasic amino acids is disturbed, but less severely than in the Type I presentation. Thus, in Type II cystinuria, some cystine uptake by jejunal mucosa prevails, but at a markedly reduced level, and oral cystine loading does not increase the plasma cystine level. In Type III cystinuria, cystine and lysine uptake by jejunal mucosa is variably reduced but not obliterated, and the increment in plasma cystine following an oral cystine load is blunted but present. Studies by Rosenberg and coworkers have disclosed that all three types of cystinuria in the homozygous state manifest with excessive renal excretion of all four dibasic amino acids.[17] However, in the heterozygous state, Type I cystinuria is characterized by normal cystine (nonelevated) excretion, whereas Type II and Type III presentations show an elevation in cystine and lysine excretion (though not quite up to the level encountered in the homozygous state), probably owing to a prevailing (though reduced) intestinal uptake of these amino acids.

Association of Cystinuria with Other Abnormalities

Approximately 30 per cent of patients with homozygous cystinuria may form stones that do not contain cystine or that contain cystine as a minor constituent of a mixed stone.[12] The mixed stone formation cannot be explained on the basis of inductive properties of cystine. No evidence exists for the heterogeneous nucleation of calcium oxalate, brushite, or hydroxyapatite by cystine.[11] Calcium phosphate stones could theoretically form, since urinary pH is often high owing to consumption of a low-methionine diet and as urinary tract infection is not uncommon from recurrent stone formation. The high urinary pH would enhance phosphate dissociation and saturation of calcium phosphate. Although low methionine levels might normally augment citrate excretion, this rise may be averted by the destruction of citrate by bacterial enzymes.

The most plausible explanation for the mixed stone formation is the coexistence of other stone-forming risks in cystinuric patients. In a recent study at Dallas,[12] hypercalciuria was disclosed in 18.5 per cent of patients, hyperuricosuria in 22.2 per cent, and hypocitraturia in 44.4 per cent. Patients with mixed stones of cystine and calcium salts had significantly higher urinary calcium and lower citrate. The exact pathophysiology of these concurrent disturbances is not known.

DIAGNOSIS

The urinary sediment (preferably in fresh first morning void) should be examined for the presence of typical hexagonal cystine crystals. The urine sample should also be screened for "qualitative" cystine by the cyanide-nitroprusside test.[18] A positive reaction suggests that cystine excretion exceeds 75 mg/liter. A false-positive test may be encountered in patients with homocystinuria and acetonuria. On roentgenologic examination, cystine calculi are radiopaque (though not as much) like calcareous calculi but are more rounded and homogeneous in appearance. They may attain the size of a staghorn.

If the preceeding studies are suggestive of the presence of cystinuria, urinary cystine excretion should be quantitated. Urinary cystine exceeding 250 mg/gram of creatinine is usually diagnostic of homozygous cystinuria. Stones passed or removed should be analyzed. The presence of cystine provides a definitive diagnosis of cystinuria.

TREATMENT (Table 9–1)

The object of treatment is to reduce the urinary concentration of cystine to below its solubility limit. Unfortunately, that solubility is hard to define in a given urine sample because of wide variability (see Fig. 9–1).[11] During a state of high fluid intake (which is a critical part of treatment), cystine solubility is likely to approach that of a 5 mM sodium synthetic solution (see Fig. 9–1) because of the reduced concentration of solubilizing macromolecules and electrolytes.[11] Thus, it is recommended that the cystine concentration in urine be kept below 200 mg/liter (irrespective of pH).

Dietary Manipulation

A low-methionine diet has often been recommended for the control of cystine nephrolithiasis because of the well-known requirement of this essential amino acid for cystine production.[19] Although this dietary maneuver may reduce cystine excretion, a rigid methionine restriction is impractical. The compliance is often poor with a diet devoid of or severely restricted in flesh meat, poultry, fish, eggs, casein, soybeans, wheat, and peanuts. Moreover, there may be long-term adverse consequences of such a diet on other organ systems, such as the skeleton. Thus, it is prudent to recommend avoiding the excessive intake of the above-mentioned food items, but not necessarily to restrict them severely.

A recent report suggests that cystine excretion is dependent on dietary sodium intake, by a mechanism poorly described.[16] Thus, a direct correlation has been described between urinary cystine and urinary sodium in four cystinuric patients. This study implied that a reduction in dietary sodium intake by 150 mEq/day (8.8 grams of sodium chloride a day) could reduce urinary cystine by 650 μmol (156 mg) a day. Although an avoidance of dietary sodium excess would be advisable on general grounds, the following points should be noted:

1. Such a rigid dietary sodium restriction is difficult to achieve practically.
2. The reduction in cystine excretion produced by sodium restriction is modest.
3. There may be an opposing effect of reduced solvent action of sodium on cystine solubility from a low-sodium diet.[11]

Moreover, this study needs to be repeated, since it was done in a small number of patients on an uncontrolled diet with a probable variable intake of proteins.

Conservative Measures

In patients with moderate cystinuria (250 to 500 mg/day) with cystine calculi, conservative measures of high fluid intake and alkali should be attempted first.

TABLE 9–1. MANAGEMENT OF CYSTINURIA

Modality	Mechanism of Action
Moderate methionine restriction	Limits substrate for cystine synthesis
Dietary sodium restriction	Reduces cystine excretion
High fluid intake	Lowers urinary cystine concentration
Potassium citrate, 30–40 mEq/day	Increases cystine solubility
Glutamine	Reduces cystine excretion (during high-sodium diet)
D-Penicillamine	Reduces cystine excretion by complexing cysteine
MPG	Reduces cystine excretion by complexing cysteine

The aim of fluid therapy is to increase urine volume sufficiently to reduce cystine solubility below the solubility limit. At least 3 liters of fluid (ten 10-ounce glassfuls) should be provided daily, including two glasses with each meal and at bedtime. The patients should be expected to awake at night to urinate; they should drink two more glasses of fluids before returning to bed. Additional fluids should be consumed if there is excessive sweating or intestinal fluid loss. A minimal urine output of 2 liters/day on a consistent basis should be sought, a goal attainable by most patients with proper and persistent instruction. Stone prevention and dissolution have been reported following a high fluid intake.[20]

All types of fluid are generally permissible, with the possible exception of milk (with high methionine content) and brewed tea (with high oxalate content, increasing the risk for calcium oxalate nephrolithiasis, which sometimes complicates cystine nephrolithiasis). Fruit juices (grapefruit, orange, cranberry, apple, and grape) may be particularly advantagenous, because they provide not only water but also alkali. For example, 900 ml of orange juice (one glassful three times a day) may provide enough potassium citrate to increase the urinary pH by 0.5 unit.

The object of alkali therapy is to increase the urinary pH to enhance cystine solubility. However, excessive alkali therapy is not indicated. Substantial increase in cystine solubility does not occur until the urinary pH exceeds 7.5. The provision of alkali, no matter how much, rarely raises the urinary pH above 7.5. When the urinary pH increases above 7.0 with alkali therapy, the complication of calcium phosphate nephrolithiasis may ensue because of the enhanced urinary supersaturation of hydroxyapatite in an alkaline environment.

It is recommended that a modest amount of alkali be provided to maintain the urinary pH in a high normal range (6.5 to 7.0). Potassium alkali preparations are advantageous over those of sodium alkali, because they do not cause hypercalciuria,[21] are less likely to cause the complication of calcium stones,[22] and are devoid of sodium-induced enhancement of cystine excretion.[16] Citrate is preferable to bicarbonate because it produces a more constant and persistent elevation in the urinary pH (see Chapter 6). The slow-release citrate preparation is probably superior to the readily available liquid preparation in this regard.[23] A common practice is to use potassium citrate (wax matrix tablets) at a typical dosage of 15 to 20 mEq twice a day. The dosage may be adjusted, depending on the results of the urinary pH.

Glutamine

In 1979, Miyagi and associates[14] reported that glutamine given orally or intravenously significantly reduced cystine excretion in a patient with cystinuria. This effect was attributed to the secretion of glutamine into the proximal tubular lumen in exchange for cystine. Unfortunately, van den Berg and coworkers were unable to confirm this finding in their study of five cystinuric patients.[15]

In a recent report, however, Jaeger and colleagues[16] showed that glutamine administration (2.1 grams/day in three divided doses orally) reduced cystine excretion when the sodium intake was high (300 mEq/day) but not when it was normal (150 mEq/day).

The reduction in cystine excretion is equivalent to that produced by an avoidance of an excessive sodium intake. Thus, glutamine has little value in patients maintained on a sodium-restricted diet.

D-Penicillamine

The object of D-penicillamine treatment is to reduce total cystine excretion by complexing cysteine, the monomeric form of cystine.[7, 24] It may be added to the conservative treatment program when the latter is ineffective in controlling stone formation in patients with moderate cystinuria. In patients with severe cystinuria (>500 mg/day), in whom the customary conservative program alone is not likely to be effective, D-penicillamine therapy (*with* conservative measures) may be begun.

D-Penicillamine (ββ-dimethyl-cysteine) shares with cysteine a free sulfhydryl group (Fig. 9–3). Thus, it readily undergoes thiol-disulfide exchange with cystine (cysteine–cysteine disulfide) to form penicillamine–cysteine disulfide, which has a much higher aqueous solubility than cystine. Following oral administration, a sufficient amount of D-penicillamine could appear in urine to complex cysteine and thereby lower cystine excretion.

The dose of D-penicillamine should not be arbitrary but should be based on that amount required to reduce urinary cystine concentration to below its solubility limit (generally <200 mg/liter). The extent of the decline in cystine excretion is proportional to the D-penicillamine dosage. Each increment in the D-penicillamine dosage of 250 mg/day might be expected to reduce urinary cystine by 75 to 100 mg/day. Accordingly, assuming that a minimal desired urine output of 2 liters/day has been achieved, the minimal effective D-penicillamine dose might be 1250 mg/day when cystine excretion is 1000 mg/day or 750 mg/day when urinary cystine is 800 mg/day. The medication is generally given in divided doses before meals, since its absorption may be impaired when it is mixed with certain foods.

There is substantial evidence that D-penicillamine can favorably modify the course of cystine nephrolithiasis. If adequate amounts of the drug could be given to lower urinary cystine to desired levels, one should expect a reduction in the

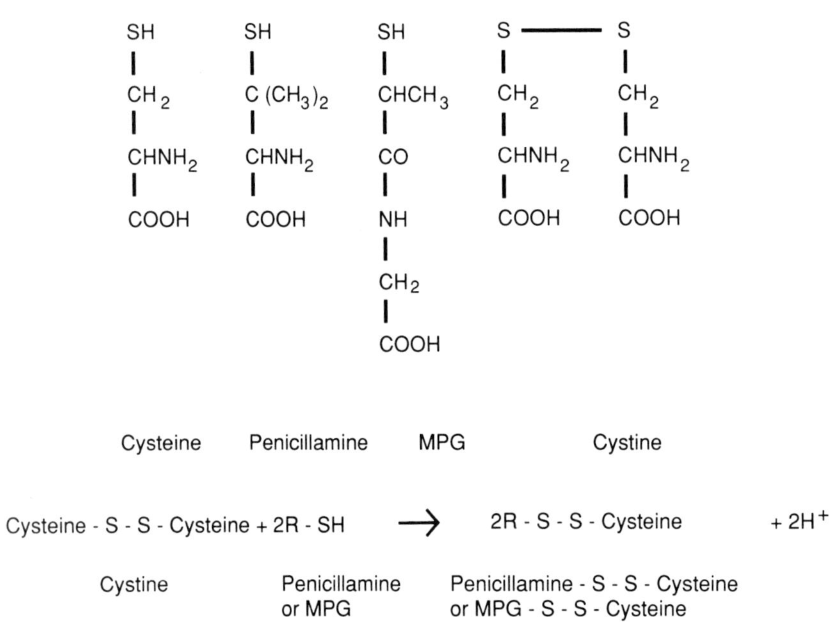

FIGURE 9–3. Reaction of cystine with penicillamine or α-mercapto-propionyl glycine (MPG).

rates of stone passage and new stone formation. When there is a sufficient fall in cystine excretion to produce urinary undersaturation, dissolution of existing cystine stones could occur.

Unfortunately, a substantial number of patients develop adverse reactions to D-penicillamine treatment. Side effects include gastrointestinal complications (nausea, emesis, diarrhea, loose stools, anorexia, abdominal pain, and bloating or flatus); impairment in taste and smell (probably due to chelation of zinc); dermatologic complications (pharyngitis, oral ulcers, rash, ecchymosis, pruritis, urticaria, pemphigus, elastosis perforans serpiginosa, and skin wrinkling); hypersensitivity reactions (laryngeal edema, dyspnea, respiratory distress, fever, chills, arthralgia, weakness, fatigue, myalgia, and adenopathy); hematologic abnormalities (leukopenia, agranulocytosis, thrombocytopenia, anemia, and eosinophilia); abnormal liver function tests; and renal complications (proteinuria, nephrotic syndrome, and glomerulonephritis). In up to 50 per cent of patients, the cessation of D-penicillamine therapy may be required because of these side effects. In some of them, D-penicillamine therapy may be reinstituted by desensitization. This technique entails restarting treatment at a low dosage of D-penicillamine of 10 to 25 mg/day, with a gradual increase in dosage at 3-day intervals until the desired dosage is reached, to be achieved over a period of about 1 month.

During long-term therapy, D-penicillamine may cause vitamin B_6 deficiency by binding pyridoxine. Before the appearance of significant symptoms (dizziness, seizures, glossitis, and seborrheic dermatitis), it may be prudent to provide pyridoxine supplementation (50 mg/day) in patients receiving large doses of D-penicillamine (>1 gram/day) chronically.

α-Mercaptopropionylglycine (MPG)

This newly approved drug (in the United States) may serve as a reasonable alternative to D-penicillamine, especially in the setting of toxicity to the latter drug.[8, 25] MPG shares chemical properties similar to those of D-penicillamine (Fig. 9–3). It undergoes thiol-disulfide exchange with cystine to form a readily soluble MPG–cysteine disulfide. The reduction in urinary cystine produced by MPG is similar to that obtained during D-penicillamine therapy. Thus, the same comments regarding dosage schedule previously given for D-penicillamine apply to the MPG treatment. Available data from Japan and Europe suggest that MPG is as effective as D-penicillamine in inhibiting cystine stone formation.

The major advantage of MPG appears to be its apparent reduced toxicity. A recent review of the literature disclosed 10 reports entailing 120 cystinuric patients undergoing clinical trial with MPG.[8] Minor gastrointestinal problems occurred in 35 patients, rash in 14, urticaria in 3, pemphigus in 1, fever in 7, and nephrotic syndrome in 2 patients. These adverse reactions were generally less common and less serious than those reported with D-penicillamine. Although serious side effects such as pemphigus and nephrotic syndrome have also been encountered during MPG therapy, they occurred less frequently. Thus, among 120 patients taking MPG, only 2 apparently had to stop taking the medication because of adverse reactions.

The experience at Dallas is compatible with the preceding findings.[8] Since 1980, the Dallas group has organized and conducted a multiclinic trial with MPG, to assess the therapeutic role of MPG as an alternative to D-penicillamine in the management of cystine nephrolithiasis. The primary objective was to determine the safety and efficacy of MPG in patients with known toxicity to D-penicillamine.

Among 49 patients who took D-penicillamine first and later received MPG, 41 patients (83.7 per cent) developed side effects from D-penicillamine and 37 (75.5 per cent) from MPG. Adverse reactions involved all organ systems. Frequent adverse reactions to D-penicillamine were nausea in 36.7 per cent of patients, proteinuria in 12.2 per cent, and fatigue in 16.3 per cent. These reactions were also observed during MPG therapy, but less frequently. Thus, nausea was encountered in 24.5 per cent of patients, emesis in 10.2 per cent, anorexia in 8.2 per cent, rash in 14.3 per cent, proteinuria in 10.2 per cent, and fatigue in 14.3 per cent.

Moreover, serious side effects were less common during MPG therapy. Thus, 69.4 per cent of patients required cessation of D-penicillamine treatment, whereas only 30.6 per cent had to stop taking MPG. Among 34 patients who could not tolerate D-penicillamine, 22 could be maintained on MPG.

MPG was effective in reducing cystine excretion. During long-term treatment with MPG (average dose of 1193 mg/day), urinary cystine was maintained at 350 to 560 mg/day, and the urinary saturation of cystine was kept undersaturated. Commensurate with these changes, MPG produced remission of stone formation in 63 to 71 per cent of patients and reduced the individual stone formation rate in 81 to 94 per cent.

Thus, MPG would seem to have a definite role in the management of cystine nephrolithiasis, especially in patients who have developed toxicity to D-penicillamine.

Captopril

There is a recent unconfirmed report that captopril reduces citrate excretion in cystinuria.[26] The basis for this action remains to be established.

REFERENCES

1. Thier SO, Segal S: Cystinuria. *In* Stanbury JB, Wyngaarden JB, Fredrickson DS (eds).: The Metabolic Basis of Inherited Disease. New York, McGraw-Hill, 1972, pp 1504–1519.
2. Wollaston WH: On cystic oxide: A new species of urinary calculus. Trans R Soc Lond 100:223, 1810.
3. Noehden GH: Scientific notices—chemistry, cystic oxide—communicated in a letter from Dr. Noehden to Mr. Children. Ann Philos 7:146, 1824.
4. Berzelius JJ: Calculus urinaires. Traite Chem 7:424, 1833.
5. Friedman E: Der Kreislauf des Schwefels in der organischen. Nature Ergeb Physiol 1:15, 1902.
6. Garrod AE: Inborn errors of metabolism. Lancet 2 (Lecture I, p 1; Lecture II, p 73; Lecture III, p 142; Lecture IV, p 214), 1908.
7. Crawhall JC, Scowen EF, Watts RWE: Effect of penicillamine on cystinuria. Br Med J 1:585, 1963.
8. Pak CYC, Fuller C, Sakhaee K, et al: Management of cystine nephrolithiasis with alpha-mercaptopropionylglycine. J Urol 136:1003–1008, 1986.
9. Dent CE, Senior B: Studies on the treatment of cystinuria. Br J Urol 27:317–332, 1955.
10. Ettinger B, Kolb FO: Factors involved in crystal formation in cystinuria: In vivo and in vitro crystallization dynamics and a simple, quantitative colorimetric assay for cystine. J Urol 106:106–110, 1971.
11. Pak CYC, Fuller CJ: Assessment of cystine solubility in urine and of heterogeneous nucleation. Invest Urol 129:1066–1070, 1983.
12. Sakhaee K, Poindexter JR, Pak CYC: The spectrum of metabolic abnormalities in patients with cystine nephrolithiasis. J Urol 141:819–821, 1989.

13. Broadus AE, Thier SO: Metabolic basis of renal-stone disease. N Engl J Med 300:839–845, 1979.
14. Miyagi K, Nakada S, Ohshiro D: Effect of glutamine on cystine excretion in a patient with cystinuria. N Engl J Med 301:196–198, 1979.
15. Van den Berg K, Jones JD, Wilson DM, Smith LH: Glutamine therapy of cystinuria. Invest Urol 18:155–157, 1980.
16. Jaeger P, Portmann L, Saunders A, et al: Anticystinuric effects of glutamine and of dietary sodium restriction. N Engl J Med 315:1120–1123, 1986.
17. Rosenberg LE, Downing S, Durant JL, Segal S: Cystinuria: Biochemical evidence for three genetically distinct diseases. J Clin Invest 45:365–371, 1966.
18. Brand E, Harris MM, Biloon S: Cystinuria: Excretion of a cystine complex which decomposes in the urine with the liberation of free cystine. J Biol Chem 86:315, 1930.
19. Kolb FO, Earll JM, Harper HA: "Disappearance" of cystinuria in a patient treated with prolonged low methionine diet. Metabolism 16:378–381, 1967.
20. Dent CE, Friedmann M, Green H, Watson LCA: Treatment of cystinuria. Br Med J 1:403, 1965.
21. Sakhaee K, Nicar M, Hill K, Pak CYC: Contrasting effects of potassium citrate and sodium citrate therapies on urinary chemistries and crystallization of stone-forming salt. Kidney Int 24:348–352, 1983.
22. Pak CYC, Sakhaee K, Fuller C: Successful management of uric acid nephrolithiasis with potassium citrate. Kidney Int 30:422–428, 1986.
23. Pak CYC, Skurla C, Brinkley L, Sakhaee K: Augmentation of renal citrate excretion by oral potassium citrate administration: Time course, dose frequency schedule and dose response relationship. J Clin Pharmacol 24:19–26, 1984.
24. Dahlberg PJ, Van den Berg CJ, Kurtz SB, et al: Clinical features and management of cystinuria. Mayo Clin Proc 52:533–542, 1977.
25. Linari F, Marangella M, Fruttero B, Bruno M: The natural history of crystinuria: A 15 year follow-up in 106 patients. *In* Smith LH, Robertson WG, Finlayson B (eds).: Urolithiasis: Clinical and Basic Research. New York, Plenum Press, 1981, p 145.
26. Sloand JA, Izzo JL: Captopril reduces urinary cystine excretion in cystinuria. Arch Intern Med 147:1409–1412, 1987.

Miscellaneous Stones

10

Charles Y.C. Pak

In Chapters 3 to 9, prominent or well-recognized causes of nephrolithiasis were considered. This chapter discusses rare types of stones and less well known causes of stones. Rare forms of stones composed of 2,8-dihydroxyadenine and xanthine are due to inborn errors of metabolism. Some stones (triamterene, silica) are a direct result of treatment. Less well known or discussed causes of stones include medullary sponge kidney, hypomagnesiuric calcium nephrolithiasis, stone disease of pregnancy, and childhood nephrolithiasis.

2,8-DIHYDROXYADENINE STONES

Normally, adenine (e.g., from a dietary source) is reutilized by conversion to adenylic acid by adenine phosphoribosyl transferase (APRT); it is not metabolized to adenosine. In 2,8-dihydroxyadenuria, there is a deficiency of the APRT enzyme occurring as an inborn error of metabolism.[1–3] With the normal salvage pathway blocked, the accumulated adenine is oxidized by xanthine oxidase (xo) to 8-hydroxyadenine and to 2,8-dihydroxyadenine (Fig. 10–1). Thus, 2,8-dihydroxyadenine, which is not a normal purine metabolite, appears in substantial amounts in urine. Because of its low aqueous solubility, 2,8-dihydroxyadenine precipitates out of urine, leading to stone formation.

There is a certain analogy between 2,8-dihydroxyadeninuria and the Lesch-Nyhan syndrome.[4] In the latter syndrome, the block in the conversion of hypoxanthine and guanine to their respective nucleotides by a deficiency of the enzyme hypoxanthine-guanine phosphoribosyl transferase (HGPRT) leads to the accumulation of hypoxanthine (Fig. 10–1) (see Chapter 7). The oxidation of hypoxanthine by xanthine oxidase leads to uric acid overproduction and stones. Both 2,8-dihydroxyadenine and uric acid stones are radiolucent, and the stone disease appears during early childhood in both syndromes. The treatment with allopurinol, a xanthine oxidase inhibitor, reduces the renal excretion of both purine metabolites.

However, certain differences exist. Whereas uric acid solubility is pH dependent (see Chapters 5 and 7), the solubility of 2,8-dihydroxyadenine is independent of pH within the physiologic range.[3] Thus, alkali therapy, which is useful in uric acid lithiasis, may actually exaggerate the course of 2,8-dihydroxyadenine stone disease. Whereas uric acid stones are smooth and pale yellow, stones of 2,8-dihydroxyadenine are rough, friable, and pale gray in appearance. The enzymatic technique for uric acid will not detect 2,8-dihydroxyadenine, and the colorimetric assay cannot distinguish the two purine metabolites. The stones of 2,8-dihydroxyadenine could be differentiated from those of uric acid by infrared spectrophotometry.

The condition of 2,8-dihydroxyadeninuria is an extremely rare disorder, with the incidence of heterozygosity placed at 0.5 to 1 per cent. Its only clinical manifestation is nephrolithiasis. Urate metabolism is intact. This condition should be suspected in any children with radiolucent stones. The only known treatment is allopurinol without alkali.

Xanthine Stones

Xanthine stones occur in about one third of patients with classic xanthinuria.[5] Classic xanthinuria is an inborn error of metabolism inherited as an autosomal recessive trait, characterized by the deficiency of xanthine oxidase. Thus, the oxidation of hypoxanthine to xanthine, and of xanthine to uric acid, is blocked (Fig. 10–1). Uric acid synthesis is severely impaired, resulting in very low serum and urinary uric acid values of 0 to 1.4 mg/dl and 0 to 8 mg/day, respectively. Conversely, the serum concentration and renal excretion of xanthine and hypoxanthine are dramatically increased. Stones of xanthine rather than hypoxanthine develop, because of the lower aqueous solubility of xanthine. In some patients, crystals of xanthine and hypoxanthine may be deposited in muscle, causing muscle cramps during exercise.

Xanthinuria may be diagnosed by radiolucency of the stone and severe hypouricemia and hypouricosuria. A high fluid intake is generally effective in controlling xanthine stone formation. When this conservative program is ineffective, allopurinol has been recommended. By inhibiting residual xanthine oxidase

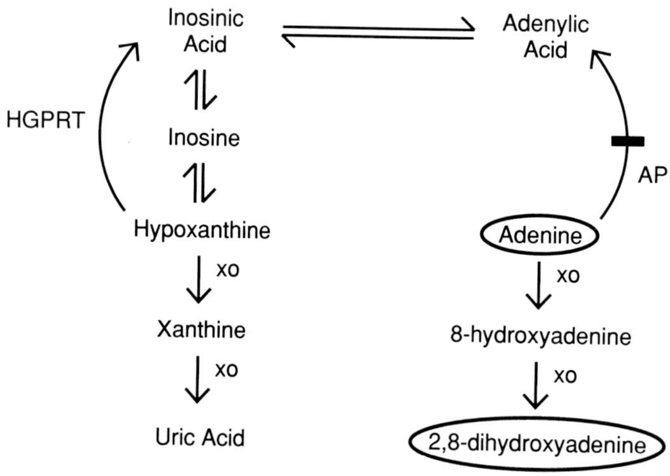

FIGURE 10–1. The metabolic pathway leading to 2,8-dihydroxyadenine.

activity, this paradoxical use of allopurinol may reduce xanthine excretion in favor of more soluble hypoxanthine excretion.

Enhanced renal excretion of xanthine and hypoxanthine is also encountered during allopurinol therapy. However, the degree of xanthinuria is far less than that found in classic xanthinuria, since allopurinol only partially inhibits xanthine oxidase at the customary dose and rarely reduces serum and urinary urate levels below 3 mg/dl and 250 mg/day, respectively. Thus, xanthine stone formation is a highly unlikely event during allopurinol therapy.

"IATROGENIC" STONES

Triamterene Stones

Triamterene is a potassium-sparing diuretic that is widely used in combination with hydrochlorothiazide for the management of fluid retention, hypertension, and hypercalciuric calcium nephrolithiasis. The presence of triamterene and its metabolite has been reported in stones passed by patients taking this drug.[6–8]

Up to 70 per cent of orally administered triamterene appears in urine, about 15 per cent in its native form, and 85 per cent as its phenolic metabolite, 6-parahydroxytriamterene. The low aqueous solubility of triamterene and its metabolite accounts for their presence in stones.

Ettinger and coworkers[6] found triamterene in 181 stones from 50,000 stones submitted to a commercial laboratory for stone analysis, for an estimated incidence of the complication of 1 per 1500 triamterene users. Triamterene was the sole or predominant component in 65 of 181 stones (36 per cent). In the remaining stones, where it occurred as a mixture with calcium oxalate or uric acid, triamterene was often present as the nucleus. Thirty-five per cent of patients who passed mixed stones containing triamterene and 19 per cent of those with pure triamterene stones had a past history of forming uric acid or calcium oxalate stones. These results suggested that triamterene could cause stones de novo or complicate the course of uric acid or calcium oxalate nephrolithiasis.

However, in a study of a large number of subjects enrolled in a prepaid health maintenance organization,[7] the incidence of hospitalization for renal stones was 0.052 per cent, not different from that encountered in those receiving hydrochlorothiazide alone of 0.055 per cent, or in the general population of 0.036 per cent. Moreover, triamterene was shown to be devoid of a promotive role in calcium oxalate crystallization.[9]

Nevertheless, it is clear that triamterene could add to a stone burden owing to its low solubility even when it occurs as adventitious deposits. Recently, unusual casts containing crystals have been found in the urine of approximately one half of patients taking triamterene, suggestive of the development of interstitial nephritis.[10] Moreover, the need for triamterene in the management of hypercalciuric nephrolithiasis has become less acute with the availability of amiloride and potassium citrate. Amiloride not only is potassium sparing, but also may itself lower urinary calcium or augment the hypocalciuric action of thiazide[11] (see Chapter 3). Potassium citrate enhances citrate (inhibitor) excretion, as well as prevents hypokalemia[12] (see Chapter 6). Thus, the use of triamterene among patients with nephrolithiasis should be discouraged.

Silica Stones

It is well known that cattle grazing in sandy areas could form silica stones. In human beings, silica stones are distinctly rare, appearing only in those taking antacids containing silicates (e.g., magnesium trisilicate).[13]

Normally, the renal excretion of silica is only 10 mg/day, representing about 5 per cent of 200 mg/day that is ingested (from vegetables, whole grains, and seafoods). This amount of silica is too low to cause stones. However, the urinary content of silica could approach 500 mg/day in subjects taking magnesium trisilicate. A large amount of silica (silicon dioxide, the major component of sand) could be formed upon the reaction of trisilicate with gastric acid. The subsequent absorption and renal excretion of silica could lead to its supersaturation and crystallization in urine.

Silica stones are radiolucent. However, they have a spiky jackstone appearance, confusing their identification with that of calcium oxalate stones. The only known treatment is the cessation of silicate therapy.

OTHER CAUSES OF STONES

Medullary Sponge Kidney

Medullary sponge kidney is an anatomic abnormality confined to the medullary portion of the kidneys. It is characterized by ectasia of the collecting ducts with small cysts. This condition is detected on intravenous pyelogram as the characteristic "paintbrush" appearance surrounding enlarged papillae, reflecting delayed drainage of dye from dilated tubules into pyramids. In its fully developed form, easily recognizable on a routine intravenous pyelogram, medullary sponge disease has been reported in 2 to 5 per cent of patients with renal calculi.[14] When special care is taken (using infusion nephrotomography and a small focal spot), medullary sponge disease has been detected in a much larger percentage (20 per cent) of patients with renal calculi, probably reflecting disclosure of milder forms of tubular ectasia.[15] The prevalence of medullary sponge kidney in the general population is unknown. The medullary sponge disease is usually diagnosed as an incidental finding in patients undergoing intravenous pyelography for a renal disease (usually stones or infection). It is likely that tubular ectasia is also present in a substantial number of subjects without symptoms or disease involving the urinary tract.

In stone-forming patients with medullary sponge kidney, several abnormalities have been reported, including primary hyperparathyroidism,[16, 17] hypercalciuria,[14, 18, 19] impaired urinary concentration ability, and defective urinary acidification. A major point of controversy has concerned the question of whether these disturbances resulted from tubular ectasia or represent epiphenomena.

Yendt has proposed that tubular ectasia may cause partial renal resistance to parathyroid hormone (PTH), producing the picture of renal hypercalciuria.[15] With prolonged parathyroid stimulation, hypercalcemic hyperparathyroidism could occur. In support of this hypothesis, Dlabal and associates[18] reported a case of a patient with medullary sponge kidney who had the clinical picture of renal hypercalciuria documented by the correction of hypercalciuria and parathyroid stimulation with thiazide. Maschio and colleagues found primary hyperparathyroidism in 36 per cent and renal hypercalciuria in 29 per cent of patients with medullary sponge kidney.[19]

In contrast, studies at Dallas[14] and at Chicago[20] disclosed that the patients with medullary sponge kidney and renal stones had the same spectrum of biochemical abnormalities as the overall population of stone formers or those without tubular ectasia. The renal leak hypothesis for the genesis of primary hyperparathyroidism is not supported by the usual finding of adenoma rather than hyperplasia in abnormal parathyroid tissue and by the long-term correction of hypercalciuria and amelioration of stone disease following surgery. The high prevalence of medullary sponge kidney in patients with stones cannot be strictly invoked for the causal role of tubular ectasia in nephrolithiasis, without knowing the prevalence data in the general population.

Thus, we would favor the view that medullary sponge kidney represents a congenital anatomic abnormality and that it is generally not a cause for metabolic derangements responsible for stone disease. It could, however, contribute to urinary tract infection and exaggerate stone disease.

Hypomagnesiuric Calcium Nephrolithiasis

There is conflicting literature regarding magnesium excretion among patients with nephrolithiasis, some reports showing reduced urinary magnesium but others reporting normal values. In an extensive series of more than 1000 patients carefully evaluated at Dallas, hypomagnesiuria with calcium stones was detected in 4.3 per cent of patients.[21]

This entity (termed hypomagnesiuric calcium nephrolithiasis), occurring in the absence of bowel disease (chronic diarrheal syndrome or malabsorption), is probably dietary in origin, for the following reasons. Magnesium metabolism, including intestinal absorption, has been reported to be normal in patients with "idiopathic" calcium nephrolithiasis.[22] In the study at Dallas, hypomagnesiuric patients gave a history of avoidance of magnesium-rich chocolates and nuts.[21] This dietary habit was probably imposed as a part of a general dietary oxalate restriction, as these food items are also rich in oxalate.

In the series at Dallas, 67 per cent of patients with hypomagnesiuria also had hypocitraturia.[21] This concurrent abnormality is probably dietary in origin as well, since many patients gave a history of a low intake of citrus fruit products.

The calcium stone formation in hypomagnesiuric patients may be attributed to the loss of "inhibitor" activity of magnesium. Magnesium complexes oxalate, thereby reducing ionic oxalate concentration and the saturation of calcium oxalate.[23] It has only a modest inhibitory effect on the crystal growth of calcium oxalate. This background probably accounts for the apparent clinical utility of magnesium oxide and magnesium hydroxide in the prevention of recurrent calcium oxalate stone formation.

Recent studies at Dallas suggest that magnesium citrate may be ideally indicated for the treatment of hypomagnesiuric calcium nephrolithiasis.[24] Compared with magnesium oxide, magnesium citrate has a much higher solubility from the intestinal tract. Moreover, by providing citrate, it is capable of overcoming hypocitraturia, which often accompanies this disorder.

Stone Disease During Pregnancy

The formation of renal stones during pregnancy is a potentially troublesome event, because of the risk of infection and the possible need for urologic instrumentation and surgical intervention. However, Coe and associates reported that stone disease "had no adverse effects upon pregnancy other than an increase in urinary infections."[25] In 78 stone-forming women of childbearing age, they examined their records for complications of pregnancy before and following the onset of stone disease. The frequency of premature delivery, spontaneous abortion, hypertensive complications, caesarean section, or gestational diabetes was equivalent when the same subjects had stones as when they were free of stones. However, infection of the urinary tract was three times more common.

A finding of considerable interest was the disclosure that the frequency of stone disease was not altered during pregnancy.[25] It is now clear that pregnancy elicits changes in various urinary risk factors for stones. However, these changes occur in opposite directions. On the one hand, an intestinal hyperabsorption of calcium could occur from the placental production of 1,25-$(OH)_2$vitamin D.[26, 27] Thus, a marked hypercalciuria could develop, especially following customary dietary calcium supplementation. On the other hand, there is substantial enhancement of the renal excretion of citrate and glycoproteins (nephrocalcin) during pregnancy.[28] Thus, the promotive effect of hypercalciuria on stone formation is opposed by the inhibitory effect of citrate and nephrocalcin.

Childhood Nephrolithiasis

It has been customary to attribute nephrolithiasis occurring in children to inherited disorders such as primary hyperoxaluria or cystinuria. However, it is becoming increasingly clear that hypercalciuria constitutes a major cause of stones in the pediatric population. Hypercalciuria was encountered in 53 per cent of children with calcium stones in the series of Moore and colleagues[29] and 81 per cent in the series by Stapleton and associates.[30]

As in adults, the hypercalciuria in children is heterogeneous in origin. From a group of 20 children with calcium nephrolithiasis, Moore and colleagues[29] concluded that 7 had renal hypercalciuria, since they had high serum PTH levels, which decreased upon thiazide therapy. Hymes and Warshaw[31] found that 3 of 12 hypercalciuric children had an increased fasting urinary calcium and cyclic adenosine monophosphate (cAMP), indicative of renal hypercalciuria. Four had absorptive hypercalciuria, since they had normal fasting urinary calcium and an exaggerated calciuric response to an oral calcium load. However, five children had fasting hypercalciuria with normal urinary cAMP. In the series of Stapleton and coworkers, 4 of 17 with hypercalciuria had absorptive hypercalciuria.[30] The remaining 13 had fasting hypercalciuria but normal serum PTH values. Thus, as in adult patients with hypercalciuric calcium nephrolithiasis (see Chapter 3), a substantial number of children with hypercalciuria presented with fasting hypercalciuria and normal parathyroid function. Further studies have not been done to isolate subgroups within this presentation (see Chapter 3). Thiazide is the treatment of choice for the hypercalciuric nephrolithiasis of children, regardless of type.

Several reports have appeared showing that hypercalciuria is present in children with gross or microscopic hematuria, without proteinuria, urinary tract infection, or stones.[32–34] The correction of hypercalciuria by thiazide resolved hematuria. Some patients with hematuria eventually progressed to develop renal stones. The exact physicochemical background by which hypercalciuria might cause hematuria is unknown.

REFERENCES

1. Barratt TM, Simmonds HA, Cameron JS, et al: Complete deficiency of adenine phosphoribosyltransferase. Arch Dis Child 54:25–31, 1979.
2. Simmonds HA, Van Acker KJ, Cameron JS, Snedden W: The identification of 2,8-dihydroxyadenine, a new component of urinary stones. Biochem J 157:485–487, 1976.
3. Simmonds HA, Sahota A, Rose GA, et al: Adenine phosphoribosyltransferase deficiency presenting with supposed "uric acid" stones: Pitfalls of diagnosis. J R Soc Med 71:791–795, 1978.
4. Nyhan WL: The Lesch-Nyhan syndrome. Adv Nephrol 3:59–70, 1973.
5. Wyngaarden JB: Xanthinuria. *In* Stanbury JB, Wyngaarden JB, Fredrickson DS (eds).: The Metabolic Basis of Inherited Disease. 3rd ed. New York, McGraw-Hill, 1972, pp 992–1002.
6. Ettinger B, Oldroyd NO, Sorgel F: Triamterene nephrolithiasis. JAMA 244:2443–2446, 1980.
7. Jick H, Dinan BJ, Huanter JR: Triamterene and renal stones. J Urol 127:224–225, 1982.
8. Patel KM: Triamterene nephrolithiasis complicating Dyazide therapy. J Urol 126:230–231, 1981.
9. Werness PG, Bergert JH, Smith LH: Triamterene urolithiasis: Solubility, pK, effect on crystal formation, and matrix binding of triamterene and its metabolites. J Lab Clin Med 99(2):254–262, 1982.
10. Spence JD, Wong DG, Lindsay RM: Effects of triamterene and amiloride on urinary sediment in hypertensive patients taking hydrochlorothiazide. Lancet 2:73–74, 1985.
11. Leppla D, Browne R, Hill K, Pak CYC: Effect of amiloride with or without hydrochlorothiazide on urinary calcium and saturation of calcium salts. J Clin Endocrinol Metab 57:920–924, 1983.
12. Pak CYC: Citrate and renal calculi. Miner Electrolyte Metab 13:257–266, 1987.
13. Levison DA, Banim S, Crocker PR, Wallace DMA: Silica stones in the urinary bladder. Lancet 1:704–705, 1982.
14. O'Neill M, Breslau NA, Pak CYC: Metabolic evaluation of nephrolithiasis in patients with medullary sponge kidney. JAMA 245:1233–1236, 1981.
15. Yendt ER, Jarzylo S, Finnis WA, Cohanim M: Medullary sponge kidney (tubular ectasia) in calcium urolithiasis. *In* Smith LH, Robertson WG, Finlayson B (eds).: Urolithiasis. New York, Plenum Press, 1981, pp 105–112.
16. Rao DS, Frame B, Block MA, Parfitt AM: Primary hyperparathyroidism: A cause of hypercalciuria and renal stones in patients with medullary sponge kidney. JAMA 237:1353–1355, 1977.
17. Gremillion DH, Kee JW, McIntosh DA: Hyperparathyroidism and medullary sponge kidney. JAMA 237:799–800, 1977.
18. Dlabal PW, Jordan RM, Dorfman SG: Medullary sponge kidney and renal-leak hypercalciuria: A link to the development of parathyroid adenoma? JAMA 241:1490–1491, 1979.
19. Maschio G, Tessitore N, D'Angelo A, et al: Medullary sponge kidney and hyperparathyroidism: A puzzling association. Am J Nephrol 2:77–84, 1982.
20. Parks JH, Coe FL, Strauss AL: Calcium nephrolithiasis and medullary sponge kidney in women. N Engl J Med 306:1088–1091, 1982.
21. Preminger GM, Baker S, Peterson R, et al: Hypomagnesiuric hypocitraturia: An apparent new entity for calcium nephrolithiasis. J Lith Stone Dis 1:22–25, 1989.
22. Danielson BG, Johansson G, Jung B, et al: Gastrointestinal magnesium absorption. Miner Electrolyte Metab 2:116–123, 1979.
23. Meyer JL, Smith LH: Growth of calcium oxalate crystals. Invest Urol 13:36–39, 1975.
24. Lindberg JS, Zobitz MM, Poindexter JR, Pak CYC: Magnesium bioavailability from magnesium citrate and magnesium oxide. J Am Coll Nutr, (accepted for publication).
25. Coe FL, Parks JH, Lindheimer MD: Nephrolithiasis during pregnancy. N Engl J Med 298:324–326, 1978.
26. Zerwekh JE, Breslau NA: Human placental production of 1α,25-dihydroxyvitamin D_3: Biochemical characterization and production in normal subjects and patients with pseudohypoparathyroidism. J Clin Endocrinol Metab 62:192–196, 1986.
27. Gertner JM, Coustan DR, Kliger AS, et al: Pregnancy as state of physiologic absorptive hypercalciuria. Am J Med 81:451–456, 1986.
28. Harvey JA, Zobitz MM, Pak CYC: The relationship of estrogen and progesterone to urinary citrate excretion. J Lith Stone Dis 1:204–208, 1989.
29. Moore ES, Langman CB, Favus MJ, et al: Secondary hyperparathyroidism in children with symptomatic idiopathic hypercalciuria. J Pediatr 103:932–935, 1983.
30. Stapleton FB, Noe HN, Roy S III, Jerkins G: Hypercalciuria in children with urolithiasis. Am J Dis Child 136:675–677, 1982.
31. Hymes LC, Warshaw BL: Idiopathic hypercalciuria. Am J Dis Child 138:176–180, 1984.
32. Stapleton FB, Roy S III, Noe HN, Jerkins G: Hypercalciuria in children with hematuria. N Engl J Med 310:1345–1348, 1984.
33. Roy S III, Stapleton FB, Noe HN, Jerkins G: Hematuria preceding renal calculus formation in children with hypercalciuria. J Pediatr 99:712–715, 1981.
34. Kalia A, Travis LB, Brouhard BH: The association of idiopathic hypercalciuria and asymptomatic gross hematuria in children. J Pediatr 99:716–719, 1981.

11

General Guidelines in Medical Evaluation

Charles Y.C. Pak

Considerable progress has been made in the differentiation of causes of nephrolithiasis. Stones can now be analyzed reliably by several commercial laboratories. Methods are available for the analysis of a wide variety of risk factors in urine. Besides elucidation of many metabolic disturbances, environmental and nutritional influences on stone formation are better understood. Reliable diagnostic protocols are available, adaptable for those with a single stone episode or those with active recurrent stone formation, involving an extensive or a relatively simple evaluation.

This chapter first considers the diagnostic value of stone composition and discusses pertinent aspects of history taking, especially as it relates to dietary abuses, which might be etiologically important in stone formation. Diagnostic protocols are then described.

HISTORICAL CONSIDERATIONS

Rapid advances in diagnostic evaluation may be illustrated by changes that have occurred in the author's own laboratory.

In 1968, a diagnostic evaluation for stones lasted 2 weeks and entailed measurement of intestinal calcium absorption (by forearm counting of radiocalcium)[1] and urinary calcium in patients on a constant dietary regimen, as well as an indirect assessment of parathyroid function from changes in phosphate excretion following calcium infusion.[2] No simple and reliable methods for assessing serum parathyroid hormone (PTH), urinary oxalate, and citrate were available; urinary uric acid was not determined.

In 1972, stone disease was considered to comprise three main entities: primary hyperparathyroidism, idiopathic hypercalciuria, and normocalciuric nephrolithiasis.[3] The last was a miscellaneous category that included causes of noncalcareous calculi.

In 1972, an immunoassay for serum PTH was established in the laboratory.

In 1974, the hypercalciuria of nephrolithiasis was classified into three major forms: absorptive, renal, and resorptive.[4]

In 1975, a fasting and oral calcium load test was developed to facilitate differentiation of hypercalciurias.[5] Routine analysis of urinary oxalate and uric acid was implemented.

In 1979, a routine assay for urinary citrate was instituted.

In 1980, an ambulatory protocol for the medical evaluation of nephrolithiasis was reported.[6] This evaluation allowed classification of nephrolithiasis into 11 causes. No "metabolic" abnormality was identified in 10.8 per cent of patients.

In 1985, a reliable urine preservation and collection kit, permitting analysis of available urinary risk factors and display of results in a graphic format, was introduced.[7]

In 1988, refinement of the ambulatory protocol permitted differentiation of stone disease into 18 causes (see Chapter 1).[8] No abnormality was detected in only 3 per cent of patients.

DIAGNOSTIC VALUE OF STONE COMPOSITION

The diagnosis of different causes of nephrolithiasis is no longer made solely on the basis of stone composition, because of increasing reliance on underlying physiologic derangements. However, stone analysis is still important and should be obtained in every stone-forming patient if a sample is available (Table 11–1).

Radiologic Appearance

Radiopaque stones include those containing calcium oxalate, calcium phosphate, and struvite. Cystine stones are also radiopaque, though less dense. Radiolucent stones include those composed solely of uric acid, 2,8-dihydroxyadenine, triamterene, xanthine, and silica. Uric acid stones may have a faint radiopacity because of the incorporation of calcium salts.

The morphologic appearance of radiopaque stones may provide clues to

TABLE 11–1. VALUE OF STONE COMPOSITION

STONE TYPE	ETIOLOGY
Radiopaque Stones	
Calcium oxalate	Hypercalciuria, hyperoxaluria, hyperuricosuria, hypocitraturia, hypomagnesiuria
Calcium phosphate (hydroxyapatite)	Primary hyperparathyroidism, renal tubular acidosis, sodium alkali therapy
Struvite or carbonate apatite	Urinary tract infection with urea-splitting organisms
Cystine	Cystinuria
Radiolucent Stones	
Uric acid	Gouty diathesis, hyperuricosuria, chronic diarrheal syndrome, dehydration
2,8-Dihydroxyadenine	2,8-Dihydroxyadeninuria
Triamterene	Triamterene therapy
Xanthine	Xanthinuria
Silica	Magnesium trisilicate therapy

their mineral composition or to the underlying disease process. Cystine stones are moderately dense and have a homogeneous rounded appearance. Struvite stones are more dense but also tend to have a rounded appearance. Cystine and struvite stones may reach staghorn size. Calcium oxalate stones often have a dense, spiculated appearance.

Cortical nephrocalcinosis suggests the diagnosis of primary hyperoxaluria. Medullary nephrocalcinosis is encountered in distal renal tubular acidosis and primary hyperparathyroidism. Medullary nephrocalcinosis should be distinguished from medullary sponge disease (Chapter 10), which represents focal dilatation of the collecting ducts containing small calcific deposits, rather than calcification in renal parenchyma.

Stone Composition

The diagnosis of stone disease is sometimes made on the basis of stone composition. Thus, the disclosure of cystine and struvite or carbonate apatite is diagnostic of cystinuria and infection with urea-splitting organisms, respectively. The presence of 2,8-dihydroxyadenine, triamterene, silica, or xanthine indicates 2,8-dihydroxyadeninuria, treatment with triamterene or magnesium trisilicate, or xanthinuria (see Chapter 10). In these conditions, the crystallographic identification is critical for the diagnosis; laboratory and clinical data provide supporting evidence.

For the remaining stones, stone composition is helpful but not conclusive for diagnosis of the underlying disease. The finding of uric acid in stones suggests undue acidity of urine or high urinary urate concentration (see Chapter 7). However, it cannot distinguish whether the stone originates from gouty diathesis or chronic diarrheal syndrome. Stones composed predominantly of hydroxyapatite could arise from distal renal tubular acidosis (see Chapter 6), primary hyperparathyroidism (see Chapter 3), or a complication of chronic sodium alkali therapy. Calcium oxalate stones could be due to a wide variety of disorders, including hypercalciuria, hyperoxaluria, hyperuricosuria, hypocitraturia, and hypomagnesiuria.

HISTORY TAKING

A careful history should be taken during the evaluation of the stone-forming patient, since it may provide clues to the underlying cause or causes of stone formation. It should include relevant demographic data, medications taken or treatments received, concurrent or other illnesses, and nutritional habits.

Demographic Data

Important demographic information that should be taken from every stone-forming patient includes sex, race, and age (current and at onset of stone disease).

Absorptive hypercalciuria and hyperuricosuric calcium nephrolithiasis are more common in men than in women and are rare among the black population. Most commonly afflicted are middle-aged white men. Renal hypercalciuria has less male preponderance than the above-mentioned conditions. Many give a history of urinary tract infection prior to stone disease. Primary hyperparathyroidism is more common in women than in men, with postmenopausal women being most prone.

Enteric hyperoxaluria and infection lithiasis are more common in women than in men. Cystinuria affects the two sexes equally. Uric acid lithiasis due to primary gout is much more common in men, but that resulting from gastrointestinal disease affects women more. Calcium oxalate stone disease in children should suggest the idiopathic hypercalciuria of childhood or primary hyperoxaluria. The latter condition should be distinguished by evidence of oxalosis and renal failure.

Some stone-forming conditions have a genetic predisposition. A careful family study of absorptive hypercalciuria has disclosed an autosomal dominant mode of inheritance. In descendants of the index patient spanning three generations, intestinal hyperabsorption of calcium was found in every relative tested.[9] Stone formation did not occur in all descendants, however, suggesting the requirement of both environmental and genetic influences for the development of clinical disease.

Medications

Certain medications could cause or exaggerate stone disease; a careful history should be obtained for all medications taken (Table 11–2).

Acetazolamide, a carbonic anhydrase inhibitor now used mainly for glaucoma and altitude sickness, induces metabolic acidosis with hypercalciuria, hypocitraturia, and high urinary pH.[10] It may cause development of calcium stones composed of calcium phosphate and calcium oxalate.

Vitamin C supplementation could augment oxalate excretion (see Chapter 4) and, in large doses, could increase urinary calcium as well. Calcium supplements, vitamin D preparations, and phosphorus-binding antacids (such as aluminum hydroxide) could raise urinary calcium. The hypercalciuric action of aluminum-binding antacids has been attributed to the reduced gastrointestinal binding of calcium by phosphate (due to aluminum phosphate precipitation), making more calcium available for absorption, and stimulated synthesis of 1,25-$(OH)_2$vitamin D (from hypophosphatemia). Theophylline and some calcium channel blockers may increase urinary calcium by a poorly understood mechanism.[11]

Triamterene therapy may result in deposition of this poorly soluble drug as a sole or a mixed stone (see Chapter 10). Though rare, allopurinol treatment may cause xanthine crystalluria (see Chapter 10). Uricosuric agents (such as

TABLE 11–2. STONE-PROVOKING MEDICATIONS

Medication	Stone Type	Mechanisms
Acetazolamide	Calcium phosphate, calcium oxalate	Metabolic acidosis with hypercalciuria, hypocitraturia
Vitamin C	Calcium oxalate	Hyperoxaluria
Calcium supplements and vitamin D preparations	Calcium oxalate, calcium phosphate	Hypercalciuria
Phosphorus-binding antacids	Calcium oxalate	Hypercalciuria
Theophylline and calcium channel blockers	Calcium oxalate, calcium phosphate	Hypercalciuria
Triamterene	Triamterene	Urinary excretion of triamterene
Uricosuric agents	Uric acid	Hyperuricosuria

probenecid) may produce transient hyperuricosuria (see Chapter 7). Marked hyperuricosuria could result during chemotherapy of malignancy owing to tissue catabolism.

A careful history should also be taken for past medical treatments of stone disease. Their failure may indicate inaccuracy of the original diagnosis or a need for a more specific therapy.

Concurrent or Other Illnesses

Renal stones may be a complication of other diseases. A careful history should be taken for them. Patients with gouty arthritis may have uric acid or calcium nephrolithiasis (see Chapter 7). Chronic diarrheal states may also cause both types of stones (see Chapter 6). They include gastric resection, pancreatitis, pancreatectomy, malabsorption, regional enteritis, blind loop syndrome, small bowel resection, and ulcerative colitis. The association of primary hyperparathyroidism with nephrolithiasis is well known (see Chapter 3). Relevant history includes pathologic skeletal fractures, peptic ulcer disease, the presence or symptoms of hypercalcemia, and neck surgery indicative of parathyroid surgery. Chronic urinary tract infection may be responsible for infection lithiasis (see Chapter 8). It may also cause tubular damage and may theoretically produce renal tubular acidosis and renal hypercalciuria. Moreover, persistent active urinary tract infection could exaggerate stone disease or cause resistance to certain treatment programs (e.g., potassium citrate and orthophosphate) by destroying urinary citrate and pyrophosphate. Useful history includes the nature of the offending organism (with urea-splitting capacity or not), age at onset, frequency of recurrence, and type of antibiotic used.

Nutritional Habit

A careful nutritional history should be taken, directing particular attention to estimated fluid intake and to ingestion of foods rich in calcium, oxalate, purines, sodium, and acid ash content. In addition, an inadequacy in the intake of fruits and magnesium should be noted. Though discussed in previous chapters, the pathogenetic role of various dietary factors in stone formation is now briefly reviewed.

Fluid Intake. Inadequate fluid intake resulting in low urine output represents one of the major risk factors, predisposing to all forms of stone disease. It enhances the urinary saturation of all stone-forming salts by increasing the concentration of constituents of the stone.[12]

The adequacy of fluid intake should be assessed relative to the estimated fluid loss occurring from sweating and bowel movements. Under normal circumstances, the "insensible loss" represents about 800 ml per day. Thus, approximately 2800 ml of total fluid must be ingested to produce a urine output of 2 liters/day. However, in an exercising individual with excessive sweating or in a patient suffering from diarrhea, much more fluid must be ingested to produce the same urine output. It is useful to obtain an estimate of total fluid intake as well as that of water. The total fluid intake includes water contained in solid food, estimated to be approximately 500 to 1000 ml/day.

Since fluids are most valuable for stone prevention if they are distributed throughout the day, a history should be taken for the customary time of ingestion of fluids.

CALCIUM. A high dietary intake of calcium may provoke hypercalciuria and stone formation in patients with intestinal hyperabsorption of calcium. A severe calcium restriction could cause hyperoxaluria (see Chapter 4).

Table 11–3 presents a list of calcium-rich food items and their approximate calcium content for an average serving. With use of this table, an approximate calcium intake may be obtained from an average weekly consumption of the food items obtained from the history. A more accurate intake may be derived from

TABLE 11–3. CALCIUM-RICH FOOD ITEMS

FOOD ITEM	SERVING (oz)	CALCIUM CONTENT (mg)
Low fat yogurt	1 cup (8 oz)	415
Milkshake	1 cup (8 oz)	362
Pizza, cheese	½ of 10-inch pizza	355
Eggnog, nonalcoholic	1 cup (8 oz)	330
Low fat yogurt with fruit	1 cup (8 oz)	314
Sardines, canned	½ cup (3½ oz)	303
Skimmed milk (½% fat)	1 cup (8 oz)	302
Whole milk	1 cup (8 oz)	291
Cheese soup made with milk	1 cup	288
Swiss cheese	1 slice (1 oz)	272
Red salmon	½ cup (3½ oz)	259
Ricotta	1 ounce	257
Soft serve ice milk	1 cup	236
Provolone	1 ounce	214
Cheddar cheese	1 slice (1 oz)	204
Pink salmon	½ cup (3½ oz)	196
Cheese sauce, homemade	¼ cup	178
Mushroom soup made with milk	1 cup	178
Ice cream or ice milk	1 cup	176
American cheese	1 slice (1 oz)	174
Tomato soup made with milk	1 cup	159
Mozzarella	1 ounce	147
Custard or pudding	½ cup	145
Mustard greens, cooked	½ cup	138
Cream pie	1 piece (⅛ pie)	137
Cottage cheese, creamed	1 cup (8 oz)	136
Sherbet	1 cup	96
Oysters, raw	5–8 medium	94
Broccoli, cooked	1 large stalk	88
Tofu	2 ounces	73
Cornbread	1 piece (2 oz)	65
Dock (sorrel), cooked	½ cup	55
Flour tortillas	1 each	46
Corn tortillas	1 each	42
½ & ½ cream	2 tablespoons	32
White bread	1 slice	30
Calcium may not be as well absorbed from these foods due to oxalate content:		
Cocoa from mix with milk	1 cup	298
Chocolate milk	1 cup (8 oz)	284
Collard greens, cooked	½ cup	152
Turnip greens, cooked	½ cup	138
Spinach, cooked	½ cup	107
Cocoa from mix with water	1 cup (8 oz)	107
Beet greens, cooked	½ cup	99
Okra, cooked	8–9 pods	92
Kale, cooked	½ cup	89
Milk chocolate bar	1 bar (1.02 oz)	55
Green beans, cooked	½ cup	31

an actual list and amount of all foods consumed during a 1-week period. An avoidance of all dairy products and dark roughages would generally leave a calcium intake of 400 to 600 mg/day.

It should be noted that the bioavailability of calcium differs considerably among different calcium-rich food items. For example, calcium from milk may be better absorbed by normal subjects than that from spinach by as much as 10-fold.[13, 14] Unfortunately, various food items cannot be quantitated with respect to their bioavailability, because of limited bioavailability data and expected variation in individual responses.

OXALATE. A high-oxalate diet could enhance oxalate excretion and contribute to or cause calcium oxalate stone formation.

A list of food items with a high oxalate content is given in Table 11–4. There

TABLE 11–4. OXALATE-RICH FOOD ITEMS

FOOD ITEM	SERVING (oz)	OXALATE CONTENT (mg)
Beet greens, cooked	½ cup	916
Purslane, leaves, cooked	½ cup	910
Rhubarb, stewed, no sugar	½ cup	860
Spinach, cooked	½ cup	750
Beets, cooked	½ cup	675
Chard, Swiss, leaves cooked	½ cup	660
Rhubarb, canned	½ cup	600
Spinach, frozen	½ cup	600
Beets, pickled	½ cup	500
Poke greens, cooked	½ cup	476
Endive, raw	20 long leaves	273
Cocoa, dry	⅓ cup	254
Dandelion greens, cooked	½ cup	246
Okra, cooked	8–9 pods	146
Potatoes, sweet, cooked	½ cup	141
Kale, cooked	½ cup	125
Peanuts, raw	⅓ cup (1¾ oz)	113
Turnip greens, cooked	½ cup	110
Chocolate, unsweetened	1 ounce	91
Parsnips, diced, cooked	½ cup	81
Collard greens, cooked	½ cup	74
Pecans, halves, raw	⅓ cup (1¼ oz)	74
Tea, leaves (4-min infusion)	1 level tsp in 7 oz water	72
Wheat germ, toasted	¼ cup	67
Gooseberries	½ cup	66
Potato, Idaho white, baked	1 medium	64
Carrots, cooked	½ cup	45
Apple, raw with skin	1 medium	41
Brussels sprouts, cooked	6–8 medium	37
Strawberries, raw	½ cup	35
Celery, raw	2 stalks	34
Milk chocolate bar	1 bar (1.02 oz)	34
Raspberries, black, raw	½ cup	33
Orange, edible portion	1 medium	24
Green beans, cooked	½ cup	23
Chives, raw, chopped	1 tablespoon	19
Leeks, raw	½ medium	15
Blackberries, raw	½ cup	13
Concord grapes	½ cup	13
Blueberries, raw	½ cup	11
Currants, red	½ cup	11
Apricots, raw	2 medium	10
Raspberries, red, raw	½ cup	10
Broccoli, cooked	1 large stalk	6
Cranberry juice	½ cup (4 oz)	6

is considerable variability in oxalate bioavailability among foodstuffs and between individual patients. Thus, an estimation of the total daily oxalate intake has a limited value. It is generally sufficient to obtain a qualitative judgment of whether oxalate intake is high and to identify an unusual preference for a specific oxalate-rich food, such as spinach.

PURINES. All meat products (beef, poultry, and fish) are rich in purines. If taken in excessive amounts, they could therefore cause hyperuricosuria and urate-induced crystallization of calcium salts in urine (see Chapter 5).

SODIUM. A high sodium intake could exaggerate stone disease by provoking sodium urate–induced calcium oxalate crystallization,[15] enhancing calcium excretion,[16] and sometimes reducing citrate excretion.

Sodium-rich food items are given in Table 11–5. Unfortunately, sodium intake calculated from such diet tables sometimes considerably underestimates the actual amount of sodium taken. It is not unusual to encounter a patient with a very high urinary sodium who professes to have avoided sodium-rich foods and salt shakers. This discrepancy may be due to the frequent use of prepared foods,

TABLE 11–5. SODIUM-RICH FOOD ITEMS

Food Item	Serving (oz)	Sodium Content mEq	Sodium Content (mEq range)
Teriyaki barbecue marinade	1 fluid ounce	198	
Salt	1 teaspoon	100	
Frozen dinners (all varieties)	1 each	76 avg.	(30–163)
Salt, onion	1 teaspoon	69	
Salt, celery	1 teaspoon	65	
Meats and fish, canned	3½ ounces	59 avg.	(27–191)
Salt, seasoning	1 teaspoon	56	
Soups, dehyd., reconstituted	1 cup	50 avg.	(32–144)
Pizza, cheese	½ of 10-inch	49	
Salt, Lite	1 teaspoon	48	
Soups, canned	1 cup	47 avg.	(28–168)
Soy sauce	1 tablespoon	45	
Smoked link sausage, pork	1 link (2½ oz)	44	
Pickles (all varieties)	1 large (3½ oz)	40 avg.	(22–62)
Cottage cheese, creamed	1 cup	37	
Vegetable juices, canned	1 cup (8 oz)	32	
Ham, cured, cooked	3½ ounces	31	
Monosodium glutamate	1 teaspoon	29	
Corn grits with imitation ham bits, instant	1 pkt (prepared)	29	
Frankfurter (all varieties)	1 frank (1½ oz)	22 average	
Sauerkraut	½ cup	22	
Bacon, Canadian, cooked	1 slice (1 oz)	19	
Cheese, processed	1 ounce	18 avg.	(17–19)
Gravies	¼ cup	16 avg.	(6–31)
Vegetables, canned with salt	½ cup	16 avg.	(5–29)
Sausage, pork, cooked	1 patty (1 oz)	15	
Bacon, cured, cooked	3 slices	15	
Salt pork, raw	1 ounce	15	
Cheese food, processed	1 ounce	14 avg.	(11–19)
Chips and snacks	1 ounce	14 avg.	(6–37)
Salami (all varieties)	1 slice (1 oz)	13 average	
Bologna (all varieties)	1 slice (1 oz)	12 average	
Cereals, ready-to-eat, salt added in processing	1 ounce	10 avg.	(4–15)
Cheeses, natural	1 ounce	9 avg.	(2–20)
Sauces and condiments	1 tbsp (½ oz)	9 avg.	(2–45)
Salad dressings, regular	1 tbsp (½ oz)	7 avg.	(3–14)
Peanut butter	2 tablespoons	7	

which are variably salted, as well as eating at restaurants where foods are often oversalted. A careful daily log of all foods consumed during a 1-week period might disclose the source of aberrant sodium intake.

ACID ASH CONTENT. Animal proteins are rich in sulfur-containing amino acids. When they are metabolized, sulfate is released. Thus, a high consumption of animal protein could reduce urinary citrate and pH, as well as augment urinary calcium and uric acid.[17]

Such food items are listed in Table 11–6. Most of the sulfur in food is available in an organic form (as sulfur-containing amino acids). Meat products are rich in sulfur, with no distinction between beef, poultry, and fish. Other

TABLE 11–6. FOOD ITEMS RICH IN ACID ASH CONTENT

FOOD ITEM	SERVING (oz)	SULFUR CONTENT (mmoles)
Goose	3½ ounces	9.95
Chicken	3½ ounces	9.29
Liver	3½ ounces	7.86
Crab	3½ ounces	7.77
Turkey	3½ ounces	7.20
Beef	3½ ounces	6.89
Haddock	3½ ounces	6.89
Pike	3½ ounces	6.67
Pork	3½ ounces	6.67
Venison	3½ ounces	6.16
Fish, all kinds	3½ ounces	6.11
Veal	3½ ounces	6.11
Mutton	3½ ounces	5.68
Rabbit	3½ ounces	5.68
Shrimp	3½ ounces	5.58
Frog	3½ ounces	5.02
Heart	3½ ounces	4.58
Kidney	3½ ounces	4.49
Mustard greens, cooked	½ cup	4.43
Brains	3½ ounces	4.05
Eel	3½ ounces	4.05
Broccoli, cooked	1 large stalk	3.93
Eggs, whole	1 large	3.65
Corn, mature	½ cup	3.49
Blackeyed peas, dried, cooked	½ cup	3.37
Kale, cooked	½ cup	3.34
Brussels sprouts	6–8 medium	3.06
Beans, dried, cooked	½ cup	3.03
Peanuts	1 ounce	2.40
Peas, mature, cooked	½ cup	2.40
Egg white	white of 1 large egg	2.18
Wheat bran	1 ounce	2.15
Lima beans, dried, cooked	½ cup	2.12
Cabbage, cooked	½ cup	1.90
Cheese, hard	1 ounce	1.87
Oatmeal (rolled oats), cooked	1 oz dry = ¾ cup ckd	1.81
Cocoa	1 ounce	1.72
Lentils, dry, cooked	½ cup	1.65
Asparagus	½ cup	1.59
Soybeans, mature, cooked	½ cup	1.59
Almonds	1 ounce	1.43
Macaroni, dry, cooked	½ cup	1.40
Barley	1 ounce	1.34
Cauliflower	½ cup	1.31
Egg yolk	yolk of 1 large egg	1.12
Rice, polished, dry, cooked	1 oz dry = ¾ cup ckd	1.12
Chocolate	1 ounce	1.00
Currants	1 ounce	0.90

sulfur-rich foods include eggs, hard cheese, nuts, beans, peas, and oatmeal. Thus, a limited intake of meat products alone may not eliminate sulfur excess.

Citrus Fruit Products. Citrus fruits are rich in citric acid and potassium, particularly in the former. They confer a biochemical action analogous to that of potassium citrate. This action, which is protective against stone formation, is characterized by a rise in urinary pH and citrate and occasionally by a fall in urinary calcium (see Chapter 6). Citrus fruits contain a modest amount of calcium (approximately 100 mg/liter) and vitamin C (<500 mg/liter). Despite an allegation to the contrary, the content of oxalate in citrus fruits is modest (0 to 21 mg/liter). The amount of calcium, ascorbate, and oxalate contained in fruit juices is probably insufficient to affect stone disease adversely. Thus, the net effect of citrus fruits is beneficial. Conversely, a low intake of citrus fruits constitutes a risk for stone formation.

The content of citrate and potassium, as well as sodium, calcium, magnesium, and oxalate, in various fruit products is shown in Table 11–7.

Magnesium. Magnesium complexes urinary oxalate, thereby reducing the urinary saturation of calcium oxalate (see Chapter 10). Low urinary magnesium thus constitutes a risk for stone formation.

Magnesium-rich foods are listed in Table 11–8. The main sources of magnesium are nuts, beans, and grains. It is noteworthy that patients with calcium oxalate nephrolithiasis are often told to refrain from ingesting nuts, which are also high in oxalate content. This practice may make them prone to develop undesirable hypomagnesiuria, however.

EVALUATION OF SINGLE-STONE FORMERS

There is considerable debate regarding the extent of diagnostic evaluation that should be applied to patients presenting with a single stone episode. The following arguments against an extensive diagnostic evaluation have been proposed.

Patients who have formed one stone may not form another. Even if they should have recurrence, it may be many years before that happens. Moreover, most single-stone formers have been reported to respond favorably to a conser-

TABLE 11–7. IONIC COMPOSITION OF CITRUS JUICES

Juice	Sodium (mEq/liter)	Potassium (mEq/liter)	Calcium (mg/liter)	Magnesium (mg/liter)	Citrate (mg/liter)	Oxalate (mg/liter)
Apple	1.6	28.4	41	43	52.1	12.1
Orange	0.5	53.3	96	110	8,140	Too low to detect
Grape	0.2	8.3	34	44	1,735	Too low to detect
Tangerine	0.5	40.2	54	97	8,523	5.5
Pineapple	None detected	30.4	105	116	5,860	20.5
Limeade	0.9	4.2	34	13	6,648	Too low to detect
Lemonade	0.1	0.5	11	10	6,189	Too low to detect
Pineapple-orange-banana	0.2	44.0	88	118	6,285	14.8
Grapefruit	0.1	37.7	101	96	14,500	8.1

TABLE 11–8. MAGNESIUM-RICH FOOD ITEMS

Food Item	Serving (oz)	Magnesium Content mg (mg range)
Peanuts, all types, roasted	½ cup	131
Tofu, raw, regular	½ cup	127
Peanuts, all types, raw	½ cup	123
Broccoli, cooked	2 large stalks	120
Spinach, cooked	½ cup	79
Chard, Swiss, cooked	½ cup	76
Soybeans, cooked	½ cup	74
Tomato paste, canned	½ cup	67
Simulated meat products, meat extender	1 ounce	61
Small white beans, cooked	½ cup	61
Sweet potato, canned, mashed	½ cup	61
Black beans, cooked	½ cup	60
Dock (sorrel), cooked	½ cup	60
Nuts & seeds, all types	1 ounce	60 avg. (9–152)
Pumpkin seeds	1 ounce	152
Chestnuts	1 ounce	9
Chili with beans, canned	½ cup	58
White beans, cooked	½ cup	57
Baked beans	½ cup	55
Navy beans, cooked	½ cup	53
Peanut butter	2 tablespoons	51
Succotash, cooked	½ cup	51
Beet greens, cooked	½ cup	49
Lima beans, baby, cooked	½ cup	49
Refried beans, canned	½ cup	49
Mung beans, cooked	½ cup	48
Artichoke, cooked	1 medium	47
Pinto beans, cooked	½ cup	47
Whole grain cereals, ready-to-eat	1 ounce	47 avg. (22–134)
Blackeyed peas, dried, cooked	½ cup	46
Okra, cooked	½ cup	46
Great Northern beans	½ cup	44
Squash, acorn, baked	½ cup cubes	43
Lima beans, large, cooked	½ cup	41
Kidney beans, all types, cooked	½ cup	40
Chickpeas, cooked	½ cup	39
Purslane, cooked	½ cup	39
Yogurt, low fat varieties	1 cup (8 oz)	37
Broadbeans, cooked	½ cup	36
Split peas, cooked	½ cup	36
Lentils, cooked	½ cup	35
Milk, fluid, all types	1 cup (8 oz)	35 avg. (28–40)

vative program of high fluid intake and avoidance of dietary excesses.[18] Thus, for an average patient with single stone formation, an extensive workup would not seem to be indicated.

On the other hand, many patients with single episodes have various metabolic and environmental disturbances, placing them at increased risk for recurrent stone formation.[19] In some patients, the metabolic derangement disclosed may be a reflection of a multisystem disease (e.g., renal tubular acidosis or renal hypercalciuria with secondary hyperparathyroidism). In such patients, medical treatments could be justified solely for the treatment of extrarenal manifestations (e.g., skeletal involvement of previously mentioned conditions).[20] Finally, the cost of medical evaluation, even when it is extensive, is low relative to the cost of stone removal or of care for renal colic.[21] Thus, medical evaluation may be construed as cost effective because of its potential for selection of an appropriate and effective prophylactic program.

The decision to investigate thoroughly a first-time stone former should ideally be shared by the physician and the patient. Some patients may elect to seek a thorough evaluation. One approach is to gauge the extent of evaluation according to the estimated potential for, or risk of, new stone formation. Patients at risk might be middle-aged white men with a family history of stones or those with intestinal disease (chronic diarrheal states), pathologic skeletal fractures, osteoporosis, urinary tract infection, or gout. In these patients, an extensive evaluation would be indicated (to be described).

In single-stone formers without risk, the following abbreviated protocol might be applied. A careful history should be taken for predisposing conditions, medications, dietary aberrations, and insufficient fluid intake. A multichannel blood screen should be performed to identify primary hyperparathyroidism (from high serum calcium concentrations), renal phosphate leak (from hypophosphatemia), distal renal tubular acidosis (from abnormal serum electrolytes), and gouty diathesis (from hyperuricemia). A fresh spot urine sample should be cultured for urea-splitting organisms (suggestive of infection stones) and examined for pH (with a pH electrode) and crystalluria. High pH (>7.5) is compatible with infection lithiasis and low pH (< 5.5) with uric acid lithiasis. Identification of a particular crystal type in the urinary sediment is compatible with but is not diagnostic of that type of nephrolithiasis. A qualitative examination of a spot urine sample for cystine (nitroprusside test) provides a clue to the presence of cystinuria. An abdominal roentgenologic examination, with oblique views when necessary, is recommended. Available stones should be analyzed for stone composition.

EXTENSIVE DIAGNOSTIC EVALUATION

A more extensive evaluation, directed at the identification of underlying physiologic derangements, should be performed in patients with recurrent nephrolithiasis as well as in single-stone formers at increased risk for further stone formation.

Several reliable protocols are available for the differentiation of different forms of nephrolithiasis. First introduced in 1976, the protocol utilized at Dallas has undergone further refinement and has now been applied in more than 1200 patients.[6]

Description of Ambulatory Protocol

This ambulatory evaluation requires three outpatient visits and may be completed within a month.[6] It depends largely on procedures that should be available in a routine clinical laboratory. Certain specialized procedures may be obtained commercially.

All medications that could affect the metabolism of calcium, uric acid, or oxalate should be discontinued before and during the period of evaluation, whenever possible. They include vitamin C, acetazolamide, calcium supplements, and antacids, as well as those that may have constituted the stone treatment program, such as thiazide, phosphate, allopurinol, or magnesium.

Briefly, three 24-hour urine samples are collected. Two (random samples) are obtained while patients adhere to their customary diet and fluid intake. The third (restricted) sample is collected on the final day of a 7-day restricted diet

(400 mg of calcium; 100 mEq sodium/day; and avoidance of oxalate-rich foods, such as nuts, brewed tea, chocolate, and dark greens). The purpose of obtaining the restricted sample is to standardize dietary factors so that hypercalciuria could be better defined. Moreover, the comparison of urinary values during a random situation with those during restriction permits an assessment of the role of environmental urinary risk factors. The week on the restricted diet also provides essential preparation for the "fast and calcium load test" that is performed on the third visit (to be described below).

On the first visit, a thorough history is taken, designed to elicit information regarding the nature and severity of stone disease and potential risk factors (Table 11–9). It includes the total number of stones passed and surgically removed; stone composition, if known; and evidence of any existing stones. A careful estimate is made of the frequency of stone episodes during the preceding 3 years to assess recent "stone activity." Specific dates and dosages of past treatment programs for the control of stone disease are obtained. Personal history is sought for predisposing medical conditions, such as gout, intestinal disease, and kidney infection. A family history is obtained for nephrolithiasis, gout, and bowel disease. A list is compiled for all medications taken (currently and during the period covering the stone disease), including vitamins and nutritional supplements. A careful diet history is obtained, directing particular attention to estimated fluid intake and to intake of foods rich in sodium, calcium, oxalate, and purines.

A kidney, ureter, and bladder (KUB) film or intravenous pyelogram, or both, should be obtained if not performed previously. Stones passed or removed should be submitted for analysis. Blood (venous) tests obtained on the first visit include complete blood count and multichannel screen (calcium, phosphorus, creatinine, uric acid, sodium, potassium, chloride, and carbon dioxide). The 24-hour random urine sample (collected on a random diet and fluid intake) is analyzed for calcium, uric acid, creatinine, sodium, oxalate, citrate, pH, total volume, and qualitative cystine.

On the second visit, another 24-hour urine sample collected on a random diet and fluid intake is analyzed for calcium, uric acid, creatinine, sodium, pH, and total volume (Table 11–9). The patient is then instructed to follow a diet restricted in calcium (400 mg/day), sodium (100 mEq/day), and oxalate, to be maintained until the third visit (at least 7 days). This instruction may be given by a trained nurse or technician, and not necessarily by a dietitian, using such information as is found in Table 11–10.

On the third visit, another 24-hour urine sample collected on the seventh day of the restricted diet is assayed for calcium, uric acid, creatinine, sodium, oxalate, citrate, pH, and total volume (Table 11–9). A fasting venous blood sample is analyzed for multichannel screen and immunoreactive PTH. The

TABLE 11–9. OUTLINE OF AMBULATORY PROTOCOL

Visit 1:	Random diet
	History
	Sequential multiple analysis (SMA)–20
	24-hr urine for stone risk factors
Visit 2:	Random diet
	Repeat 24-hr urine for stone risk factors
	Instruction on a diet restricted in calcium, sodium, oxalate
Visit 3:	Restricted diet
	SMA-20 and PTH
	24-hr urine for stone risk factors
	Fast and calcium load test

TABLE 11–10. DIET LIMITING CALCIUM, SODIUM,* AND OXALATE

Food Group	Foods Allowed	Foods not Allowed
Beverages	Carbonated drinks; coffee; decaffeinated coffee; fresh lemonade; limeade; instant tea	*All milk*, including buttermilk, canned milk, eggnog, malted milk, milkshakes, and powdered milk; hot chocolate, cocoa mixes; lemonade made from frozen concentrate; brewed tea
Bread and cereals	Biscuits, bread, cornbread, hamburger buns, and muffins; pancakes; sweet rolls; waffles; cooked and dry cereals without added salt (check labels)	Bread, crackers, and rolls with salt topping; corn tortillas; flour tortillas; cooked and dry cereals with salt added
Cheese	*None*	*All cheeses*, including American, cheddar, cottage cheese, cream cheese, Gouda, mozzarella, Parmesan, provolone, ricotta, and Swiss; cheese crackers; cheese foods; cheese puffs; cheese sauces and spreads; cheese sticks; dips; processed cheese
Desserts and sweets	Fruit cobblers, fruit pies, gelatin desserts; white and yellow cake with sugar icing; shortcake; tapioca; cookies; bread pudding (no milk); lemon sauce with cornstarch; vanilla wafers; graham crackers; fruit ices and popsicles; honey, jam, jelly, marmalade, preserves, syrup, and sugar	*All chocolate* in cakes, icings, pies, candy, cookies, and puddings; chocolate chips; chocolate syrup; Boston cream pie; custards; puddings; rice pudding; yogurt; *All ice cream*, including mellorine, frozen custard, frozen yogurt, ice milk, sherbet, and "dietetic" ice cream; chiffon pie and cream pie; molasses
Fats	Butter, margarine, vegetable oil, and most salad dressings; powdered or liquid nondairy creamer; nondairy whipped topping	Sour cream; salad dressings made with cheese, yogurt, or sour cream; ½ and ½ cream, whipping cream
Fruits and juices	Fresh, canned, and frozen fruit and fruit juice; dried fruits	Canned carrot juice, tomato juice, and vegetable cocktail juice; powdered fruit juice substitutes; electrolyte replacement drinks (Gatorade); rhubarb
Meats and meat substitutes	*Two average meat portions per day* of baked, boiled, broiled, or fried beef, chicken, fresh-water fish, fresh pork, seafood, tuna, turkey, veal, or venison; homemade chili, meat pies, and stews; eggs	Barbecued, cured, salty, canned, or smoked meats and fish: anchovies, caviar, herring, salmon, sardines, corned beef, chili, tamales, and stews; dried chipped beef; frankfurters; ham; luncheon meats; pizza; salt pork; bacon; sausage; meat pies; TV dinners
Starches	Corn, macaroni, noodles, potatoes, rice, and spaghetti; dried beans and dried peas in moderation	Macaroni and cheese; potato chips; corn chips; tortilla chips; corn pudding
Vegetables and soups	Fresh, canned*,† and frozen vegetables; homemade soups without added salt; lettuce	Sauerkraut and other vegetables prepared in brine; canned pork and beans; hominy; *All greens*, such as beet greens, collard greens, mustard greens, polk greens, spinach, and turnip greens; cheese soup; all canned soup (unless low sodium content is indicated); bouillon cubes; canned broth
Miscellaneous	Spices, herbs, and extracts; unsalted peanut butter; *small amounts* of meat tenderizer, brown gravy and sauces such as catsup, chili sauce, spaghetti sauce, steak sauce, and Worcestershire Sauce because these *do contain salt*!	*Added salt*; seasoned salt; monosodium glutamate (MSG); prepared horseradish and mustard; olives; pickles; salted nuts; salted popcorn; regular peanut butter; soy sauce; cream gravies and white sauce; hollandaise; newburg sauce
Supplements	NONE unless recommended by physician	Vitamin D; vitamins plus minerals; vitamin C
Medications	Only as directed by physician	

**Instructions for limiting salt:*

1. Use no salt or seasoned salt at the table.
2. Eat foods only lightly salted during preparation.
3. Do not add salt in the preparation of foods to which salt is added in processing—for example, canned vegetables.
4. When preparing food from a recipe, use half the amount of salt specified.

†Canned vegetables should be drained and rinsed to decrease salt.

patient undergoes "fast and calcium load test" on the morning of the third visit.[5] The essential requirements of this test are as follows:

1. Patients are kept on a low-calcium, low-sodium diet for at least 1 week and fasted for 10 to 12 hours to eliminate the effect of absorbed calcium on fasting calcium excretion.
2. Ample fluid intake (as distilled water) is provided to ensure adequate hydration.
3. A 1-gram calcium load is given orally in a standard meal, the response to which has been well characterized in normal subjects.
4. Urine samples are collected as accurately as possible (with patients urged to empty the bladder as completely as possible) for 2 hours before and for 4 hours after a 1-gram calcium load (representing fasting and postload samples).

Although the exact timing may vary to accommodate the special requirements of the laboratory or patients, the following schedule has been found to be suitable. Patients fast for 12 hours from 9 PM of the seventh day of the restricted dietary regimen. Distilled water (300 ml each time) is provided at 9 PM and midnight. At 7 AM of the following day, patients completely empty their bladder (discarding urine) and then drink an additional 600 ml of distilled water (while fast is continued). Urine is collected from 7 AM to 9 AM (fasting sample). At 9 AM, after collection of the fasting urine sample, 1 gram of calcium (elemental) is mixed in a liquid synthetic meal (250 ml) and is given orally. A urine sample (postload) is collected from 9 AM to 1 PM over a 4-hour period. Fasting and postload samples are analyzed for calcium and creatinine. The liquid synthetic diet may be substituted by other standard meals such as milk. If so, it is advised that normal control data be obtained separately, rather than relying on the control values obtained with the synthetic meal.

Interpretation of Tests

Assessment of the Effect of Environmental Influences. Results in urine samples obtained during a random diet, especially when compared with those in urine samples collected during a restricted diet, permit an assessment of environmental risk factors.

When urinary calcium in random samples exceeds that in restricted samples, one should suspect that the normal intake of calcium is excessive or that the intake of other factors (such as sodium, carbohydrate, or acid ash) is exaggerated. Under steady-state conditions in the absence of diarrhea or excessive sweating, urinary sodium approximates the dietary intake by less than 20 mEq/day. Thus, the finding of urinary sodium exceeding 150 mEq/day suggests that sodium intake is high. In patients with normouricemia without a history of gout, a high urinary uric acid excretion (>700 mg/day) indicates a high purine intake. A history of preference for animal proteins supports this suspicion. In the absence of bowel disease, high urinary oxalate (>44 mg/day) indicates that the consumption of oxalate-rich foods (spinach, nuts, chocolate, and brewed tea) is high or that vitamin C supplements (substrate for oxalate synthesis) are taken. The finding of normal urinary oxalate during the restricted diet supports this conclusion. Low urinary volume suggests an inadequate fluid intake, excessive fluid loss, or profuse sweating. In the absence of abnormal gastrointestinal fluid loss or sweating, urine volume is less than the total fluid intake by approximately 500 to 1000 ml/day.

Results During Restricted Diet and Response to Fast and Calcium Load. The measurement of urinary calcium on the restricted diet permits a definition of hypercalciuria. The finding of urinary calcium exceeding 200 mg/day is indicative of hypercalciuria, irrespective of age, sex, and body size. The response to the fast and calcium load test allows differentiation of varying forms of hypercalciuria. A high calcium excretion during the fasting state in the setting of normocalcemia (and hence normal renal filtered load of calcium) denotes that an impaired renal tubular reabsorption of calcium (renal calcium leak) is present. The simultaneous occurrence of high serum PTH with fasting hypercalciuria supports the diagnosis of renal hypercalciuria with secondary hyperparathyroidism. It should be emphasized that the value of fasting urinary calcium depends on the preparation of patients on a diet limited in calcium and sodium before the test. In patients with intestinal hyperabsorption of calcium, abnormally high values for fasting urinary calcium may be found if they are not prepared properly, owing to the delayed clearance of absorbed calcium and persistent parathyroid suppression (and hence inhibited renal tubular reabsorption of calcium).[22] Fasting hypercalciuria with normal serum PTH following adequate preparation suggests occurrence of primary 1,25-$(OH)_2$ vitamin D excess, renal phosphate leak, or combined disturbances in renal proximal tubular function (Chapter 3). Fasting urinary calcium is best expressed as milligrams per deciliter of glomerular filtrate (GF), since it is reflective of renal function rather than of muscle mass or body size. This measure may be obtained by simply multiplying urinary calcium in milligrams per milligram of creatinine by the corresponding serum creatinine in milligrams per deciliter.

The extent of renal calcium excretion after an oral load of calcium provides an indirect assessment of intestinal calcium absorption. In patients with normal fasting urinary calcium (<0.11 mg/dl GF), a urinary calcium postcalcium load of more than 0.2 mg/mg creatinine indicates that intestinal calcium absorption is high and suggests the diagnosis of absorptive hypercalciuria. The urinary calcium postcalcium load is best expressed in milligrams per milligram of creatinine, since it is a function of a fixed oral calcium load.

Assessment of Accuracy of Urine Collection. A major drawback to the proper interpretation of tests is the improper collection of urine. It is essential that at the start of collection the bladder be completely emptied and the specimen discarded. At the conclusion of a collection, the bladder must be completely emptied again and the specimen saved. A careful instruction on urine collection procedure should be given to every patient without a consideration of the initial perception of the patient's understanding. It is often the seemingly intelligent persons who make the mistake of overcollecting or undercollecting urine.

The accuracy of urine collection could be assessed from urinary creatinine values and body weight. In a carefully studied population on a metabolic dietary regimen in whom the accuracy of urine collection was ensured, the mean urinary creatinine in men was 22.1 ± 4.7 (SD) mg/kg, whereas it was 17.2 ± 3.8 mg/kg in women. Thus, a value substantially below these figures would indicate undercollection, and a value far exceeding these numbers would suggest overcollection.

Diagnostic Criteria

Diagnostic criteria for the major forms of nephrolithiasis in their pure presentations, constructed from results of the ambulatory protocol, are presented in Table 11–11. Detailed characteristics were defined in previous chapters.

TABLE 11–11. DIAGNOSTIC CRITERIA

Criterion	AH-I	AH-II	RH	PHPT	PL	1,25	EH	HUCN	Idiop Hypocit	RTA	GD
Serum calcium	N	N	N	↑	N	N	N	N	N	N	N
Phosphorus	N	N	N	↓	↓	N	N	N	N	N	N
PTH	N	N	↑	↑	N	↓	↑	N	N	N	N
Urinary calcium											
fasting	N	N	↑	↑	↑	↑	↓	N	N	↑	N
1-gram calcium load	↑	↑	↑	↑	↑	↑	↓	N	N	N	N
	↑	N	↑	↑	↑	↑	↓	N	N	↑	N
24-hr (restricted diet)											
Oxalate	N	N	N	N	N	N	↑	N	N	N	N
Uric acid	N	N	N	N	N	N	↓	↑	N	N	N/↑
Citrate	N	N	N	N	N	N	↓	N	↓	↓	N
pH	N	N	N	N	N	N	↓	N	N	↑	↓

AH-I = absorptive hypercalciuria Type I; AH-II = absorptive hypercalciuria Type II; RH = renal hypercalciuria; PHPT = primary hyperparathyroidism; PL = renal phosphate leak; 1,25 = primary 1,25-$(OH)_2$ vitamin D excess; EH = enteric hyperoxaluria; HUCN = hyperuricosuric calcium nephrolithiasis; idiop hypocit = idiopathic hypocitraturia; RTA = renal tubular acidosis; GD = gouty diathesis; N = normal; ↑ = increase; ↓ = decrease.

A SIMPLIFIED AMBULATORY EVALUATION

The previously described ambulatory protocol is worthy of consideration for the evaluation of patients with recurrent nephrolithiasis or with high risk, because of its high diagnostic yield and reliability. Unfortunately, this protocol may be too cumbersome for ready adoption by some practicing physicians. A simplified approach has therefore been devised.

The StoneRisk Profile[7]

Recent advances in analytical technology now allow reliable determination of various urinary constituents that could influence renal stone formation. These assays include calcium, oxalate, and citrate (stones could result from disturbed metabolism of these substances), as well as total volume and sodium (the result of environmental or dietary influences). From such determinations, it is possible to calculate urinary saturation with respect to stone-forming salts. Thus, a profile of stone-forming risks can now be constructed and depicted graphically for easy recognition. This service is available commercially in the United States.

Essential Elements of the StoneRisk Profile. A 24-hour urine collection kit, containing a volume marker and appropriate preservatives, is provided by the physician to the patient. After collection of a 24-hour urine sample, two small (30-ml) aliquots are sent via regular mail to a central laboratory. The laboratory then calculates the total volume from the dilution of the volume marker and analyzes urinary "metabolic risk factors" (calcium, oxalate, uric acid, citrate, and pH) as well as "environmental risk factors" (total volume, sodium, sulfate, phosphorus, and magnesium).[7] From these analyzed values, "physicochemical risk factors" are computed.[7]

Display of Data.[7] To provide a visual display of all available data in a single report, each risk factor is assigned a vertical line with linear or logarithmic scales. Risk factors are grouped into metabolic, environmental, or physicochemical risks. A horizontal line intersecting each vertical scale at the approximate midpoint represents the upper or lower normal limit. The direction of increasing values is appropriately adjusted, so that values below the horizontal line represent normal values (reduced risk) and those above the line represent abnormal values (increased risk). For example, values for urinary calcium increase upward, whereas those for citrate increase downward on the scale. For metabolic and environmental risks, values above the horizontal dashed line indicate abnormally high or abnormally low determinations. For physicochemical risks, values above the horizontal dashed line represent relative supersaturation (greater degree of supersaturation than in normal subjects) with respect to specified stone-forming salts.

A sample display in a patient with recurrent calcium nephrolithiasis is shown in Figure 11–1. The results are sent to the requesting physician[3] to assist them in making the diagnosis.

Value and Limitations of the StoneRisk Profile

The StoneRisk Profile has an obvious diagnostic utility. In this display, wider normal limits were sometimes employed to reflect the presentation of the usual stone-forming population. Urinary calcium exceeding 250 mg/day is indicative of the presence of one of the varying forms of hypercalciuria. Urinary uric acid of greater than 700 mg/day is indicative of hyperuricosuric calcium nephrolithiasis; oxalate exceeding 45 mg/day, hyperoxaluria; citrate less than 320 mg/day, hypocitraturic calcium nephrolithiasis; pH less than 5.5, gouty diathesis; pH

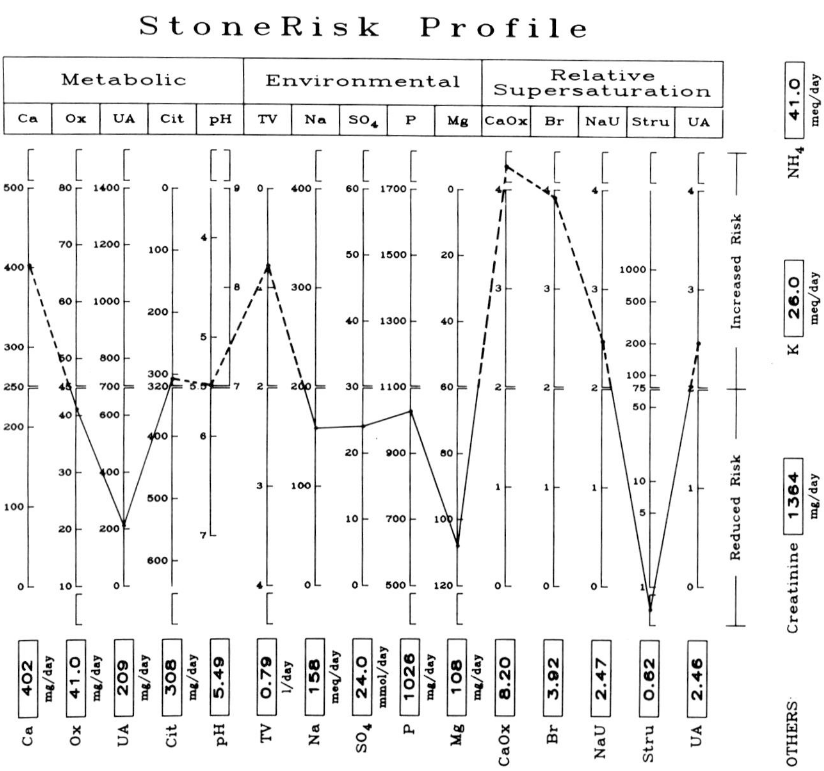

FIGURE 11–1. Graphic display of urinary risk factors in a patient with recurrent nephrolithiasis.

greater than 7.5, infection stones; and volume less than 2 liters/day, low urine volume. The association of relative supersaturation of uric acid with low urinary pH further supports the diagnosis of gouty diathesis. A finding of relative supersaturation of struvite with high urinary pH is almost diagnostic of infection stones.

However, a definitive diagnosis of a particular underlying derangement generally cannot be made without additional information (clinical history, radiograph, stone analysis, and blood chemistry). In some instances, it might be desirable to confirm the presence of various abnormalities on repeat measurements. Moreover, the StoneRisk Profile does not permit differentiation of different forms of hypercalciuria.

Acknowledgment

The author would like to thank Linda Brinkley for formulation of diet tables.

REFERENCES

1. Wills MR, Zisman E, Wortsman J, et al: The measurement of intestinal calcium absorption by external radioisotope counting: Application to study of nephrolithiasis. Clin Sci 39:95–106, 1970.
2. Pak CYC, East D, Sanzenbacher L, et al: A simple and reliable test for the diagnosis of hyperparathyroidism. Arch Intern Med 129:48–55, 1972.
3. Pak CYC, East C, Sanzenbacher LJ, et al: Gastrointestinal calcium absorption in nephrolithiasis. J Clin Endocrinol Metab 35:261–270, 1972.
4. Pak CYC, Ohata M, Lawrence EC, Snyder W: The hypercalciurias: Causes, parathyroid functions and diagnostic criteria. J Clin Invest 54:387–400, 1974.
5. Pak CYC, Kaplan RA, Bone H, et al: A simple test for the diagnosis of absorptive, resorptive and renal hypercalciurias. N Engl J Med 292:497–500, 1975.
6. Pak CYC, Britton F, Peterson R, et al: Ambulatory evaluation of nephrolithiasis: Classification, clinical presentation and diagnostic criteria. Am J Med 69:19–30, 1980.
7. Pak CYC, Skurla C, Harvey J: Graphic display of urinary risk factors for renal stone formation. J Urol 134:867–870, 1985.
8. Pak CYC: Medical management of nephrolithiasis: Update 1987. J Urol 140:461–467, 1988.
9. Pak CYC, McGuire J, Peterson R, et al: Familial absorptive hypercalciuria in a large kindred. J Urol 126:717–719, 1981.
10. Parfitt AM: Acetazolamide and sodium bicarbonate induced nephrocalcinosis and nephrolithiasis. Arch Intern Med 124:736–740, 1969.
11. Colin AA, Kraiem Z, Kahana L, Hochberg Z: Effects of theophylline on urinary excretion of cyclic AMP, calcium, and phosphorus in normal subjects. Miner Electrolyte Metab 10:359–361, 1984.
12. Pak CYC, Sakhaee K, Crowther C, Brinkley L: Evidence justifying a high fluid intake in treatment of nephrolithiasis. Ann Intern Med 93:36–39, 1980.
13. Recker RR, Bammi A, Barger-Lux MJ, Heaney RP: Calcium absorbability from milk products, an imitation milk, and calcium carbonate. Am J Clin Nutr 47:93–95, 1988.
14. Brinkley L, McGuire J, Gregory J, Pak CYC: Bioavailability of oxalate in foods. Urology 17:534–538, 1981.
15. Pak CYC, Holt K, Zerwekh JE: Attenuation by monosodium urate of the inhibitory effect of glycosaminoglycans on calcium oxalate nucleation. Invest Urol 17:138–140, 1979.
16. Wills MR, Gill JR, Bartter FC: The interrelationships of calcium and sodium excretions. Clin Sci 37:621–630, 1969.
17. Breslau NA, Brinkley L, Hill KD, Pak CYC: Relationship role of animal protein-rich diet to kidney stone formation and calcium metabolism. J Clin Endocrinol Metab 66:140–146, 1988.
18. Hosking DH, Erickson SB, Van Den Berg CJ, et al: The stone clinic effect in patients with idiopathic calcium urolithiasis. J Urol 130:1115–1118, 1983.
19. Pak CYC: Should patients with single renal stone ocurrence undergo diagnostic evaluation. J Urol 127:854–858, 1982.

20. Preminger GM, Sakhaee K, Pak CYC: Hypercalciuria and altered intestinal calcium absorption occurring independently of vitamin D in distal renal tubular acidosis. Metabolism 36:176–179, 1987.
21. Pak CYC: Role of medical prevention. J Urol 141:798–801, 1989.
22. Pak CYC, Galosy RA: Fasting urinary calcium and adenosine 3′-5′-monophosphate: A discriminant analysis for the identification of renal and absorptive hypercalciuria. J Clin Endocrinol Metab 48:260–265, 1979.

12

General Guidelines in Management

Charles Y.C. Pak

The primary objective of medical management is the prevention of recurrent stone formation. The medical approach may be fully justified because of the high rate of recurrence characterizing most forms of stone disease.

Recently, major strides have been made in the medical management of nephrolithiasis. Many treatment programs have been developed that are known to correct the underlying metabolic or environmental disturbances in urine. By using them, it is now possible to prevent recurrence of stone formation in most patients. Moreover, there is emerging evidence that medical treatment may be effective in causing dissolution of stones in vivo (including calcium stones under certain circumstances) and in averting adverse extrarenal manifestations of certain stone diseases.

Despite this progress, there is no evidence that a short-term application of medical treatments produces a "cure" or a permanent correction of underlying abnormalities and occurrence of stone formation.[1] Thus, the current prophylactic approach mandates a long-term commitment, requiring a continuous prolonged adherence to the treatment program.

The type of medical treatment chosen and the rigor of its application are dependent on several factors: severity of stone disease (single or recurrent stone formation, inactive or active), presence of extrarenal manifestations, availability of selective treatment program (capable of correcting underlying derangements), efficacy and safety of treatment, ability of treatment to avert extrarenal manifestations and cause dissolution of existing stones, and anticipated compliance of the patient with a long-term treatment program. A simple and less rigorous program might be applied for single or inactive disease, without extrarenal manifestations. More aggressive treatments would be indicated for recurrent active disease, particularly when correctable extrarenal manifestations are present and when there are existing stones that might be amenable to dissolution.

These questions are explored in this chapter.

HISTORICAL CONSIDERATIONS

In antiquity, considerable mysticism surrounded the medical management of nephrolithiasis. The Assyrians and Babylonians used black saltpeter, shell of ostrich egg, and pine turpentine.[2] In 1500 BC, the Rig-Veda prescribed spells and incantations. The Greeks emphasized shaking on wagons or ships, milk of the mother of a male child, and baths.[3]

However, the value of high fluid intake has long been appreciated. Celsus instructed his patients to drink a lot of water.[4] Cyprian, a famous lithotomist, claimed that he never operated on a beer drinker.[2]

In 1826, Sir Astley Cooper[2] prescribed "liquor potassae," potassium carbonate, and sodium carbonate for uric acid stones.

In 1962, Howard and colleagues[5] introduced the concept of "good" and "evil" urine. The good urine from normal subjects presumably contained an inhibitor of stone formation, whereas the evil urine from patients with stones was devoid of or deficient in it. Treatment with orthophosphate was shown to restore the goodness and retard stone formation. In 1964, Fleisch and coworkers[6] showed that the inhibitor activity of orthophosphate treatment was due to enhanced pyrophosphate excretion.

In 1970, Yendt and associates[7] found that thiazide lowered urinary calcium and prevented recurrent calcium nephrolithiasis.

In 1973, Coe and Raisen[8] reported that allopurinol was effective in inhibiting calcium stone formation in patients with hyperuricosuria.

In 1982, sodium cellulose phosphate was approved by the Food and Drug Administration (FDA) for the management of absorptive hypercalciuria in the United States.[9]

In 1983, acetohydroxamic acid was approved for the treatment of infection stones.[10]

In 1985, potassium citrate was approved for the prevention of uric acid lithiasis and for the management of hypocitraturic calcium nephrolithiasis.[11]

In 1988, α-mercaptopropionylglycine was approved for the treatment of cystinuria.[12]

TREATMENT OF SINGLE STONE OR INACTIVE DISEASE

Patients presenting after their stone episode may be stone free for several years before the appearance of another episode. Some of them may not form another stone again. If initial exploratory diagnostic studies (as outlined in Chapter 11) fail to disclose alarming biochemical derangements, adverse extrarenal manifestations, or the presence of secondary disease for stone formation (such as primary hyperparathyroidism, chronic diarrheal state, or gout), it may be prudent to offer conservative treatment measures first before applying specific treatment.[13] Available data suggest that an application of conservative therapy could considerably delay the development of the second stone in single-stone formers.

It is acknowledged that conservative measures should be useful in all patients with nephrolithiasis. Thus, they should be applied together with a specific medical treatment program in patients with recurrent active stone disease.

Some conservative programs are applicable to all forms of stone disease, whereas others are useful for particular causes. It is apparent that the extent to which certain dietary indiscretions contribute to stone formation often depends on the particular physiologic derangement identified. Thus, some dietary modifications should not be made universally but selectively applied according to the cause of stone disease. Inappropriately used dietary change may be ineffective or may cause harm.

Conservative treatment measures comprise an avoidance of stone-provoking drugs, high fluid intake, and dietary modification, as described further on.[14] The reader is referred to Chapter 11 for additional descriptive material.

Avoidance of Stone-Provoking Drugs

As discussed in Chapter 11, acetazolamide, vitamin C supplementation, calcium supplements, vitamin D preparations, and triamterene may cause or aggravate stone formation. If their pathogenetic role can be established, these drugs should be stopped or their dose reduced, if possible.

High Fluid Intake

High fluid intake is the only nutritional modification that is universally agreed to be useful in all forms of nephrolithiasis.[15]

The objective of treatment is to drink a sufficient amount of fluid to achieve a minimal urine output of at least 2 liters/day. During normal activity, approximately 3 liters of fluid must be drunk daily to reach this goal. A higher intake is required when there is excessive sweating or gastrointestinal fluid loss. Fluid intake should be distributed throughout the day to ensure a consistently high urine output. Any form of fluids is acceptable, except for milk in absorptive hypercalciuria and tea in calcium oxalate nephrolithiasis. Although citrus fruit juices may contain vitamin C and oxalate, the beneficial effect of the provision of fluid predominates over any potential increase in oxalate excretion. There is probably no special advantage of cranberry juice over any other citrus fruit juice. Besides provision of fluid, citrus juices may possess citraturic action, further offsetting the propensity for stone formation (see Chapter 6).

Ideally, the patient should develop a habit of drinking two glasses (20 ounces) of fluid with every meal, one glass between meals and at bedtime, and, if he or she should get up at night to urinate, one to two glasses. If 50 per cent of the fluid is taken as water, then the other half can be fluids of the patient's choosing.

Dietary Oxalate Restriction

Although the dietary restriction of oxalate may be beneficial in any cause of calcium oxalate nephrolithiasis, it is particularly indicated when there is increased intestinal absorption of oxalate. These conditions include enteric hyperoxaluria, absorptive hypercalciuria, and therapy with sodium cellulose phosphate (see Chapter 4).

Only a moderate oxalate restriction is generally necessary in controlling hyperoxaluria in patients with absorptive hypercalciuria. Such a diet comprises avoidance of dark green roughages, rhubarb, tea, chocolate, and nuts. A more rigid oxalate restriction, involving avoidance of other oxalate-rich foods (see

Chapter 11), may be necessary in enteric hyperoxaluria and during sodium cellulose phosphate therapy.

Dietary Calcium Restriction

Rigid calcium restriction (< 400 mg/day) is ill advised even in patients with absorptive hypercalciuria who have a high intestinal calcium absorption, since it is difficult to follow, may adversely affect general nutrition, and may cause negative calcium balance. However, a moderate calcium restriction (400 to 600 mg/day) may be useful in absorptive hypercalciuria, since it alone may control the hypercalciuria in the Type II presentation[16] or may permit reduction of the dosage of medication necessary to restore normal urinary calcium in the Type I presentation.

Calcium restriction is neither necessary nor indicated in patients with nephrolithiasis with *normal* intestinal absorption of calcium. However, an excessive intake of calcium (>1 gram/day) should be avoided in these patients, since it may produce hypercalciuria of sufficient magnitude to be promotive of stone disease even when intestinal calcium absorption is normal.

If dietary calcium restriction is to be applied, a simultaneous limitation of oxalate intake is recommended to avoid enhancement of oxalate excretion. Such a diet (moderately restricted in calcium and oxalate) may be followed by the patient with relative ease, without impairing general nutrition, by the avoidance of dairy products, excessive amounts of dark green vegetables, tea, chocolate, and nuts.

Dietary Sodium Restriction

A sodium restriction (< 200 mEq/day and preferably 100 mEq or 5.85 grams of sodium chloride) may be helpful in all patients with idiopathic calcium urolithiasis. It may be indicated particularly in patients with hypercalciuria. A moderate sodium restriction may usually be achieved by the avoidance of obviously salty foods, such as prepared broths, soups, and processed vegetables, and by restricting the use of the salt shaker at mealtime. Salt substitutes may be used. It may sometimes be necessary to have the patient keep a daily log of all foods consumed to find the incriminating salty food item.

Dietary Restriction of Animal Proteins

In patients whose intake of animal proteins is excessive, a moderate limitation of animal protein ingestion may be attempted, for example, by omitting animal protein products in one meal each day or reducing the size of such servings. A more rigid restriction of animal proteins is often not practical. The advantage of a vegetarian diet over a meat diet, with respect to protection against stone formation, has not been clearly established. The institution of a vegetarian diet may induce other alterations in the urine, including increased oxalate excretion that may oppose the beneficial effects of reduced calcium and uric acid and of increased urinary citrate and pH. At this point it would seem important to eliminate dietary excesses of animal proteins (>1.7 grams per kilogram of body weight per day) or of vegetables and to advise moderate consumption of all food types. Stone formers often consume an inadequate quantity of fruits. It may be helpful to advise them to consume a moderate amount (10 ounces daily) of citrus fruit juices on a daily basis. This practice may be beneficial, since it would neutralize the acid load from animal protein ingestion, augment citrate excretion, and provide fluids.

TREATMENT OF RECURRENT ACTIVE DISEASE

A more specific medical treatment program is indicated in patients who continue to form stones, who are recalcitrant to a conservative treatment program, who present with extrarenal manifestations, or who have existing stones that might be responsive to dissolution.

Continued Application of a Conservative Program

A conservative program of increased fluid intake and dietary modification should be maintained even when specific treatments are applied. Certain conservative measures are critical for the success of some specific treatments.

Sodium restriction is often necessary in patients who require thiazides for the control of hypercalciuria (see Chapter 3). If the dietary sodium is high (>150 mEq/day), the hypocalciuric action of thiazide can be attenuated. When sodium cellulose phosphate is used in the treatment of absorptive hypercalciuria, dietary restriction of oxalate is critical to the success of the program, as mentioned previously. When this precaution has not been followed along with magnesium supplementation and moderate calcium restriction, sodium cellulose phosphate may have limited effectiveness in controlling stone formation. When allopurinol is used to treat hyperuricosuria, the reduced intake of animal protein should be continued if possible.

Selective Therapy for Nephrolithiasis

Elucidation of the pathophysiology and formulation of diagnostic criteria for different causes of nephrolithiasis have made feasible the adoption of selective or optimal treatment programs.[16, 17] Such programs should achieve the following:

1. Reverse the underlying physicochemical and physiologic derangements.
2. Inhibit new stone formation.
3. Overcome nonrenal complications of the disease process.
4. Be free of serious side effects.

The rationale for the selection of certain treatment programs is the assumption that the particular physicochemical and physiologic aberrations identified with the given disorder are etiologically important in the formation of renal stones and that the correction of these disturbances will prevent stone formation. Moreover, it is assumed that such a selected treatment program would be more effective and safer than a "random" treatment.[18] Despite a lack of conclusive experimental verification, these hypotheses appear reasonable and logical. It is recommended that selective therapy be applied initially in patients with active stone disease who have definable physiologic abnormalities amenable to correction by medical treatment. Selective treatment would also be indicated in patients who continue to form stones while receiving conservative treatment.

Table 12–1 summarizes selective therapies for various causes of stone disease. Mechanism of drug action, dose schedule, and side effects have been described in detail in previous chapters.

Nonselective Treatment of Nephrolithiasis

It has not been known whether a rigorous selective treatment program is more effective than a less selective one. Ettinger and colleagues[19] found chlor-

TABLE 12–1. SELECTIVE TREATMENT PROGRAM

CONDITION	TREATMENT	PHYSIOLOGIC ACTION	PHYSICOCHEMICAL ACTION
Absorptive hypercalciuria Type I	Sodium cellulose phosphate	↓ Intestinal calcium absorption ↓ Urinary calcium	↓ Urinary saturation of calcium salts
	Thiazide	↓ Urinary calcium	↓ Urinary saturation of calcium salts
Absorptive hypercalciuria Type II	Low-calcium diet	↓ Intestinal calcium absorption ↓ Urinary calcium	↓ Urinary saturation of calcium salts
Renal hypercalciuria	Thiazide	↓ Urinary calcium (sustained) ↓ Intestinal calcium absorption	↓ Urinary saturation of calcium salts
Primary hyperparathyroidism	Parathyroidectomy	↓ Parathyroid hormone (PTH) ↓ Urinary calcium	↓ Urinary saturation of calcium salts ↑ Inhibitor activity
Renal phosphate leak	Orthophosphate	↓ $1,25(OH)_2D$ ↓ Urinary calcium ↑ Urinary citrate and pyrophosphate	↓ Urinary saturation of calcium oxalate ↑ Inhibitor activity
$1,25(OH)_2D$ excess Combined defect	Thiazide	↓ Urinary calcium	↓ Urinary saturation of calcium salts
Hyperuricosuric calcium nephrolithiasis	Allopurinol	↓ Urinary uric acid	↓ Urate-induced crystallization of calcium salts
	Potassium citrate	↑ Urinary citrate ↑ Urinary pH	↓ Urinary saturation of calcium oxalate ↓ Urate-induced crystallization of calcium salts
Chronic diarrheal syndrome	↓ Oxalate intake	↓ Urinary oxalate	↓ Urinary saturation of calcium oxalate
	Potassium citrate	↑ Urinary citrate ↑ Urinary pH	↓ Urinary saturation of calcium oxalate and uric acid ↑ Inhibitor activity
	Magnesium citrate	↑ Urinary magnesium and citrate	↓ Urinary saturation of calcium oxalate
Hypocitraturic calcium nephrolithiasis, including renal tubular acidosis (RTA)	Potassium citrate	↑ Urinary citrate ↑ Urinary pH	↓ Urinary saturation of calcium salts ↑ Inhibitor activity
Hypomagnesiuric calcium nephrolithiasis	Magnesium citrate	↑ Urinary magnesium and citrate	↓ Urinary saturation of calcium oxalate
Gouty diathesis	Potassium citrate	↑ Urinary pH ↓ Undissociated uric acid	↓ Urinary saturation of uric acid
Cystinuria	D-penicillamine or MPG	Mixed disulfide with cystine ↓ Urinary cystine	↓ Urinary saturation of cystine
Infection stones	Acetohydroxamic acid	↓ Urease activity ↓ NH_4^+ ↓ pH	↓ Urinary saturation of struvite
Low urine volume	High fluid intake	↑ Urine volume	↓ Urinary saturation of stone-forming salts

thalidone to be more effective than placebo in inhibiting new stone formation in patients with idiopathic calcium oxalate nephrolithiasis, noncategorized with regard to the cause of hypercalciuria and without distinction between normal and excessive renal excretion of calcium or uric acid. However, a study at Dallas[18] indicated that a more selectively applied potassium citrate therapy in patients with hypocitraturia provided a better clinical response than in those with normocitraturic calcium nephrolithiasis. Thus, in the hypocitraturic group, the stone formation rate declined from 4.14 stones to 0.4 stone per patient-year following potassium citrate treatment; 82.3 per cent of patients had remission, and the group stone formation rate declined by 90.3 per cent. In contrast, the normocitraturic group showed a reduction in the stone formation rate from 3.33 stones to 0.75 stone per patient-year, a remission rate of 74 per cent and a decline in the group stone formation rate of 77.5 per cent. The less favorable response in the normocitraturic group probably reflected the presence of other metabolic abnormalities not corrected by potassium citrate therapy.

ADVANTAGES OF SELECTIVE THERAPY (Table 12–2)

Side Effects of Nonselective Therapy

Treatment of renal hypercalciuria with sodium cellulose phosphate may exaggerate secondary hyperparathyroidism and aggravate or produce bone disease.[9] The use of this calcium-binding agent in patients with normal calcium absorption could cause a negative calcium balance. Similarly, a diet limited in calcium in patients other than those with high calcium absorption may produce a calcium-deficient state.

The sequelae of nonselective use of thiazide in absorptive hypercalciuria Type I include transient retention of calcium in the skeleton and eventual loss of the hypocalciuric response.[20] Thiazide may cause hypercalcemia in patients with resorptive hypercalciuria.

Parathyroidectomy is not "curative" for renal hypercalciuria. There may be recurrence of renal hypercalciuria and nephrolithiasis after surgery.[21]

Orthophosphate therapy for normophosphatemic absorptive hypercalciuria may cause calcium retention, since high intestinal calcium absorption is maintained despite a reduction in urinary calcium.[22] As noted, there are reports of parathyroid stimulation and soft tissue calcification during orthophosphate use.[23]

There is no evidence that the use of potassium citrate in normocitraturic states at customary dosages (< 80 mEq/day) would be harmful. However, if this drug is used in the presence of urinary tract infection, it may aggravate the infection and promote calcium phosphate precipitation.

We would consider the substitution of potassium citrate with sodium alkali to be nonselective. When sodium alkali is given, it may increase urinary calcium and sodium.[24] Thus, the urinary saturation of calcium salts may increase, and

TABLE 12–2. ADVANTAGES OF SELECTIVE THERAPY

1. More effective control of stone recurrence
2. Avoidance of side effects of nonselective therapy
3. Correction of extrarenal complications
4. Reduced requirement for stone surgery
5. Dissolution of existing stones

urate-induced crystallization of calcium salts may be promoted.[24] These effects may override the citraturic response of the alkali therapy. Hence, the complication of calcium stones may occur during sodium alkali therapy. In five patients with documented uric acid lithiasis studied by us recently, treatment with sodium bicarbonate or sodium citrate caused calcium stones (calcium oxalate, calcium phosphate, or both) in all five.[25] When potassium alkali was provided, no new stones were formed.

These potential complications of nonselective treatments attest to the value of the selective approach.

Correction of Extrarenal Manifestations by Selective Therapy

Even if conservative treatments inhibit stone formation, additional therapies may be indicated for the prevention of extrarenal complications. Nephrolithiasis should be considered as potentially representing a multisystem disease in which stone formation is only one manifestation. Selective treatment of nephrolithiasis may also correct attendant nonrenal complications.

In renal hypercalciuria there may be skeletal involvement, as indicated by a reduced bone density noted on photon absorptiometry.[26] Selective treatment with thiazide may avert this complication by restoring normal parathyroid function,[27] as shown by stable bone density during long-term follow-up.

Primary hyperparathyroidism is manifested clinically by peptic ulcer disease and bone disease, as well as by nephrolithiasis. Parathyroidectomy typically prevents all three manifestations.

Although controversial, there is some evidence that bone may be affected adversely in patients with renal phosphate leak because of hypophosphatemia.[28] Orthophosphate therapy may retard this development.

Various cardiac and musculoskeletal side effects may accompany the hypokalemia resulting from renal tubular acidosis, chronic diarrheal states, and thiazide-induced hypocitraturia. Potassium citrate may correct this complication unless there is severe chloride deficiency.

In renal tubular acidosis (distal), there is subnormal intestinal calcium absorption and hypercalciuria. Bone disease may develop. Potassium citrate therapy improves calcium balance by increasing intestinal calcium absorption and reducing calcium excretion and thus averts bone loss.[29]

These examples, showing the ability of selective treatments to overcome nonrenal complications, further justify the adoption of the selective treatment approach.

Reduced Requirement for Stone Surgery

In 89 patients participating in a long-term clinical trial at Dallas, an analysis was made of surgeries required for removal of stones. All surgeries were for symptomatic calculi associated with obstruction, intractable bleeding, pain, or fever.

During the 3 years preceding treatment, the 89 patients participating in the study required 61 surgeries for removal of stones (45 "open," 16 "basket").[30] During an average of 2 years of potassium citrate treatment, only 10 surgeries were required (8 open, 2 basket), all for stones that had been present when the treatment was started. The results provide supporting evidence that potassium citrate treatment inhibited new stone formation.

Dissolution of Existing Calcium Stones

In approximately 40 per cent of patients with existing calcium nephrolithiasis, potassium citrate therapy (>9 months) caused reduced stone mass, often not accounted for by stone passage.[31] A similar apparent dissolution of existing calcium stones has not been reported with placebo or a conservative program.

SUGGESTED GUIDELINES FOR FOLLOW-UP

A careful follow-up is mandatory after initiation of therapy, for the following reasons. First, not all patients respond uniformly to a given treatment program. The recommended dose may be too much or too little for some patients. Second, the severity of stone disease often fluctuates during the course of the disease in the same patient in an unpredictable fashion. Sometimes the disease becomes less severe, other times worse. Thus, the dose of a given treatment may need to be altered to accommodate the changing severity of stone disease. Third, all treatments may potentially cause side effects. Some complications are reflected in abnormal biochemistry or laboratory tests, without appearance of symptoms, such as abnormal liver function tests during allopurinol therapy or parathyroid stimulation during sodium cellulose phosphate therapy. Finally, many patients may become less compliant with recommended therapy, especially when the memory of renal colic wanes.

It is therefore recommended that patients be followed at regular intervals while on medical prophylactic therapy. In the program at Dallas, patients are routinely followed every 4 months after initiation of therapy. When a satisfactory correction of the abnormal urinary biochemical and physicochemical condition and control of the stone disease have been achieved, patients can be followed at less frequent intervals (e.g., every 6 to 12 months).

At each visit, a careful history should be taken for stone episodes, complications of treatment, and compliance with the recommended drug therapy and dietary recommendation. In patients with calcium or uric acid nephrolithiasis, the following tests are recommended: serum multichannel screen (including calcium, phosphorus, creatinine, potassium, carbon dioxide, creatinine, and uric acid) and 24-hour urinary calcium, oxalate, uric acid, citrate, pH, total volume, and sodium. Additional tests could be added as indicated.

StoneTrack

In Chapter 11, the StoneRisk Profile was described for the assay and graphic depiction of urinary risk factors, designed for the initial evaluation of patients with nephrolithiasis. The StoneTrack is a modified version of the StoneRisk Profile, developed to "track" patients on medical prophylactic programs. It has the same simple urine collection kit and a reliable preservation system, permitting access to any patient residing anywhere in the country.

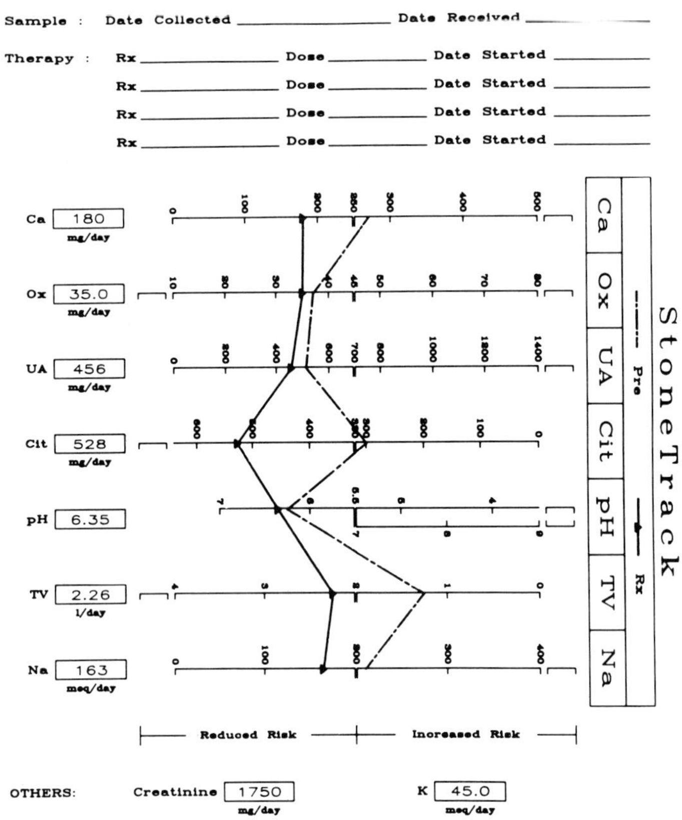

FIGURE 12–1. StoneTrack for following the response to medical therapy.

Graphic Display. From the aliquots of a 24-hour urine shipped via regular mail by the patient, the central laboratory performs analysis for calcium, oxalate, uric acid, citrate, pH, total volume, and sodium. The results obtained while the patient is receiving treatment are compared with pretreatment values on the same plot using the same graphic display as was used in the StoneRisk Profile (Fig. 12–1).

Interpretation. The data should first be examined for adherence to the conservative treatment program. Urine volume less than 2 liters/day suggests inadequate fluid intake and the need to drink more fluids. Sodium restriction should be urged if urinary sodium exceeds 200 mEq/day. In patients without bowel disease or primary hyperoxaluria who present with mild-to-moderate hyperoxaluria (45 to 80 mg/day), dietary oxalate restriction and avoidance of vitamin C supplementation should be instituted.

The results should then be evaluated for the adequacy of drug therapy. The knowledge of the customary urinary biochemical response to various treatments (see Table 12–1) should allow determination of the adequacy of a given treatment. When the response is inadequate, the data should be examined and the patient closely questioned for compliance with the treatment program.

Certain laboratory tests provide clues to compliance with the treatment program. Urinary potassium (also provided in the StoneTrack as an ancillary test) usually increases by the amount of potassium contained in the medication during potassium citrate treatment; a subnormal value indicates that a full dose was not taken. Urinary phosphorus increases substantially during orthophosphate therapy and modestly during sodium cellulose phosphate therapy. Serum uric acid concentration declines by about 2 mg/dl during allopurinol therapy.

If there is an inadequate response to treatment (i.e., the expected results of treatment are not obtained), and there is reason to question compliance, patients should be urged to take the full dose of the drug or drugs as recommended and to adhere to appropriate dietary restrictions and adequate fluid intake. It is important to remember that certain dietary indiscretions could blunt the effect of drug treatment. A high sodium intake, indicated by urinary sodium exceeding 200 mEq/day, could attenuate the hypocalciuric action of thiazide. An exaggerated intake of calcium or animal proteins could obviate the calcium-binding capacity of sodium cellulose phosphate or the hypouricosuric action of allopurinol, respectively. When there is insufficient biochemical response despite adequate compliance, a consideration should be given to altering the treatment dosage.

It is critical that side effects of treatment are carefully sought at each visit. If hyperoxaluria develops during sodium cellulose phosphate therapy, a more rigid dietary oxalate restriction is required. When serum parathyroid hormone (PTH) is high or bone density declines, the dose of sodium cellulose phosphate should be reduced. Hypokalemia caused by thiazide therapy should be treated with potassium supplementation, preferably as potassium citrate. The appearance of abnormal liver function tests requires cessation of allopurinol or thiazide therapy.

REFERENCES

1. Pak CYC: Medical management of nephrolithiasis: Update 1987. J Urol 140:461–467, 1988.
2. Wesson MB: Renal Calculi: Etiology and prophylaxis. J Urol 34:289, 1935.
3. Fuchs R: Geschichte der Heilkunde bei den Griechen. *In* Neuburger M, Pagel J (eds): Handbuch der Geschichte der Medizin. Jena, German Democratic Republic, G. Fischer, 1902, pp 153–402.
4. Hippocrates: The Genuine Works of Hippocrates, translated from the Greek with a Preliminary Discourse and Annotations by Francis Adams. Vol I. *In* On Airs, Waters and Places. New York, William Wood & Company, 1849, No 9, pp 165–166.
5. Howard JE, Thomas WC Jr, Mukai T, et al: The calcification of cartilage by urine, and a suggestion for therapy in patients with certain kinds of calculi. Trans Assoc Am Physicians 75:301–305, 1962.
6. Fleisch H, Bisaz S, Care AD: Effect of orthophosphate on urinary pyrophosphate excretion and the prevention of urolithiasis. Lancet 1:1065–1067, 1964.
7. Yendt ER, Guay GF, Garcia DA: The use of thiazides in the preparation of renal calculi. Can Med Assoc J 102:614–620, 1970.
8. Coe FL, Raisen L: Allopurinol treatment of uric-acid disorders in calcium-stone formers. Lancet 1:129–131, 1973.
9. Pak CYC: A cautious use of sodium cellulose phosphate in the management of calcium nephrolithiasis. Invest Urol 19:187–190, 1981.
10. Griffith DP, Osborne CA: Infection (urease) stones. Miner Electrolyte Metab 13:278–285, 1987.
11. Pak CYC: Citrate and renal calculi. Miner Electrolyte Metab 13:257–266, 1987.
12. Pak CYC, Fuller C, Sakhaee K, et al: Management of cystine nephrolithiasis with alpha-mercaptopropionyl-glycine (Thiola). J Urol 136:1003–1008, 1986.
13. Hosking DH, Erickson SB, Van Den Berg CJ, et al: The stone clinic effect in patients with idiopathic calcium urolithiasis. J Urol 130:1115–1118, 1983.
14. Pak CYC, Smith LH, Resnick MI, Weinerth JL: Dietary management of idiopathic calcium urolithiasis. J Urol 131:850–852, 1984.
15. Pak CYC, Sakhaee K, Crowther C, Brinkley L: Evidence justifying a high fluid intake in treatment of nephrolithiasis. Ann Intern Med 93:36–39, 1980.
16. Pak CYC, Peters P, Hurt G, Kadesky M, et al: Is selective therapy of recurrent nephrolithiasis possible? Am J Med 71:615–622, 1981.
17. Pak CYC: Medical management of nephrolithiasis. J Urol 128:1157–1164, 1982.

18. Pak CYC: Role of medical prevention. J Urol 141:798–801, 1989.
19. Ettinger B, Citron JT, Livermore B, Dolman LI: Chlorthalidone reduces calcium oxalate calculus recurrence but magnesium hydroxide does not. J Urol 139:679–684, 1988.
20. Preminger GM, Pak CYC: Eventual attenuation of hypocalciuric response to hydrochlorothiazide in absorptive hypercalciuria. J Urol 137:1104–1109, 1987.
21. Barilla DE, Pak CYC: Pitfalls in parathyroid evaluation in patients with calcium urolithiasis. Urol Res 7:117–182, 1979.
22. Barilla DE, Zerwekh JE, Pak CYC: A critical evaluation of the role of phosphate in the pathogenesis of absorptive hypercalciuria. Miner Electrolyte Metab 2:302–309, 1979.
23. Dudley FJ, Blackburn CRB: Extraskeletal calcification complicating oral neutral-phosphate therapy. Lancet 2:628–630, 1970.
24. Sakhaee K, Nicar M, Hill K, Pak CYC: Contrasting effects of potassium citrate and sodium citrate therapies on urinary chemistries and crystallization of stone-forming salt. Kidney Int 24:348–352, 1983.
25. Pak CYC, Sakhaee K, Fuller C: Successful management of uric acid nephrolithiasis with potassium citrate. Kidney Int 30:422–428, 1986.
26. Lawoyin S, Sismilich S, Browne R, Pak CYC: Bone mineral content in patients with primary hyperparathyroidism, osteoporosis, and calcium urolithiasis. Metabolism 28:1250–1254, 1979.
27. Pak CYC: Physiological basis for absorptive and renal hypercalciurias. Am J Physiol 237:F415–F423, 1979.
28. Bordier P, Ryckewart A, Gueris J, Rasmussen H: On the pathogenesis of so-called idiopathic hypercalciuria. Am J Med 63:398–409, 1977.
29. Preminger GM, Sakhaee K, Pak CYC: Hypercalciuria and altered intestinal calcium absorption occurring independently of vitamin D in distal renal tubular acidosis. Metabolism 36:176–179, 1987.
30. Pak CYC, Fuller C, Sakhaee K, et al: Long term treatment of calcium nephrolithiasis with potassium citrate. J Urol 134:11–19, 1985.
31. Pak CYC, Sakhaee K, Fuller CJ: Physiological and physicochemical prevention of calcium-stone formation by potassium citrate therapy. Trans Assoc Am Physicians 96:294–305, 1983.

13

Chemolysis

Martin I. Resnick
J. Patrick Spirnak

The ideal chemolytic agent would be nontoxic, orally administered, inexpensive, and able to dissolve the stone in question within a relatively short time (e.g., within days). Though in many instances this ideal is nearly reached (e.g., alkaloid agents used to dissolve uric acid stones), for the majority of urinary calculi, safe, easily administered, and rapid-acting agents are nonexistent. The ideals desired are easily conceived, but unfortunately progress has been slow in the development of this treatment modality.

HISTORY

Most medical historians credit Crowell with the first successful application of chemolysis in treating urinary stones.[1] In 1924, he reported the successful dissolution of two cystine stones by irrigating the renal pelvis in a retrograde manner with merbromin (Mercurochrome). The patient was also administered oral alkylating agents during the period of irrigation. Approximately two decades later in 1943, Suby and Albright reported the successful dissolution of phosphate calculi by irrigating with a magnesium and citrate solution administered through a nephrostomy tube.[2] The solutions found to be most effective (B and G) were acidic (pH 4.2) and contained magnesium to reduce mucosal irritability and a citrate buffer. A recent report supports this observation that magnesium tends to protect the urothelium.[3] Only calcium phosphate, magnesium ammonium phosphate, and calcium carbonate stones were found to be susceptible to these solutions. In 1962, Keyser and associates attempted to dissolve the outer colloid coating of stones by using enzymes (ferment solution) in combination with Suby's solution G.[4] The solution was applied to the stones via two ureteral catheters. It is of interest that they noted that a 0.5 per cent urease solution was most efficacious. In 1959, Mulvaney reported on the dissolution of urinary tract stones with local irrigation using 10 per cent hemiacidrin, a solution containing a mixture of gluconic and citric acid and their magnesium salts.[5, 6] The solution probably functions by a magnesium-calcium ion exchange in the calculus, thus forming a more soluble salt. In 1962, Kohler reported a death associated with hemiacidrin irrigation, and the patient's autopsy revealed extensive renal damage.[7] A year later in 1963, four deaths were reported in patients experiencing septic shock and severe pulmonary edema.[8] Because of these observations, hemiacidrin was withdrawn from clinical use in the United States, and the utilization of chemolytic solutions generally fell into disfavor.

With the development of endourology and the refinement of percutaneous techniques, in addition to the utilization of extracorporeal shock wave lithotripsy, there has been a renewed interest in these techniques. Not only have attempts been made to improve the methods of dissolution of uric acid and cystine stones, but also new techniques and solutions have been applied to the traditionally more resistant stones—magnesium ammonium phosphate and calcium oxalate.

INDICATIONS

Chemolysis can be utilized as the initial or primary treatment of a stone, or it may be used secondarily, usually following a surgical or fragmentation procedure (percutaneous nephrolithotomy, extracorporeal shock wave lithotripsy). The choice of the most appropriate approach is primarily dependent on stone type and location, the clinical status of the patient, and the availability of methods of treatment. Therapy can also vary with regard to whether it is systemic or local. An example of the former is the administration of an oral alkylating agent in an attempt to dissolve a uric acid stone, and an example of local therapy would be administration of hemiacidrin solution through a nephrostomy tube to assist in dissolution of a struvite or infection stone. Typically, uric acid and cystine stones are treated with systemic agents, but at times cystine stones can also be treated by local irrigation as well. Struvite stones will often respond to local therapy. Unfortunately, the most common stones, calcium oxalate–calcium phosphate stones, do not respond well to any form of chemolysis.

SYSTEMIC ALKALINE THERAPY

In most instances, administration of alkylating agents to obtain systemic alkalinization is the initial form of therapy for treating both cystine and uric acid stones. In both cases, the principle of chemolysis is based on the physical laws of urinary saturation and dissolution-crystallization. Associated with the administration of alkylating agents is the recommendation to increase fluid intake so that 24-hour urinary volumes are increased to 2 to 4 liters. This practice is often particularly recommended in attempts to dissolve cystine stones. It is this combination of urinary alkalinization and dilution that often has significant impact on the ability to achieve total stone dissolution.

Uric Acid Stones

Uric acid stones typically form in the presence of an acidic urine (pH less than 5.5), and in most instances hyperuricosuria is not present. Uric acid is a weak organic acid with a pKa of 5.35 in urine at 37°C. Stone formation occurs because uric acid is in the nondissociated form in the presence of acidic urine and supersaturation and subsequent crystallization results. Similarly, when urinary pH approaches 7.0, more than half of the uric acid is in the dissociated form, and not only is crystallization unlikely but also dissolution often occurs.[9–13] On the basis of the solubility curve of uric acid, there is little advantage in attempting to raise the urine pH to greater than 7.0. In addition, attempts to decrease uric acid excretion by dietary restriction or by administration of allopurinol, an xanthine oxidase inhibitor, may be of benefit.[11]

Sodium bicarbonate in a daily dose of 0.5 to 1.5 mEq/kg is the least expensive and therefore the most popular of the alkylating agents. When it is administered in this dosage evenly throughout the day (usually four times daily), urinary pH can often be elevated to the therapeutic range. Sodium bicarbonate tablets are generally composed of 12 mEq of base in each gram of sodium bicarbonate or 7.5 mEq in the readily available 10-grain tablet. It is unusual to require more than 4 grams of sodium bicarbonate. Sodium bicarbonate can be interspersed between potassium alkalinizing salts, but it is unusual to require more than 4 grams of sodium bicarbonate for the usual dose of 75 to 100 mEq of potassium salts. The disadvantage of this approach is the high sodium load administered to patients, and if this becomes a problem, a mixture of sodium–potassium citrate and citric acid can be substituted.[14, 15] Many patients with uric acid stones have concomitant hypertension or other cardiovascular problems; therefore, it is desirable to avoid a large sodium load if possible.

Another oral preparation being used with increasing frequency is potassium citrate. The average dose varies from 15 to 20 mEq three or four times a day, and sustained levels of alkalinization are readily achieved. The absorbed citrate is metabolized to bicarbonate, and it is the alkaline load that induces citrate production and excretion by the kidney. Studies indicate that it is only a small percentage of the orally administered citrate that reaches the kidney in its unmetabolized form. Potassium citrate is also available in wax-impregnated tablets, which results in delayed release and subsequently more sustained levels of alkalinization.

Acetazolamide, a carbonic anhydrase inhibitor, has also been used to assist in urinary alkalinization. The agent is particularly helpful when a large sodium load is to be avoided. The dosage used is 250 to 500 mg/day. Side effects are few but can include formation of calcium stones caused by the occurrence of secondary renal tubular acidosis.

Systemic alkalinization could also be achieved with intravenous solutions of bicarbonate and sodium lactate. Because the former solution is associated with a high sodium load, the tendency has been to use intravenous infusions of the latter as a means of achieving systemic alkalinization.[16, 17] Sodium lactate is a racemic salt in which the levo form is oxidized to bicarbonate and the dextro form is converted to glycogen. In addition, the glycogen provides an antiketogenic effect, and the sodium ion has an acid-neutralizing action. A one-sixth molar lactate solution is isotonic and, when metabolized in the normal manner, has the potential for acid neutralization equivalent to 340 ml of a 5 per cent sodium bicarbonate solution and an antiketogenic effect equivalent to 1000 ml of a 3 per cent dextro solution. Sodium lactate is converted completely to bicarbonate in only 1 to 2 hours.[18]

The use of a one-sixth molar lactate infusion at a rate of 500 ml every 6 to 10 hours is as safe and effective as direct irrigation with a sodium bicarbonate solution. A rapid change in urinary pH is achieved and remains constant. This form of systemic therapy provides an alternative approach in patients with obstructive and nonobstructive uric acid stones. Since interventional techniques are avoided, the chances of infection or complications are minimized. The rapid and effective achievement of sustained alkalinization is a particular advantage for the hospitalized patient, affording the opportunity for rapid stone dissolution. Success rates approaching 90 per cent have been achieved with this form of therapy.

A decided disadvantage of intravenous infusion therapy is the requirement for hospitalization during the period of administration. The current high cost of hospitalization makes this approach impractical for most patients, and it is therefore typically used in the patient with uric acid stones for whom hospitalization is required because of associated problems, such as pain or renal obstruction. Experience indicates that this approach is most effective in rapidly dissolving or assisting in the passage of uric acid ureteral stones. The passage of stones likely occurs because of the reduction in stone size related to treatment. Experience also indicates that the partially obstructed kidney produces an alkaline urine, and in association with lactate infusion, stone dissolution can often be accomplished with this approach.[19] Obviously, if hospitalization is not required, systemic alkalinization can be achieved with oral agents, as previously described.

It is well recognized that in most instances the formation of uric acid stones is associated with a persistently acidic urine because of an inability of the kidney to excrete base, and it is only the minority of patients who have associated abnormalities in pure metabolism with resultant hyperuricosuria.[20–23] Though restriction of dietary purines can be effective in preventing stone recurrence, more rapid reduction in urinary levels is usually required to aid in dissolution. Allopurinol, a xanthine oxidase inhibitor, is often very effective in potentiating the effect of alkylating agents. Administration of this agent in association with a high fluid intake to achieve an increased urinary volume (>2 liters/24 hr) is often very beneficial. This agent inhibits both xanthine oxidase and hyoxanthine oxidase and decreases the conversion of these two amino acids to uric acid. The agent is usually administered as a single dose of 300 mg. The drug is relatively safe, and side effects include rash, bone marrow suppression, hepatitis, vasculitis, formation of xanthine stones, and hypersensitivity reactions. The overall incidence of side effects is approximately 20 per cent, but the agent must be discontinued in only 5 per cent of patients.[15, 24]

Cystine Stones

Systemic alkalinization can also be utilized to dissolve cystine stones effectively. Approximately 1 to 3 per cent of all urinary stones are composed primarily of cystine,[25, 26] and stones occur in individuals homozygous for cystinuria. They generally have an early onset in the first or second decade of life, often occur bilaterally, typically are diagnosed after several episodes, and are associated with a high rate of recurrence.[27, 28]

As with uric acid stones, cystine stones are more soluble in an alkaline medium, and the attainment of a dilute alkaline urine is the primary goal of therapy for both dissolution and prevention. The pKa of cystine is 8.3; therefore, the solubility of stones of this type increases greatly above pH 7.5. In addition, the presence of high-volume (4 liters/24 hr) dilute urine favors dissolution of existing stones and greatly assists in preventing new stone formation. Alkalinization can be achieved with either sodium bicarbonate (250 to 500 mg/day in four divided doses) or potassium citrate (15 to 20 mEq three or four times a day).

The former medication is being recommended with decreasing frequency because of the high sodium load, the tendency to induce calcium stones because of the increased calcium excretion associated with a high salt intake, and the recent evidence suggesting a reduction in cystine excretion associated with a sodium-restricted diet.[29, 30] An additional advantage of the latter agent, potassium citrate, is that new delayed-release formulations tend to provide more sustained elevations in urinary pH.

One-sixth molar sodium lactate intravenous infusions can also be effective in dissolving cystine stones. The agent is administered as has been described for treating uric stones. As noted previously, problems exist because of the high sodium load and the need for hospitalization during the period of infusion. This approach is used if hospitalization is required because of associated pain or infection. It is also very useful following extracorporeal shock wave lithotripsy or, more commonly, percutaneous nephrolithotomy in helping to dissolve any residual stone fragments. Unlike uric acid stones, cystine stones are radiopaque and therefore cannot be monitored with routine radiographs (kidney, ureter, and bladder [KUB] films and nephrotomograms without injection of contrast agents).

Other agents that act systemically and are most effective are the thiol-disulfide exchangers. D-Penicillamine is the original agent in this category, but another that has recently gained approval by the U.S. Federal Drug Agency (FDA) is 2-mercaptoproprionylglycine (2-MPG).[31–34] These agents act at the disulfide bond of the cystine molecule and convert it to two molecules, each containing cystine and the exchanger-thiol residue. The resulting thiol-cystine complex is 50 times as soluble as the cystine molecule alone. Addition of these agents greatly enhances dissolution, but long-term maintenance is usually not recommended because of associated side effects, which include bone marrow suppression, proteinuria and resultant nephrotic syndrome, and maculopapular skin eruptions. Fortunately, all are reversible when the drug is discontinued. Vitamin B_6 (pyridoxine) is often administered in association with D-penicillamine to reduce the incidence of side effects.

Thiols are more effective when present in an alkaline medium; therefore, these drugs are administered in association with an alkylating agent of the types previously described. It is important to monitor urinary pH during therapy. In addition, decreases in cystine excretion can be monitored by quantitative amino acid analysis of urine. Though it has been reported that a low-methionine diet can also effect dissolution, compliance is poor, and therefore it is not often practical.

Systemic alkalinization in association with oral administration of a thiol exchanger is effective in dissolving only approximately 50 per cent of cystine stones and complete failures occur owing to poor compliance by the patient with a strict medical regimen but also owing to other noncystine crystalline elements associated with the stone.[28] Studies indicate that approximately 25 to 30 per cent of these stones contain calcium oxalate, calcium phosphate, and/or struvite, which interfere with attempts at chemolysis.[35, 36] These stones often appear more radiopaque than the pure cystine calculus, and this occurrence can often be predicted on a careful review of appropriately obtained radiographs.

The use of systemic agents in the treatment of other stone types—calcium oxalate, calcium phosphate, and struvite—is generally ineffective. Appropriate agents are not available for dissolution of calcium oxalate and calcium phosphate stones, and attempts at dissolution have usually been carried out by direct infusion of an appropriate agent onto or around the stone. This can be accomplished by placement of retrograde ureteral catheters but is more commonly performed by use of a nephrostomy tube. Exceptions always exist, and it has been observed that some patients with renal tubular acidosis receiving treatment with potassium citrate will clear their burden of multiple small stones, but whether this finding represents spontaneous asymptomatic passage or true dissolution remains unknown. Struvite stones are amenable to local irrigation with an appropriate agent, as are cystine and uric acid stones. Finally, chemolysis of struvite stones can occasionally be accomplished with administration of acetohydroxamic acid, a urease inhibitor, or an appropriate antibiotic, or both, but these approaches are often very time consuming and unreliable.[37, 38] These approaches are discussed in more detail in Chapter 8.

LOCAL THERAPY

Typically, local therapy is used as adjunctive treatment for dissolution of stone fragments remaining after extracorporeal shock wave lithotripsy, percutaneous nephrolithotomy, or open surgery. Though often used in the treatment of struvite stones, this technique is applicable for uric acid and cystine stones as well. Occasionally, local chemolysis can be used as primary therapy. This is particularly true in the association of struvite stones in patients with intractable infections or in those who are a poor surgical risk (e.g., those with spinal cord injury, myelomeningocele, or urinary diversion). This approach is appealing because it avoids an invasive procedure in the patient in whom the likelihood of stone recurrence is high.

To be effective, local chemolysis must maximally expose the stone to the irrigating solution. In addition, adequate drainage of the kidney is essential not only to provide for ready egress of the solution but also to prevent significant elevations in intrarenal pelvic pressure so as to minimize intravenous resorption of the particular agent. It is also imperative to maintain a sterile urine, and if infection is detected, the infusion should be immediately discontinued.

Many systems have been devised for irrigation. Some are planned, and others tend to conform to the particular clinical situation, but all should adhere to the principles as outlined previously. Irrigation via ureteral catheters is of limited value, since the patient must remain at bedrest because repositioning of the catheter is frequently necessary and because only small amounts of solution can be administered at a slow rate, thereby prolonging the time required for stone dissolution.

In most instances, the irrigating solution is administered via a nephrostomy catheter, and various systems of renal drainage have been devised (Fig. 13–1).

Universal stent techniques are shown in Figure 13–1*A*. This technique, described by Smith, utilizes a nephrostomy tube positioned at the stone. A universal stent is also placed in the kidney and positioned with its drainage holes in the renal pelvis. Outflow is provided by the stent, thus avoiding the requirement of a urethral catheter and making the system more comfortable for the patient. An additional advantage of this technique is that if fragments change position, the flow can be reversed by infusing through the stent, with drainage provided by the nephrostomy tube.[39–41]

Another system, described by Hare and McOmish, utilizes a 12F or 14F coaxial sheath (Fig. 13–1*B*).[42] Irrigation fluid is administered via a polyethylene catheter that can be manipulated to administer the solution in the most appropriate portion of the kidney. Outflow is provided by the outer Teflon sheath.

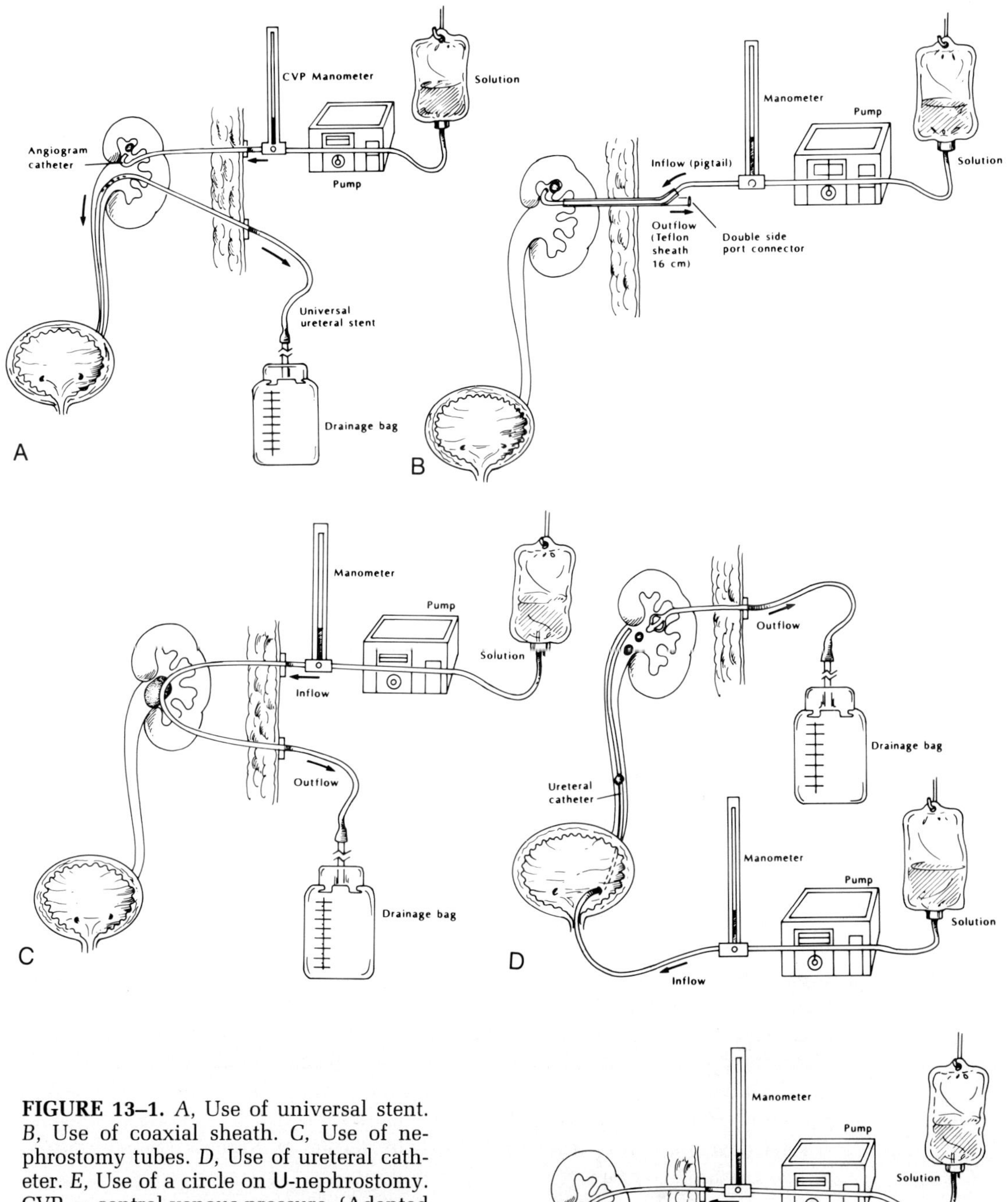

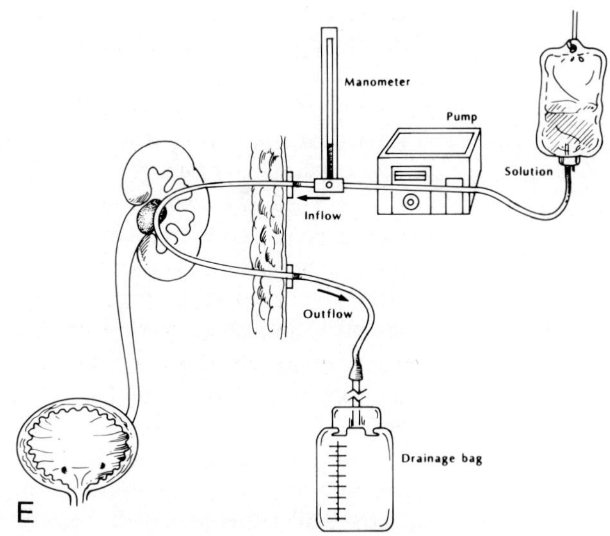

FIGURE 13–1. *A,* Use of universal stent. *B,* Use of coaxial sheath. *C,* Use of nephrostomy tubes. *D,* Use of ureteral catheter. *E,* Use of a circle on U-nephrostomy. CVP = central venous pressure. (Adapted from Eshaghi M, Smith AD: Chemolysis of calculi: Systemic and direct approaches. *In* Smith AD, Castaneda-Zuniga WR, Bronson JG (eds): Endourology: Principles and Practice. New York, Thieme, 1986, pp 173–202.)

The infusion-drainage system can also be reversed if it is believed that this would be more effective in a given clinical situation.

Two nephrostomy tubes can also be utilized: one for infusion and the other for drainage (Fig. 13–1*C*). Effective drainage is provided with this approach, but it does necessitate two nephrostomy tracts. In addition, the unprotected ureteropelvic junction and ureter may become occluded owing to dislodged stone fragments.

Adequate drainage of the kidney can also be obtained with a ureteral catheter (Fig. 13–1*D*). The advantage of this technique is that placement of only one nephrostomy tube is necessary, but the significance of this advantage is the potential for obstruction and poor drainage often associated with a small ureteral catheter. As noted previously, the presence of the urethral catheter is often uncomfortable to the patient and significantly limits mobility. With these systems, it is imperative that intrapelvic pressures be carefully monitored, and the irrigation should be discontinued if drainage is believed to be inadequate.

Another commonly used system utilizes a circle or U-nephrostomy tube (Fig. 13–1*E*). The holes in the catheters are positioned in the renal pelvis, and the inflow and outflow ports can be alternated. A significant disadvantage with this approach is the inability to position the point of infusion to be in direct contact with the stone. In addition, these tubes tend to slip, and the central holes can be displaced from within the renal pelvis, thus interfering with inflow and outflow.

Another ingenius but relatively simple technique is the use of a computer to provide both inflow and outflow through a single ureteral catheter (Fig. 13–1*F*).[43] A ureteral catheter is positioned in the renal pelvis and connected to a pressure monitor with a computer-controlled valve. An automatic shut-off valve activates, should the intrapelvic pressure become greater than 15 cm water. It is believed that the system of intermittent irrigation with associated turbulence of the infusion solution may be more effective than continuous systems. The system is experimental but is most promising as being a safe and effective means of achieving stone dissolution.

When irrigating solutions are used to effect stone dissolution, the patient must be treated with appropriate antibiotics to eradicate any infection and to render the urine sterile. The sterility of daily urine cultures obtained from the irrigation catheter must also be confirmed. In addition, irrigation should not be performed in the presence of urinary obstruction. Continuous monitoring of intrapelvic pressures is essential, and levels should not be allowed to exceed 20 to 25 cm water. It has been demonstrated that if these pressures are allowed to exceed venous pressures, systemic resorption occurs and the patient becomes at risk for development of sepsis and of toxicity secondary to the systemic infusion of the irrigating solution.[44]

To ensure that intrapelvic pressures do not exceed venous pressures, various devices have been developed, and they are shown in Figure 13–1. A manometer is positioned so that zero pressure is recorded at the level of the kidney, and a cut-off valve is set at the desired pressure (e.g., 25 cm water). The system is left open via a stopcock-type valve, so spontaneous decompression of the system occurs should the desired maximal pressure be exceeded. It is important to emphasize that if the patient is repositioned, the zero point should be reestablished.

Prior to irrigation with the desired chemolytic solution, the renal pelvis should be irrigated with a sterile saline solution for 24 to 48 hours. It is imperative that the collecting system be completely intact before irrigation is instituted.

Plain radiographs, nephrograms, and nephrotomograms should be obtained prior to initiating dissolution to document the integrity of the collecting system and to document the position and size of stones to be dissolved. The leakage of contrast material must be resolved before irrigation is initiated. When complete healing has occurred and the patient tolerates saline infusion, the appropriate irrigating solution can then be administered. Generally, the infusion rate should not exceed 120 ml/hr, and it should obviously be discontinued if intrapelvic pressures are high. If the patient experiences any discomfort, fever, or evidence of extravasation, irrigation should be discontinued immediately. If nursing or monitoring personnel are limited at any time, dissolution should not be carried out (e.g., 11 PM to 7 AM). It is also useful to instruct the patient about the mechanics of the system so that he or she can also stop the irrigation if indicated (e.g., if pain occurs). Follow-up plain radiographs and nephrotomograms should be obtained every 3 to 5 days, as they are helpful in monitoring stone dissolution. Irrigation should be continued for 24 to 48 hours after the patient is stone free radiographically because small undetectable fragments may remain.

As noted, urine obtained from nephrostomy tubes must be cultured daily. In addition, daily serum samples should be obtained for complete blood count, creatinine, blood urea nitrogen (BUN), and electrolytes. Specific parameters (e.g., serum magnesium and calcium levels) should be obtained based on the irrigating solution being used (e.g., hemiacidrin).

Should the patient develop sepsis, the urine culture become positive, and/or blood chemistries become abnormal, the irrigation should be immediately discontinued. All tubes should be maintained on dependent drainage, and if any evidence of obstruction is suspected, they should be replaced. When the problem resolves and the patient stabilizes, infusion can again be resumed.

STRUVITE OR INFECTION STONES

Infection stones are composed primarily of magnesium ammonium phosphates (struvite) and carbonate apatite and occur in approximately 15 to 25 per cent of the stone-forming population. The ratio of men to women is 1:2, and in all instances these stones are associated with urease-producing bacteria.[45, 46] Urealysis results in an elevation of urinary pH to greater than 7.0 and a subsequent increase in the concentration of carbonate ions. The enzymatic breakdown of urea produces an increase in urinary alkalinity and in bicarbonate and ammonia concentration, all of which conditions favor precipitation of magnesium ammonium phosphate and carbonate apatite. Normally, sterile urine is undersaturated with respect to magnesium ammonium phosphate and carbonate apatite; however, with the breakdown of urea and the resultant chemical changes in the urine, the urine rapidly becomes supersaturated with these products. Urease production by bacteria occurs most commonly in the species of *Proteus*, *Pseudomonas*, *Klebsiella*, and *Staphylococcus*. *Escherichia coli* organisms do not produce urease and, when associated with a struvite stone, likely represent a superimposed infection. It is also important to remember that urinary tract infections with urease-producing bacteria superimposed on metabolic stone disease can result in the deposition of struvite stones on a noninfectious calculus; therefore, careful evaluation of patients with "infection stones" for an underlying metabolic disorder should be carried out.[47]

Acidifying Solution

Hemiacidrin is composed of the following: D-glucuronic acid, 0.3 per cent; glucuronolactone, 0.1 per cent; citric acid, 0.6 per cent; magnesium citrate, 5.9 per cent; magnesium gluconocitrate, 1.2 per cent; magnesium carbonate, 0.8 per cent; and calcium carbonate, 0.2 per cent. It is used in a 10 per cent solution at pH 4.0. As noted previously, hemiacidrin was withdrawn from use within the kidney because of reported deaths from sepsis associated with its use in the early 1960s.[7, 8] Investigative studies regarding the effects of this agent were carried out in the 1970s. Cunningham noted radiographic changes in the upper tract urothelium with development of ulcerations and nodule formation in patients treated with this agent.[48] It was also demonstrated that significant absorption could occur, as demonstrated by elevations in serum magnesium levels during irrigation at the rate of 80 ml/hr.[49] Others have shown in animal experiments (dogs) that direct intravenous infusion could be carried out at rates up to 200 ml/liter before death occurred.[50] Further experience suggested that toxicity associated with these early reports was secondary to infection and related sepsis, and it has been repeatedly emphasized that the urine must be sterile both before and during irrigation.[51] Another commonly available acidifying agent is Suby's solution G, which contains citric acid monohydrate, magnesium citrate, and sodium citrate maintained at pH 4.[2, 4]

Acidifying solutions are primarily buffered citric acid solutions, and the mechanism of action in the dissolution of struvite stones relates to the acidity of the solution and the formation of soluble calcium citrate complexes. The presence of magnesium in these solutions increases chemolysis by ion exchange with calcium in addition to decreasing the irritative effect of citric acid on the urothelium. Direct irrigation is performed as previously described. Careful daily monitoring of urine cultures and the serum levels of BUN, creatinine, and magnesium is essential during the period of infusion. The complications of infusion of these agents include hypermagnesemia, which results in peripheral vasodilation or respiratory depression.[49, 52] Sepsis is associated with the infusion of the agent in an infected system.

Though used primarily for adjunctive dissolution of remaining fragments following surgery, percutaneous nephrolithotomy, or extracorporeal shock wave lithotripsy, hemiacidrin irrigation has been used for primary treatment as well.[53–66] Success rates have varied, and when used following open surgical procedures for removal of struvite stones, the incidence of recurrent stone disease in patients rendered stone free varies from 0 to 25 per cent over a mean follow-up period of 17 to 84 months. Similarly, the incidence of recurrent infection in patients rendered stone free after irrigation varies from 0 to 28 per cent over a similar period of follow-up. As expected, recurrent infection was often associated with recurrent stone formation. In most instances, when utilized as an adjunct to other methods of stone removal, more than 75 per cent of remaining stone fragments can be effectively dissolved. Reviews of reports documenting the efficacy of percutaneous nephrolithotomy and extracorporeal shock wave lithotripsy often mention the adjunctive use of hemiacidrin irrigation with these procedures, but unfortunately the success rates and the time required for irrigation are often not documented.

Success following irrigation as a form of primary therapy has been greater than 80 per cent, but few data are available regarding the follow-up period of stone recurrence. The period of time of irrigation varies but ranges from 5 to 90 days. Because of the significant amount of time required for irrigation and the need for close monitoring of the patient, this approach is primarily utilized in individuals who are poor candidates for a more invasive procedure or in those who have a high likelihood of developing recurrent disease because of the presence of intractable urinary tract infections or cutaneous urinary diversion.

CYSTINE STONES

As noted, in most instances, pure cystine stones can be adequately dissolved by the combined administration of systemic alkalinizing agents and thiols. At times, particularly following surgery or percutaneous nephrolithotomy, direct irrigation of the stone may be a more efficient means of rendering these patients stone free. Alkalinizing agents and thiols are often also used in this manner.

Alkalinizing agents are composed primarily of sodium bicarbonate, tromethamine, and tromethamine E. The first-named solution is usually prepared by adding four ampules of sodium bicarbonate to 1N saline, resulting in a final concentration of 178 mEq/liter. Tromethamine E (THAM-E) is an organic amine buffer of pH 10.6. When reconstituted from its powdered form, the solution has an osmolarity of 367 osm/liter. THAM-E raises the pH of the irrigating solution to 10.5, making it a very effective means of dissolving cystine stones.[67, 68] It has long been established that the solubility of cystine rises with increasing urinary pH.[69, 70] Solubility is increased by 50 per cent at pH 7.5. At pH 9.0, the solubility increases 1400 per cent. An 80 per cent success rate has been achieved with this approach, but in one report an average of 29 days of treatment was required.

Cystine stone dissolution has also been found to be enhanced by the addition of acetylcystine to the irrigating solution. Mulvaney first advocated oral administration of acetylcystine in daily doses of 20 to 500 mg/kg of body weight, but further studies revealed that only a small percentage of the compound reached the circulation in its acetylated form.[71–74] Acetylcystine binds with the cysteine molecule, creating a highly soluble complex. Studies by Saltzman and Gittes demonstrated that the combination of acetylcystine with a strong alkalinizing agent, such as tromethamine, at a pH of approximately 9.0 yielded a very effective solution for cystine dissolving stones.[75] With alkaline solutions containing acetylcystine, successful primary dissolution occurs in greater than 60 per cent of cases, with the period of irrigation ranging from 5 to 90 days.[76–78] Experimentally, it has been demonstrated that shock wave lithotripsy enlarges the surface area of cystine stones, thereby increasing the efficacy of dissolution with acetylcystine-alkylating solutions.[79]

URIC ACID STONES

Systemic alkalinization is often very effective in dissolving uric acid stones, but irrigating these calculi is also successful. A variety of alkalinizing agents have been shown to be effective, including sodium bicarbonate and tromethamine.[80–88] Success with these solutions, when used either as primary therapy or as adjunctive therapy, has been greater than 90 per cent. In contrast to other stones undergoing chemolysis, uric acid stones dissolve relatively quickly, and the time needed for irrigation has ranged from 3 to 21 days, with the majority of stones requiring less than 10 days of irrigation to achieve complete dissolution.

CALCIUM OXALATE–CALCIUM PHOSPHATE STONES

Unfortunately, the common calcium oxalate–calcium phosphate stones are not readily amenable to chemolysis. When the procedure is attempted, chelating agents have been utilized more than alkalinizing or acidifying agents, which have been successfully used for stones of other compositions.[89, 90] Unfortunately, ethylenediaminetetraacetic acid (EDTA), an effective chelating agent, has been found to be ineffective in dissolving these stones.[39] Experimental studies performed in vitro identified various chelating agents that appear to be effective in dissolving calcium oxalate and calcium phosphate stones at pH 8, but their clinical efficacy and toxicity remain unknown.[91]

CONCLUSION

Chemolysis is an effective means of treating stones of specific chemical composition. Alkalinizing agents are very effective in dissolving uric acid stones, and when combined with thiols, cystine stones can be dissolved as well. Administration can be either systemic or by local irrigation. Struvite stones have been found to be effectively dissolved with acidifying solutions, but usually treatment is carried out in association with percutaneous nephrolithotomy or extracorporeal shock wave lithotripsy. Calcium oxalate–calcium phosphate stones unfortunately are not readily amenable to chemolytic agents.

When chemolysis is performed, particularly with local irrigation, careful monitoring of the patient is required to avoid problems related to metabolic disturbances and sepsis. When carried out in a carefully planned manner in the appropriate patient, this form of therapy can be most effective and can render many patients stone free.

REFERENCES

1. Crowell AJ: Cystine nephrolithiasis: Report of case with roentgenographic demonstration of disintegration of stone by alkalinization. Surg Gynecol Obstet 38:87, 1924.
2. Suby HI, Albright F: Dissolution of phosphatic urinary calculi by the retrograde introduction of a citrate solution containing magnesium. N Engl J Med 228:81, 1943.
3. Reckler J, Rodman JS, Jacobs D, et al: Urothelial injury to the rabbit bladder from various alkaline and acidic solutions used to dissolve kidney stones. J Urol 136:181, 1986.
4. Keyser LD, Scherer PC, Claffey LW: Studies in the dissolution of urinary calculi: Experimental and clinical studies. J Urol 59:826, 1962.
5. Mulvaney WP: A new solvent for certain urinary calculi: Preliminary report. J Urol 82:546, 1959.
6. Mulvaney WP: The clinical use of renacidin in urinary calcifications. J Urol 84:206, 1960.
7. Kohler FP: Renacidin and tissue reaction. J Urol 87:102, 1962.
8. Fostvedt GA, Barnes RW: Complications during lavage therapy for renal calculi. J Urol 89:329, 1963.
9. Fried FA, Vermuelen CW: Artificial uric acid concretion and observations on uric acid solubility and supersaturation. Invest Urol 2:131, 1964.
10. Atsman A, deVries A, Lazebnik J, Salinger H: Dissolution of renal uric acid stones by oral alkalinization and large fluid intake in a patient suffering from gout. Am J Med 27:167, 1959.
11. Rodman JS, Williams JJ, Peterson CM: Dissolution of uric acid calculi. J Urol 131:1039, 1984.
12. Burns JR, Ganthier JF, Finlayson B: Dissolution kinetics of uric acid calculi. J Urol 131:708, 1984.
13. Sadi MV, Saltzman N, Feria G, Gittes RF: Experimental observations on dissolution of uric acid calculi. J Urol 134:575, 1985.
14. Gill WB: Urolithiasis update. Am J Kidney Dis 1:66, 1983.

15. Rudman D, Afforah H, Tuttle EP, Glenn JF: Medical management of the patient with renal calculi. AUA Update 2. Houston, American Urological Association, 1983.
16. Kursh ED, Resnick MI: Dissolution of uric acid calculi with systemic alkalinization. J Urol 132:286, 1984.
17. Lewis RW, Roth JK Jr, Polanco EJ, Roberts JA: Molar lactate in the management of uric acid renal obstruction. J Urol 125:87, 1981.
18. Alkalinizing agents in American hospital formulary service. Am Soc Hosp Pharmacol 40:8, 1959.
19. Libert MH, Wart F: Management of uric acid renal obstructin by intravenous lactate. Eur Urol 11:22, 1985.
20. Henneman PH, Wallach S, Dempsey EF: The metabolic defect responsible for uric acid stone formation. J Clin Invest 41:537, 1962.
21. Yu TF, Gutman AB: Uric acid nephrolithiasis in gout: Predisposing factors. Ann Intern Med 67:1133, 1967.
22. Barzel US, Sperling O, Frank M, deVries A: Renal ammonium excretion and urinary pH in idiopathic uric acid lithiasis. J Urol 92:1, 1964.
23. Armstrong WA, Greene LF: Uric acid calculi: With particular reference to determinations of uric acid content of blood. J Urol 70:545, 1953.
24. May P, Schindler E: Methods and results of conservative treatment of uric acid stones in urinary calculi. *In* Cifuentes Delatte L, Rapado A, Hodkinson A (eds): Recent Advances in Etiology, Stone Structure and Treatment. Basel, S Karger, 1973, p 111.
25. Menon M, Krishman CS: Evaluation and medical management of the patient with calcium stone disease. Urol Clin North Am 10:4, 1983.
26. Prien EL: Crystallographic analysis of urinary calculi: A 23-year study. J Urol 89:917, 1963.
27. Cifuentes JM, Pourmand G: Mineral composition of 103 stones from Iran. Br J Urol 55:465, 1983.
28. Evans WP, Resnick MI, Boyce WH: Homozygous cystinuria—evaluation of 35 patients. J Urol 127:707, 1982.
29. Dahlberg PF, Van Den Berg CJ, Kurtz SB, et al: Clinical features and management of cystinuria. Mayo Clin Proc 52:533, 1977.
30. Martelle WA, Norman RW: Dietary restriction of sodium as a means of reducing urinary cystine. Urol Res 16:264, 1988.
31. Jaeger P, Portmann L, Saunders A, Rosenberg LE, Thier SO: Anticystinuric effects of glutamine and of dietary sodium restriction. N Engl J Med 315:1120, 1986.
32. Kallistratos G: Physiochemical principles and clinical results concerning the conservative treatment of kidney stones. Urol Int 29:93, 1974.
33. Kallistratos G: Litholytic agents: Preventive and curative drugs for nephrolithiasis. Drug Design 4:237, 1973.
34. Koide T, Konoshita K, Takemoto M, et al: Conservative treatment of cystine calculi: Effect of oral alpha-mercaptoproprionylglycine on cystine stones, dissolution and/or prevention of stone recurrence. J Urol 128:513, 1982.
35. Dent CE, Senior BS: Studies on the treatment of cystinuria. Br J Urol 27:317, 1955.
36. Shaw DG, Sutor DJ: Cystine stone dissolution. Br J Radiol 45:664, 1972.
37. Rodman JS, Williams JJ, Peterson CM: Partial dissolution of struvite calculus with oral acetohydroxamic acid. Urology 22:410, 1983.
38. Lewis GA, Schuster GA, Cooper RA: Dissolution of renal calculi with dicloxacillin. Urology 22:401, 1983.
39. Smith AD, Lee WJ: Percutaneous stone removal procedure including irrigation. Urol Clin North Am 10:719, 1983.
40. Sheldon CA, Smith AD: Chemolysis of calculi. Urol Clin North Am 9:121, 1982.
41. Eshghi M, Smith AD: Chemolysis of calculi: Systemic and direct approach. *In* Smith AD, Castaneda-Zuniga WR, Bronson JG (ed): Endourology: Principles and Practice. New York, Thieme, 1980, pp 173–202.
42. Hare WSC, McOmish D: Nephrostomy lavage set for dissolving renal stones. Radiology 144:932, 1982.
43. Kuwahara M, Kambe K, Takahashi K, et al: Intermittent irrigation system for dissolution of renal calculi: Monitored by computer. J Urol 128:1379, 1982.
44. Mulvaney WP: The hydrodynamics of renal irrigations: With reference to calculus solvents. J Urol 89:765, 1963.
45. Nemoy NJ, Stamey TA: Surgical, bacteriological and biochemical management of "infection stones." JAMA 215:1470, 1971.
46. Griffith DP: Struvite stones. Kidney Int 13:372, 1978.
47. Resnick MI: Evaluation and management of infection stones. Urol Clin North Am 8:265, 1981.
48. Cunningham JJ, Friedland GW, Stamey TA: Radiologic changes in the urothelium during renacidin irrigations. J Urol 109:556, 1973.
49. Cato AR, Tulloch AGS: Hypermagnesemia in a uraemic patient during renal pelvis irrigation with renacidin. J Urol 111:313, 1974.
50. Rosen DI, Nemoy NJ, Wolf PL, et al: Intravenous infusion of renacidin in dogs. Invest Urol 9:31, 1977.

51. Nemoy NJ, Stamey TA: Use of hemiacidrin in management of infection stones. J Urol 116:693, 1976.
52. Jenny DB, Goris AB, Urwiller RD, et al: Hypermagnesemia following irrigation of renal pelvis: Cause of respiratory depression. JAMA 240:1378, 1978.
53. Sant G, Blaivas JG, Meares EM Jr: Hemiacidrin irrigation in the management of struvite calculi: Long-term results. J Urol 130:1048, 1983.
54. Jacobs SC, Gittes RF: Dissolution of residual renal calculi with hemiacidrin. J Urol 115:2, 1976.
55. Royle G, Smith JC: Recurrence of infected calculi following postoperative irrigation with stone solvent. Br J Urol 48:531, 1976.
56. Low AI: The use of hemiacidrin in the management of staghorn calculi. *In* Brockis JG, Finlayson B (eds): Urinary Calculus. Littleton, MA, PSG Publishing Company, 1981, p 427.
57. Silverman DE, Stamey TA: Management of infection stone: The Stanford experience. Medicine 62:44, 1983.
58. Dretler SP, Pfister RC: Primary dissolution therapy of struvite calculi. J Urol 131:861, 1984.
59. Pfister RC, Dretler SP: Percutaneous chemolysis of renal calculi. Urol Radiol 6:138, 1984.
60. Palmer JM, Bishai MB, Mallon DS: Outpatient irrigation of the renal collecting system with 10 per cent hemiacidrin: Cumulative experience of 365 days in 13 patients. J Urol 138:262, 1987.
61. Spirnak JP, DeBaz BP, Green HY, et al: Complex struvite calculi treated by primary extracorporeal shock wave lithotripsy and chemolysis with hemiacidrin irrigation. J Urol 140:1356, 1988.
62. Kleine RS, Cattolica EV, Rankin KN: Hemiacidrin renal irrigation: Complications and successful management. J Urol 128:241, 1982.
63. Brock WA, Nachtsheim DA, Parsons CL: Hemiacidrin irrigation of renal pelvic calculi in patients with ileal conduit diversion. J Urol 123:345, 1980.
64. Uhlir K: The peroral dissolution of renal calculi. J Urol 104:239, 1970.
65. Fam B, Rossier AB, Yalla S, et al: The role of hemiacidrin in the management of renal stones in spinal cord injury patients. J Urol 116:696, 1976.
66. Dretler SP: Chemolysis of urinary calculi. AUA Update Series 5: Lesson 21. Houston, American Urological Association, 1986.
67. Tseng CH, Talmalker YB, Tank ES, et al: Dissolution of cystine calculi by pelvicaliceal irrigation with tromethamine-E. J Urol 128:1281, 1982.
68. Crissey MM, Gittes RF: Dissolution of cystine ureteral calculus by irrigation with tromethamine. J Urol 121:811, 1979.
69. Lewis HB: Cystinuria: A review of some recent investigations. Yale J Biol Med 4:437, 1932.
70. Weinberg SR, Tabenkin PA: Observations on therapy of cystine calculus disease. Mich Intern Med 90:850, 1952.
71. Mulvaney WP, Quilter T, Mortera A: Experiences with acetylcystine in cystinuric patients. J Urol 114:107, 1975.
72. Collini WR, Mattern SR, Shapiro P, et al: Methods of diminishing cystine excretion in cystinuria. J Urol 93:729, 1965.
73. Thomas J, Landier JF, Capentier C, et al: Cystinic lithiasis and its treatment. *In* Roth RA, Finlayson B (eds): Stones: Clinical Management of Urolithiasis. Baltimore, The Williams and Wilkins Company, 1982, pp 248–266.
74. North DS, Peterson RG, Krenzelok EP: Effect of activated charcoal administration in acetylcystine serum levels in humans. Am J Hosp Pharmacol 38:1022, 1981.
75. Saltzman N, Gittes RF: Chemolysis of cystine calculi. J Urol 136:846, 1986.
76. Smith AD, Lange PH, Miller RP, et al: Dissolution of cystine calculi by irrigation with acetylcysteine through percutaneous nephrostomy. J Urol 13:422, 1979.
77. Dretler SP, Pfister RC: Percutaneous dissolution of renal calculi. Annu Rev Med 34:359, 1983.
78. Weirich W, Ackermann D, Riedmiller H, et al: Die Auflosurg von Cystin-Steinen mit N-Acetylcystein nach perkutaner Nephrostomies. Alt Urol 12:224, 1981.
79. Schmeller NT, Kersting H, Schuller J, et al: Combination of chemolysis and shock wave lithotripsy in the treatment of cystine renal calculi. J Urol 131:434, 1984.
80. Gordon RL, Verstandig AG, Shapiro A: Salvage of an obstructed single kidney by combined percutaneous nephrostomy and percutaneous stone extraction and alkalinization. Eur Urol 9:50, 1983.
81. Hedglock MW, Eisenberg RL, Williams RD: Antegrade catheter technique to dissolve uric acid ureteral calculi. Urology 19:40, 1982.
82. Hardy B, Klein LA: In situ dissolution of ureteral calculus. Urology 8:444, 1976.
83. Spatars RF, Linke CA, Barbaric ZL: The use of percutaneous nephrostomy and urinary alkalinization in the dissolution of obstructing uric acid stones. Radiology 129:629, 1978.
84. Eason AA, Sharlip ID, Spaulding JO: Dissolution of bilateral uric acid calculi causing anemia. JAMA 240:670, 1978.
85. Nummi P: Dissolution of uric acid stones by local lavage. Scand J Urol Nephrol 7:172, 1973.
86. Sadi MV, Saltzman N, Feria G, et al: Experimental observations on dissolution of uric acid calculi. J Urol 134:575, 1985.
87. Blaivas JS, Pais UM, Spellman RM: Chemolysis of residual stone fragment after extensive surgery for staghorn calculi. Urology 6:680, 1975.

88. Ansari ER, Kazim E, Husain I: Management of choked ureter in obstructive renal failure due to uric acid lithiasis. J Urol 128:257, 1982.
89. Gittes RF, Raymond S: A new chemical approach to the dissolution of urinary calculi. J Urol 65:474, 1951.
90. Heap GJ, Perrin DD, Cliff WJ: Dissolving urinary stones with a chelating agent. Med J Aust 1:714, 1976.
91. Verplaetse H, Verbeek RMH, Minnaert H, et al: Screening of chelating agent for chemolysis. Eur Urol 12:190, 1986.

14

Surgery of Kidney and Ureteral Stones

Martin I. Resnick
J. Patrick Spirnak

The treatment of both renal and ureteral calculi has undergone significant changes over the past two to three decades. In the mid and late 1960s, major advances were made in a variety of interrelated areas. Newly developed antibiotics have enhanced all forms of medical care but are particularly applicable to the patient with urinary calculi and associated urinary tract infections. In addition, improved understanding of the pathogenesis of stone formation and the development of management programs to prevent stone growth and recurrence have also had significant impact on improved success. A better understanding of renal ischemia and the role of hyperthermia, the development of fine suture material and microsurgical procedures, as well as improved methods of detecting stones intraoperatively, all have had a cumulative but major impact. In the late 1960s and early 1970s, open surgical procedures, particularly anatrophic nephrolithotomy, were perfected, and improved results following removal of these large stones were realized. Percutaneous techniques were developed in the late 1970s, and extracorporeal shock wave lithotripsy (ESWL) became a reality in the early 1980s. These last two techniques, used either alone or in combination, have been successfully employed in the treatment of large staghorn calculi.

The role of open surgery for removal of both renal and ureteral stones is certainly diminished. Though most calculi are small and pass spontaneously, a select minority are too large and become lodged in the renal pelvis, calyx, infundibulum, or ureter. Currently, most are managed with ESWL or percutaneous nephrolithotomy, and understandably there is a tendency to forget the significant improvements that have been made in open surgery over the past several decades. Although it is apparent that the role of open surgery will not be as prominent in the future as it once was, urologists must maintain proficiency in and knowledge of a variety of open renal techniques. Traditional surgery will most likely continue for the management of complete staghorn calculi associated with intrarenal scarring and associated infundibular and calyceal stenosis, a condition in which intrarenal reconstruction is required. Similarly, other open procedures, such as partial nephrectomy, would at times also be necessary.

Ureterolithotomy will occasionally be performed in those patients in whom treatment with other less invasive modalities has failed. It is important that the clinical urologist not only be adept at the performance of these procedures but also be knowledgeable about their indications and the appropriate measures that are required in the management of these patients both preoperatively and postoperatively.

HISTORICAL OVERVIEW

Hippocrates is credited with being the earliest physician to describe the first surgical procedure on the kidney. As was commonplace at that time, surgery was performed to provide drainage of a lumbar or perirenal abscess, and the kidney was inadvertently incised during this procedure. Hippocrates noted that urinary fistulas were not infrequent following surgical drainage of perirenal abscesses, and he graphically described the procedure in his writings on the four diseases of the kidney:[1]

> . . . the urine, scalding and turbid is painful to pass, and leaves a thick sediment like flour or reddish, if bile predominates; if it is phlegm, it is white and thick. The disease lasts about a year and separation may develop; in this case an incision is made down to the kidney and the pus is evacuated.

It is not known whether Hippocrates deliberately performed nephrotomy for stone removal, but it is more likely that infected hydronephrotic kidneys were incised, as were perirenal abscesses. Calculi were probably extracted through these incisions or passed spontaneously during the postoperative period. Celsus, Galen, and other early physicians mentioned kidney stones in their writings, but none believed surgical extraction to be either safe or feasible. For hundreds of years, reports of stone surgery were few and poorly described. For example, a report by Cardan of Milan in 1501 described the purposeful opening of a renal or perirenal abscess with the extraction of 18 stones. In 1581, Rousset used the term "nephrotomy" in reporting the development of a urinary-cutaneous fistula in two patients, following an attempt to drain a presumed perirenal abscess with cautery and silver wire.

During the 1700s and early 1800s, various European surgeons had isolated experiences utilizing renal parenchymal incisions to remove intrarenal stones. Though success was varied, many patients evidently were relieved of their pain, infection, and abscess. During this time, most surgeons agreed that nephrotomies be limited to those cases in which the stone-containing kidney was distended with purulent matter and the stone was not palpable through a sinus tract. They recommended complete drainage of the kidney and either removal of the stone at the time of surgery or leaving them to be expelled spontaneously at a later time. In 1775, Hevin, who was believed to have been the first to use the term "nephrolithotomy," also concluded that renal operations be limited to infected kidneys.[2, 3]

On the basis of autopsy findings in 1869, Thomas Smith reported a "novel method for removing stones"; he proposed that the removal of branched calculi could be effected through a nephrotomy and described the technique in detail. Finally, in 1872 Marduel pointed out that the term "nephrotomy" did not accurately describe an operation in which the substance of the kidney was incised to effect removal and suggested that nephrolithotomy was more accurate to describe the intent of the procedure. He believed that the procedure could be performed safely, but better and more reliable means were required for accurate determination of the presence of stones so that the indications for the procedure could be more accurately defined.

Though reported 12 years following its performance, credit for the first deliberate nephrolithotomy can be attributed to Dr. William Ingalls at Boston City Hospital on October 8, 1872. Ingalls performed the procedure on a 31-year-old female patient in whom he had earlier drained the perirenal abscess. The postoperative course was complicated by sepsis. The patient eventually recovered and was in good health 8 years after the procedure. In 1880, Sir Henry Morris, an English surgeon, performed the first nephrolithotomy on a healthy kidney free of abscesses. In 1898, he reported his results on 34 nephrolithotomies and recorded only one death. Successful results helped to disprove the dangers of nephrolithotomy and showed the feasibility of removing renal stones before the kidney was converted into an abscess sac.

It is of interest that incisions in the renal pelvis, the pyelolithotomy, followed many of the descriptions regarding nephrotomy and nephrolithotomy. It was recognized in the late 1800s that incisions of the renal parenchyma were accompanied by bleeding both intraoperatively and postoperatively. Heieke, in 1879, employed the pyelolithotomy for removal of stones. This operation became very successful, and because it was associated with fewer complications, it rapidly became the preferred method of open stone removal. In 1880, Vincenz Czerny also described the pyelolithotomy and in 1887 was the first to use catgut to reapproximate the incision in the renal pelvis.

Controversy developed over which method of stone removal was preferable. Nephrolithotomy offered the major advantage of visualizing the entire collecting system directly, and it evolved into the conservative procedure of choice. With the development of useful clinical radiography in the early 1900s, accurate stone localization became possible and resulted in a renewed interest in pyelotomy for stone removal. In 1913, Lower advocated pyelolithotomy as the procedure of choice for simple pelvic stones.

Initial attempts at the surgical removal of ureteral calculi were directed at those stones located at the ureteral meatus. In 1732, LaDran used forceps to remove a tapering ureteral stone of which only a portion projected through the meatus. In 1788, Desault designed a specific blade with which he incised the ureteral meatus of a female patient and removed the stone. Dogon proposed the performance of a ureterotomy in 1856, and in 1879 Emmet operated upon two women for distal stones. During this period, many surgeons described removing stones located in the ureter. Generally, these were distal, and the approach used was extraperitoneal. Intraperitoneal approaches were often associated with significant complications and were discarded about the turn of the century.

It is also of interest to review methods of stone localization. Prior to the development of modern radiographic techniques, clinicians had difficulty in establishing the diagnosis of renal calculi with any degree of certainty. Indications for the surgical removal of stones were based mainly on clinical impressions of stone identification, and localization was performed with seemingly crude and imprecise methodology. In 1880, Barker, an English surgeon, described the technique of needling the kidney percutaneously in an effort to document the presence of a stone. The patients so studied generally presented with a flank mass likely due to perirenal abscess, and the needle was inserted into the flank at a point midway between the twelfth rib and the iliac crest. The presence of the point was documented when the point of the needle grated against the surface.[4] Evidently, this method never became popular, but similar techniques were also reported.

Surgeons of the late 1800s described the importance of carefully inspecting the surgically exposed kidney, with special attention given to areas having variations in contour or consistency or both. Other techniques devised to localize stones intraoperatively included probing the pelvis and calyces, performing a pyelotomy, and passing instruments to the lower pole of the kidney into the lowest calyx and bluntly probing for the stone. Most surgeons agree that if the stone could not be located by these maneuvers a nephrotomy should be done. The poor results of these approaches were brought out in the 1880s by the study of Dickenson, in which he reviewed a number of surgical procedures performed for stone removal.[5] He found that the expected stone was not present in 8 of 22 nephrotomies or in 7 of 16 nephrectomies. It is likely that all surgeons agreed that other and more precise techniques were needed.

Following Rankin's description of the surgical applications of radiographs in 1895, the possibility of their use in the diagnosis of renal calculi was raised. In 1896, MacIntyre was the first to use this new method to diagnose a urinary calculus.[6] In 1899, Albarran demonstrated examples of radiographic evidence of calculi, and in the same year Abbe collected additional cases from the literature.[7, 8] In an effort to increase diagnostic accuracy, the use of an opaque ureteral catheter was described by Von Illyes in 1902, and retrograde pyelography was introduced by Voelcher and von Lichtenberg in 1906.[9, 10] These techniques provided a major advance for diagnosing disorders of the kidney. Robson was the first to suggest a possible application of intraoperative radiographs to aid in stone localization.[11] The procedure was first described by Braasch and Carmen in 1919.[12, 13] Renal fluoroscopy was used intraoperatively, and small stone fragments that were not detected by palpation alone were localized. Quinby described the use of a static x-ray cassette for the purpose of obtaining films at the time of surgical intervention for stones.[14] Southerland reported that the combined intraoperative use of roentenography and fluoroscopy would largely eliminate the failure to find and remove all stones and stone fragments and advocated the routine use of these techniques in all stone surgery.[15, 16] Southerland also introduced the technique of placing needles into the kidney at the time of surgery and prior to taking radiographs in an effort to aid in stone localization. Others have described the use of wide grids or radiopaque threads to mark the kidney so that the stone could be localized with respect to the margins of the kidney.[17, 18] The eventual introduction and use of commercially available films in sealed plastic bags has greatly facilitated the technique for obtaining intraoperative radiographs on a routine basis. New techniques utilizing radioisotopes and ultrasound have been reported to aid in stone localization, but none is as popular or as practical as the method of static intraoperative roentgenography.[19, 20]

INDICATIONS FOR OPEN SURGICAL REMOVAL OF CALCULI

Although the procedures have changed over the years, the objectives of them have remained unchanged. These include removal of all stones, improvement of intrarenal drainage with reconstruction of the collecting system when necessary; preservation of maximal renal function; and eradication of upper urinary tract infections, when present, to reduce the rate of stone recurrence.

Today most small stones can be satisfactorily treated with ESWL or percutaneous nephrolithotomy or a combination of these two techniques. The role of open surgery is certainly reduced and in some respects remains controversial.

In light of recent developments, the indications for open renal surgery, especially anatrophic nephrolithotomy for removal of large staghorn calculi, include the following: the presence of extensive stone disease, which would necessitate multiple procedures, either percutaneous techniques or ESWL; the necessity for intrarenal reconstruction to improve intrarenal drainage; the presence of very hard stones that are not amenable to ESWL or percutaneous procedures; and the experience, expertise, and preference of the surgeon. Other indications for open surgical procedures for stone removal are not specifically related to anatrophic nephrolithotomy and include partial nephrectomy when required, the presence of coexisting problems in the kidney (e.g., ureteropelvic junction obstruction), and the presence of an infected, nonfunctioning kidney that necessitates nephrectomy. The inability to remove ureteral stones by ureteroscopic percutaneous or ESWL techniques is an obvious indication for ureterolithotomy.

In most instances, surgery can be delayed until a preliminary metabolic evaluation is completed. However, if severe obstruction or sepsis occurs, prompt temporizing urinary drainage is indicated. This drainage can be accomplished by retrograde catheter placement, percutaneous nephrostomy drainage, or, at times, formal open surgical removal.

PREOPERATIVE EVALUATION

Prior to surgery, all patients should have a thorough preoperative metabolic evaluation in an effort to identify predisposing factors leading to stone formation, and, unless an emergency situation exists, surgical intervention should be delayed until complete metabolic evaluation has been completed.[21, 22]

Hyperparathyroidism, hypercalciuria, hyperuricosuria, renal tubular acidosis, and cystinuria are but a few of the detectable metabolic causes of stone disease that are associated with stone formation. Measurements of serum and urinary calcium, phosphorus, uric acid, citrate, oxalate, creatinine, and electrolytes and the qualitative nitroprusside test for cystine are screening tests that often alert the physician to the existence of various metabolic disorders. In an effort to assess renal function, at least two 24-hour urine specimens should be obtained and measured for creatinine clearance. New computerized radionuclide studies have also been shown to be useful in the assessment of renal function and offer the advantage of providing specific data on each renal unit.

Urinalysis, urine culture, and antibiotic sensitivity studies of all cultured organisms are essential in documenting the presence and type of urinary tract infection and in the planning of appropriate antibacterial therapy. If patients are infected with multiple bacterial species, each organism should be adequately identified and appropriate antibiotic sensitivity studies performed. Stone cultures are also of value, since it is well recognized that the bacteria become deeply embedded within the interstices of the stone and are protected from the action of antibacterial agents. Occasionally, it is helpful to localize the urinary infection with the use of selected ureteral catheterization.

Analysis of previously removed or passed stones is also essential in the management of these patients. If possible, the nucleus of the stone should be analyzed separately from the periphery. The information gained may indicate the initiating factors responsible for stone formation (e.g., calcium oxalate, cystine, or uric acid in the nucleus), whereas analysis of the outer layer may reveal factors responsible for its growth (e.g., magnesium ammonium phosphate and infection).

Radiographic studies are indispensable in evaluating patients with renal calculi. Large staghorn stones often fill the renal pelvis and extend to the infundibulum and calyces, and because they may be poorly mineralized and relatively nonopaque, they are difficult to visualize adequately on routine radiographic studies. Plain nephrotomograms prior to injection of any contrast agents are most helpful in detecting the presence of small fragments in calyceal extensions of seemingly uniform calculi. Excretory urograms with oblique views, coupled with tomography, are also essential in revealing the presence, size, and location of stones. In addition, contrast studies in evaluating the contralateral kidney and lower urinary tract to detect the presence of anatomic or functional abnormalities or both is necessary. Retrograde pyelograms are frequently of value not only in evaluating the site of obstruction of a nonfunctioning kidney but also in assessing strictured infundibula and dilated calyces that may not be visualized with the usual excretory urographic procedures. The information gained is invaluable in planning the necessary intrarenal reconstructive procedures that are often required. Precise localization of ureteral stones is also mandatory. Patients coming to surgery generally have not had their condition corrected by prior interventional techniques, and the stones will be fixed in their place. Ureteroscopy or retrograde pyelography or both are often essential. Voiding cystourethrography, cystometrics, and cystoscopy are also essential studies that are often helpful in detecting functional and anatomic abnormalities of the urinary tract that may predispose a patient to urinary tract infection and subsequent stone formation.

In the presence of suspected radiolucent stones, computerized tomography (CT) performed without contrast injection will prove diagnostic and delineate the extent of renal and ureteral involvement.[23] Renal angiography is not routinely obtained but may be helpful in providing a "renal roadmap" in the patient with a staghorn calculus who has undergone prior renal surgery and in whom an anatrophic nephrolithotomy is planned. Individuals with an anomalous urinary tract, including the presence of renal fusion anomalies such as horseshoe kidneys or crossed fused ectopia, may likewise benefit from presurgical renal angiography.

RENAL SURGERY

Surgical Approaches to the Kidney

A number of different surgical approaches to the kidney have been described.[24, 25] Gustav Simon, in 1869, performed the first nephrectomy utilizing what he believed to be the most direct and atraumatic route to the kidney—the vertical lumbar incision.[26] As the art of renal surgery progressed, surgeons often reached the kidney through an anterior transperitoneal approach. This incision was useful in the days prior to the development of current radiographic techniques in that it allowed for the complete exploration of both kidneys. With the development of sophisticated radiographic techniques, the need for gross inspection of both kidneys became obsolete, and the anterior transabdominal approach was replaced by the lumbar or flank incision. By surgically exploring the kidney through an extraperitoneal incision, the morbidity associated with the transabdominal approach was avoided. We currently utilize all three surgical approaches to the kidney and believe it essential for the surgeon operating on patients with renal calculi to be well versed in all techniques.

Posterior Vertical Lumbotomy

The posterior approach to the kidney remains the most direct route to the renal fossa and avoids the trauma and postoperative pain associated with other muscle-transecting incisions.[25–29] When properly performed, it also avoids entry into either the peritoneal or the pleural cavity, averting the potential associated complications when these areas are entered. We currently use this approach for all simple renal pelvic stones not amenable to removal by percutaneous techniques.

After anesthetizing and intubating are accomplished, the patient is placed prone on the operating table. To allow effective ventilation and promote venous return, the abdomen and anterior chest are elevated off the operating table by placing the patient on two laterally placed, rolled bed sheets. The table is flexed slightly to increase the distance between the twelfth rib and the posterior iliac crest.

To maximize the exposure, the incision is started at the lower margin of the twelfth rib, directly over the sacrospinalis muscle, and is extended caudally to the level of the posterior iliac crest in a gentle curve. In the obese patient or in a high-positioned kidney, additional exposure can be achieved by removing a small segment of the twelfth rib. The incision is deepened through the posterior lumbodorsal fascia, revealing the sacrospinalis muscle group (Fig. 14–1). This muscle is retracted medially using broad retractors, and the anterior lumbodorsal fascia is incised. The quadratus lumborum muscle is identified and is likewise medially retracted, exposing the retroperitoneal space. To facilitate exposure further, the costovertebral ligamentous attachment of the twelfth rib is incised.

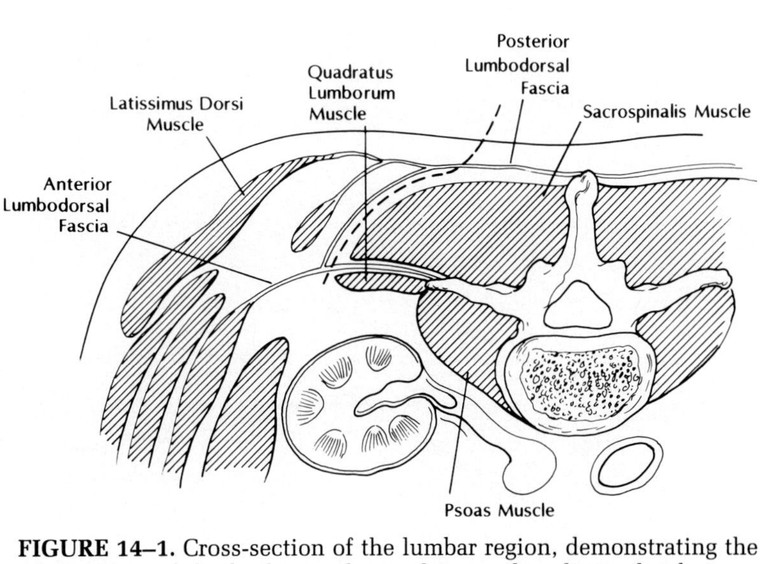

FIGURE 14–1. Cross-section of the lumbar region, demonstrating the relationship of the back muscles to the muscle-splitting lumbotomy incision.

A self-retaining retractor is then placed. While making the incision, care should be taken to avoid traumatizing the iliohypogastric nerve. With the use of sponge sticks, the kidney contained within Gerota's fascia is mobilized downward and laterally. Gerota's fascia is incised, and the kidney, pelvis, and upper ureter are dissected. After removing the stone and closing the pelvis, the fascial layers are closed.

Flank Approach

The lateral flank incision is probably the most frequently utilized approach to the kidney. Depending on the position of the kidney, a subcostal incision, twelfth or eleventh rib resection, or intercostal incision can be effectively employed. This incision, when properly performed, avoids entry into both the peritoneal and the pleural cavities. Unfortunately, unlike the posterior approach, exposure gained through the flank depends on transection of the latissimus dorsi, the external and internal oblique muscles, and the transversus abdominus muscle. Nerves to these muscles may also be traumatized, resulting in an unsightly postoperative bulge in the flank.

After obtaining a suitable level of anesthesia, the patient is placed on the operating table in the flank position, with the iliac crest positioned over the kidney rest (Fig. 14–2). The bottom leg is flexed at the hip and knee, and the upper leg remains straight and is supported on a pillow. The patient's back should be parallel to the edge of the operating table and should be as close to the side as possible. The kidney rest is slowly elevated while the blood pressure is carefully monitored. After completely elevating the kidney rest, the table is flexed to increase further the distance between the lower rib and the iliac crest. A rolled sheet is placed beneath the lower axilla to remove pressure from the brachial plexus and prevent postoperative neuropathy. The head is likewise supported. The uppermost extremity is extended and supported on an armboard. The patient is taped to the table with 3-inch adhesive tape. A standard flank incision is then performed.

We use this approach in all kidneys previously operated on and when complete mobilization of the kidney is required, as in anatrophic nephrolithotomy.

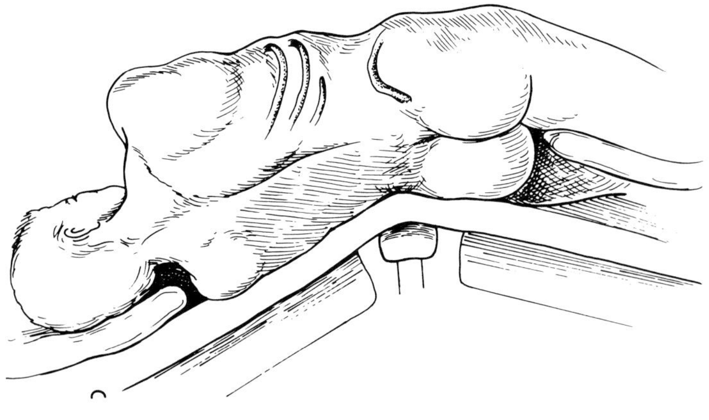

FIGURE 14–2. Patient in standard flank position with the kidney rest elevated.

Anterior Approach

The anterior transperitoneal approach to the kidney is reserved for those patients with physical deformities who could not tolerate the flank position. It is also useful in patients with renal fusion anomalies, such as a pelvic or horseshoe kidney. We utilize either a standard midline or chevron incision, depending on the position of the kidney.

PYELOLITHOTOMY

Simple pyelolithotomy is used for the removal of calculi confined to the renal pelvis. Minimal dissection of the renal sinus is usually needed, and exposure of the entire kidney is generally not required. The procedure has limitations. Large trapped calyceal stones are difficult to remove completely. Attempts to remove large branched stones are usually difficult and ill advised.

The incision selected depends on the anatomic position of the kidney, the previous surgical procedures performed, and the personal experience of the surgeon. A retroperitoneal approach provides good access to the kidney by a route avoiding major vessels and important adjacent organs. Dependent extraperitoneal urinary drainage is easily achieved postoperatively. Most simple pyelolithotomies can be performed through a subcostal or twelfth rib incision, but the approach that allows initial identification of structures in previously unoperated upon areas should be chosen.

After exposing the retroperitoneal space, Gerota's fascia is incised longitudinally along the posterior aspect of the kidney. Frequently, localization of the renal pelvis is made easier by first identifying the upper ureter and dissecting proximally until the renal hilus is exposed. Dissection of the pelvis is confined to the posterior surface. After the pelvis is identified, the hilar fat is dissected to expose the posterior surface and the margin of the renal sinus (Fig. 14–3*A*). The stone can usually be palpated at this time. Two traction sutures of 4–0 chromic catgut are placed to stabilize the edges of the planned pyelotomy. With use of a No. 12 hooked scalpel blade, a transverse pyelotomy is made parallel to the renal axis (Fig. 14–3*B*). The incision is made high in the renal sinus to avoid injury to the ureteropelvic junction and to facilitate prompt, watertight healing. The stone is then grasped with a forceps and extracted (Fig. 14–3*C*). Irrigation of the renal pelvis and infundibula with normal saline helps to remove small remaining fragments. The collecting system is inspected utilizing stay sutures and vein retractors; at times, an illuminated nasal speculum assists in visualization. Exploration with a small dissecting sponge will occasionally assist in the delivery of small residual stones. If any question exists concerning persistent sizable stone fragments, operative radiographs are indicated. A soft red rubber catheter, No. 8 to 10F, passed down the ureter helps to ensure adequacy of the ureteropelvic junction and absence of ureteral obstruction. After all stone fragments have been removed and the absence of distal ureteral obstruction has been demonstrated, the pyelotomy is closed loosely with interrupted sutures of 4–0 chromic catgut on an atraumatic needle (Fig. 14–3*D*). Neither stents nor vents are generally used. A Penrose or small suction drain is placed at the pyelotomy site and brought out through the posterior angle of the incision or through a stab wound. The fascial layers are reapproximated with interrupted chromic catgut sutures. Drains are secured with nonabsorbable sutures, and sterile dressings are applied.

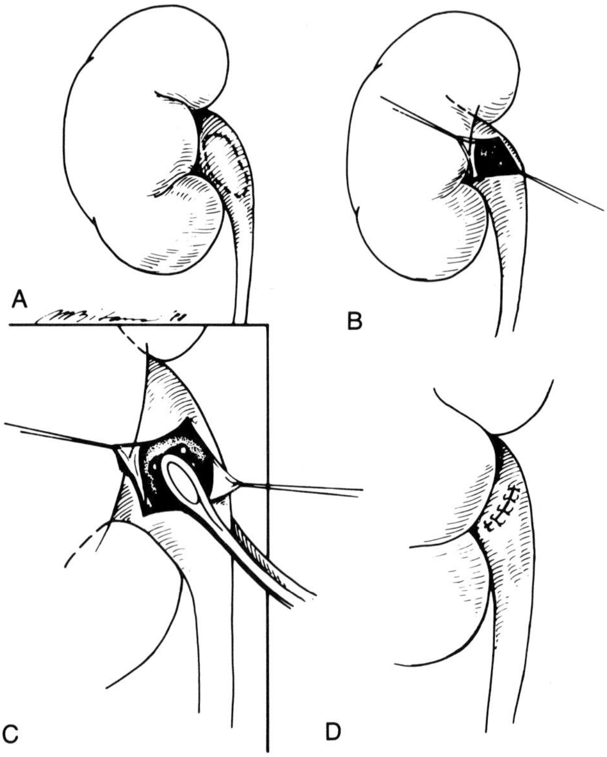

FIGURE 14–3. *A*, The hilar fat is dissected off the posterior surface of the pelvis, and the margin of the renal sinus is freed. *B*, Two traction sutures are placed to stabilize the edges of the pyelotomy. *C*, The stone is grasped with a forceps and extracted. *D*, The pyelotomy is closed loosely with interrupted 4–0 chromic catgut sutures.

EXTENDED PYELOLITHOTOMY

In 1965, Gil-Vernet described the modification of the simple pyelotomy incision, which allowed additional exposure of the intrarenal collecting system.[30] This procedure facilitates the removal of branched calculi without the added inherent risks of blood loss associated with parenchymal incisions.

Trapped calyceal and branched calculi cannot usually be adequately removed through a simple pyelotomy. Dissection of the renal sinus and exposure of the infundibula permit access to these larger stones. Advocates of the extended pyelolithotomy feel it is superior to anatrophic nephrolithotomy because it is less traumatic to the renal parenchyma. Operative blood loss is usually minimal, so that occlusion of the renal vessels is rarely required.

Gil-Vernet originally utilized a posterior vertical lumbotomy incision for extended pyelolithotomy. However, repeated episodes of infection associated with inflammation and scarring characteristic of kidneys with staghorn calculi make adequate exposure through this incision difficult. A flank incision located to maximize exposure of the kidney and its contained stone is generally preferred. Adequate exposure of the upper pole calyces is usually needed, thus requiring the incision to be higher than the one used when performing a simple pyelolithotomy. An eleventh or twelfth rib incision or an eleventh interspace incision is generally adequate, but as emphasized previously, the approach should be tailored to the individual requirements of the operation and the experience of the surgeon. Preoperative knowledge of the location and configuration of the renal arteries, provided by an angiogram, aids in planning the approach to the kidney and the stones, but this study is not required in most instances.

Upon entering the retroperitoneal space and opening Gerota's fascia longitudinally, the renal pelvis and ureteropelvic junction are exposed posteriorly. In branched calculi, the renal pedicle should be located and exposed to a sufficient degree to allow rapid digital or clamp compression to control unexpected bleeding. After determining the accessibility of the major vessels, peripelvic fat is dissected to expose the posterior pelvis and the edge of the renal sinus (Fig. 14–4*A*). Using blunt and sharp scissor dissection, the adventitia overlying the pelvis is opened where it is adherent to the posterior edge of the kidney. This procedure allows access to the renal sinus. The plane between the posterior surface of the pelvis and the renal hilar tissue is developed by blunt dissection, using small vein retractors to retract the posterior edge of the kidney anteriorly and medially and stay sutures to retract the pelvis posteriorly and laterally. A Kutner dissector is gently introduced into the sinus to aid in the deeper dissection until the entire posterior portion of the kidney is freed from the underlying collecting structures. With good retraction, the infundibula come easily into view (Fig. 14–4*B*). Further exposure can be facilitated by gentle lateral retraction of the pelvic-infundibular junction with a vein retractor or a blunt-nose right-angle

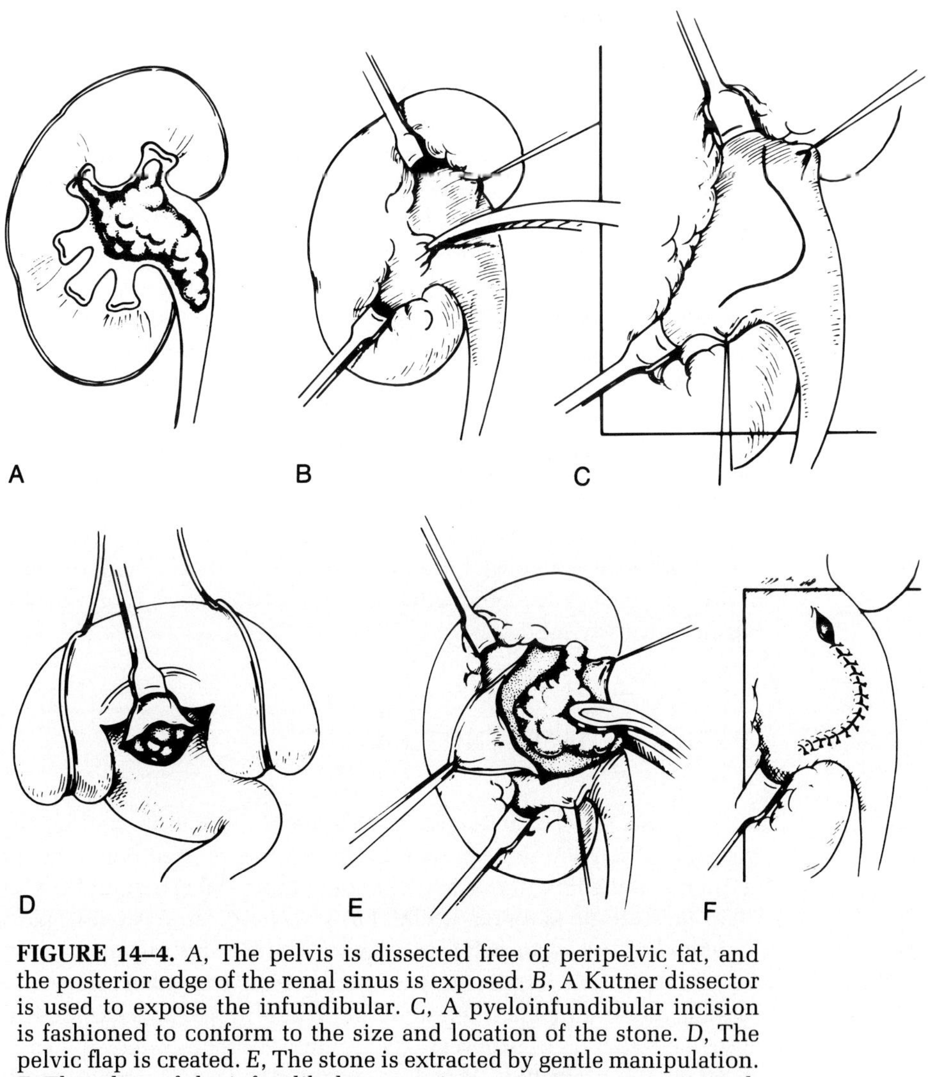

FIGURE 14–4. *A*, The pelvis is dissected free of peripelvic fat, and the posterior edge of the renal sinus is exposed. *B*, A Kutner dissector is used to expose the infundibular. *C*, A pyeloinfundibular incision is fashioned to conform to the size and location of the stone. *D*, The pelvic flap is created. *E*, The stone is extracted by gentle manipulation. *F*, The edges of the infundibular extensions are now reapproximated, and the pelvis is closed loosely with interrupted sutures.

clamp. If performed correctly, the dissection is bloodless. In instances in which the tissue planes have been obliterated by inflammation, the dissection is performed subadventitially because the adventitia is adherent to the peripelvic fat.

A pyeloinfundibular incision fashioned to conform to the size and location of the stone is made using a hooked scalpel blade and curved or angled scissors (Fig. 14–4*C*). The incision, which should be located to maximize exposure and manipulative opportunities, can extend into the infundibulum to the level of the calyx, permitting its exposure (Fig. 14–4*D*). The stone is freed by gentle manipulation; if it is necessary to fracture the calculus, this should be done cleanly at a site that can be visualized with ease. Following delivery of the first branch, the remaining extensions are usually easily freed (Fig. 14–4*E*). If a calyceal extension is larger than the infundibulum, dilation or preferably longitudinal incision through the obstructing infundibulum will be required.

Calyceal fragments can frequently be removed under direct vision. All calyces should be explored using traction sutures, vein retractors, or a nasal speculum to improve vision and irrigation. Dissectors, stone forceps, scoops, and digital probing aid in locating and removing stones. Bimanual palpation of the kidney may assist in localizing large trapped calculi. Some calyceal or bell-shaped stones cannot be removed in this manner and require a small nephrotomy in the overlying renal parenchyma. Usually, these stones are readily palpable on the outer surface of the kidney because the parenchyma in the region of the stone is thinned and scarred. Intraoperative radiographs of the kidney are essential in performing surgery on branched calculi to ensure that all fragments are removed. Thorough irrigation with normal saline is performed to assist in the removal of small fragments. A soft red rubber catheter is passed in the distal ureter to detect obstruction.

The infundibular incision is usually not reapproximated or is closed transversely with interrupted sutures of 4–0 chromic catgut. If a stricture is present, a flap or dismembered procedure may be used to correct the abnormality. At times, incised infundibula may be joined to each other and the pelvis to ensure an adequate lumen. The pelvis is closed loosely with interrupted catgut sutures (Fig. 14–4*F*). The posterior portion of the kidney falls against the infundibular incision after the retractors are removed. Penrose or small plastic suction drains are placed at the renal hilum and near any distant nephrotomy sites. Fascial layers are reapproximated with interrupted 0 chromic catgut sutures. Leakage of urine is usually minimal.

PYELONEPHROLITHOTOMY

Because of the anatomic distribution of the inferior and posterior segmental arteries, it is possible to perform a lower pole nephrotomy without endangering either vessel and without first clamping the renal artery and cooling the kidney. This procedure is often useful for removing large stones, particularly those confined to the renal pelvis and lower infundibular system.

A lower pole nephrotomy is indicated for removal of branched calculi located within the lower pole infundibulum. When properly performed, this procedure provides adequate exposure for complete stone removal. The procedure is particularly useful in those situations in which a simple pyelotomy is not applicable, such as in a kidney with a small intrarenal pelvis.

Once the kidney has been anesthetized and placed in a flank position, an incision is made at the eleventh or twelfth rib, which is generally satisfactory for exposing the kidney. This incision is performed in a standard manner. After all muscles are incised and Gerota's fascia is identified, it is preferable to incise this fascial plane carefully in a cephalad-caudad direction. This maneuver preserves the structure to which the kidney should be returned following completion of the nephrotomy. The fatty layer overlying the kidney is sharply dissected from the renal capsule, and the kidney is suspended with 1-inch umbilical tapes.

Following complete exposure of the kidney, it is useful to identify the main renal artery and, if possible, its branches. Control of the pedicle is important, but clamping of the main renal artery with the use of hypothermia is not necessary with parenchymal incisions into the lower pole. The renal pelvis is then identified, and the kidney is positioned so that the entire renal pelvis and posterior surface of the kidney are in the operative field. Often, the calculus can be palpated within the renal pelvis.

It is useful to identify the distribution of the posterior segmental artery in this region. This can easily be accomplished by administering 20 ml of methylene blue intravenously while the posterior segmental artery is temporarily occluded. The posterior segment will blanch, whereas the remaining portion will be stained blue. Though it is not mandatory to perform the lower pole nephrotomy along the division between the posterior and inferior segments, hemostasis will be easier to maintain if this is done.

A pyelotomy is then made and directed so that it will extend in the direction of the lower pole infundibulum (Fig. 14–5). It is useful to direct the more distal portion of the pyelotomy away from the ureteropelvic junction so that if tears occur during stone extraction, they will not extend into this region.

The nephrotomy is made along the renal tissue overlying the lower pole infundibulum (Fig. 14–6). Initially, the renal capsule is incised sharply, but the renal parenchyma is separated by blunt dissection, usually with the back of the scalpel handle. This practice minimizes injury to the intralobular arteries that lie

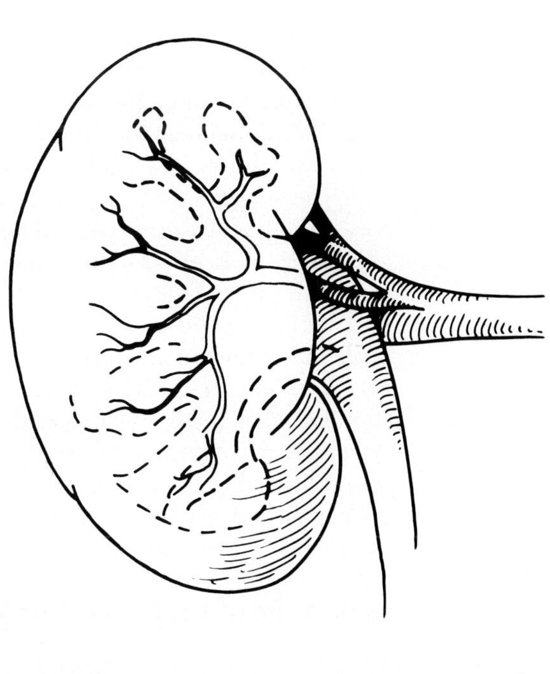

FIGURE 14–5. The pyelotomy incision is placed so that it will extend into the lower pole infundibulum.

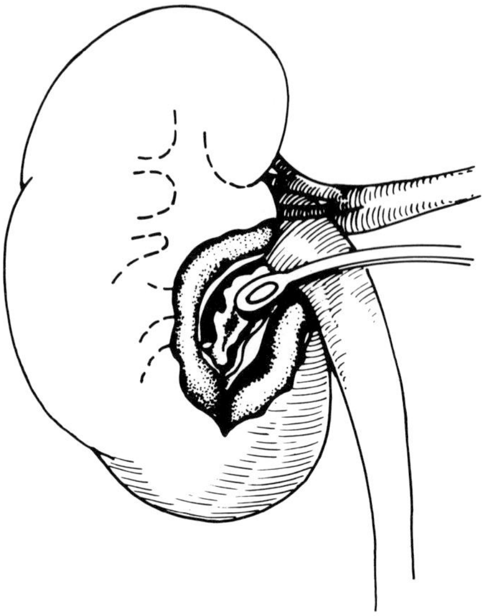

FIGURE 14–6. The nephrotomy is made along the renal tissue overlying the lower pole infundibulum.

near the infundibulum. Small vessels are usually readily identifiable and are ligated with 5–0 or 6–0 chromic catgut suture and transected. The incision should extend into the lower pole infundibulum and calyces. With appropriate exposure, the calculus lying within the lower pole can be extracted; should calyceal extensions exist, these should be opened individually prior to stone manipulation. When the stone has been removed, each calyx should be explored and irrigated to ensure the complete removal of all small fragments.

Nonreactive Silastic ureteral stents are used and typically are passed from the renal pelvis into the bladder early in the procedure. This prevents migration of stone fragments down the ureter and provides good drainage postoperatively, so that the incidence of postoperative urinary extravasation is minimized.

The use of intraoperative radiographs is important to ensure complete stone removal. An important step in the procedure is to obtain an intraoperative plain radiograph prior to performing the nephrotomy. Frequently, small calculi or lines of cleavage between seemingly solidly staghorn stones may be identified on plain films but may not be apreciated on previous pyelograms or tomograms. This initial radiograph also permits comparison with those taken later in the procedure and frequently is most helpful in deciding whether any stone fragments have been retained. Similarly, a radiographic study should be obtained routinely prior to renal closure to document removal of all fragments. All fragments must be removed if urinary tract infection is to be eradicated and recurrent stone formation prevented.

Following the complete removal of all stones, the renal pelvis and lower pole infundibulum are closed with a running 6–0 chromic catgut suture (Fig. 14–7). A running 4–0 catgut suture is used to close the renal capsule (Fig. 14–8). Parenchymal renal veins should be suture ligated, and hemostasis should be ensured after suturing the renal capsule and before wound closure. No mattress-type parenchymal sutures are used because they are likely to result in tissue ischemia and eventual hemorrhage. At the completion of the procedure, the kidney is returned to Gerota's fascia, which is closed with an interrupted chromic catgut suture. The lower pole of the kidney and upper ureter are also covered with perirenal fat. By surrounding the kidney and upper ureter with fat, the

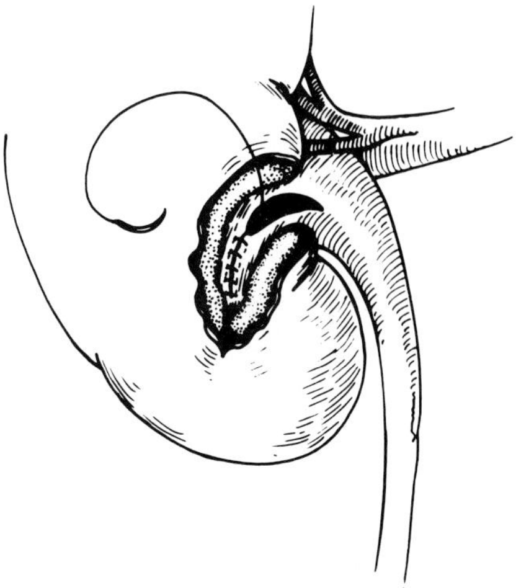

FIGURE 14–7. The renal pelvis and lower pole infundibulum are closed with running 6–0 chromic catgut suture.

risks of adhesion formation and perineal scarring are reduced. If Gerota's fascia has been obliterated because of chronic inflammation or prior surgical procedures, an omental flap is mobilized and used to cover the kidney and upper ureter.

The flank wound is closed in layers with interrupted chromic catgut sutures. A small Penrose drain is left within Gerota's fascia and brought out through a separate stab incision to provide a drainage tract for fluid collections. This drain is left in place until all drainage subsides, usually within 72 hours.

COAGULUM PYELOLITHOTOMY

Coagulum pyelolithotomy, described by Dees,[31] did not gain widespread urologic acceptance until being rediscovered by Patel 30 years later.[32] Since then, in an effort to simplify the technical aspects of the procedure, decrease the

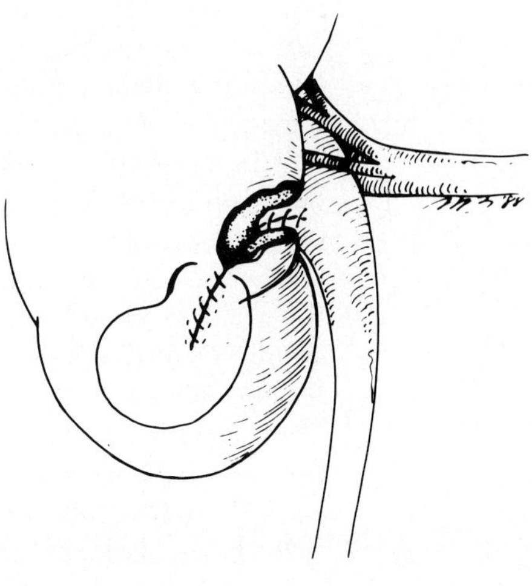

FIGURE 14–8. The renal capsule is closed with a running 4–0 chromic catgut suture.

associated morbidity, and improve the surgical results, the coagulum recipe has undergone a number of modifications.[33–39] Prior to the development of percutaneous and extracorporeal shock wave techniques, coagulum pyelolithotomy had gained an accepted role in the removal of multiple renal stones.

The clot, or coagulum, on which the procedure is based is formed by a reaction between local fibrinogen and thrombin. Fibrin monomers organize to form stable fibrin in the presence of both calcium and thrombin. Cryoprecipitate, readily available in most blood banks, is routinely used as the source of fibrinogen and, when combined with calcium and thrombin, will form a clot of great tensile strength. Calcium chloride serves to neutralize the anticoagulant (citrate) present in the cryoprecipitate and acts as a cofactor to facilitate the conversion of prothrombin to thrombin.[40]

The ideal candidate for coagulum pyelolithotomy has a large extrarenal pelvis with multiple small calculi contained in the intrarenal collecting system. It may also be helpful in the patient with multiple calyceal stones who is undergoing anatrophic nephrolithotomy or pyelonephrolithotomy.

Prior to performing the coagulum procedure, it is essential that all materials be readily available in the operating room. The kidney is exposed in the usual fashion, and the upper ureter is identified and occluded with a soft vessel loop. Topical thrombin (5000 units) is reconstituted with 5 ml of normal saline. Ten ml of a 10 per cent calcium chloride solution is placed in a small sterile basin, and to it is added 0.25 ml of the reconstituted thrombin solution. Four units of cryoprecipitate (40 to 60 ml) and a few drops of methylene blue, useful in facilitating future identification and removal of the entire clot, are placed in a separate sterile container. Heating the solution does not increase the tensile strength; therefore, the entire procedure is performed at room temperature.

A 19-gauge butterfly needle or angiocath is positioned in the renal pelvis, and all urine is aspirated and measured (Fig. 14–9). The cryoprecipitate is aspirated in a 50-ml syringe, and to this is added 1 ml of the thrombin–calcium chloride solution. If the capacity of the renal pelvis is larger than 50 ml, 2 ml of the thrombin–calcium chloride solution are used. Further addition of calcium chloride acts only to reduce the set time without increasing the tensile strength and is not recommended.[41] The solution is then briefly mixed, and the volume corresponding to the predetermined pelvic capacity is injected into the renal pelvis. Overdistention resulting in pyelovenous backflow should be avoided. Clotting typically occurs 30 to 45 seconds after mixing the solution. After 5 minutes, the renal pelvis is incised, and the coagulum with the entrapped stones is removed. Burns and Finlayson[41] showed that waiting an additional 5 minutes results in no further significant increase in tensile strength and is therefore not warranted. Radiographs are routinely obtained to confirm complete stone removal.

In an effort to simplify the procedure further, Kalash and associates[36] rely on tissue levels of thromboplastin to provide the necessary thrombin and obtain excellent results by injecting only cryoprecipitate and calcium chloride. Marshall[37] has further revised their technique and performs the procedure by first injecting the predetermined amount of cryoprecipitate into the renal pelvis and then adding 1 ml of 10 per cent calcium chloride. Pyelotomy is performed 5 to 7 minutes later.

Coagulum pyelolithotomy has generally been considered to be a safe procedure. However, at least one case of a fatal pulmonary embolism directly related to the procedure has been reported.[42] The pulmonary embolism is believed to have occurred as a result of overdistending the renal pelvis, with

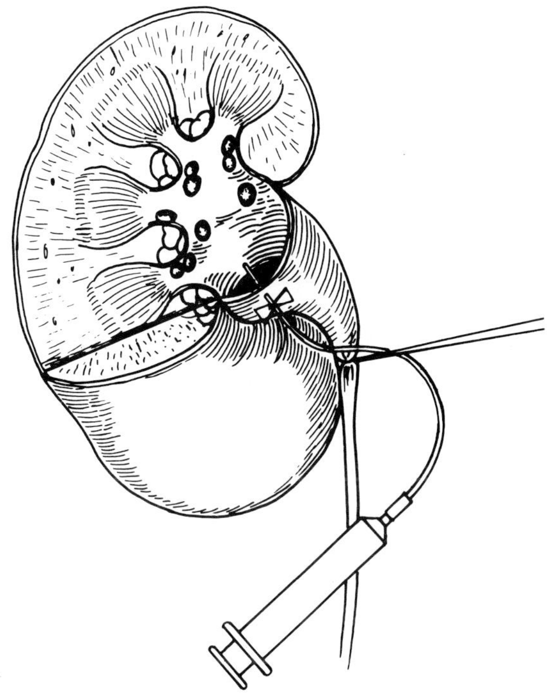

FIGURE 14–9. The desired coagulum recipe is injected via a butterfly needle placed in the renal pelvis. Note the vessel loop tightened around the proximal ureter.

subsequent pyelovenous backflow and dissemination of the thrombogenic material into the systemic circulation. Studies on dogs have confirmed this theory.[42] To avoid this potentially lethal complication, one must carefully measure the pelvic capacity and avoid overdistention of the renal pelvis. Deleting thrombin from the coagulum recipe might further enhance the safety of this procedure.[42] The risk of hepatitis and allergic reactions has been minimized with the use of cryoprecipitate. Retained clots pose little threat to the patient and will usually be dissolved within 24 to 48 hours by the urokinase/plasmin–mediated mechanism of clot lysis.[34]

ANATROPHIC NEPHROLITHOTOMY

Anatrophic nephrolithotomy is indicated when the surgeon must remove branched or staghorn calculi associated with infundibular stenosis or when prior stone surgery has been performed, making dissection of the renal sinus difficult, if not impossible. The term "anatrophic" was coined by Boyce and relates to the segmental distribution of the intrarenal artery. Division in these vessels results in atrophy of the parenchyma supplied by that vessel; incisions in the renal parenchyma that do not transect these vessels spare this tissue and are therefore not atrophic, hence the term "anatrophic."[43, 44]

The presence of an untreated staghorn calculus is associated with significant morbidity resulting from persistent urinary tract infection or obstruction or both. Survival of patients is often also reduced if the stone is left in situ, with overall mortality rates ranging from 28 to 50 per cent over a 10-year period.[43, 44] In approximately 50 per cent of patients with unoperated on staghorn calculi, renal function will deteriorate even in the absence of progressive radiographic changes in the size of the stone.

Intrarenal Anatomy

A certain knowledge about intrarenal anatomy and the relationship of the collecting system to the renal vasculature is essential in the performance of anatrophic nephrolithotomy. Surgeons practicing in the early 1900s had an excellent understanding of the gross renal anatomy and the renal blood supply. However, they lacked in knowledge of the intrarenal anatomy and vasculature. Josef Hyrtl, a nineteenth century Viennese anatomist, was the first to study the intrarenal vasculature.[45] In an effort to study the ramifications of blood vessels, he developed a technique of corrosion preparations that consisted of injection of the blood supply of different organs and their digestion by acid. Hyrtl can be credited as the first to study intrarenal arteries, and in 1882, 19 years prior to a similar report by Brödel, he described the presence of a relatively avascular plane between the anterior and posterior vascular segments. In 1901, Brödel, a medical artist working at the Johns Hopkins Medical School, published his classic report, "The Intrinsic Blood Vessels of the Kidney and Their Significance in Nephrotomy."[46] Using a method similar to that of Hyrtl, Brödel injected kidneys with celloidin, digested the specimens to obtain a cast of the arteries, and studied their distribution in relationship to the collecting structures. Brödel accurately described the branching of the main renal artery and emphasized the segmental distribution and the lack of free anastomosis between the segmental branches.

Probably the most discussed and quoted concept to be derived from this work is that of the relatively avascular plane between the anterior and posterior arterial segments. Unfortunately, this point has become confused in the literature owing to the interchange of terms "Brödel's white line" and "Brödel's line," the former being a white line overlying the vascular longitudinal columns of Bertin and the latter being the division between the anterior and posterior segments and the recommended line of incision for the posterior longitudinal nephrotomy. The distinction has been clearly described by Myers in 1971.[41] With Brödel's assistance as a medical illustrator, Kelly further expanded on Brödel's previous studies and clearly showed the importance of an appreciation of the renal anatomy when performing not only nephrolithotomy but other types of renal operative procedures as well.[48]

The divisions of the renal pelvis and the number and distribution of the calyces and papillae are the most variable components of the renal anatomy (Fig. 14–10). The renal calyces drain the renal papillae and are in immediate apposition. The total number of calyces is usually 8 but can range from 4 to 12. A single calyx may drain one papilla, whereas a composite calyx may drain multiple papillae. The polar calyces demonstrate the greatest variation in size and shape and are generally compound. The calyces drain into the infundibula, which are the primary divisions of the renal pelvis and are usually two or three in number. The infundibula, or primary divisions, then empty into the renal pelvis.

The calyx of the uppermost primary division is usually single but often receives multiple papillae and is therefore referred to as a compound or composite calyx. The remainder of the calyces are usually paired and are arranged anterior or posterior to an imaginary line that divides the kidney longitudinally into an anterior and a posterior half. The anterior group of calyces is irregularly arranged but usually lies at an angle of 70 to 75 degrees from the frontal plane. The

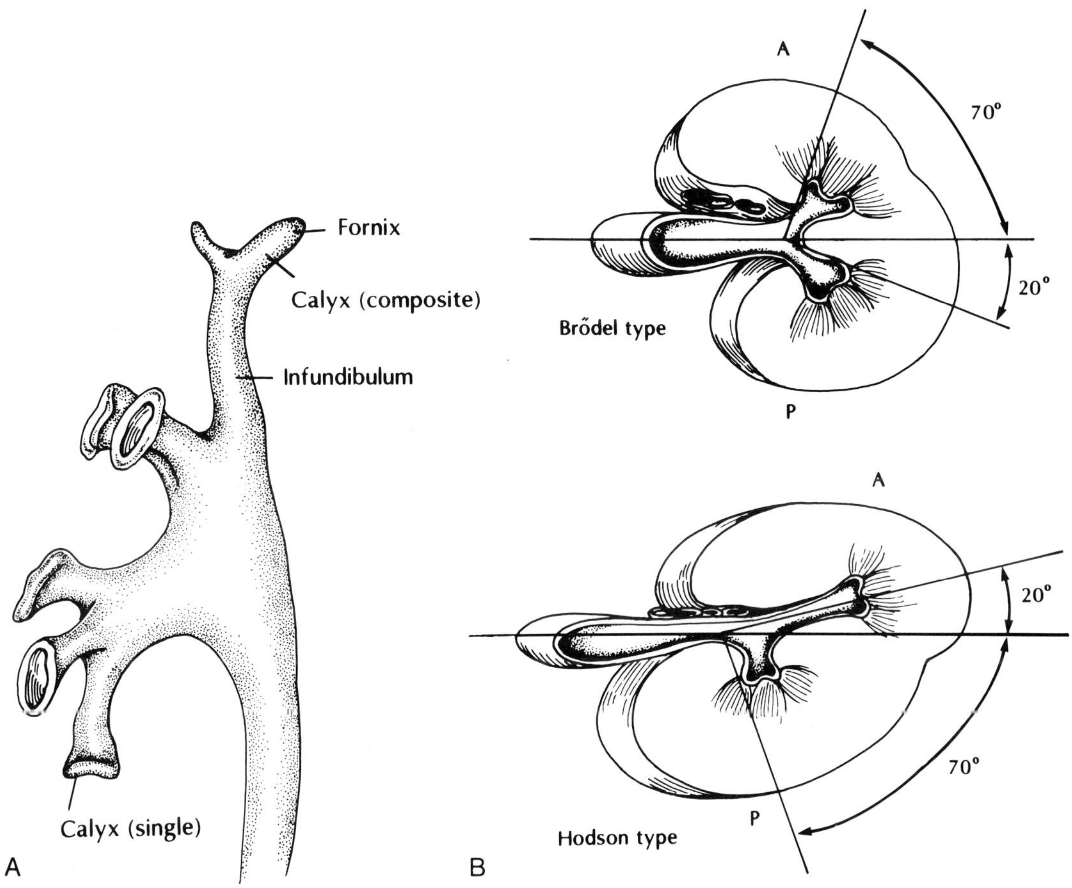

FIGURE 14–10. *A*, Renal pelvis and its primary and secondary divisions. *B*, Relationship of anterior and posterior calyces.

posterior calyces are arranged more regularly and form a 20-degree angle with the frontal plane.

On the basis of the arterial distribution, the kidney is divided into four vascular segments: anterior, posterior, superior, and inferior. In 70 to 80 per cent of kidneys, the renal artery divides into its primary branches before entering the renal hilum. Approximately 50 per cent of the time, the first branch is the posterior division of the renal artery, which supplies the posterior renal segment. In about one third of kidneys, the first branch is the vessel to the lower pole segment. In the remaining instances, either the artery to the upper pole segment will be the first branch or the posterior branch will arise simultaneously with the anterior segmental artery.

The anterior division represents the main continuation of the renal artery and will typically divide into the superior, anterior, and inferior segmental arteries as well as the apical artery of Graves. This vessel usually branches either immediately before or within the superior aspects of the renal hilum. The posterior division proceeds without further significant branching to vascularize the posterior segment.

Further branching of the four segmental arteries occurs in an orderly fashion (Fig. 14–11). Eight to 12 paracalyceal arteries arise from the segmental branches

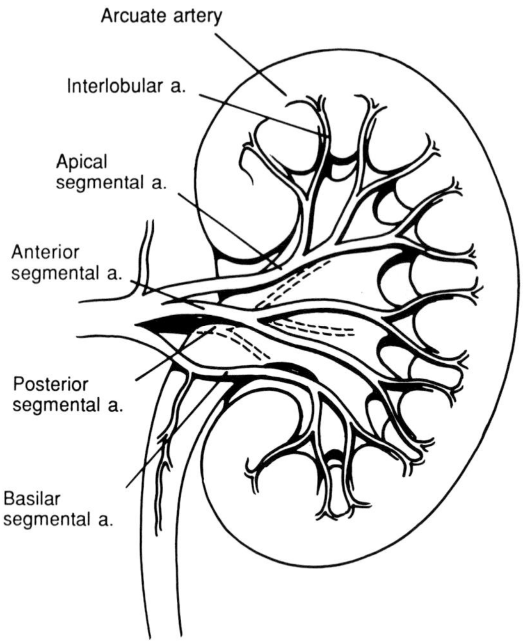

FIGURE 14–11. Successive branching of main renal artery.

and course along opposite margins of the infundibula toward the papillae. Transmedullary arteries arise as third-order branches, near the point where the vessels enter the renal parenchyma at the level of the calyceal cup, and are usually paired. They pass through the medulla in the interpapillary spaces to reach the cortex, where they either subdivide or continue to form the arcuate arteries. Each calyx receives a group of nephrons from a distinct portion of the kidney, and each can be supplied by more than one arterial segment (Fig. 14–12).

From a surgical standpoint, the kidney is divided into four surgical segments that correspond to the distribution of the four segmental arteries (Fig. 14–13).

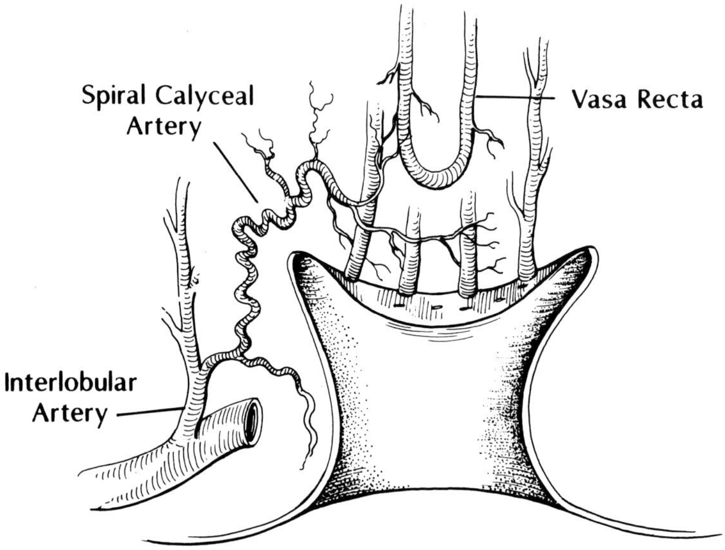

FIGURE 14–12. Blood supply to papilla.

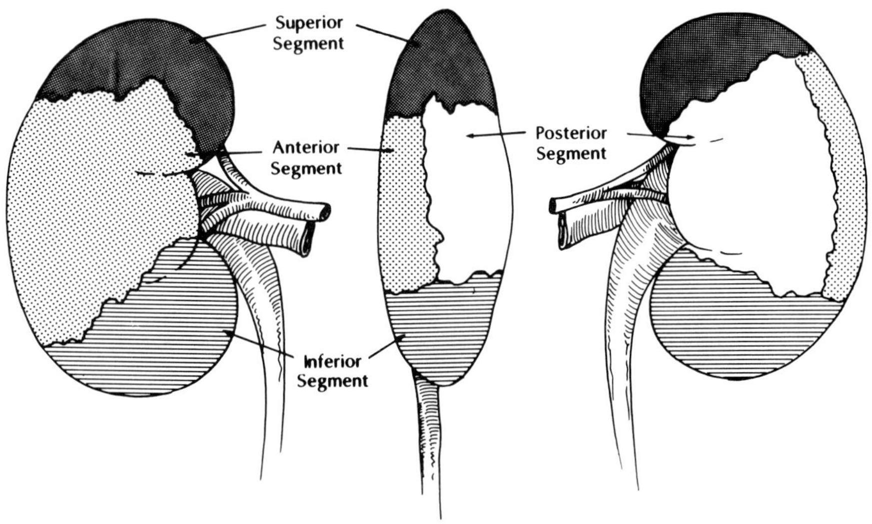

FIGURE 14–13. Four distinct renal vascular segments.

The upper and lower pole segments include a single polar calyceal system. The double row of pyramids between these polar segments comprises the anterior and posterior renal segments.

The artery to the superior renal segment has an extrahilar source of origin in nearly all cases. It supplies the anterior surface of the upper superior segment and, in approximately 50 per cent of kidneys, will also provide blood supply to the posterior surface of the superior pole. In the remaining cases, the posterior surface will be supplied by a superior polar extension of the posterior segmental artery.

The artery to the inferior renal segment also originates before the anterior segmental artery enters the hilum and is therefore easily isolated at the time of surgery. The artery passes in front of the renal pelvis and descends obliquely to its lower border, where it then crosses the renal pelvis and divides into anterior and posterior branches.

The artery to the anterior segment arises as the direct continuation of the anterior division of the renal artery. In about one half of all kidneys, a single artery will supply the entire anterior segment. Variation will depend on the vascular supply to the superior and inferior pole segments.

The anterior vascular segment is the largest of the four renal segments and occupies the entire anterior midportion of the kidney and extends laterally over the convex border to include a variable amount of posterior parenchyma. Included in this segment are the anterior and posterior surfaces of the anterior row of calyces, as well as the anterior surface of the posterior row of calyces.

The posterior artery in 50 per cent of kidneys is the first branch of the main renal artery. It usually is extrahilar in origin and supplies the entire posterior renal segment. Unlike the other branches of the renal artery, it runs posterior to the renal pelvis in the superior renal hilum. The size of the posterior segment is highly variable and cannot be predicted on the basis of external tomography. The posterior segment can be delineated by injecting methylene blue after first clamping the posterior segmental artery. In about one third of kidneys, the posterior segment will extend to include the lateral convex border of the kidney or even beyond, and onto the anterior surface. In these instances, the posterior artery will provide more of the blood supply to the posterior row of calyces;

however, it is rare for this vessel to supply both the anterior and the posterior surfaces of these calyces.

Brödel's white line is the linear whitish depression located on the posterior lateral surface of the kidney that overlies the highly vascular longitudinal columns of Bertin. This landmark should not be confused with the relatively avascular plane, or Brödel's line, which is the proper site of incision for anatrophic nephrolithotomy and overlies the division between the anterior and posterior renal segments (Fig. 14–14).

The renal venous vasculature does not follow the corresponding arterial segmental distribution. The venous system demonstrates free anastomosis between the intrarenal veins, and therefore occlusion of venous channels can be performed without the threat of jeopardizing the renal parenchyma. In general, the main renal vein that enters the vena cava may arise from as many as four main trunks that leave the hilum and then join prior to emptying into the vena cava.

Surgical Techniques

The intersegmental anatrophic nephrolithotomy is indicated for the removal of multiple branched calculi with associated infundibular stenosis. When properly performed, the procedure provides maximal exposure of the intrarenal collecting system, so that complete stone removal can be accomplished. If necessary, reconstructive procedures can be performed on scarred and strictured infundibula and calyces, so that optimal urinary drainage is obtained. In addition, the

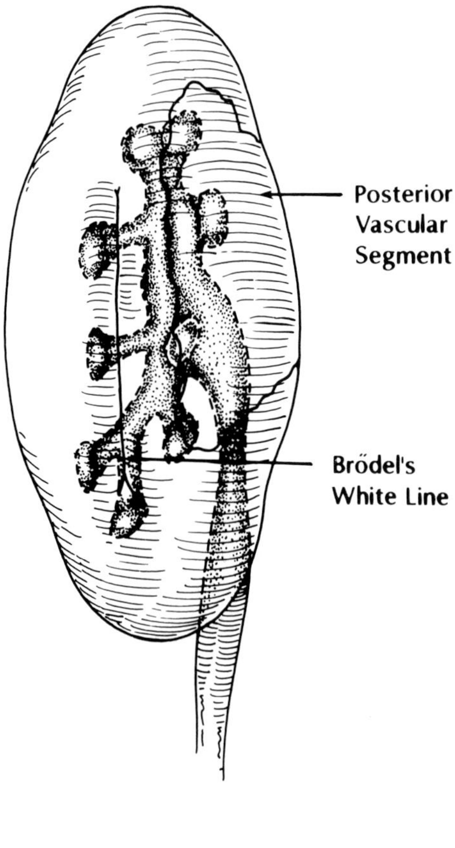

FIGURE 14–14. Posterior vascular segment and Brödel's white line.

procedure is useful in those situations in which pyelolithotomy is not applicable, such as in a kidney with a small intrarenal pelvis and in those instances in which previous surgery has been performed and proper dissection of the renal sinus is difficult, if not impossible.

Once the patient has been anesthetized and the endotracheal tube positioned, a Foley catheter is inserted into the bladder and placed to facilitate gravity drainage. Urine output is monitored continually during the operative procedure. The patient is then placed in the lateral position, the lower extremity is flexed, and the upper limb is kept straight and supported on a pillow. The kidney rest is raised, and the table is flexed to provide maximal separation of the lower ribs and iliac crest. After the patient is fixed in position on the operating table with wide adhesive tape, the skin is prepped, and the patient is draped in a standard manner.

Generally, the kidney can be satisfactorily exposed through an eleventh or twelfth rib incision. If previous renal surgery has been performed, it is preferable to approach the kidney through an incision placed above the area of prior surgery. This permits initial access to the kidney through unscarred tissue. After all muscles are incised and Gerota's fascia is identified, it is desirable to incise with care this fascial plane posteriorly in a cephalad-caudad direction. This maneuver preserves this "fatty envelope" to which the kidney should be returned following closure of the nephrotomy. The fatty layer overlying the kidney is then sharply dissected from the renal capsule, and the kidney is suspended with 1-inch umbilical tapes.

After complete exposure of the kidney, the main renal artery and its branches are carefully dissected and identified. Care should be taken to preserve the pelvic branch of the renal artery in an effort to avoid ischemic damage to the renal pelvis and upper ureter. The division between the anterior and posterior arterial segments (avascular plane) is identified by administering 20 ml of methylene blue through a peripheral vein while the posterior segmental artery is temporarily occluded (Fig. 14–15). The posterior segment blanches while the

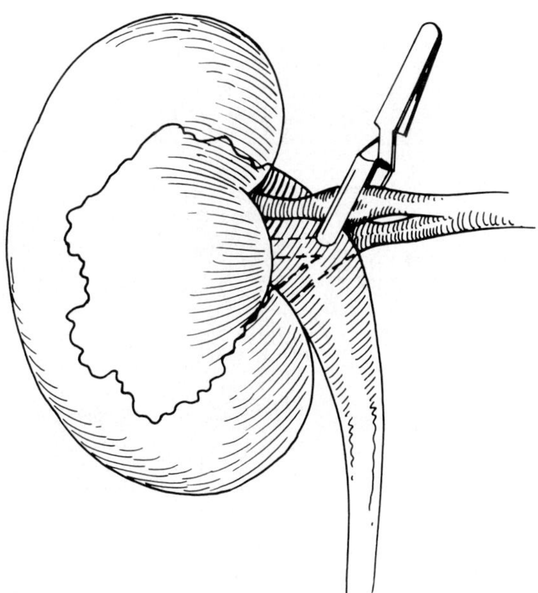

FIGURE 14–15. Intraoperative definition of posterior vascular segment. Methylene blue is administered peripherally while the posterior segmental artery is occluded.

remaining portion of the kidney is stained blue. The main renal artery is then occluded with an avascular clamp, a waterproof drape is placed around the kidney, and the kidney is packed in an ice slush prepared from a physiologic salt solution. To prevent excessive cooling of the intraabdominal structures, dry abdominal packs are placed between the rubber drape and the reflected peritoneum. Five to 10 minutes prior to clamping the main renal artery, 25 grams of mannitol is instilled intravenously to increase the osmolarity of the glomerular filtrate and intratubular fluid and thus prevent ice crystal formation during hypothermia.

The nephrotomy is made along the avascular plane, as defined with methylene blue (Fig. 14–16). Initially, the renal capsule is incised sharply, but the renal parenchyma is separated by blunt dissection, usually with the back of the scalpel handle. This practice minimizes injury to the intralobular arteries lying near the infundibula. Small vessels are usually readily identifiable and are ligated with 5–0 or 6–0 chromic catgut suture and transected.

Should venous "back bleeding" be a problem, the renal vein is occluded at this point and is maintained in this state until the completion of the procedure. The nephrotomy incision should remain within the avascular plane, and it is helpful to try to angle the incision toward the midportion of the renal hilum. Ideally, it should transect the collecting structures at the base of the posterior infundibula. Recent anatomic studies have indicated that a renal papilla may be supplied by branches of two distinct segmental arteries.[49] The important surgical application of this finding is that when the nephrotomy incision in the plane between the anterior and posterior segmental vessels approaches a papilla, it is less traumatic to bisect the papilla than to carry the incision around it. Circumferential incisions in these instances tend to result in partial ischemia and necrosis of these structures, as opposed to incisions that continue along natural vascular planes.

If large posterior calyceal stones are present, occasionally a dilated calyx

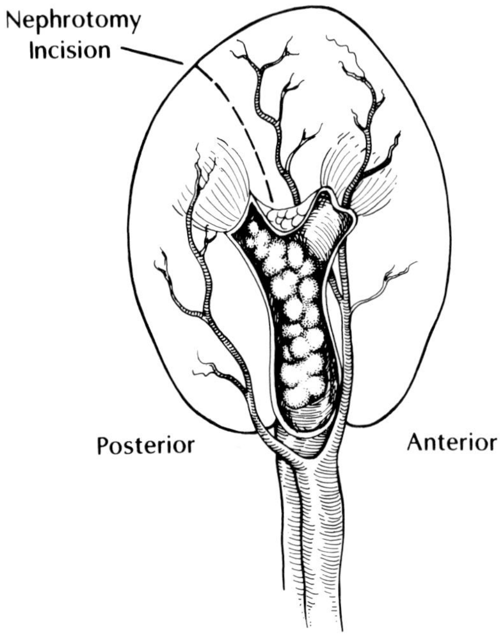

FIGURE 14–16. Nephrotomy incision is placed on a plane between the anterior and posterior vascular segments.

may be entered initially. This maneuver is often helpful in identifying the remaining collecting structures. It is important to emphasize that great care and precision should be observed in exposing these structures, and the areas of the collecting system to be incised (infundibula, calyces) should be dictated by the location of the stones and the degree of scarring or obstruction present. It is important that all calyceal extensions of the stone be identified and that the stone be manipulated only after it is completely freed of all surrounding structures. This approach will tend to minimize stone fractures and thus reduce the incidence of retained calculi. After the body of the stone is removed, the renal pelvis and calyces are carefully inspected, and all debris and small stone fragments are removed by irrigation.

When strictured and scarred infundibula and calyces are encountered, intrarenal reconstruction of these structures is required to promote optimal drainage and prevent urinary stasis. Calyorrhaphy signifies repair of a single calyx, and calycoplasty indicates repair of adjacent strictured calyces. Both are performed after all stone fragments have been removed. Calyorrhaphy is accomplished by incising the calyx along its appropriate margin and suturing the walls to the membranes of the renal pelvis (Fig. 14–17). Posterior calyces are opened along anterior margins, and anterior ones are opened posteriorly. Polar calyces are opened along their appropriate lateral margin. This maneuver shortens and widens the lumen and provides free drainage of urine. Calycoplasty is performed by initially incising adjacent stenotic calyces along their appropriate margins (Fig. 14–18). The borders are then approximated, and, in effect, two calyces are converted into a single structure. All repairs are performed with 6–0 chromic catgut suture. Only the epithelium and muscularis should be included in the repair because deeper sutures will inadvertently damage the underlying interlobular arteries. The ultimate goal of both procedures is to obtain a mucosa-lined passageway from the renal papilla directly into the renal pelvis. No definite rules can be applied to all forms of repair, since the type of repair of severely scarred, long, or, at times, completely obstructed calyces is determined by the particular anatomic deformity and by the ingenuity and expertise of the surgeon.

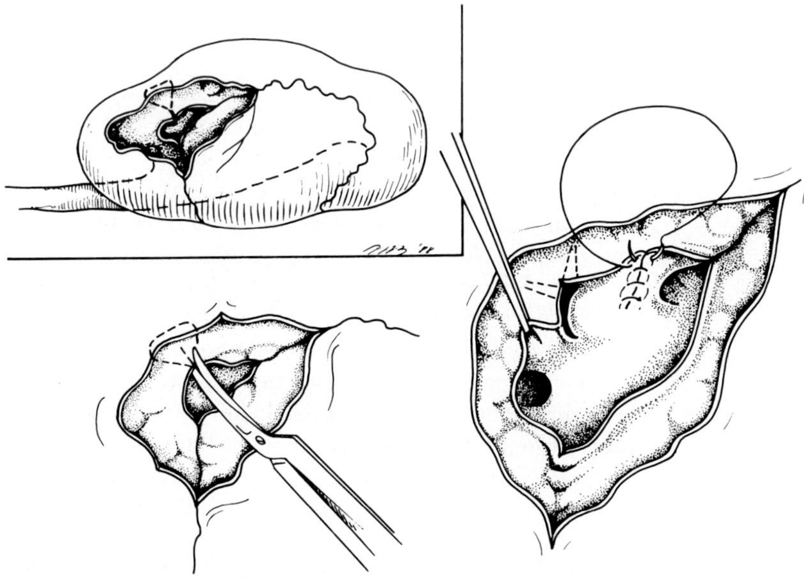

FIGURE 14–17. Calyorrhaphy for repair of single stenosed calyx.

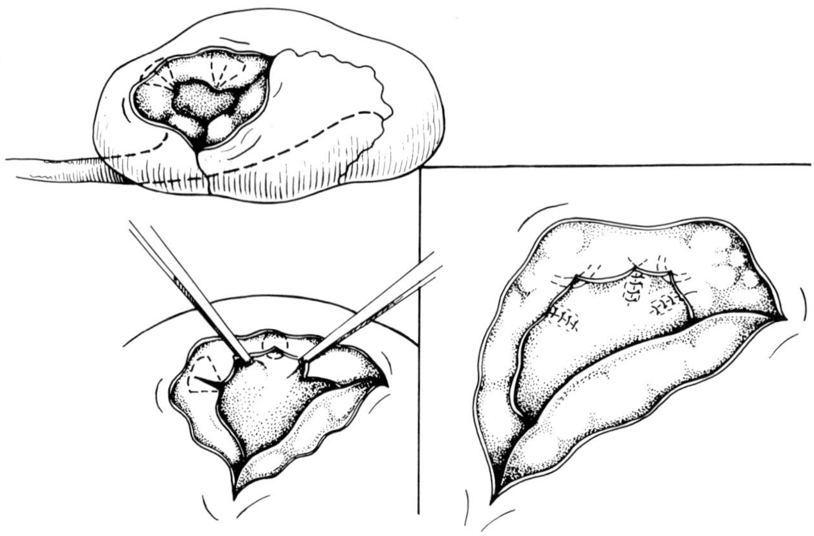

FIGURE 14–18. Calycoplasty for repair of adjacent strictured calyces.

Nonreactive stents are routinely used and typically are passed from the renal pelvis into the bladder early in the procedure. This practice prevents the migration of small stone fragments down the ureter during the procedure and provides good drainage postoperatively, so that the incidence of postoperative urinary extravasation is minimized. Following the complete removal of all stones and the performance of all necessary reconstructive procedures, the renal pelvis is closed with a running 6–0 chromic catgut suture (Fig. 14–19), and a running 4–0 chromic catgut suture is used to close the renal capsule (Fig. 14–20). Parenchymal renal veins are suture ligated, and hemostasis should be assured completely after closure of the renal capsule and before wound closure. No mattress-type parenchymal sutures are used because they are likely to result in tissue ischemia and eventual hemorrhage.

At the completion of the procedure, all slush is removed from the kidney, and the clamp is removed from the renal artery. The kidney is returned to Gerota's fascia, which is closed with an interrupted 0 chromic catgut suture. The lower pole of the kidney and upper ureter are also covered with perirenal fat. By surrounding the kidney and upper ureter with fat, the formation of adhesions and perirenal scarring is reduced. If Gerota's fascia has been obliterated because of chronic inflammation or prior surgical procedures, an omental flap is mobilized and used to cover the kidney and upper ureter. The omentum can usually be easily mobilized by opening the peritoneum as it is reflected along the medial aspect of the kidney. Usually, adequate omentum can be brought through the opening to cover the desired structures easily. The omentum is sutured to the kidney and is also brought around the upper ureter and sutured to itself. It is also important to suture the walls of the peritoneal opening to the omentum to prevent herniation of the abdominal contents.

The flank wound is closed in layers with interrupted 0 chromic catgut sutures, and a small Penrose drain is left within Gerota's fascia and brought out through a separate stab incision to provide a tract for any fluid collection. This drain is left in place and removed when all drainage subsides—usually within 72 hours. Nephrostomy and pyelostomy tubes are not used in that they have been

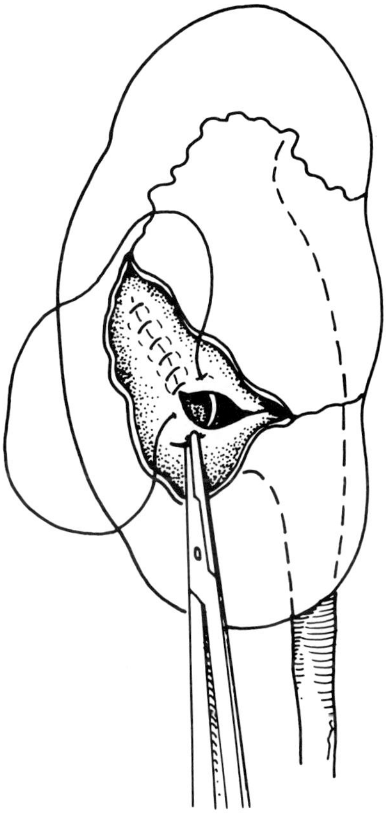

FIGURE 14–19. Closure of renal pelvis.

found not only to be unnecessary but also to result in loss of functional renal parenchyma and to provide a nidus for further infection.

Auxiliary Details

Renal Hypothermia

The significant advance contributing to the success of the anatrophic nephrolithotomy was the demonstration that the adverse effects of renal ischemia could be avoided by local organ cooling.[50–54] Renal cooling reduces cellular metabolic activity so that the parenchymal cells, particularly those of the proximal convoluted tubule, are able to tolerate a period of ischemia. Controversy has surrounded the optimal temperature needed to prevent ischemic changes, but experimental studies and clinical experience indicate that the kidney maintained at approximately 15 to 20°C will be best protected from ischemic injury. There does not appear to be any clinical difference in the mechanism of cooling, whether it be by packing the kidney in the ice slush prepared from physiologic salt solutions or by the application of external cooling coils or other cooling capsule devices.

Intraoperative Radiographs

The use of intraoperative radiographs is important to ensure complete stone removal[55] (Fig. 14–21). An essential step in the procedure is to obtain an

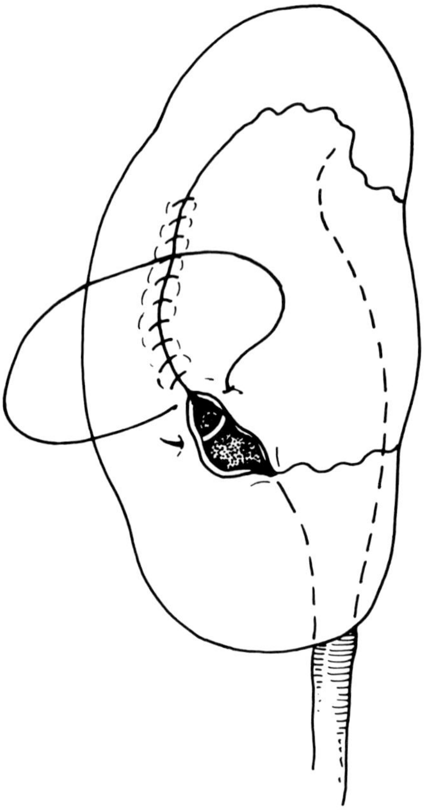

FIGURE 14–20. Closure of renal capsule.

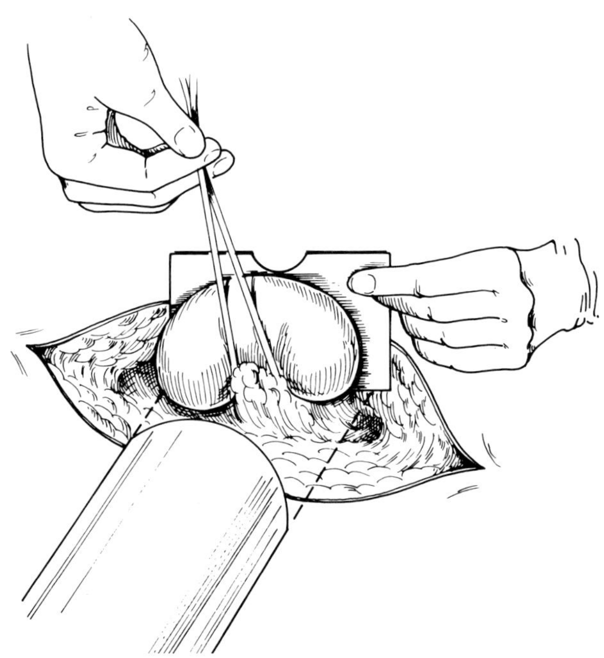

FIGURE 14–21. Intraoperative radiograph.

intraoperative plain radiograph prior to performing the nephrotomy. Not infrequently, small calculi or lines of cleavage between apparently solid staghorn stones (or both) that were not appreciated on previous pyelograms or tomograms will be identified. This initial film also permits comparison with radiographs taken later in the procedure and frequently is most helpful in deciding if stone fragments have been retained. Similarly, a radiograph should be obtained routinely prior to renal closure to ensure that all fragments have been removed. Residual small stones can serve as nidi for reinfection, for studies have shown that these fragments must be removed if the urinary tract infection is to be eradicated and recurrent stone formation prevented. Such techniques as coagulum pyelolithotomy, operative nephroscopy, intraoperative ultrasonography, and pulsatile irrigation have all been reported helpful in reaching this goal.

Microsurgical and Special Instrumentation

The surgical instruments and suture material used in making the nephrotomy and subsequent calycoplasty deserve comment. Microsurgical instrumentation consisting of optical loupes, suture holders, scissors, and scalpel is most important and is utilized routinely throughout the procedure. A Penfield retractor, nerve hooks, and Ragnel retractors are useful in exposing and opening calyces for detection and removal of stone fragments and aid in the exposure of these structures during the reconstructive procedure. Probably one of the most useful adjuncts is in the development of fine suture material. Sutures of 6–0 chromic catgut dyed blue to aid in visualization are invaluable in the suturing of calyces and pelvis. A plastic disposable bulldog clamp is used to occlude the renal artery. The clamp should cause no damage to the arterial wall, since intimal tears lead to vascular thrombosis with resultant renal damage.

Preoperative Medications—Antibiotics and Steroids

Antibiotics are usually administered prior to surgery, and preferably the agent should have high urinary and serum levels and should be nonnephrotoxic.[56] Penicillin or one of its synthetic analogues is usually adequate in controlling most infections and is administered to most patients in high dosages (sodium penicillin, 60 million units daily in a continuous intravenous infusion; ticarcillin, 200 mg/kg/24 hr in four to six divided intravenous doses) 48 to 72 hours preoperatively. Many of the bacterial isolates from this group of patients are also sensitive to cephalosporins, and these agents can be used in full dosage when penicillin allergies exist. It is important to remember that approximately 10 to 15 per cent of patients experience a cross penicillin allergy and that in combination with other antibacterials these agents, specifically aminoglycosides, should be avoided and utilized only when administration of other agents is not suitable because of either the patient's allergy or a specific bacterial sensitivity. When used, aminoglycosides should not be administered within 24 hours prior to or after surgery, and the dosage should be reduced accordingly if renal function is impaired. When these and other agents are administered during the postoperative period, urine is cultured periodically and renal function is continually monitored.

Heparin administration, either systemically or intraarterially, at the time of renal exposure has not been practiced. However, in an effort to reduce venous sludging in the small intrarenal veins, methylprednisolone (900 to 1000 mg) is administered intramuscularly approximately 2 hours prior to surgery. The true effectiveness of this approach requires further studies, but no adverse effects have been noted and venous thrombosis has not been a problem in our population of patients.

RADIAL NEPHROTOMY

Single or multiple radial nephrotomy incisions may be extremely useful as a primary procedure to remove peripherally located stones or, as is more often the case, as a complementary or adjunctive procedure useful in combination with any of the surgical techniques already described. The segmental divisions of the main renal artery as well as their branches progress to the periphery of the kidney in radial fashion[57] (Fig. 14–22). This radial distribution allows for parenchymal incisions to be made parallel to the renal vessels with a minimal loss of functioning parenchyma.

The kidney is exposed through a flank incision and completely mobilized, as in anatrophic nephrolithotomy. The renal artery is identified and controlled with a vessel loop. An intraoperative radiograph is obtained, and the stone is accurately localized. It is not unusual for peripheral calculi to be easily palpated through areas of thinned-out renal cortex. If the stone is not easily palpated, the use of ultrasound may be helpful in localizing its exact position. Stones associated with normal parenchymal thickness are often not readily palpable; therefore, clamping the renal artery will soften and shrink the kidney and may facilitate stone removal. The kidney can tolerate warm ischemic times of 10 to 15 minutes without permanent loss of function[58]; however, if multiple nephrotomies or a prolonged ischemic time is anticipated, the kidney should be cooled. Clamping

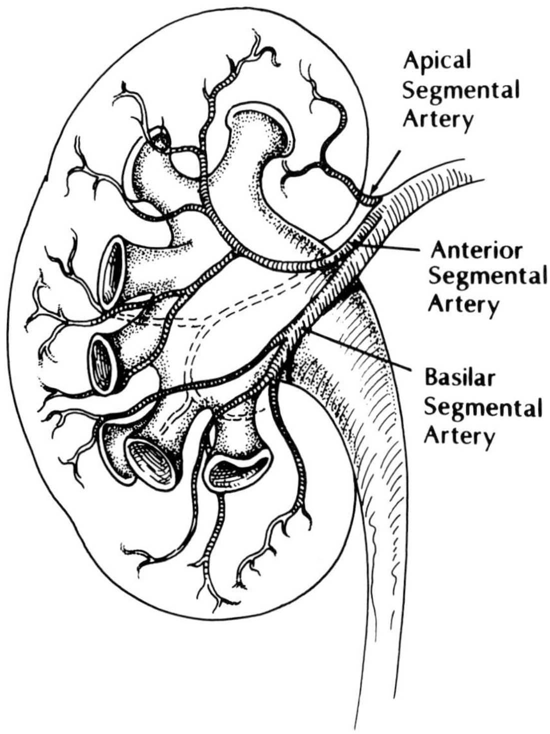

FIGURE 14–22. Radial distribution of the renal vasculature.

the renal artery not only facilitates stone localization but also allows parenchymal dissection to proceed in a bloodless field.

As with anatrophic nephrolithotomy, the renal capsule is sharply incised, and the parenchyma is bluntly dissected either with the back of a scalpel handle or with small brain or malleable retractors (Fig. 14–23). Often the intralobar arteries will be identified, and these may be spared by gentle retraction as the parenchymal incision is deepened. The blunt dissection is continued until the pericalyceal fat is identified. The calyx is sharply incised directly over the stone. The stone is carefully mobilized and removed intact.

To avoid the major renal vasculature, the parenchymal incision is made on the convexity of the posterior renal surface. Most calyces can be approached in this manner, and large venous branches crossing on the anterior surface will be avoided.[59] The use of the intraoperative Doppler stethoscope may further decrease the chance of ischemic injury.

The calyx is irrigated and then directly visualized to ensure complete stone removal. Radiographs are obtained to identify residual fragments. If no stones remain, the calyx is closed with fine absorbable sutures. If this is not technically possible, simple closure of the capsule, including 1 to 2 mm of parenchyma, with fine absorbable suture will suffice. Again, deep mattress sutures are to be avoided. The area is drained, and the incision is closed in the usual fashion. With use of the vessel-sparing principles just described, it is possible to perform multiple radial nephrotomies with very little trauma to the renal parenchyma.[60]

PARTIAL NEPHRECTOMY

Partial nephrectomy is a therapeutic procedure for many localized renal conditions, including vascular lesions, localized carcinoma in a solitary kidney, trauma, segmental obstruction or infection, and renal stone disease localized to

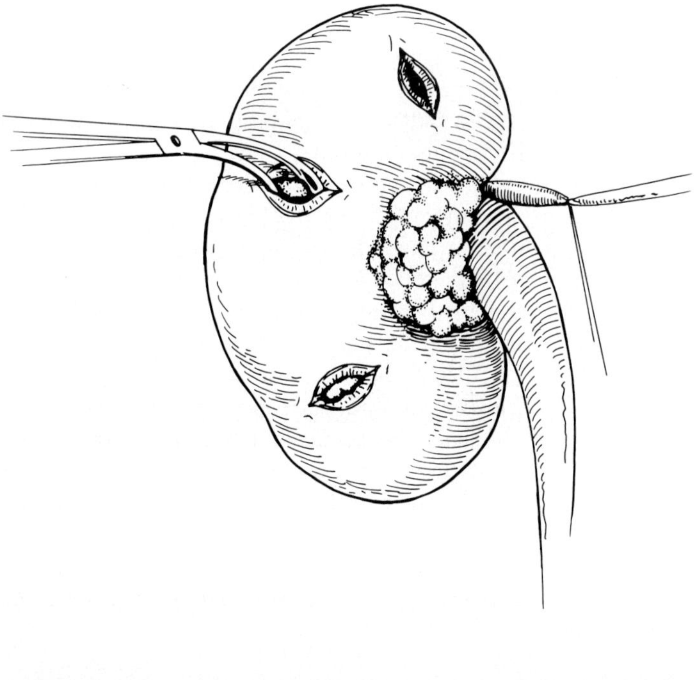

FIGURE 14–23. Radial distribution of the multiple nephrotomies and the vessel loop placed around the renal artery.

either pole.[61] This procedure, when first introduced, was embraced with great enthusiasm, and stone disease became one of the major indications for its use. Advocates believed stone recurrence rates to be reduced when the stone and associated abnormal renal parenchyma were surgically removed. We now know that although partial nephrectomy meets many of the proposed criteria for a suitable stone procedure, in most instances it needlessly sacrifices functioning renal parenchyma and does not necessarily reduce the incidence of further stone formation.

In 1884, Wells is credited with performing the first inadvertent partial nephrectomy in a patient with a perirenal lipoma.[62] It was not until 1889 that Kummell performed the first deliberate partial nephrectomy for stone disease.[62] At the turn of the century, surgeons, frustrated by the frequent complications of hemorrhage and urinary fistula, all but abandoned the procedure.[63] Stewart resurrected interest in the procedure when he demonstrated that about 75 per cent of all stones were formed in either radiographically or histologically abnormal lower pole calyces.[64] In 1960, he published the first large series of more than 200 patients treated by partial nephrectomy and noted a 6.4 per cent incidence of ipsilateral stone recurrence in patients followed from 1 to 8 years.[65] Other studies with similarly short follow-up periods appeared in the literature, corroborating Stewart's low recurrence rate.[66, 67] These results, when compared with the 58 per cent ipsilateral recurrence rate reported by Williams, appear remarkable at best and suggest a significant place for partial nephrectomy in the treatment of stone disease.[68]

It was not until 1971, when Myrvold and Fritjofsson reported a 57 per cent recurrence rate after partial nephrectomy in 65 patients followed for an average of 9 years, that the procedure began to fall into disfavor.[69] Rose and Fellows reexamined the initial population of patients reported by Stewart, only now with a 20-year follow-up period, and found essentially no difference in the recurrence rate for the operated on and nonoperated on kidneys.[70] Marshall and associates also found no difference in the stone recurrence rate when they compared the various surgical procedures, including pyelolithotomy, nephrolithotomy, and partial nephrectomy for the single small polar stone.[71]

In general, partial nephrectomy most often needlessly sacrifices salvageable renal tissue and should be reserved for those patients with severe obstruction associated with parenchymal damage in whom recovery of renal function is expected to be negligible or the rare individual with calyceal stones associated with a polar diverticulum. It is the rare patient with stones who benefits from partial nephrectomy.

Although several different techniques have been advocated for the performance of partial nephrectomy,[62, 72–76] no procedure is clearly superior to any of the others. The kidney is approached through a standard flank incision and mobilized sufficiently to allow complete access to the involved pole and hilar vessels. The proximal ureter is identified and traced to the renal pelvis. It is important to mobilize the pelvis sufficiently so as not to leave diseased tissue behind. The vascular pedicle is dissected, and the branch to the involved pole is identified. Ligating the branch to the involved segment not only reduces the blood loss but also facilitates tissue resection by identifying the margins of excision. The capsule over the involved pole is incised and bluntly peeled back beyond the proposed margins of excision. Preserving the capsule will later facilitate closure. The parenchyma is bluntly transected with the back of a scalpel handle, and encountered vessels are sequentially ligated. The collecting system is sharply transected, and the diseased segment is removed. Manual compression of the remaining parenchyma will allow identification and ligation of bleeding vessels with 5–0 chromic catgut. The collecting system is closed in a watertight fashion with a running 4–0 absorbable suture. The capsule is trimmed, and the edges are closed over the remaining parenchyma with a 4–0 absorbable suture. If, after ligating all obvious bleeding vessels, the cut parenchymal surface continues to bleed, it is helpful to place a piece of Gelfoam on the raw surface and reapproximate the cut edges with horizontal mattress sutures of 2–0 chromic catgut. These sutures are placed only a few millimeters from the edge of the surface in an attempt to limit ischemic necrosis of the remaining parenchyma. Prior to closing, a radiograph is obtained to confirm complete stone removal. The area is well drained, and the incision is closed.

NEPHRECTOMY

Nephrectomy, although meeting many of the objectives of stone surgery, cannot be endorsed as routine treatment for renal stone disease. Nephrectomy needlessly sacrifices renal tissue, and in as many as one third of patients with stones, calculi will develop in the contralateral kidney.[70] Nephrectomy should be reserved for the rare patient with chronic obstruction and a nonfunctioning kidney, as determined by radionuclide renal scan using one of the glomerular isotopes. If the involved kidney demonstrates a clearance of greater than 20 ml/min, recognizing the fact that renal scanning techniques frequently underestimate renal function in the obstructed kidney, attempts should be made to preserve that kidney by removing the stone if the patient is a reasonable surgical candidate. In addition, the patient with a solitary kidney and less than a 10 ml/min clearance deserves an attempt at stone removal, as it is well known that relief of obstruction will frequently result in a dramatic improvement in renal function.[77, 78] Nephrectomy is indicated in the elderly or debilitated patient with a complex renal stone, recurrent infection, and a normally functioning contralateral kidney who is thought to be a poor candidate for a difficult and possibly prolonged operative procedure.

POSTOPERATIVE COMPLICATIONS

In addition to pulmonary complications for open surgery, cardiovascular changes should be considered as well. In the flank position, decreased venous return can result and hypotension may be encountered. It is therefore important to add flexion gradually and raise the kidney while continuing to monitor the blood pressure.

Stone migration during the intraoperative manipulation of the kidney, with the resultant inability to localize, is a serious problem when encountered. The placement of a Silastic stent often obviates the passage of fragments down the ureter, and, as noted, it is for this reason that it is passed early in the procedure. In addition, intraoperative radiographs are essential for the same reason.

Though complete surgical removal of the stone and eradication of infection are attempted by all renal surgeons, these goals are often not reached. The residual stone rate based on various authors' reports varies from 5 to 26 per cent. Not all patients are cleared of urinary tract infection, and only approximately 60 to 80 per cent will have their infection eradicated following stone removal and intensive treatment with appropriate antibiotics. The stone recurrence rate is also variable and based on a review of many surgeries—approximately 30 per cent within 6 years. A recent review of Boyce's experience revealed an overall recurrence rate of 22 per cent within 10 years.[79] Of interest was the difference in the rate of recurrence between women (9 per cent) and men (43 per cent). Half of the male patients' recurrent stones were infected preoperatively with *Pseudomonas* organisms. The high recurrence rate in this group is likely related to the difficulty in treating these infections with antibiotics that were available in the late 1960s. Aminoglycosides and other newer agents were just being developed, and it is likely that the persistent and subsequent stone recurrence will be reduced in patients treated with modern agents. The remaining male patients with recurrent disease were found to have undiagnosed metabolic disorders that likely contributed to new stone formation. The findings in female patients revealed that only two recurrences were related to persistent urinary tract infection.

Another report of interest is that of Segura and associates, who followed 75 patients with infection stones and found that 25 per cent developed recurrent infections alone and only 9 per cent developed recurrent stones and infection.[80] Others have also demonstrated a low recurrence rate following surgical removal of struvite stones. When combined with postoperative irrigation with hemacidrin, the stone recurrence rate varied from 3 to 25 per cent over a mean follow-up period of 17 to 66 months.[81] As expected, the incidence of recurrent urinary tract infection was also reduced in these patients and varied from 0 to 28 per cent. These studies clearly emphasize the need for continued follow-up and reevaluation of patients in an effort to detect recurrent infection and identify any metabolic disorder that may predispose to recurrent disease.

Retained stone fragments also represent a major concern in terms of nidus for further calculus formation unassociated with infection. Residual stone fragments are probably of less concern for calcium oxalate, cystine, and uric acid stones than for struvite stones. Stones of these former compositions may grow in size but are influenced by the concentration of the active products in the urine and the formation product of these substances and not by the presence of the stone fragments. Sleith and Wickham reported that 70 per cent of retained infection stones increase in size but only 30 per cent of infected stones did so.[82]

Postoperative Renal Hemorrhage

Fewer than 10 per cent of patients will experience postoperative hemorrhage significant enough to require blood transfusion. The low rate of postoperative bleeding is likely secondary to the carefully placed nephrotomy incision, which avoids large intrarenal vessels, and the precise closure of the calyces, renal pelvis, and capsule so that sufficient tamponade is provided to occlude small intrarenal vessels adequately.[83] Bleeding usually occurs on the seventh to fourteenth postoperative day and is likely to be secondary to the failure of the sutures used to close the intrarenal structures. At times, postoperative renal hemorrhage has been associated with the chronic administration of steroids for the treatment of sarcoidosis and other specific disorders.

Patients are initially managed with fluids and blood transfusion as is clinically indicated. Passage of a nonreactive ureteral stent has also been found to be useful in managing this problem. Oral administration of aminocaproic acid (Amicar) is being used with increasing frequency, with excellent results. This antifibrinolytic agent has been very effective in managing this problem, and complications secondary to intrarenal clot development or systemic hematologic problems have not been encountered. The agent is generally effective within 12 hours and is discontinued 24 hours after the bleeding has subsided. One patient has been encountered who developed an arteriovenous fistula of the type and configuration typically observed after needle biopsy of the kidney. Because of persistent hematuria, reexploration was undertaken, and the involved blood vessels were ligated. Postoperatively, the patient did well, and radiographic and renal function studies demonstrated a satisfactory result.

Pulmonary Complications

Between 5 and 10 per cent of patients undergoing nephrolithotomy will experience postoperative difficulties related to pulmonary dysfunction.[84] Though the spectrum of ages of patients is quite broad, at least one third are greater than 50 years old, and the presence of chronic pulmonary disorders is not uncommon. Preoperatively, all patients are evaluated by an anesthesiologist, and, when indicated, pulmonary function studies are obtained. Postoperatively, all patients are encouraged to cough and deep breathe, and intermittent positive-pressure breathing is often used in an effort to decrease the incidence of pulmonary complications.

Of concern is the effect of the lengthy operative procedure on the "down lung" while the patient is in the flank position. Average anesthesia time for each procedure is approximately 5 hours, and it is expected that expansion of the dependent lung would be diminished; it is interesting that clinical experience has shown that the dependent lung is not at increased risk for development of atelectasis, for previous studies have shown that though 31 per cent of patients will have some degree of pulmonary congestion early in the postoperative period, these changes are present in both lung fields to an equal degree. With experience, anesthesiologists have found that it is beneficial to hyperventilate the patient briefly prior to removal of the endotracheal tube. This hyperventilation is performed while the patient is on the operating table but is placed in a supine position. It is their belief that vigorous reexpansion of the lungs is very helpful in reducing postoperative atelectasis and other pulmonary problems.

Pneumothorax is another pulmonary complication that occurs in fewer than 5 per cent of patients. Many patients have had multiple surgical procedures in addition to the presence of chronic urinary tract infection, and not unexpectedly the diaphragm and overlying pleura are adherent to the upper pole of the kidney. When the pleura is opened inadvertently, it is promptly closed with running chromic catgut sutures. It is imperative to maintain positive pressure on the lungs during the final stages of the repair, and chest tubes are not used. No detectable postoperative problems have been attributed to pleural injury when such injury is promptly recognized and repaired; however, chest radiographs are routinely obtained promptly after the patient returns to the recovery room.

In more than 400 nephrolithotomies performed at the Bowman Gray School of Medicine, there have been two deaths secondary to massive pulmonary embolism occurring during the postoperative period. A small number of patients have had nonfatal pulmonary emboli, and these have been effectively managed with systemic anticoagulation. Occasionally, vena caval plication has been necessary to reduce the chance of further emboli in predisposed patients. In an effort to decrease the rate of venous thrombosis and associated pulmonary emboli, all patients are fitted with full-length elastic support hose preoperatively, and all patients continue to wear the hose for at least 4 to 5 days postoperatively. In addition, ambulation is encouraged during the first postoperative day.

The potential for developing or aggravating preexisting hypertension should be of concern with any surgical procedure on the kidney. The complication appears to be unusual. Boyce reviewed 100 patients with nephrotomy and noted that only 2 became moderately hypertensive postoperatively.[85] Whether the hypertension was directly related to the surgical procedure rather than being an unrelated development could obviously be debated. On careful dissection of the renal artery and accurate mapping of the plane of incision, the use of hypothermic ischemia of the kidney can be minimized.

Despite following all the techniques to preserve renal function that have been previously described, trauma to the renal parenchyma can still occur, and some patients will demonstrate diminished renal function postoperatively. Boyce noted that of 100 patients undergoing anatrophic nephrolithotomy only 2 had a decrease in renal function postoperatively and 1 of the patients subsequently required nephrectomy.[86] Experience with anatrophic nephrolithotomy in patients with a solitary kidney also revealed that the average preoperative renal function equaled the average postoperative function.[87, 88] Though diminution in function was noted in some patients, in others there was marked improvement. In this latter group, the relief of obstruction and resolution of infection associated with stone removal likely contributed to this result. The careful dissection of the renal artery, atraumatic clamping of the artery when necessary, and the use of methylene blue to identify vascular segments and hypothermia enable one to use this method with excellent results.

Pyelocutaneous fistula following prolonged urinary leakage represents another complication associated with renal stone surgery. Distal ureteral obstruction and infection with foreign bodies are the main causes and generally resolve spontaneously within 2 or 3 weeks postoperatively. Intervention is rarely required, but, when necessary, placement of an indwelling ureteral stent will often suffice. Routine placement of a ureteral stent is suggested after pyelonephrolithotomy and anatrophic nephrolithotomy and procedures requiring extensive dissection of the renal collecting system or in the presence of infection. Urinoma formation is a rare complication resulting from premature removal of operative drains. In the presence of urinary infection, sepsis can result. Placement of ureteral stents will be helpful in managing this problem, and percutaneous or open drainage may be required.

If metabolic disorders contributing to stone formation are discovered in the preoperative period, direct medical therapy is begun to prevent stone recurrence. Long-term follow-up includes periodic urine cultures and treatment of all urinary infections. Repeat 24-hour urine collections are also required because with the clearing of urinary obstruction and infection, abnormalities of excessive calcium excretion may become evident postoperatively. If metabolic problems are diagnosed during this period, they should be treated appropriately. Intravenous urography, including nephrotomography without injection of contrast agents, is performed 3 months postoperatively and repeated if clinically indicated. These patients require many years of follow-up to prevent the development of recurrent disease.

Mortality

Though the average age of patients undergoing renal procedures is in the midforties, a significant number of patients have multisystem disease. Approximately 20 per cent of patients are azotemic, and urinary tract infections with resistant organisms are present in more than half. In more than 900 patients having nephrolithotomy, 4 have died during the postoperative period (within 3 months of the operative procedure). One patient died of a myocardial infarction and three of pulmonary emboli.[85] Current mortality statistics are less than 1 per cent, which compares favorably with the experience of open renal surgery.

URETERAL SURGERY

The management of ureteral stones has changed greatly over the past several years. Associated with the development and refinement of percutaneous techniques, ureteroscopy, and ESWL has been the emergence of a variety of proven approaches for removing upper and lower ureteral calculi. Prior to these developments, upper ureteral stones usually required surgical removal, and in most instances lower ones were manipulated by a variety of techniques. These many changes have occurred over a relatively short time.

The evolution of modern techniques in the management of ureteral stones has been dependent upon the development of both radiographic and endoscopic techniques. Obviously, both are required to assist in stone removal. Prior to the development of these techniques, the diagnosis of ureteral stones had been largely based on clinical signs and symptoms. As noted, the development of radiographic techniques had significant impact on both the diagnosis and the treatment of these stones.

Ureteral stones vary with regard to composition, location, size, and general configuration. The stones generally occur in patients ranging in age from 20 to 25 years, and they tend to predominate in men (male/female, 3:1) and whites (whites/blacks, 4:1). Ureteral stones have their origin in the kidney; therefore, the cause of their formation is similar to that of renal stones. Stones occurring primarily in the ureter are unusual, and when they do occur, they are usually associated with ureteral obstruction caused by such conditions as ureterocele, malignancy, and atonic segments.

Because most ureteral stones have their origin in the kidney, the composition is similar to that of renal stones. Calcium oxalate–calcium phosphate stones predominate and occur in approximately 70 per cent of individuals. Cystine, uric acid, and struvite stones can also occur in the ureter, but, as with renal stones of these compositions, they are relatively infrequent. It is important to remember that knowledge of the composition of the stone is important. For example, uric acid stones (radiographically radiolucent) can effectively be managed with alkalinization of the urine, and experience has shown that this approach often results in relatively rapid stone passage and complete dissolution.[89] Similarly, knowledge of the presence of a calcium oxalate dihydrate stone (often evident on a radiograph as having medium density and hazy borders) would suggest a satisfactory outcome with ESWL because these stones fragment very well with this technology. In contradistinction, cystine and calcium oxalate monohydrate stones are not as readily amenable to ESWL, and if stones of these types are suspected, other approaches, such as ureteroscopy with direct extraction or in association with fragmentation (electrohydraulic, ultrasonic, or laser), may be more appropriate.

Knowledge of the natural history of ureteral stones is also very important when attempting to predict the specific outcome in individual patients. It is only with this information that the various available approaches can be planned and subsequently initiated. Ureteral stones occur with equal frequency on the right and left, and the points of impaction are also similar on both sides. Those points in the ureter that result in relative constriction include the ureteropelvic junction; the point at which the ureter crosses the iliac vessels; the region of the vas deferens in men and the broad ligament in women; and the intramural ureter and ureteral meatus. It is at these points that progression of ureteral stones usually stops and impaction occurs.

It has been reported that at the time of presentation most ureteral stones will be located in the lower one third of the ureter (75.3 per cent), followed in order of frequency by the upper one third or ureteropelvic junction (15.5 per cent) and the middle one third (9.2 per cent).[90] Others have reported similar experiences.[91–93] The size of the stone is also related to the chance of impaction and its location. Most impacted stones have at least one diameter greater than 2 mm, and generally stones greater than 10 mm are unlikely to pass. Ninety per cent of stones located in the distal one third of the ureter and measuring less than 4 mm in diameter will pass spontaneously, whereas only 50 per cent of stones 4.0 to 5.9 mm in diameter will be expected to pass spontaneously.[93, 94] Only 20 per cent of stones greater than 6 mm in diameter will pass without intervention. Stones located in the proximal two thirds of the ureter are less likely to pass. On the basis of the data reviewed, it is evident that most ureteral stones will occur in the distal one third of the ureter, and of those doing so, most will pass spontaneously if they are less than 4 to 5 mm in their greatest diameter. Similarly, of those stones in the upper two thirds of the ureter, spontaneous passage is unlikely, and some form of intervention is usually required. Expectant management consists of hydration and the liberal use of analgesics, but if the patient develops fever associated with urinary tract infection, severe ureteral colic unresponsive to oral medications, severe nausea and vomiting, complete obstruction of a solitary kidney, or impaction of the stone, hospital admission and surgical or manipulative intervention are usually indicated. Typically, stones located in the upper two thirds of the ureter are treated with ESWL, and those in the lower ureter are managed ureteroscopically. With newer ESWL instrumentation, stones in the lower ureter are becoming amenable to ESWL fragmentation as well. Though attempts have been made to remove upper ureteral stones ureteroscopically, the failure rate is higher in stones in this location when compared with those located more distally. Indications for ureterolithotomy include unsuccessful endoscopic removal, unsuccessful ESWL, stones in infants and children, and the presence of associated anatomic abnormalities.

Ureterolithotomy

Prior to discussing ureterolithotomy, a review of the related anatomy would be appropriate. The ureter originates from the mesonephric ducts early in gestation. As it ascends along the dorsal wall of the embryo, it is known as the ureteral bud. During its cephalad migration, it encounters the mesonephric blastema, which differentiates into the renal parenchyma. The ureteral bud forms the collecting system and ureter. Without the influence of the ureter, the mesonephric blastema will not differentiate properly. The blood supply to each renal unit ascends with the developing structure. Approximately 25 per cent of the population has more than one renal artery supplying a single kidney, the lower pole most frequently receiving the accessory branch. The origin of accessory vessels is commonly believed to be attributable to a delay in resorption of embryonic arteries, and these structures also result in the ureteral blood supply. The major sources include the superior vesical artery, a branch from the common iliac artery, and a descending branch from the renal artery. Anastomotic branches are in the periureteral adventitia (Fig. 14–24).

The ureter begins at the distal portion of the renal pelvis. Histologically, the three layers include an outer serosal covering, a smooth muscle layer, and an inner mucosal lining. The smooth muscle layer has three groupings of muscle spindles; two circular groups are separated by a longitudinal group. The upper half of the ureter lies atop the psoas muscle. On the right, the vena cava, sympathetic plexus, and vertebral column are in close proximity; on the left, the aorta is medial to the ureter. The colon is anterolateral, and the remainder of the small bowel is anterior and separated by a layer of peritoneum. At the inlet to the pelvis, the ureter crosses anterior to the iliac vessels. Because of this relationship, a recognized hazard of iliac artery reconstruction is ureteral injury.

The ureter continues dorsally and slightly lateral in its approach to the bladder while remaining retroperitoneal. In approaching the trigone, it is posterior to the superior vesical artery and broad ligament in women. At this level, the iliac vessels are lateral, as are the obturator vessels and nerve. The sigmoid colon eventually crosses the left ureter and becomes posterior to it. All female reproductive organs are anterior. Upon entering the posterolateral portion of the bladder, assuming normal anatomy, the ureter courses through the detrusor for a varying length and eventually drains into the bladder through an orifice at the trigone.

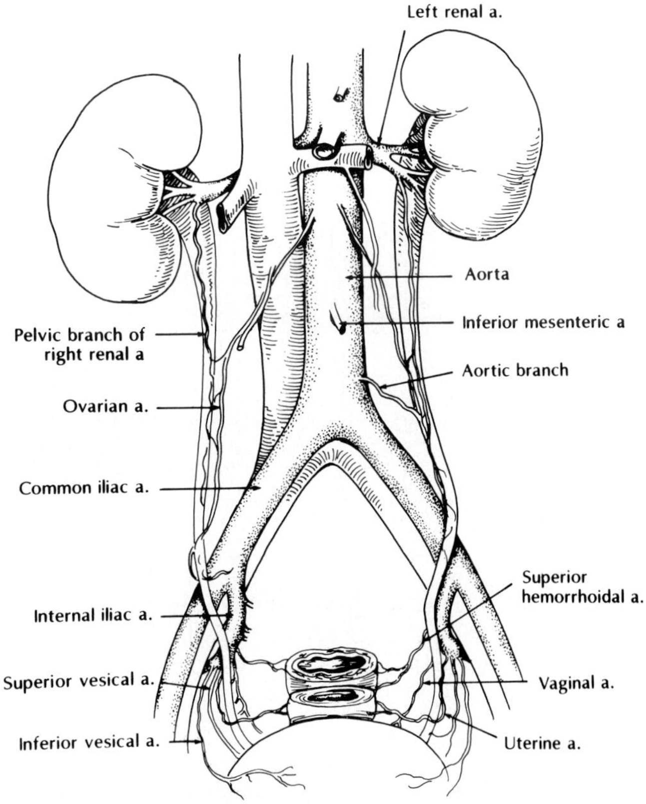

FIGURE 14–24. Anatomy of renal vessels and ureteral blood supply.

Surgical Approaches

Traditionally, the surgical approach to remove a ureteral stone that is judged unlikely to pass spontaneously has been either a ureterolithotomy or endoscopic manipulation. Recently, antegrade extraction through percutaneous avenues offers an alternative to surgery.

The 25-cm course of the adult ureter stretches from the lower pole of the kidney at L2 to the level of the symphysis pubis. Because of this broad anatomic distribution, approaches to ureteral surgery are many and varied. Once the decision has been made to proceed with surgical intervention, the choice of incision and approach must be based upon the location and shape of the stone.

A midline incision from the umbilicus to the symphysis pubis can be utilized for the removal of lower ureteral or intramural stones (Fig. 14–25). After the incision is made, the rectus abdominis muscles are divided at the midline, and a self-retaining retractor is placed after the peritoneum overlying the bladder is reflected cephalad.[95] A Pfannenstiel incision is preferred by other surgeons and also offers satisfactory exposure of the lower ureter. Several avenues can be followed to remove the stone. An intravesical or extravesical approach to the stone largely depends on its location. The more cephalad portion of the pelvic ureter should be secured to prevent the inadvertent migration of a stone, for even the most longstanding fixed ureteral stone can become dislodged during gentle ureteral manipulation.

If the stone is impacted in the intramural or distal extramural ureter, a number of surgeons will make their approach through the bladder. If the stone is palpable through the vesical mucosa, a small incision can be made and the stone can be extracted. The incision is then reapproximated with interrupted 5–0 chromic catgut suture. The advantage of this approach is that the ureteral orifice is not disturbed.

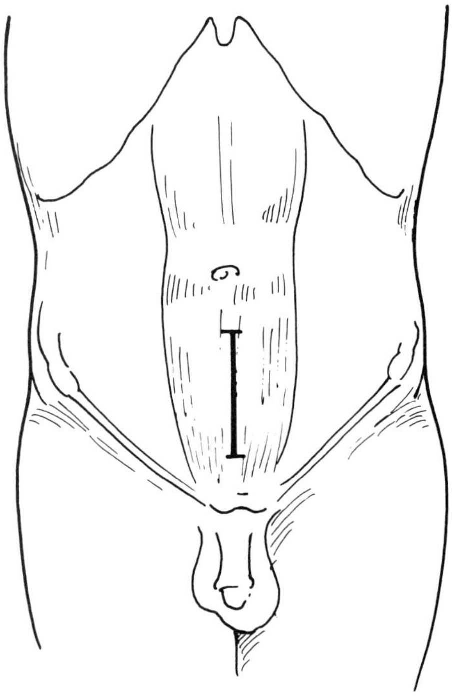

FIGURE 14–25. Midline incision from umbilicus to symphysis pubis for removal of lower ureteral or intramural stones.

When the stone has been in the distal extravesical or transmural ureter for an extended period, the periureteral tissue can sustain significant damage, and the distal ureter may be unsuitable for repair. In these instances, it may be necessary occasionally to remove the stone and ureter together. The ureteral orifice is identified and secured with a figure-of-eight silk suture. The ureter is then dissected free of its intramural attachments to a point distal to the stone. When nonreactive ureter is encountered, the ureter is transected. The bladder hiatus is usually closed, and a more lateral end-to-side anastomosis is made, taking care not to free much of the ureter and possibly embarrass its distal blood supply. The major drawback of this procedure is the creation of a freely refluxing system, but many reports indicate that sterile reflux does not cause renal damage.

A Pfannenstiel incision can be modified to approach distal ureteral stones. Limiting the size of the incision on the unaffected side or extending the lateral margin into a Gibson-type incision, which allows for greater exposure of the middle and upper ureter, makes this a viable alternative. All the intravesical and extravesical manipulation previously described for the suprapubic approach can be accomplished through this incision. The advantage of additional exposure makes this an attractive alternative.

The Gibson incision provides access to the lower ureter (Fig. 14–26*A*), and its major benefit is in providing additional exposure to the midureter (Fig. 14–26*B*). The patient is placed in a modified flank position at approximately a 45-degree angle to the table. The incision is made obliquely, extending from a midpoint 2 to 3 cm cephalad to the anterior iliac crest. The distal and proximal limits of the incision are extended according to the amount of exposure required. This practice allows adequate exposure to the ureter from the sacral promontory

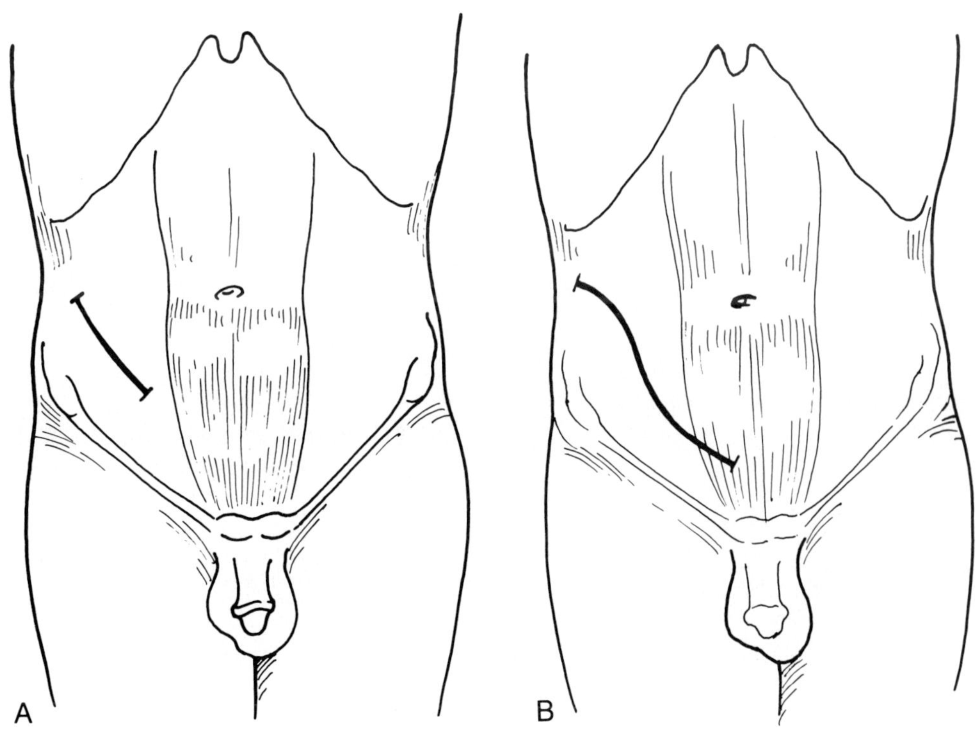

FIGURE 14–26. Gibson incision. *A*, For access to lower ureter. *B*, With additional exposure to midureter.

to the lower pole of the kidney. After the incision is made, the muscle fibers of the external oblique muscle are split along their axis and the peritoneum is reflected medially. As the intraperitoneal contents are retracted medially, the ureter is visualized. Proximal and distal control of the stone is required prior to ureterotomy. A longitudinal ureterotomy is made and closed with interrupted 5–0 chromic catgut suture. Prior to this, an 8F ureteral catheter is passed proximally and distally to ensure the patency of the ureter. A drain is left in the retroperitoneum and brought out through the wound. The wound is closed in the standard fashion. Postoperatively, patients require minimal analgesia and recuperate quickly. Once drainage subsides, the drain is removed.

The flank incision is a more extensive incision and should be reserved for proximal ureteral stones. Through this incision, the kidney can be excised if required. Ureteral reconstruction, as well as interposition of bowel, can also be accomplished through this approach (Fig. 14–27). Once the patient is in a full decubitus (flank) position, the kidney rest is elevated and the table is flexed so that the apex of the table is slightly cephalad to the anterior iliac crest. This practice helps to provide maximal exposure once the incision is made. Depending upon the site of the stone and the anticipated procedure, an incision is made and the external and internal oblique muscles are divided. Care is taken to preserve the iliohypogastric nerve, as it lies between the internal oblique and transversus abdominis muscles.

Once the internal oblique muscle is divided, the lumbodorsal fascia is incised sharply, and the transversus abdominis muscle is separated by blunt dissection. The peritoneum should be swept medially to prevent inadvertent entry. At this point, Gerota's fascia is in view, and medial retraction of the peritoneum and its contents exposes the upper ureter. In removing upper ureteral stones, all attempts should be made to keep the ureteropelvic junction intact. In addition, minimal ureteral dissection should be performed to avoid inadvertent devascularization. A longitudinal ureterotomy is made, the stone is extracted, and closure is made with absorbable suture. The transversus abdominis muscle and the

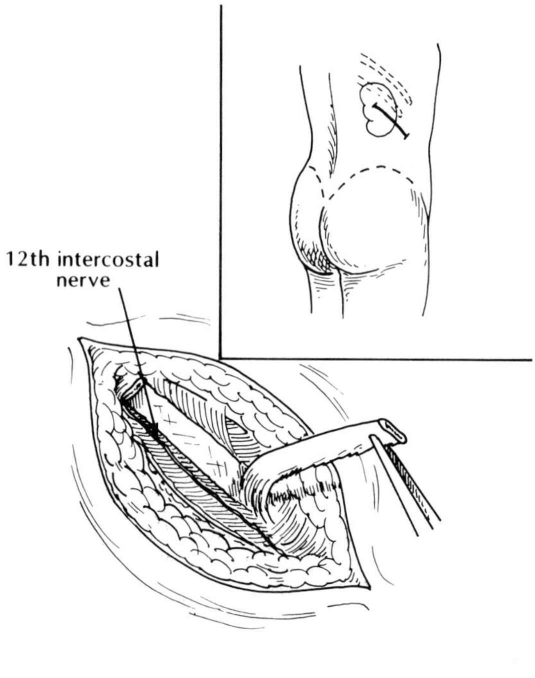

FIGURE 14–27. More extensive flank incision should be reserved for proximal ureteral stones.

external and internal oblique muscles are reapproximated with running 0 chromic catgut suture. A drain is placed in close proximity to the ureterotomy and brought out through the wound.

Care should be taken when removing a rib or dissecting a kidney that has previously been infected. Adhesions to the diaphragm can easily lead to opening the pleura, with resultant pneumothorax. If this occurs, closure over a large-bore tube (18F to 20F) should be performed. The tube is brought out through the incision and placed on water seal or suction once the incision is closed. After satisfactory reinflation of the lung is accomplished, the tube is removed and the exit site is sealed with petroleum jelly (Vaseline) gauze. Formal thoracostomy drainage may be required if the pneumothorax fails to resolve.

A midline approach is another alternative to exposing the ureter through most of its course. If the anticipated procedure is a transureteroureterostomy or a contralateral ureteropyelostomy, this approach offers satisfactory exposure. Another incision that offers a similar exposure is the chevron incision, which can be extended on both sides to offer better exposure bilaterally. Its disadvantage is that it requires the division of muscles, whereas the midline incision spares muscles. At times, postoperative pain can increase the patient's morbidity.

Once a midline incision has been made, a transperitoneal or extraperitoneal approach can be utilized.[96] The advantage of the latter is a reduction in subsequent intraabdominal adhesions. If the abdomen has been entered previously, this approach becomes more difficult. Once the layers of the rectus abdominis muscle have been separated, the posterior rectus sheath is carefully divided, taking care to preserve the peritoneum. When applying appropriate traction and counter-traction, the plane between the peritoneum and posterior rectus fascia can be sharply dissected. The peritoneum is retracted medially until the retroperitoneal structures are exposed. With this approach, the ureter can often be exposed in its entirety. A ureterotomy is made and closed, as previously described. The area is drained with a Penrose drain, which is brought out laterally through either the wound or a separate stab incision. The wound is closed with interrupted absorbable suture.

The posterior approach to upper ureteral stones is another useful technique (Fig. 14–28). With the patient in the flank position, a small incision is made over the lumbodorsal fascia between the twelfth rib and the iliac crest posteriorly. Minimal muscle transection is used, thus reducing postoperative pain. The major disadvantage is that this approach is good only for upper ureteral and pelvic stones. Closure is easily accomplished. The drain is brought out through the incision.

Percutaneous manipulation of ureteral stones is in the early stage of development. Upper ureteral stones can be grasped with special stone baskets, especially if there is some dilatation secondary to obstruction. Further evaluation of this technique is required, so that its proper place in the operative management of ureterolithiasis can be determined.

When actually incising the ureter, it is important to realize that the blood supply travels in the periureteral tissue. The longitudinal axis of the ureter is parallel to its vascular supply, which is the major reason for making longitudinal ureterotomies. The chance of disrupting the ureteral blood supply is less likely with a longitudinal incision than with a tranverse one. The anastomotic vascular network of periureteral vessels becomes critically important during healing.[97] Compounding the problem is the associated inflammation and scarring that may exist from prior surgeries for stones.

The muscular sheath that composes the middle layer of the ureter tends to

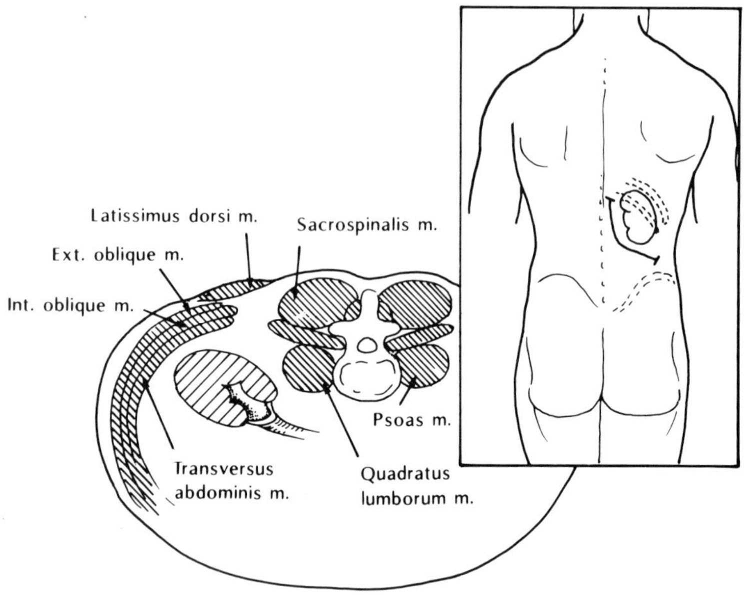

FIGURE 14–28. Posterior approach to upper ureteral stones.

heal better after a longitudinal incision than it does after a transverse incision. The mucosal defect appears to heal within 8 to 10 days whether a transverse or longitudinal incision is made. However, the more extensive the transverse incision, the greater the disruption of muscle, and the less likely adequate closure will ensue.

The proponents of transverse ureterolithotomy believe that less postoperative urinary extravasation occurs with this incision than with the longitudinal incisions. Without proper location and immobilization, the stone can be dislodged inadvertently during ureteral dissection. Before the incision is made, a radiograph should be obtained routinely to identify the location of the stone.

During surgery, a minimum of ureteral manipulation will help to prevent dislodging the stone. Once the section of ureter containing the stone is encountered, proximal and distal control is obtained. Two techniques currently employed involve occluding the ureteral lumen with vessel loops or Babcock clamps. Either technique will occlude the lumen to prevent migration, avoid injury to the ureter, and necessitate only a minimal amount of periureteral mobilization.

When stones migrate during surgery from their preoperative position, the first requirement is to relocate the stone. The use of intraoperative ureterograms is usually of little help. Tactile exploration with ureteral catheters and retrieval with a stone basket occasionally are helpful. In addition, extension of the incision, if possible, or use of a counterincision should be attempted if the stone is located. If all measures fail, it is paramount to maintain patency of the ureter. Often, the use of a stent is helpful in these situations. Prolonged urinary extravasation associated with a distally migrated stone is an unwelcome complication of ureterolithotomy.

Once the stone is removed, the ureter is intubated proximally and distally with a red rubber catheter and irrigated. This practice ensures patency of the lumen and, it is hoped, identifies stone fragments. Whether or not a stent should be used is a matter of personal choice. Stents tend not to be used with simple ureterotomies. In more extensive ureterotomies or in those associated with significant infection, a self-retaining Silastic catheter is often used to minimize urinary extravasation and decompress the proximal renal unit.[98]

Closure of the ureter is effected with several interrupted sutures of an absorbable material, such as 5–0 chromic catgut.[99] The suture approximates the outer serosal margins. Evidence suggests a shorter postoperative drainage period with no evidence of ureteral strictures on long-term follow-up.

Postoperative Complications

General postoperative complications related to pulmonary dysfunction, pulmonary emboli, and general nutrition are similar to those encountered with renal procedures and other surgical procedures as well. Management of specific problems as they relate particularly to complications are discussed below.

One of the most frequent complications is the loss of the stone intraoperatively. This complication can be limited by the use of a preoperative abdominal radiograph. As previously described, once the stone is located in the ureter, it should be immobilized. If the stone is lost, all reasonable attempts at removal should be made. Should these fail, ureteral patency should be maintained with the use of indwelling stents.

Sepsis is an inherent risk in any urologic manipulation. The judicious use of preoperative antibiotic coverage is necessary. If a specific organism can be cultured from urine or blood, then appropriate antibiotic coverage should be employed preoperatively. In many patients, this information is not available, thereby necessitating broad-spectrum coverage. An aminoglycoside and cephalosporin administered intravenously or intramuscularly will eradicate most organisms responsible for sepsis, such as enteric gram-negative pathogens. Mention of the immunocompromised, diabetic, or nutritionally debilitated patient must be made with regard to the offending organism. Yeast and unusual gram-negative organisms are most likely to be recovered in these individuals.

Inadvertent removal of periureteral tissue may result in ureteral necrosis and may lead to urinary drainage and the formation of a stricture. A minimal amount of dissection should be employed in the presence of inflammation and infection in an attempt to reduce the incidence of devascularization.

Ureterocutaneous fistulas are another complication of ureteral surgery. Distal obstruction, infection, the presence of a foreign body, or devascularization of ureteral segments all predispose to this complication. Identification and correction of the underlying cause will usually lead to resolution; treatment may be as simple as the removal of a stone fragment distal to the ureterotomy. Excessively prolonged drainage necessitates further evaluation.

Any ureteral manipulation carries with it the long-term risk of the formation of a stricture.[100] With a ureterolithotomy, transurethral stone manipulation, or percutaneous stone extraction, the possibility of ureteral damage is present. Usually, these injuries are silent and are detected only at the time of postoperative evaluation. Unexplained hematuria can alert the examiner to unsuspected obstruction, but in experience this has been a rare occurrence.

REPAIR OF SURGICAL COMPLICATIONS

The complications of ureterolithotomy involve disruption of ureteral continuity or obstruction caused by formation of a stricture. Corrective procedures are designed to reestablish the continuity of the ureter or eliminate obstruction. The procedures described are designed to accomplish these goals.

Ureteral Reimplantation

Distal ureteral injury can be managed by direct end-to-side ureteroneocystostomy. This procedure requires a ureter of sufficient length to create an anastomosis without tension. Only distal lesions are suitable for this form of correction.

This technique requires exposure of the distal third of the ureter. An infraumbilical midline incision is best for the surgical approach. The ureter is transected proximal to the lesion at a site where the blood supply is believed to be adequate. The peritoneum is then mobilized from the bladder so that the entry site of the ureter is extraperitoneal. The ureter is brought into the bladder and sutured end-to-side to the bladder wall. Prior to anastomosis, the ureter is spatulated, and no attempt is made at creating an antirefluxing anastomosis. The apical ureteral suture (5–0 chromic catgut) anchors it to the detrusor muscle; other sutures are interrupted and contain bladder mucosa and full thickness of the ureteral wall. A Silastic stent is used, and a Penrose drain is left in the extraperitoneal perivesical space.

Bladder Flap (Boari Flap)

The diseased lower third of the ureter can be replaced by a pedicle of bladder in the shape of a tube.[101] Difficulties in mobilizing the bladder are encountered if the bladder has been previously operated upon, has been irradiated, or has been traumatized.

A Gibson incision is used to expose the ureter and bladder. Once isolated, the defect in the ureter is measured, and a flap of bladder 2 to 4 cm longer than the measured ureteral defect is raised. In creating the flap, the base at the cephalad portion of the bladder measures 2 to 5 cm (Fig. 14–29). The distal portion of the flap gradually narrows and can be angulated across the bladder surface to gain length. Individual preference dictates whether the ureterocystos-

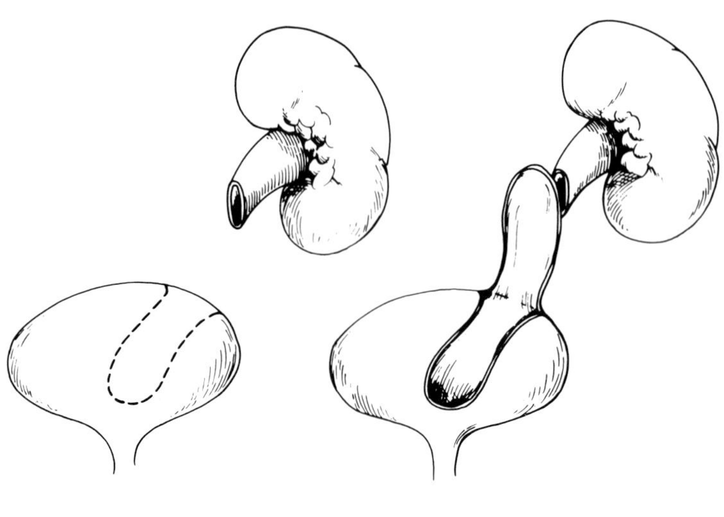

FIGURE 14–29. Creation of Boari flap.

tomy is antirefluxing. Results from both approaches are good and comparable. The bladder is repaired with interrupted 0 chromic catgut suture, and the flap is tubularized in a similar fashion (Fig. 14–30). Ureteral stents tend to be used more liberally owing to bladder mucosal edema. As in any ureteroneocystostomy, tension on the anastomosis can lead to further complications.

A bladder suspension on the ipsilateral psoas muscle can often reduce tension on the anastomosis and preserve the repair.[102] The technique requires mobilization of the bladder bilaterally. This will be difficult in a previously irradiated or operated upon bladder. Once mobilized, 2–0 chromic catgut is used to attach the bladder serosa to the psoas muscle. In performing this procedure, an extra few centimeters of length can be obtained. Often this approach is all that is required to compensate for distal ureteral loss.

Ileal Ureter

Ileal ureters in patients with stone disease are typically used either to replace a damaged ureter or in patients who have intractable stone disease and have pain and complications secondary to multiple stone passage. In 1959, Goodwin and associates used the ileal ureter in a patient with bilateral staghorn calculi and severe infection to eliminate obstruction and provide maximal drainage of the renal pelvis and lower calyces.[103] Further successful experience with the ileal ureter has suggested that it might be considered a primary form of treatment in patients with evidence of multiple renal calculi and obstruction.[104–106] The key to this operation is adequate exposure, which can be obtained through a midline abdominal incision. In most instances, the entire ureter is damaged, and the intent of the procedure is the creation of a proximal ileopyelostomy and distal ileovesicostomy.

Preoperatively, the patient is administered a bowel preparation, including

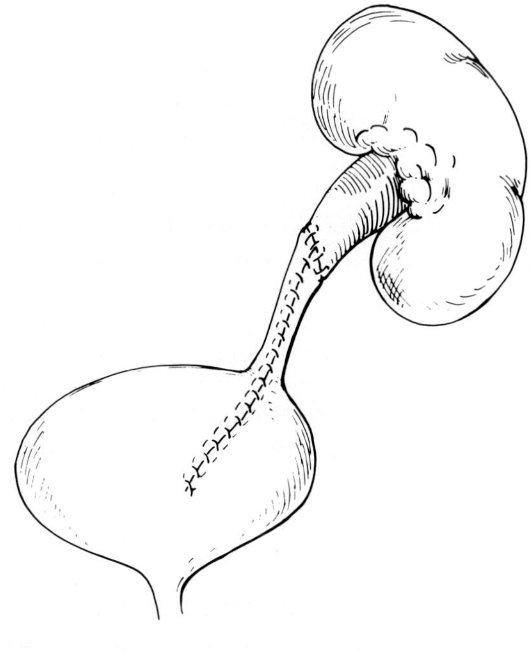

FIGURE 14–30. Anastomosis of ureter to bladder flap in a refluxing manner.

enema, cathartic, and antibiotics, as well as given a low-residue diet. Contraindications for creation of an ileal conduit is ileal disease, renal failure with creatinine greater than 2.0 to 2.2 mg/dl, neurogenic bladder dysfunction with inability to empty the bladder, and bladder outlet or distal obstruction. Typically, nonabsorbable antibiotics are administered preoperatively, and parental antibiotics are administered in the immediate preoperative and postoperative periods.

Many of these patients have impaired renal function, and the placement of bowel in close contact with urine can result in systemic acidosis. It is important also to note that if significant renal failure is observed preoperatively, this procedure is contraindicated. A long midline incision extending from the xiphoid process to the symphysis pubis affords the adequate exposure that is often necessary. This exposure is particularly important if bilateral procedures are being carried out. Performance of the procedure through an extended flank incision is useful for unilateral procedures, but generally the midline approach is preferred. After the peritoneal cavity is entered and inspected, an adequate length of ileum is identified, with the distal portion being approximately 20 cm above the ileocecal valve. The segment is isolated on its mesentery, and continuity of the intestine is restored appropriately. It is important to remember to close the mesentery adequately to avoid internal hernia formation. When choosing the bowel segment, only excessive length should be avoided. The bowel segment is placed retroperitoneally by passing it through an opening in the mesentery of the colon. This opening should be adequate to avoid compromising the blood supply to the isolated segment.

The proximal end of the ileum is then anastomosed to the exposed renal pelvis using 3–0 interrupted chromic catgut sutures. After the renal pelvis is opened widely on its anterior surface, the distal end of the ileum is anastomosed to the renal pelvis. Reinforcement sutures are often helpful. The ureter is generally left intact, and transection is not necessary. A wide anastomosis is usually obtainable, and stricture formation is uncommon. Care must be taken to ensure that the flow of urine is in an antegrade manner and that rotation of the ileal segment has not occurred. The distal portion of the ileal segment is sutured to the urinary bladder. Typically, the segment is placed on the dome or lateral segment of the bladder; therefore, it is important to fix the bladder to the psoas muscle with interrupted sutures of 1–0 chromic catgut (Fig. 14–31). Fixation will prevent movement of the bladder and also will allow for a reduction in the length of the bowel segment utilized. A generous opening is made in the bladder, and direct mucosal-to-mucosal anastomosis is performed with interrupted sutures of 4–0 chromic catgut or polyglycolic acid. Reinforcing sutures are added using 3–0 chromic catgut sutures. The use of a nipple to prevent reflux has been described, but this is generally unsuccessful in accomplishing this goal.[107, 108] Bowel is resected prior to the anastomosis with the bladder. Drains are left extraperitoneally and brought out through separate sites.

A major problem with this procedure is the absorption of filtered renal solids through the enteric mucosa. Postoperative monitoring is necessary to establish a baseline. The production of mucus from the enteric mucosa can be a problem; it is minimized through adequate fluid intake. Urinary mucus formation is also a cause of problems to patients; however, with time, experience indicates that mucus production declines.[109]

Autotransplantation

Autotransplantation can be useful in positioning the kidney to the renal pelvis by reestablishing the blood supply to the hypergastric vessel. The distal

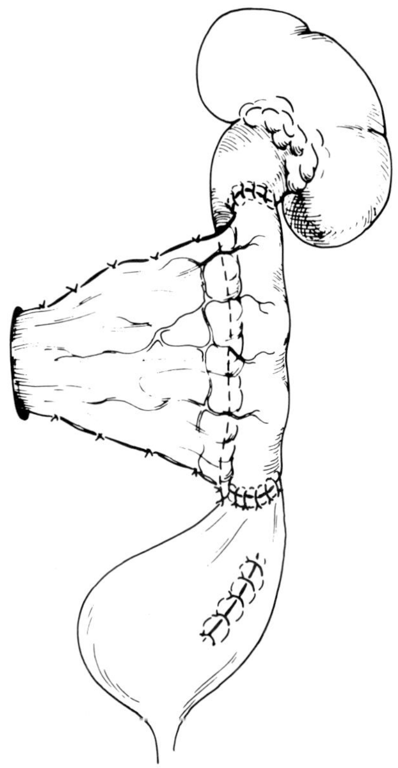

FIGURE 14–31. Typical appearance of an ileal ureter.

ureter or entire ureter can be replaced, if required, and the bladder can be anastomosed directly to the renal pelvis. This measure will allow adequate drainage of the kidney and passage of stone fragments in those patients who have intractable stone formation. The advantages of the procedure are multiple. There is no absorption of urinary solutes, as in the ileal ureter, nor is there any production of mucus. If desired, an antirefluxing anastomosis can be created using any of the standard techniques available. If the entire ureter requires replacement, a vesicopyelostomy can be created, as noted. Though experience is limited, long-term follow-up indicates that little damage to the kidney occurs because of reflux alone.[109, 110]

The procedure is contraindicated in patients with significant inflammation surrounding the renal pelvis, particularly the hilum. Preoperatively, arteriography should be performed to determine the number and location of renal arties and the extent of arteriosclerotic changes in the pelvis. Obviously, the surgeon performing such a procedure should be well versed in vascular and surgical techniques and should also have significant experience with homotransplantation. The procedure is performed similarly to those described for homotransplantation.

REFERENCES

1. Hippocrates, quoted by Murphy LJT: The History of Urology. Springfield IL, Charles C Thomas, 1972, p 22.
2. Murphy LJT: The History of Urology. Springfield IL, Charles C Thomas, 1972, p 191.
3. Ballenger EG, Frontz WA, Hamer HG, Lewis B: American Urological Association: History of Urology, Baltimore, The Williams and Wilkins Company, 1933, p 279.

4. Barker AE: A means of diagnosing renal calculi. Lancet 1:621, 1880.
5. Dickenson WH: On Renal and Urinary Affections. Vol III. London, Longmans and Green, 1885.
6. MacIntyre J: Rankin rays: Photography of renal calculus. Lancet 2:18, 1896.
7. Albarran J: Radiographie des calculs du rein. A Farnc d'Urol 4:569, 1899.
8. Abbe R: Observation on the detection of small renal calculi by Rankin rays. Ann Surg 30:178, 1899.
9. Von Illyes G: Ureterkatheterismus und radiographie. Deutsch Z Chir 62:132, 1902.
10. Voelcker F, von Lichtenberg A: Pyelographie (röntgenographie des Nierenbeckens nach kollargolfulleng). Munch Med Wochenschr 53:05, 1906.
11. Robson AWM: A method of exposing and operating on the kidney without division of muscles, vessels or nerves. Lancet 1:1315, 1898.
12. Braasch WF, Carmen RD: Renal fluoroscopy at the operating table. JAMA 73:1751, 1919.
13. Braasch WF, Carmen RD: Renal fluoroscopy at the operating table. Radiology 2:222, 1924.
14. Quinby WC: A note on the localization of renal calculi by the aid of x-ray films made during operation. J Urol 13:59, 1925.
15. Southerland CG: Renal roentgenoscopy at the operating table. J Urol 33:1, 1935.
16. Southerland CG: Roentgenoscopy and roentography of the kidney at the operating table. Surg Clin North Am 19:1041, 1939.
17. Hanley HG: Flexible renal grid-sling for localizing stones during lithotomy. Lancet 1:661, 1967.
18. Boyce WH: The localization of renal calculi during surgery. J Urol 118:152, 1977.
19. Cook JH III, Lytton B: Intraoperative localization of renal calculi during nephrolithotomy by ultrasound scanning. J Urol 117:543, 1977.
20. Berte M, Resnick MI: Intraoperative imaging of renal calculi in renal calculus surgery. Urol Radiol 6:144, 1984.
21. Drach GW: Perioperative aspects of renal stone surgery. Urol Clin North Am 1:299, 1974.
22. Pitts GW, Resnick MI: Urinary stone formation: Patient evaluation and management. Urol Clin North Am 7:45, 1980.
23. Resnick MI, Kursh ED, Cohen AM: Computerized tomography in delineation of uric acid calculi. J Urol 131:9, 1984.
24. Bodner H, Briskin H: Subdiaphragmatic renal exposure by resection of the eleventh rib. Urol Cutan Rev 54:272, 1950.
25. Kropp KA: Surgical approaches to renal and ureteral calculi. Urol Clin North Am 10:617, 1983.
26. Gil-Vernet JM: Pyelolithotomy. *In* Roth RA, Finlayson B (eds): Stones: Clinical Management of Urolithiasis. Baltimore, The Williams and Wilkins Company, 1983, pp 297–331.
27. Bensimon G, Bresette JF, Maxted WC, et al: Misconceptions about posterior approach for renoureteral surgery. Urology 19:462, 1982.
28. Novick AC: Posterior surgical approach to the kidney and ureter. J Urol 124:192, 1980.
29. Pansadoro V: The posterior lumbotomy. Urol Clin North Am 10:573, 1983.
30. Gil-Vernet JM: New surgical concepts in removing renal calculi. Urol Int 20:255, 1965.
31. Dees JE: The use of an intrapelvic coagulum in pyelolithotomy: Preliminary report. South Med J 49:503, 1943.
32. Patel JJ: The coagulum pyelolithotomy. Br J Surg 60:230, 1973.
33. Broecker BH, Hackler RH: Simplified coagulum pyelolithotomy using cryoprecipitate. Urology 14:143, 1979.
34. Burns JR, Finlayson B: Coagulum pyelolithotomy. *In* Resnick MI (ed): Current Trends in Urology. Baltimore, The Williams and Wilkins Company, 1982, pp 31–44.
35. Fischer CP, Sonda CP III, Diokno AC: Use of cryoprecipitate coagulum in extracting renal calculi. Urology 15:6, 1980.
36. Kalash SS, Young JD, Harne G: Modification of cryoprecipitate coagulum pyelolithotomy technique. Urology 19:467, 1982.
37. Marshall S, Lyon RP, Scott MP Jr: Further simplifications for coagulum pyelolithotomy. J Urol 119:588, 1978.
38. Roth RA: Surgery of renal calculi. Semin Urol 2:45, 1984.
39. Sherer JF: Cryoprecipitate coagulum pyelolithotomy. J Urol 123:621, 1980.
40. Marshall S: Coagulum pyelolithotomy. Urol Clin North Am 10:659, 1983.
41. Burns JR, Finlayson B: Coagulum pyelolithotomy: Tensile strength of coagula as a function of variables. Urology 19:381, 1982.
42. Pence Jr II, Airhart RA, Novicki DE, et al: Pulmonary emboli associated with coagulum pyelolithotomy. J Urol 127:572, 1982.
43. Blandy JP, Singh M: The case for a more aggressive approach to staghorn stones. J Urol 115:505, 1976.
44. Singh M, Chapman R, Tresidder GC, et al: The fate of the unoperated staghorn calculus. Br J Urol 45:581, 1973.
45. Hrtyl J: Handbuch der topographischen Anatomie. Vol 1. Vienna, Braumuller, 1882.
46. Brödel M: The intrinsic blood vessels of the kidney and their significance in nephrotomy. Bull Johns Hopkins Hosp 12:10, 1901.
47. Myers RP: Brödel's line. Surg Gynecol Obstet 132:424, 1971.

48. Kelly HA, Burnam CF: Diseases of the kidneys, ureters and bladder. New York, D Appleton, 1914.
49. Boyce WH, Russell JM, Webb R: Management of the papillae during intrarenal surgery. Trans Am Assoc Genito-Urin Surg 71:76, 1979.
50. Wickham JEA, Coe N, Ward JP: One hundred cases of nephrolithotomy under hypothermia. J Urol 112:702, 1974.
51. Marberger M, Eisenberger F: Regional hypothermia of the kidney: Surface or transarterial perfusion cooling? A functional study. J Urol 124:179, 1980.
52. Wickham JEA, Hanley HG, Joekes AM: Regional renal hypothermia. Br J Urol 39:727, 1967.
53. Stubbs AJ, Resnick MI, Boyce WH: Anatrophic nephrolithotomy in the solitary kidney. J Urol 119:457, 1978.
54. Wickham JEA: The surgical treatment of renal lithiasis. *In* Wickham JEA (ed): Urinary Calculous Disease. Edinburgh, Churchill-Livingstone, 1979, pp 145–198.
55. Boyce WH: The localization of intrarenal calculi during surgery. J Urol 118:152, 1977.
56. Harrison LH, Whitehurst AW, Boyce WH: Adjunct antimicrobial therapy with renal calculus surgery. J Urol 118:233, 1977.
57. Graves FT: The anatomy of the intrarenal arteries and its application to segmental resection of the kidney. Br J Surg 42:132, 1954.
58. Wickham JEA, Hanley HG, Joekes AM: Regional renal hypothermia. Br J Urol 39:727, 1967.
59. Resnick MI: Surgery of renal calculi. AUA Update Series 2:29, 1983.
60. Wickham JEA: Paravascular multiple nephrotomy. *In* Roth RA, Finlayson B (eds): Stones: Clinical Management of Urolithiasis. Baltimore, The Williams and Wilkins Company, 1983, pp 333–347.
61. Coleman CH, Witherington R: A review of 117 partial nephrectomies. J Urol 122:11, 1979.
62. Kim SK: New techniques of partial nephrectomy. J Urol 102:165, 1969.
63. Redman JF: Partial nephrectomy. Urol Clin North Am 10:677, 1983.
64. Stewart HH: Partial nephrectomy in the treatment of renal calculi. Ann R Coll Surg 11:32, 1952.
65. Stewart HH: The surgery of the kidney in the treatment of renal stones. Br J Urol 32:392, 1060.
66. Papathanassadis W, Swinney J: Results of partial nephrectomy compared with pyelolithotomy and nephrolithotomy. Br J Urol 38:403, 1966.
67. Puigvert A: Partial nephrectomy for renal lithiasis: Experience with 208 cases. Int Surg 46:555, 1966.
68. Williams RE: Long term survey of 538 patients with upper tract stones. Br J Urol 35:416, 1963.
69. Myrvold H, Fritjofsson JA: Late results of partial nephrectomy for renal lithiasis. Scand J Urol Nephrol 5:57, 1971.
70. Rose MB, Fellows OJ: Partial nephrectomy for stone disease. Br J Urol 49:605, 1977.
71. Marshall VR, Singh M, Tresidder GC, et al: The place of partial nephrectomy in the management of renal calyceal calculi. Br J Urol 47:759, 1975.
72. Goldstein AE, Abeshouse BS: Partial resections of the kidney: A report of 6 cases and a review of the literature. J Urol 38:15, 1937.
73. Semb C: Partial resection of the kidney: Operative technique. Acta Chir Scand 109:360, 1955.
74. Wein AJ, Carpiniello VL, Murphy J: A simple technique for partial nephrectomy. Surg Gynecol Obstet 146:621, 1978.
75. Poutasse EF: Partial nephrectomy: New techniques, approach, operative indication and review of 51 cases. J Urol 88:153, 1962.
76. Williams DF, Schapiro AE, Arconti JS, et al: A new technique of partial nephrectomy. J Urol 97:955, 1967.
77. Stubbs AJ, Resnick MI, Boyce WH: Anatrophic nephrolithotomy in the solitary kidney. J Urol 119:457, 1978.
78. Witherow R, Wickham JE: Nephrolithotomy in chronic renal failure: Saved from dialysis! Br J Urol 52:419, 1980.
79. Russell JM, Webb RT, Harrison LH: Long term follow-up of 100 anatrophic nephrolithotomies. *In* Brockis JG, Finlayson B (eds): Urinary Calculus. Littleton, MA, PSG Publishing Company, 1981, p 405.
80. Segura JW, Erickson SB, Wilson DW, et al: Infected renal lithiasis: Results of long-term surgical and medical management. *In* Smith LH, Robertson WG, Finlayson B (eds): Urolithiasis: Clinical and Basic Research. New York, Plenum Press, 1981, p 195.
81. Sant GR, Blaivas JG, Meares EM Jr: Hemiacidrin irrigation in the management of struvite calculi: Long term results. J Urol 130:1048, 1983.
82. Sleith MW, Wickham JEA: Long term follow-up of 100 cases of renal calculi. Br J Urol 49:601, 1977.
83. Boyce WH, Harrison LH: Complications of renal stone surgery. *In* Smith RM, Skinner DG (eds): Complications of Urologic Surgery: Prevention and Management. Philadelphia, WB Saunders Company, 1976, pp 87–105.
84. Birch AA, Mims GR: Anesthesia considerations during nephrolithotomy with slush. J Urol 113:433, 1975.
85. Boyce WH: Surgery of urinary calculi in perspective. Urol Clin North Am 10:585, 1983.

86. Boyce WH, Elkins IB: Reconstructive renal surgery following anatrophic nephrolithotomy: Follow-up of 100 consecutive patients. J Urol 111:307, 1974.
87. Boyce WH, Stubbs AJ, Resnick MI: Intrarenal nephrolithotomy and reconstruction of the solitary kidney. Trans Am Assoc Genito-Urin Surg 69:118, 1978.
88. Stubbs AJ, Resnick MI, Boyce WH: Anatrophic nephrolithotomy in the solitary kidney. J Urol 119:457, 1978.
89. Resnick MI, Kursh ED: Dissolution of uric acid calculi with systemic alkalinization. J Urol 132:329, 1984.
90. Higgins CC: Factors in recurrence of renal calculi. JAMA 113:1460, 1939.
91. Throck GW: Transurethral ureteral stone manipulation. Urol Clin North Am 10:709, 1983.
92. Fox M, Pyrah LN, Raper FP: Management of ureteric stone: Review of 292 cases. Br J Urol 37:660, 1965.
93. Carstensen HE, Hansen TS: Stones in the ureter. Acta Chir Scand [Suppl] 433:66, 1973.
94. Uenoa Kawamura T, Ogawa A, Takaysu H: Relation of spontaneous passage of ureteral calculi. Urology 10:544, 1977.
95. Bistol JB, Smith PJB: Transperitoneal ureterolithotomy for stones in the lower third of the ureter. Br J Urol 54:220, 1982.
96. Bose TK, Shaw RE: Transperitoneal ureterolithotomy. Br J Urol 47:613, 1975.
97. Persky L, Hoch W, Kursh ED: Surgical management of the ureter. *In* Harrison JH, Gittes RF, Perlmutter AD (eds): Campbell's Urology. 4th ed. Philadelphia, WB Saunders Company, 1979.
98. Persky L: Splinting versus non-splinting in ureteral surgery. *In* Bergman J (ed): The Ureters. New York, Harper and Row, 1967.
99. Androulakakis P, Deliveliotis A: Ureteric stone formed upon polyester suture: Case report. Int Surg 67:83, 1982.
100. Altebarmakian VK, Caldamone AA, Davis RS, et al: Stricture of ureter caused by stone basket manipulation. Urology 19:13, 1982.
101. Williams JL, Porter RW: The Boari bladder flap in lower ureteric injuries. Br J Urol 38:528, 1966.
102. Turner-Warwick R, Worth PHL: The psoas bladder-hitch procedure for the replacement of the lower third of the ureter. Br J Urol 41:701, 1969.
103. Goodwin WE, Winter CC, Turner RD: Replacement of the ureter by small intestine: Clinical application and results of the "ileal ureter." J Urol 81:406, 1959.
104. Goodwin WE, Cockett ATK: Surgical treatment of multiple recurrent branched renal "staghorn" calculi by pyelo-nephro-ileo-vesical anastomosis. J Urol 85:214, 1961.
105. Skinner DG, Goodwin WE: Indications for the use of intestinal segments in the management of nephrocalcinosis. J Urol 113:436, 1975.
106. Tveter KJ, Goodwin WE: The use of ileum as substitute for the ureter. *In* Resnick MI (ed): Current Trends in Urology. Vol 2. Baltimore, The Williams and Wilkins Company, 1981, p 1.
107. Tscholl R, Tettamatt IF, Sing GE: Ileal substitute of ureter with refluxplasty by terminal intussusception of bowel. Urology 9:385, 1987.
108. Turner RD, Goodwin WE: Experiments with intussuscepted ileal valve and ureteral substitution. J Urol 81:526, 1959.
109. Olson CA: Ileal ureter and renal autotransplantation. Urol Clin North Am 10:685, 1983.
110. Olson CA, Idelston B: Renal autotransplantation for recurrent renal colic. J Urol 123:467, 1980.

15 Ureteroscopy

J. Patrick Spirnak
Martin I. Resnick

HISTORICAL ASPECTS

The development of the modern ureteroscope is integrally related to many of the technologic advances in endoscopy and particularly cystoscopy that have occurred over the past 180 years. The concept of viewing the interior of the urinary bladder was attractive to many early clinicians and was first attempted by Bozzini in 1806.[1, 2] He utilized a candle and a silver mirrored tube, but because of poor distal illumination, the instrument never gained wide acceptance. Over the ensuing years, others, including Segalas (1826), Fischer (1827), Desormeaux (1853), and Cruise (1865), also developed endoscopes, but it was the instrument of Nitze (1877) that provided excellent illumination and direct vision. Refinements in both the instrumentation and the light delivery systems continued over the remainder of the nineteenth century and into the twentieth century.

The development of fiberoptic transmission of light resulted from the work of many investigators—most notably Hopkins, Curtiss, and Van Heel.[3–8] Hopkins made additional contributions, including the development of the rigid rod lens system, which provided for enhanced light transmission and subsequent visualization through rigid endoscopes. Directly associated with the refinement in fiberoptic technology was the development of flexible instruments, initially used in gastroscopy and later adapted to other forms of endoscopy, including cystoscopy and ureteroscopy. The proximal and distal spatial arrangement of the optical fibers allowed for the transmission of excellent images of the mucosal lining of viscous structures.

Young is credited with performing the first rigid ureteroscopic examination in 1929, when he passed a rigid cystoscope into the dilated ureter of a patient with valves.[9] In 1962, McGovern and Walzak performed the first flexible ureteroscopy when they passed a 9F flexible fiberscope 9 cm up a dilated ureter and visualized a stone.[10] Although these two early reports described successful ureteroscopy, both were performed in patients with dilated ureters, which facilitated passage of the instruments. It was not until the late 1970s, when Goodman[11] and Lyon[12] reported successful techniques to dilate the distal ureter, that routine endoscopic evaluation of the ureter became practical.

Early ureteroscopic examinations performed by Lyon in female patients utilized 11F pediatric cystoscopes, while 13F juvenile cystoscopes were used in male patients.[13] Owing to the shortness of these instruments, only the distal 3 to 4 cm of the ureter were visualized. In 1980, Perez-Castro[14] reported the successful visualization of the renal pelvis with a specially designed 40-cm-long rigid ureteropyeloscope passed transurethrally. In 1981, Das[15] reported the first successful ureteral stone manipulation performed under direct vision. Today, rigid ureteropyeloscopy has become an invaluable urologic procedure useful in diagnosing and treating a variety of ureteral and renal pelvic abnormalities.[16]

The early use of flexible instruments was restricted to diagnostic studies. Because of limitations in instrument design, irrigation or transurethral manipulation could not be performed. These limitations were recognized, and technologic improvement was attempted. Imaging and photography of the renal pelvis via a 2.7-mm flexible fiberoptic endoscope passed intraoperatively via a ureterotomy were performed by Takagi and associates in 1966, and Bush and associates reported their experience with flexible instruments passed under cystoscopic control in 1970. These latter workers utilized induced diuresis as a means of irrigation and passed instruments besides the ureteroscope to perform manipulations under direct vision.[17–19] Further development continues in an attempt to provide a small-caliber instrument with satisfactory visualization that allows for irrigation, visual manipulation, and a flexible tip. The ideal instrument has yet to be developed; however, remarkable progress has been made over the past 2 to 3 years.

INSTRUMENTATION

The initial reports of successful ureteroscopy utilized existing cystoscopic equipment.[12, 13] However, the preexisting equipment was not ideally suited for use in the ureter, and once ureteroscopy was recognized as a potentially useful diagnostic and therapeutic procedure, major manufacturers of endoscopic equipment (Wolf, Rosemont, IL; ACMI, Stamford, CT; Storz, Tuttlingen, W. Germany, US distributor—Culver City, CA) developed instruments designed specifically for use in the ureter. Rigid ureteroscopes are typically 40 to 45 cm in length and vary in size from 10F to 14F.[20] (See reference 20 for additional and more detailed information regarding the available rigid ureteroscopes.) Controversy exists over the actual size of these instruments, as they are not perfectly round, and the actual size is probably larger than that stated by the manufacturer. The smaller-sized instruments are best suited for diagnostic procedures, as the smaller sheaths will accommodate only the telescope. The rigid instruments best suited for stone manipulation are 11.5F to 14.0F in size and have at least a 5F working port.

The initial rigid ureteroscopes utilized rod-lens optics, which afforded the endoscopist vision equal to that of the best cystoscope. First-generation instruments were constructed similarly to cystoscopes and utilized interchangeable lenses (0 degrees and 70 degrees) placed directly down the center of the sheath (Fig. 15–1). These early instruments had a 5F working channel, which allowed stone baskets and forceps to be used under direct vision. Although an ultrasonic probe was available, it could be passed only through the center of the sheath with the telescope removed (Fig. 15–2*A* and *B*). Thus, to perform stone fragmentation, the stone had to be basketed, and the telescope had to be

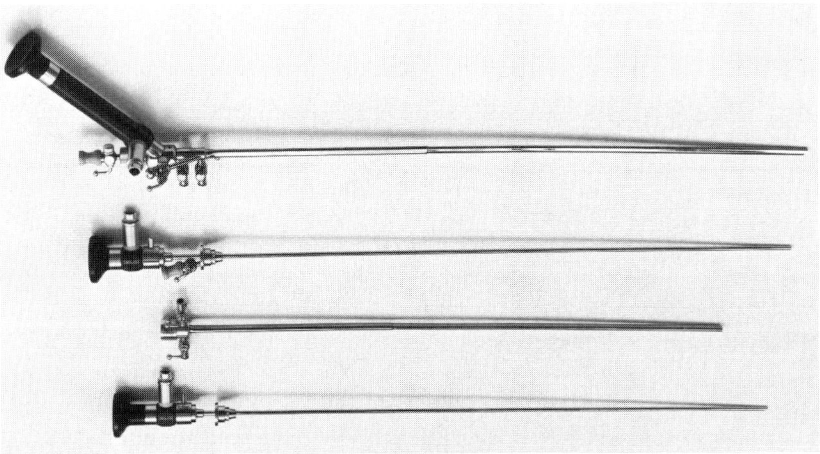

FIGURE 15–1. First- and second-generation rigid ureteroscopes (Storz). Second-generation instrument (offset lens) allowed ultrasonic stone disintegration under direct vision. First-generation instrument utilized an interchangeable lens system (0 degrees and 70 degrees).

removed and replaced with the ultrasonic probe. Stone fragmentation proceeded under fluoroscopic guidance and was often traumatic as well as unsuccessful.

Second-generation instruments were designed with the eyepiece offset either 30 or 90 degrees. The lens was an integral part of the instrument and could not be removed (Fig. 15–3*A*). These instruments had two working ports that allowed the simultaneous placement of a stone basket and ultrasound probe (Fig. 15–3*B*). Thus, stone fragmentation could be performed under direct vision.

Recently, shorter instruments (33 cm) that facilitate use in the distal ureter and midureter have become available.[21] Although rigid instruments are somewhat

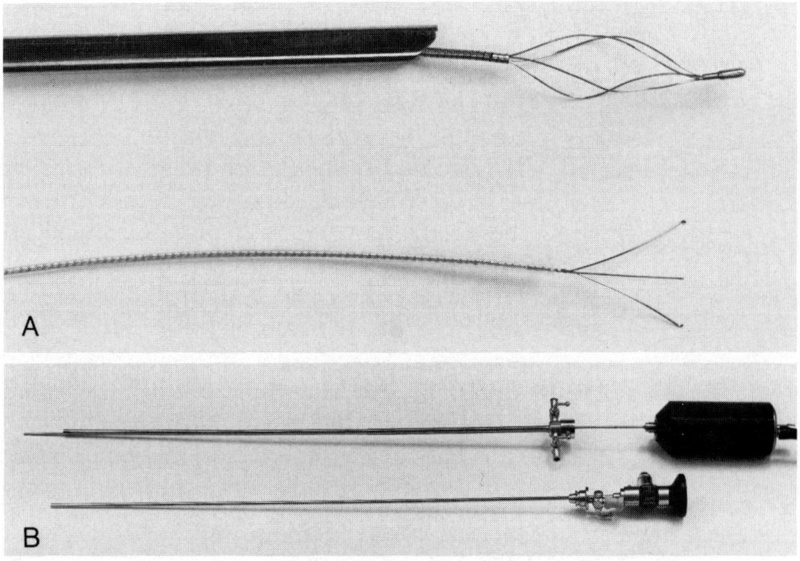

FIGURE 15–2. *A*, First-generation ureteroscope allowed stone grasping and basketing to proceed under direct vision. *B*, Ultrasonic stone fragmentation required removal of the lens and replacement with the ultrasound probe.

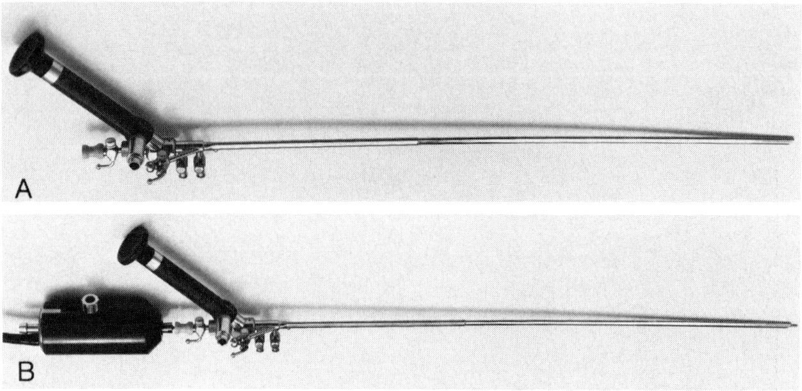

FIGURE 15–3. *A*, Second-generation Storz ureteroscope with fixed offset lens system and two working ports, which allowed simultaneous placement of a stone basket and ultrasound probe. *B*, Sonotrode passed through central working port. Stone fragmentation proceeded under direct vision.

flexible and can accommodate mild curvatures, the field of vision becomes distorted as the instrument bends. Recently, more flexible semirigid instruments have become available and can accommodate greater degrees of curvature without compromising the visual field. In 1988, the Candela Corporation (Wayland MA) introduced a 7.2F semirigid ureteroscope. This instrument differs from other rigid instruments in that it utilizes fiberoptics rather than the Hopkins rigid rod-type lens system. Its semirigid construction allows up to 2 inches of passive flexion at the distal end, while preserving a sharp, clear image without compromising the visual field. Separate operating channels (0.025 inch) allow for simultaneous passage of a laser fiber while maintaining maximal irrigation. The small 7.2F diameter virtually eliminates the need for ureteral dilation. Storz has recently introduced a similar, although larger (9.5F), semirigid ureteroscope with a 3F working channel.

Flexible instruments (6.5F to 14.4F) using fiberoptic imaging are also available.[22] A distinct advantage of these instruments is the ability to negotiate curves and kinks in the ureter, which might not be possible with rigid instruments. Distinct disadvantages include inferior optics, small irrigating channel, and small size of the working channel. The smaller instruments (6.5F to 10F) are usually passed over a guidewire placed through the working port of a large cystoscope and are nondeflecting (Fig. 15–4*A*). Although these instruments are probably best suited for diagnostic purposes, small 3F electrohydraulic probes and laser probes less than 1F in diameter are currently available and may be used to fragment calculi. A variety of small 3F stone baskets and forceps are also available (Fig. 15–4*B*). Although the larger (9.5F to 14.4F) instruments may be actively deflected and have larger irrigating and working channels, they are more difficult to pass up the ureter and require ureteral dilation, thus offering no distinct advantage over the rigid ureteroscopes in the management of ureteral stones. With continued advances in instrument design, it is anticipated that one day a small (6F to 7F), actively deflectable ureteroscope will become available.

INDICATIONS

It has been estimated that more than 80 per cent of all ureteral stones pass spontaneously.[23] Sandegard[24] has noted that a small (<4 mm) stone located in

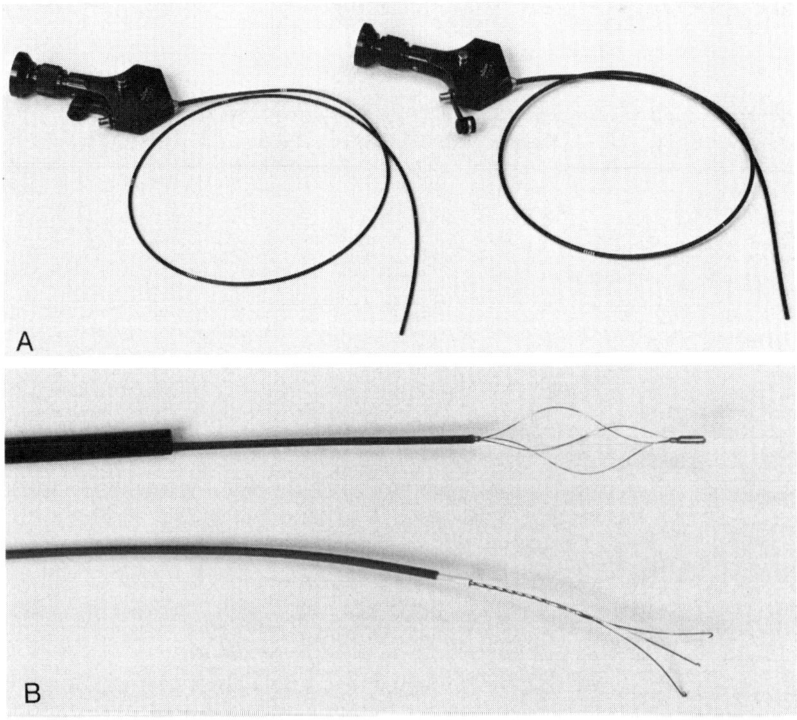

FIGURE 15–4. *A*, Number 7F and 9F passive flexible ureteroscopes (Reichert). *B*, A variety of small instruments are available for use with the 9F instrument.

the distal ureter has a 93 per cent chance of spontaneous passage when observed for 6 weeks from the onset of symptoms. A similar stone in the proximal ureter has only an 81 per cent chance of passage. Stones between 4 and 6 mm in their largest diameter have a 50 per cent chance of passage from either the proximal or the distal ureter. The vast majority of stones greater than 6 mm in size are likely to require surgical intervention. Similar findings were reported by Ueno and associates.[25] They noted that a 5-mm stone had a 55 per cent rate of passage when followed for 1 year, a 6-mm stone had a 35 per cent chance of passage, and a 7-mm stone had only a 25 per cent likelihood of spontaneous passage. No ureteral stone greater than 8 mm passed without surgical intervention. Although stone size by itself is never an absolute indication for immediate surgical intervention, from the above two studies, it is clear that calculi greater than 6 mm in their smallest diameter are unlikely to pass. Patients with recurrent ureteral colic, who have passed stones in the past, are more likely to pass stones of larger diameter and may be given a trial of observation regardless of stone size, provided no other indications for intervention exist.

The indications for ureteroscopic stone removal are similar to those for either attempted stone basketing or ureterolithotomy and include the following: severe ureteral obstruction, uncontrollable pain, urosepsis, persistent gross hematuria, lack of stone progression, and the occupation of the patient.[26]

Stones located throughout the ureter are accessible to the ureteroscope (Fig. 15–5). However, results show a poorer retrieval rate and higher incidence of complications when ureteroscopy is performed for proximal ureteral calculi.[27–29] Extracorporeal shock wave lithotripsy (ESWL) has also proved effective in treating proximal ureteral calculi without the potential morbidity associated with ureter-

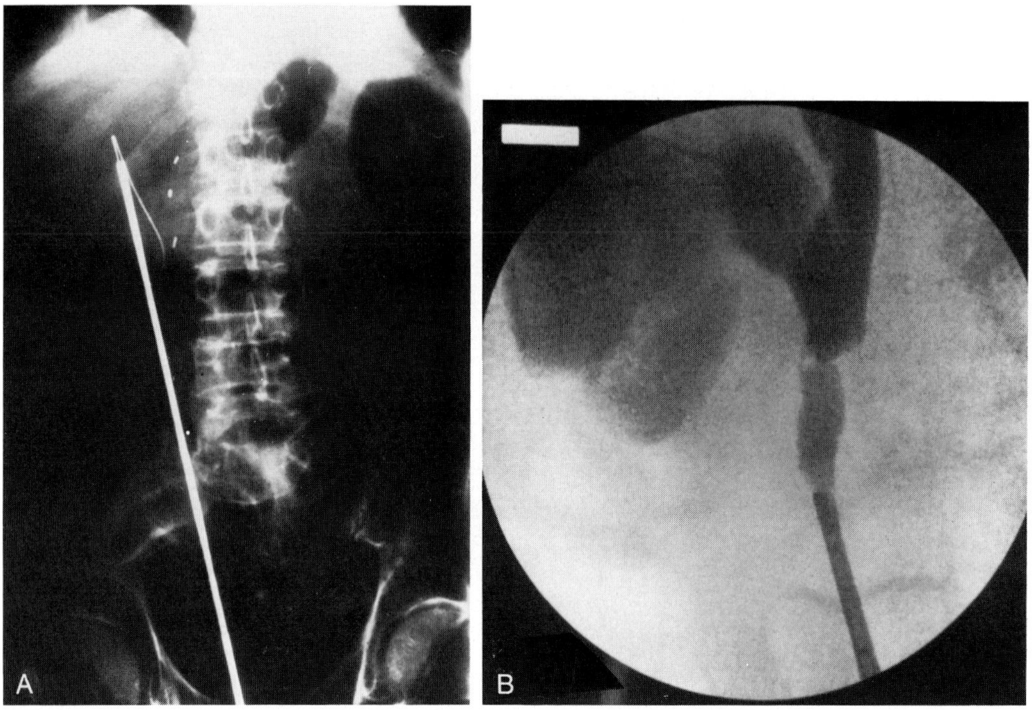

FIGURE 15–5. *A*, Rigid 11.5F ureteroscope positioned in the renal pelvis. *B*, Impacted proximal ureteral stone refractory to in situ ESWL and unable to be repositioned back into the pelvis is successfully managed using the rigid ureteroscope.

oscopy. Ureteroscopy is therefore reserved for those patients in whom primary ESWL has failed. Midureteral stones may be managed by either ESWL or ureteroscopy. However, many stones located over the sacroiliac joint are refractory to shock wave therapy and are best managed by ureteroscopy. Distal ureteral calculi are much more accessible to the ureteroscope, and when surgical intervention is indicated, ureteroscopy is the preferred treatment.

Stone composition is considered important only in identifying those patients with uric acid calculi, as dissolution remains the primary method of management. Surgical intervention is reserved for those unusual instances in which chemolysis has failed.

There are no absolute contraindications to attempted ureteroscopic stone manipulation; however, patients with anatomic abnormalities of the lower extremities that do not allow for placement in the lithotomy position are poor candidates for this procedure. Significant intravesical prostatic hypertrophy or severe urethral abnormalities make successful passage of the ureteroscope unlikely. Patients who have undergone prior pelvic surgery or who have received pelvic irradiation are more likely to have fixation of the ureter to the pelvic wall, thus making it difficult or impossible to straighten the ureter sufficiently for passage of the rigid ureteroscope. Urinary tract infections are treated with culture-specific antibiotics prior to attempting ureteroscopic stone manipulation. Prophylactic antibiotics are routinely used.

TECHNIQUE

Ureteroscopy is usually performed with the patient under general anesthesia. Although spinal or epidural anesthesia provides adequate analgesia and pelvic muscle relaxation, it does not allow for complete control of respiratory movement. A sudden cough or deep, unexpected inspiration may result in ureteral perforation.

The patient is placed in a modified dorsal lithotomy position with the leg opposite the involved ureter abducted while the ipsilateral leg is adducted. Perez-Castro has found lowering the contralateral leg further facilitates ureteral dilation and instrument passage.[30] Smith, on the other hand, has found that elevating the contralateral leg while keeping the ipsilateral leg down will decrease the vertical angle of entry of the ureteroscope into the ureter and decrease the incidence of iatrogenic injury[31] (Fig. 15–6). An endoscopy table equipped with a fixed fluoroscopy unit, or one that allows the use of a portable C-arm fluoroscope, is routinely used. Fluoroscopy is considered essential to help monitor ureteral dilation and facilitate passage of the ureteroscope.

Cystoscopy is performed with a large (23F to 25F) cystoscope. If the ureter has not been well visualized on preoperative studies, a retrograde pyelogram is obtained to define the course and configuration of the ureter distal to the stone. A minimal amount of contrast (3 to 5 ml) is injected under gentle pressure through a soft angled end-hole ureteral catheter. Successful stone removal depends on the surgeon's ability to achieve and maintain ureteral access. Multiple manipulations of the orifice enhance the likelihood of the procedure's ending in ureteral trauma; therefore, the angled end-hole catheter is used. It allows for both diagnostic studies and guidewire placement without removal of the catheter from the orifice, thus minimizing the chance of trauma to the ureteral orifice. It is also used at the end of the procedure to provide short-term drainage following atraumatic procedures. After the retrograde pyelogram, a 0.035- or 0.038-inch 140-cm-long floppy tip guidewire (Bentson) is advanced through the ureteral catheter and fluoroscopically positioned above the stone. The purpose of the

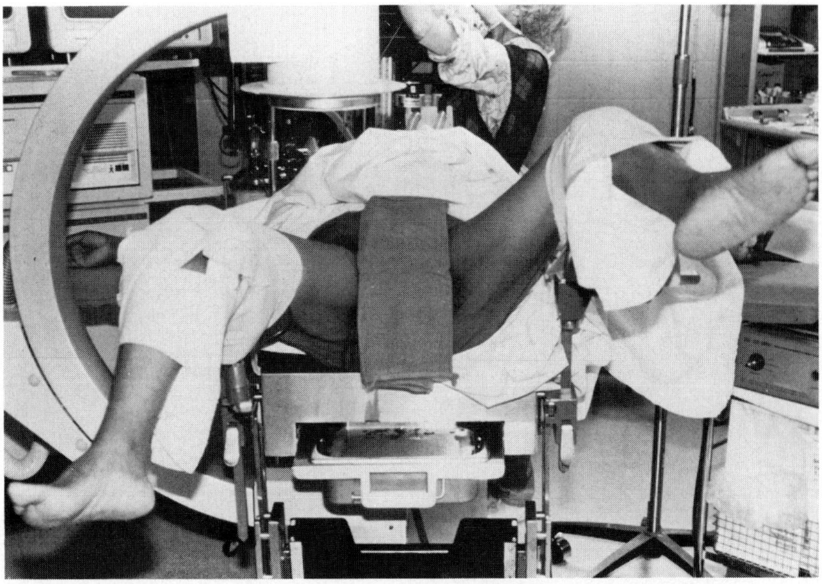

FIGURE 15–6. Favored position for right-sided ureteroscopy. The patient is in a modified lithotomy position with the ipsilateral leg adducted while the opposite leg is abducted. Elevating the contralateral leg while keeping the ipsilateral leg lowered facilitates passage of the rigid ureteroscope. Note the presence of the C-arm, a prerequisite for successful ureteroscopy.

guidewire is to facilitate ureteral dilation and passage of the ureteroscope. Once the guidewire has been positioned above the stone, it is left as a safety wire until the procedure has been successfully completed and the final ureteral catheter has been positioned. If the guidewire will not pass beyond the stone, the ureteral catheter is advanced to the stone, and while gently pushing and twisting the catheter, the guidewire is advanced (Fig. 15–7). Generally, if contrast will pass beyond the obstruction, so too will the guidewire.

The performance of successful ureteroscopy depends on adequate dilation of the ureteral orifice and intramural ureter. A number of different ureteral dilators, each requiring a slightly different technique, are currently available. Each technique has its own advantages and disadvantages,[32] and each endoscopist has his or her own preference. It is recommended that several types of dilators be available, as clinical circumstances will arise that favor one type of dilator over another. Advantages and disadvantages of each system have been reviewed by Eshghi.[32]

Ureteral dilation is performed over the guidewire under fluoroscopic guid-

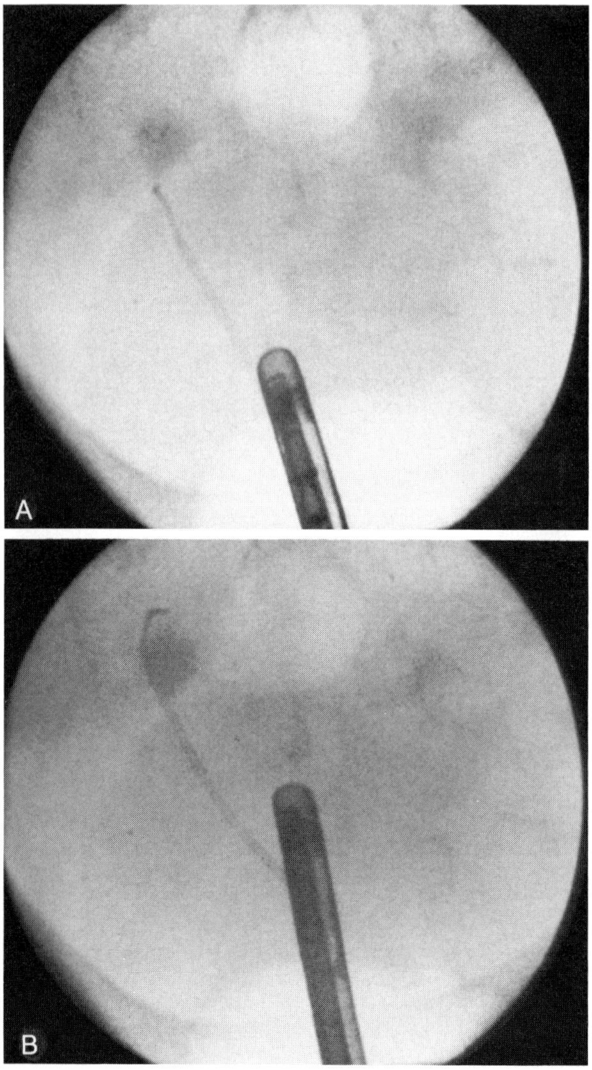

FIGURE 15–7. *A*, Floppy tip 0.035-inch guidewire (Bentson) is advanced through the angled end-hole catheter to the level of the stone. *B*, Advancement of the ureteral catheter to the level of the stone and continued gentle manipulation of the guidewire allow even impacted calculi to be bypassed and the wire to be safely positioned in the renal pelvis.

ance. The ureteral orifice and intramural ureter are tightly fixed to the bladder wall and, under normal circumstances, are quite indistensible—therefore the need for dilation. The ureter above the bladder wall readily distends with irrigation fluid and usually does not require manual dilation to allow successful passage of the ureteroscope. Olive tip metal bougies, angiographic-type balloon catheters, long fascial dilators, and the Finlayson[33, 34] ureteral access system all may be passed over a guidewire (Fig. 15–8).

Routine nonguided ureteral dilation performed without a guidewire is not recommended. However, the presence of an impacted ureteral calculus in the intramural ureter may require nonguided ureteral dilation. Under such circumstances, dilation is performed with sequential metal bougies or Braasch bulb catheters. In selected cases in which acute ureteral dilation is anticipated as being difficult owing to anatomic abnormalities of the prostate or ureter, or in patients with urosepsis due to ureteral obstruction, indwelling ureteral stents placed prior to ureteroscopy will, in many cases, dilate the ureter sufficiently to allow atraumatic passage of the ureteroscope without the added trauma of further ureteral dilation.[35] The use of continuous irrigation under pressure has also been described as an atraumatic alternative method of dilating the ureter.[30, 36]

Mechanical dilation of the ureter to facilitate stone removal is not a new concept. Bransford Lewis,[37] in 1904, described a two-blade ureteral dilator that he used to facilitate stone passage. In 1913, Buerger was the first to report using olive-tip bougies to dilate the ureter actively to 20F.[38] Illievitz,[39] in 1925, reported successful dilation of the distal ureter to 16F without complications. Several years later, Ravitch[40] balloon dilated the distal ureter to 18F. Dourmashkin[41] reported successful ureteral dilation to 54F without complication. Green[42] dilated canine ureters to 9F to 11F (comparable to 16F to 18F in humans) and noted temporary hypotonicity and diminished peristalsis. Wide dilation to 14F to 16F resulted in temporary ureteral hypertonicity, which acted as a functional obstruction and produced acute pyelectasis and ureterectasis. On the basis of these early reports, it would appear that the ureter may be acutely dilated to facilitate passage of the ureteroscope without significant risk of long-term complications. In an attempt to define the maximal extent of acute dilation a human ureter can safely tolerate, Finlayson and associates, in 1987, studied 43 human pelvic ureters and successfully dilated all to an average of 21.2F (range of 16F to 30F) without significant immediate trauma.[43] Similarly, Clayman showed no long-term histologic changes in pig ureters dilated acutely to 24F.[44] On the basis of the above clinical and experimental investigations, it would appear that the normal ureter should tolerate acute dilation to 18F without significant risk, provided the dilation is carefully and atraumatically performed.

As in any surgical procedure, there are many alternative ways to dilate the ureter successfully,[32] and it is left up to each endoscopist to identify and adopt the technique that will prove most effective in his or her hands. As in all new procedures, a definite learning curve exists where initial attempts to perform the procedure may be frustrating, time consuming, and fraught with complications.[45] We have found the Finlayson ureteral access system to provide atraumatic access to all levels of the ureter[46] (Fig. 15–9). In addition, it is easy to teach to residents unfamiliar with ureteroscopic techniques. However, there are clinical circumstances in which alternative techniques must be employed. Two widely used techniques are now described in detail.

All of the components necessary to achieve ureteral access with the Finlayson ureteral access system come in a prepackaged form (Cook Urologic, Spencer, IN). Over the guidewire, the 8F Teflon catheter is fluoroscopically positioned to

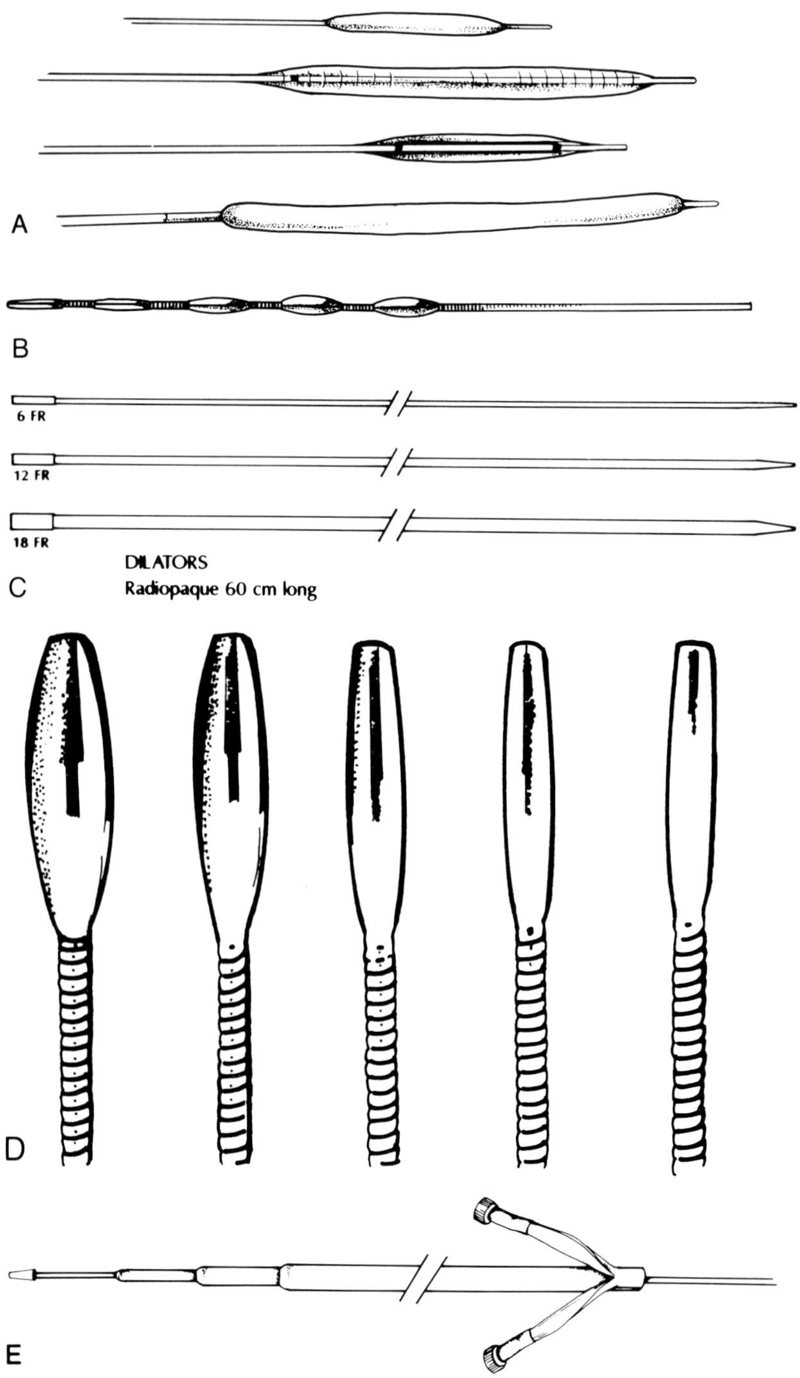

FIGURE 15–8. A variety of ureteral dilators designed to be passed over a guidewire are currently available. *A*, Balloon dilators. *B*, Smith dilators. *C*, Fascial dilators. *D*, Metal bougies. *E*, Finlayson ureteral access system.

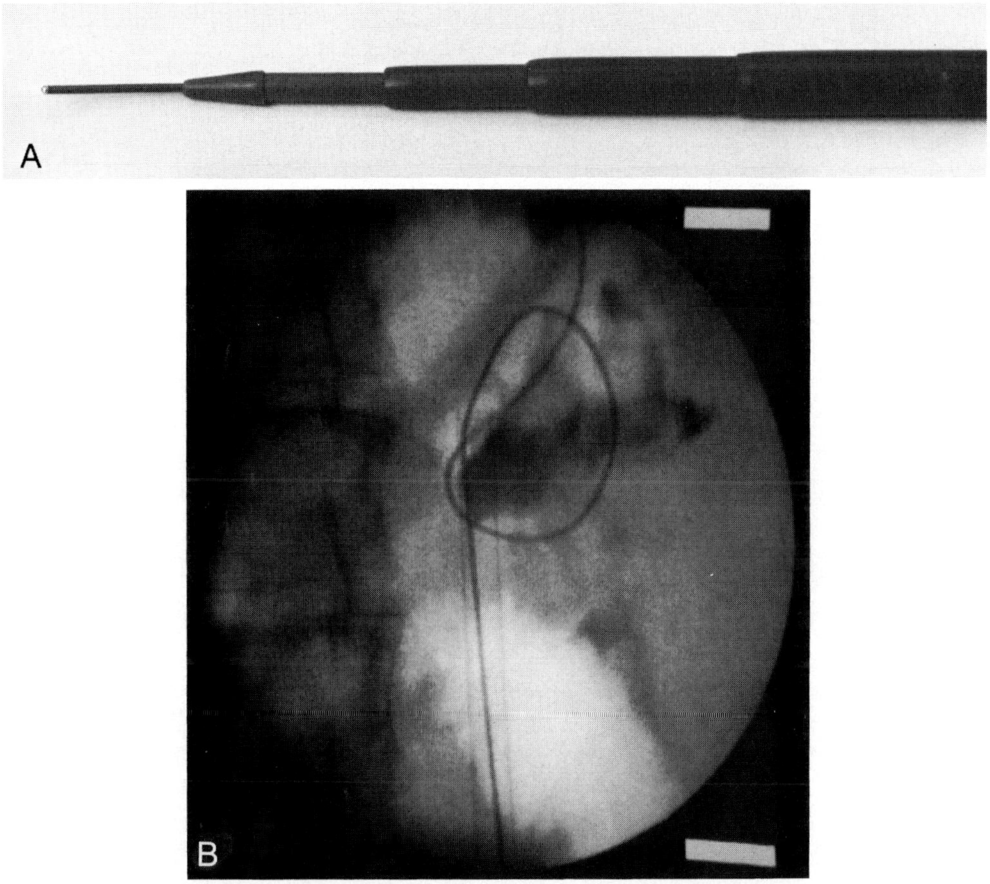

FIGURE 15–9. *A*, Finlayson ureteral access system. Note telescoping design, which allows for rapid and atraumatic ureteral dilation, and built-in Teflon stop as part of the 8F dilator, which prevents passage of the larger dilators beyond the tip. *B*, Finlayson sheath positioned in the renal pelvis.

the level of the stone (Fig. 15–10). The cystoscope is removed, leaving the wire and 8F dilator in place. The three remaining dilators, 12F, 16F, and 18F, are coaxially assembled and individually passed over the 8F catheter. Fluoroscopy is used to keep the 8F dilator at the level of the stone and to monitor the passage of the three large dilators. A built-in Teflon stop just proximal to the tip of the 8F catheter prevents slippage of the larger dilators beyond the stone (Fig. 15–11). After the 18F dilator-sheath is fluoroscopically positioned at the level of the stone, the 8F, 12F, and 16F dilators are removed, leaving the 18F sheath and guidewire in position (Fig. 15–12). The ureteroscope is then passed through the 18F sheath to the level of the stone (Fig. 15–13). In women, this may be rapidly performed under fluoroscopy. By avoiding the use of irrigation, the possibility of proximal stone migration is minimized, as is the risk of significant pyelovenous backflow. In men, the thin-walled sheath tends to kink as it passes through the prostatic urethra; in these patients, the scope is best placed under vision. The kinks may be overcome by applying gentle forward pressure as the scope is advanced. We are unaware of any complication related to kinking of the sheath and forceful passage of the scope in this manner. A recent addition to the ureteral access system is a 20F splinting sheath that fits over the 18F working sheath and

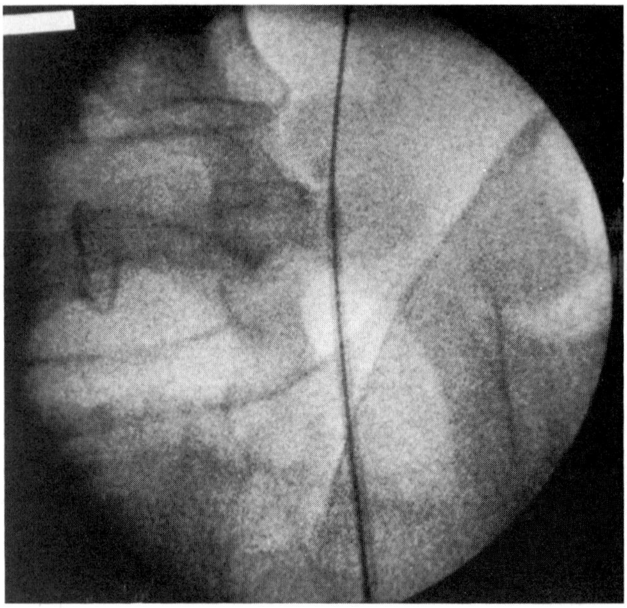

FIGURE 15–10. Initial ureteral dilation proceeds with placement of the 8F dilator over the guidewire to the level of the stone.

extends through the urethra to the ureteral orifice. This 20F sheath helps stabilize the 18F sheath and decreases the degree of kinking.[47] A second site of kinking may occur in patients with proximal and midureteral stones and is commonly found where the ureter angles to enter the bladder. Kinking in this area may also be overcome by exerting constant gentle pressure while advancing the instrument under direct vision.

When performing diagnostic ureteroscopy or in those patients with stones in whom it is not technically possible to pass the Finlayson ureteral access system, the ureteroscope is passed under direct vision. After adequate dilation of the ureterovesical junction using any of the currently available dilators (see Fig. 15–8), the ureteroscope is introduced. In male patients, it is passed into the bladder under direct vision. The guidewire serves as a valuable landmark and helps identify the ureteral orifice. It is left in place throughout the procedure, thus assuring successful placement of a ureteral stent, should ureteral perforation occur. After identifying and immediately before entering the ureteral orifice, the instrument is rotated 180 degrees so that the beveled tip of the instrument is pointing upward as the ureteroscope slides under the roof of the orifice. Once the ureter has been entered, the scope is returned to its normal position. Normal saline is used as the irrigant. To avoid excessive fluid absorption while minimizing the possibility of proximal stone migration, the height of the irrigant above the patient's kidney is kept at 30 cm or less. However, there are occasions when additional fluid pressure is required. In those situations, hand irrigation via a 12-ml syringe attached to the side port of the ureteroscope with intravenous tubing will usually improve the vision while distending the ureter sufficiently to allow advancement of the instrument (Fig. 15–14). Keating has reported no complications using this technique.[48] Once the intravesical ureter has been traversed, the flow of irrigant can usually be decreased as the normal pelvic ureter dilates readily. The ureteroscope is advanced only when the proximal ureteral lumen is clearly seen. Placing the patient in a reverse Trendelenburg position helps further limit the possibility of proximal stone migration. As one nears the iliac

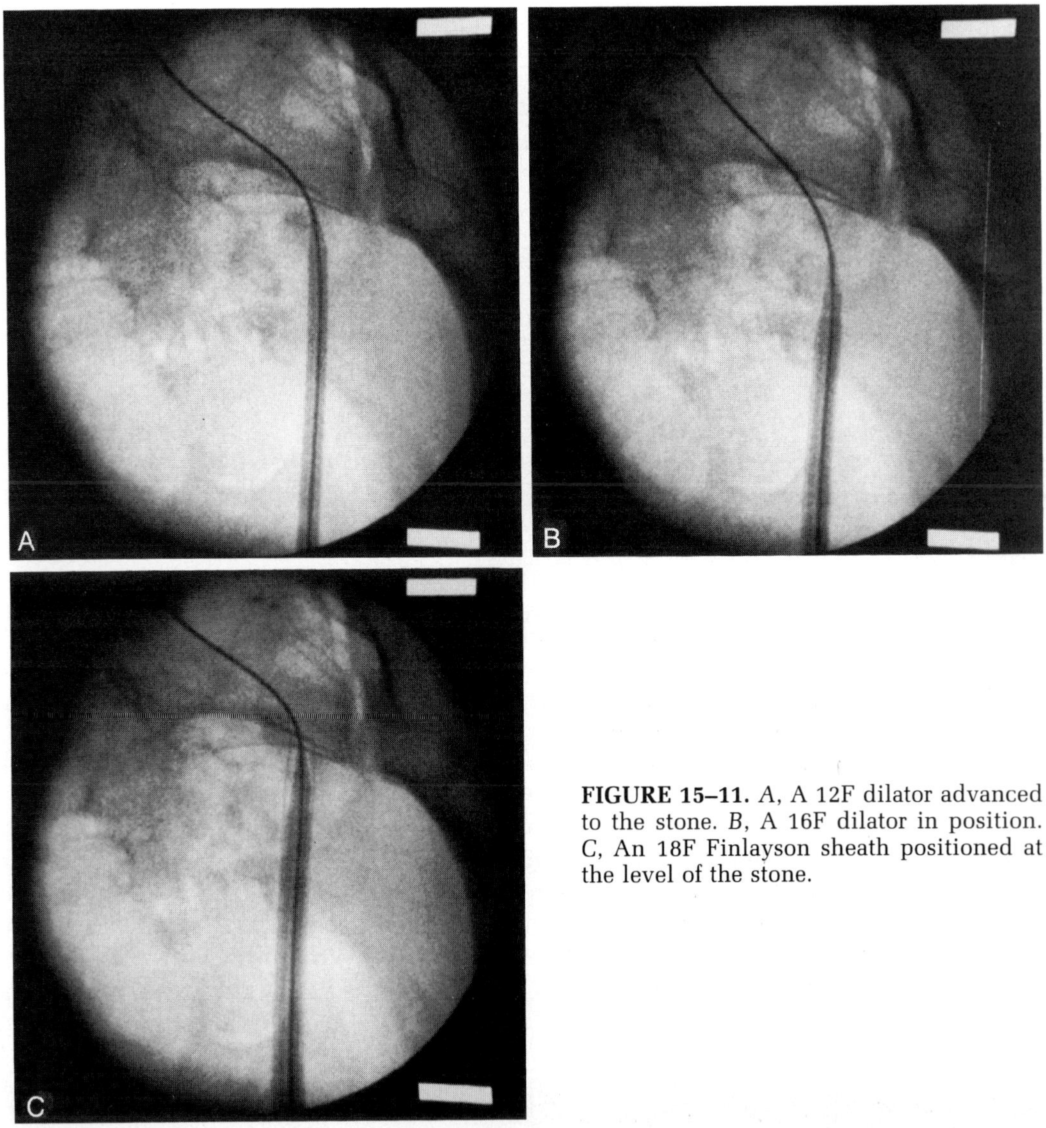

FIGURE 15–11. *A*, A 12F dilator advanced to the stone. *B*, A 16F dilator in position. *C*, An 18F Finlayson sheath positioned at the level of the stone.

artery, its pulsations are frequently noted. At this point, the ureteral lumen might also be slightly compressed. Extreme care should be taken so that perforation does not occur at this site. By using extreme care and advancing the scope only when the proximal lumen is clearly seen, one can safely negotiate the entire length of the ureter to reach stones located in the proximal ureter (see Fig. 15–5). If at any point vision becomes obscured and cannot be restored by manual irrigation, it is prudent to leave a stent indwelling and terminate the procedure.

Once the stone is visualized, a decision must be made about the safest and most expeditious way to extricate the calculus. Stones less than 6 mm (18F) in size are generally removed intact, while larger stones usually require fragmentation with ultrasound, electrohydraulic, or laser probes.

A variety of stone baskets designed for use through the ureteroscope are currently available. Baskets vary in both the number (three to eight) and the

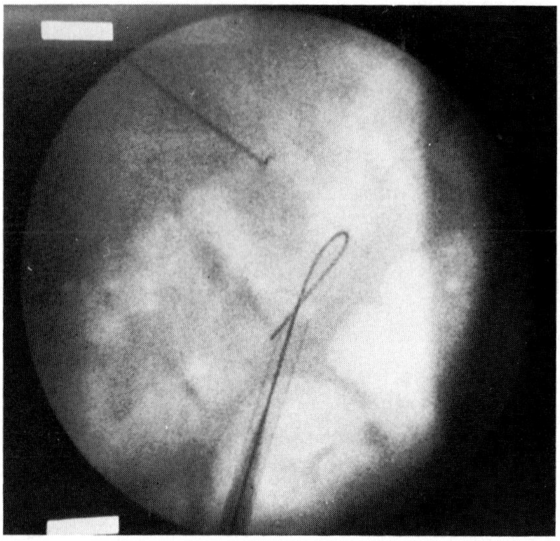

FIGURE 15–12. Coaxially assembled dilators being removed while the 18F sheath is left at the level of the stone.

shape (flat versus helical) of the wires constituting the entrapment mechanism. When manipulating large stones, a basket with three or four wires is selected. The baskets must be less than 5F in size to be passed through the working port of the currently available rigid ureteroscopes. It is recommended that several different stone baskets be available, as a second basket may succeed where a favorite has failed. In contrast to baskets designed for blind or fluoroscopic passage, filiform tips offer no advantage and may actually impede passage of the basket above the stone. Baskets designed for passage over a guidewire offer the advantage of maintaining ureteral access even while the stone is being actively manipulated. Stone removal under direct vision may also be performed with 3- or 4-prong wire-grasping forceps. There are advantages and disadvantages to each technique, and selection is usually based on the preference of the physi-

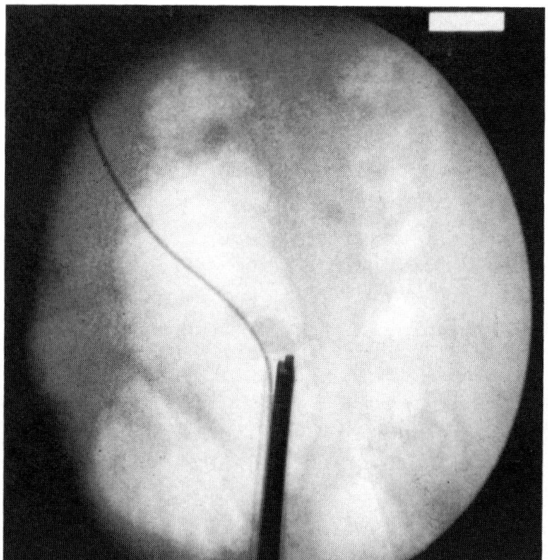

FIGURE 15–13. The rigid ureteroscope is advanced through the 18F sheath and is positioned at the level of the stone. Note the safety wire alongside the ureteroscope.

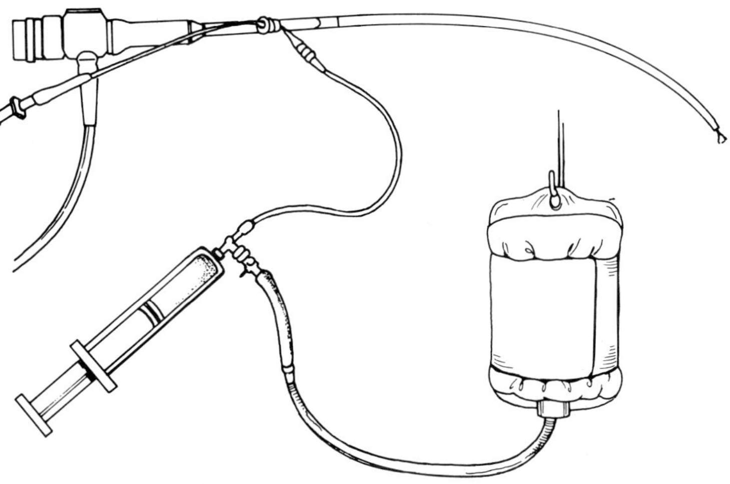

FIGURE 15–14. Technique of manual irrigation to facilitate scope advancement.

cian.[49, 50] To use the stone basket successfully, it must be passed next to or beyond the stone. Stones that are tightly impacted and adherent to the ureteral wall may be best managed by grasping forceps, as it may not be possible to pass the basket beyond the calculus successfully.

While the stone is being visualized, the basket is passed between the wall of the ureter and the stone. The position of the basket above the stone is confirmed by fluoroscopy, and the basket is opened. Under direct vision, the wires of the basket are placed around the stone, and the basket is slowly closed. The firmly entrapped stone basket and ureteroscope are slowly removed as a single unit under direct vision (Fig. 15–15). If the Finlayson sheath is used, the instrument and entrapped stone may be rapidly removed once the stone has entered the proximal sheath. If the stone does not move freely owing to a discrepancy in size between the stone diameter and lumen of the ureter, it must not be forcibly extracted for fear of lacerating or avulsing the ureter. Under these circumstances, it is best to fragment the stone using ultrasound, electrohydraulic, or laser energy.

Stones larger than 6 mm in diameter generally require fragmentation (Fig. 15–16). Transureteral ultrasonic lithotripsy is the most readily available technique. When the stone is freely mobile in a dilated ureter, it is first engaged in a stone basket to prevent proximal migration and to allow firm contact between the probe and stone. If the stone is impacted and cannot be basketed, lithotripsy may still be performed, provided the ultrasound probe can be placed against the surface of the stone with firm pressure; however, once the stone fragments, the pieces are likely to migrate proximally.

Second-generation rigid ureteroscopes are constructed with an offset lens system that allows ultrasonic lithotripsy to be performed under direct vision. The stone is fragmented by a jackhammer-type effect, which occurs when the probe is placed firmly on the stone and the energy is applied. To prevent overheating and thermal damage to the ureteral wall,[51] continuous saline irrigation is run through the probe while suction is simultaneously applied. Ideally, the stone is fragmented to a sandlike consistency, and all of the particles are aspirated through the hollow center of the probe. More likely, the stone will fragment into several pieces, which are then removed.

Ultrasonic fragmentation may also be performed using the first-generation

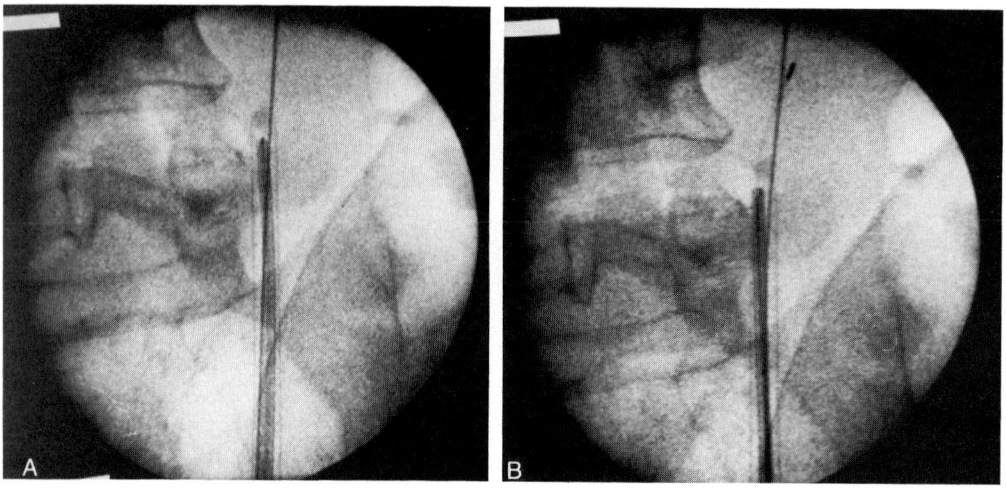

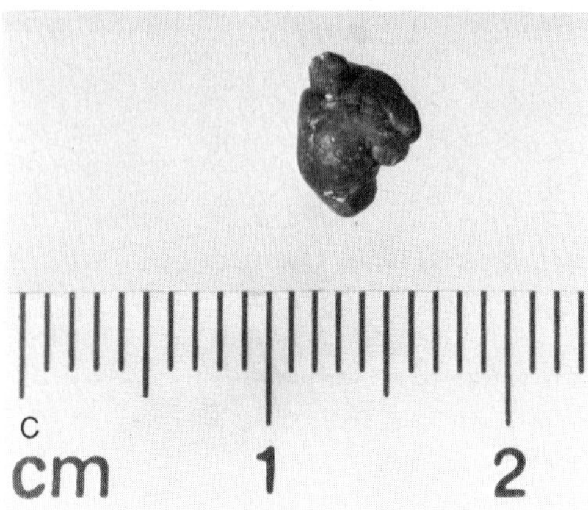

FIGURE 15–15. *A*, Ureteroscope advanced through the Finlayson sheath to the level of the stone. *B*, The stone basket is advanced beyond the stone, the entrapment mechanism is opened, and the stone is basketed under direct vision. *C*, Extracted intact stone.

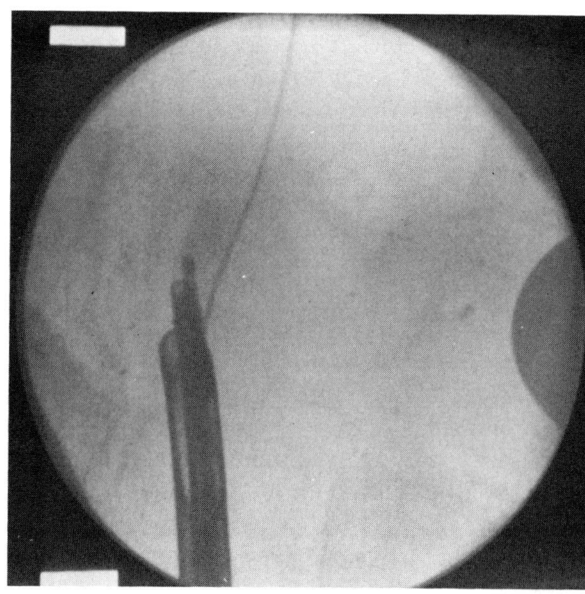

FIGURE 15–16. Stones larger than 6 mm in diameter may be safely fragmented using the ultrasonic probe. Note the tip of the probe positioned against the stone. Initial entrapment with a stone basket is required when the stone is not impacted.

rigid ureteroscope. These instruments were constructed very much like a cystoscope with a removable telescope. Since there is only one port through which the telescope or probe may be placed, the fragmentation is performed blindly. The stone is first basketed and, under direct vision, is brought into contact with the tip of the ureteroscope. The telescope is removed and replaced by the ultrasound probe. Gentle traction on the basket is maintained to keep it at the tip of the ureteroscope. Contact of the stone with the probe must be felt and maintained fluoroscopically. Suction is applied through the probe, and saline irrigation is maintained through the normal inflow channel to prevent overheating.[51] Frequent short bursts of energy are applied to the stone. Fragmentation is monitored both fluoroscopically and by frequent looking through the telescope. The procedure is terminated after the stone has been reduced sufficiently to allow safe removal.

The first use of electrohydraulic energy to fragment a ureteral calculus was reported by Reuter and Kern in 1973.[52] Since that initial report, electrohydraulic lithotripsy has become an accepted alternative to the use of ultrasound energy. The use of electrohydraulic energy in the ureter must be employed with extreme caution and only under optimal conditions, as ureteral perforation may occur if the probe is discharged when in contact with the ureteral wall. Electrohydraulic lithotripsy is reserved for stones refractory to ultrasound disintegration or those rare cases in which the stone may be viewed only with a flexible or a small-caliber rigid ureteroscope. In addition to being associated with a potentially greater risk of ureteral injury, fragments produced by electrohydraulic lithotripsy must be manually removed, as the probe is not equipped with a suction mechanism. Once the stone is visualized and it has been determined that electrohydraulic lithotripsy is required to fragment the stone, the irrigation is changed to one-sixth normal saline. To be effective, the tip of the probe must be placed on or within 1 mm of the stone's surface. To avoid damaging the optics of the lens, the probe should extend a minimum of 5 mm beyond the end of the ureteroscope. Because of the possibility of a spark generated by the probe being transmitted to the wires of a stone basket with ensuing damage to the ureteral wall, the stone should not be held in position with a metallic stone basket. Instead, a ureteral occlusion catheter may be passed proximal to the stone to prevent fragment migration. The lowest possible voltage (60 V) with the shortest possible time of discharge is initially used. Short bursts of current are applied to the stone only when the tip of the probe is clearly seen to be in contact with the stone. If the stone does not crack after five or six discharges, the voltage is increased (a maximum of 80 to 90 V).[49] The goal of electrohydraulic lithotripsy is to fragment the stone into several pieces, which may then be removed with forceps. A third technique to perform intraureteral lithotripsy has recently become available. Early clinical reports indicate that laser lithotripsy is a safe alternative to either ultrasound or electrohydraulic lithotripsy.[53–55] Reported advantages include the small size of the probe—250 μm, or 0.25 mm (0.75F)—which allows passage through a small flexible ureteroscope and the fact that it may be safely discharged directly onto the urothelium without any tissue-damaging effect. One major disadvantage is the high cost of the laser unit. The small size of the laser fiber and the large working ports of the rigid ureteroscopes require the fiber to be passed through a 4F ureteral catheter to stabilize it and allow direct placement on the stone. When a smaller ureteroscope (7 to 9F) is used with a smaller working port, the fiber may be passed directly to the stone. Stones likely to migrate are first stabilized by passing a hollow-core stone basket around the calculus or by passing a balloon catheter above the stone to occlude the ureteral lumen. The quartz fiber is placed directly on the stone, and the laser is activated. Dretler[54] has reported successful fragmentation using a tunable dye laser that emits a wavelength of 504 nm. He uses 25 to 40 mJ of energy delivered in 1-μsec pulses at 5 pulses per second. Fragmentation is continued until the remaining stone can be safely extracted.

After the stone has been removed, a ureteral catheter is routinely placed. If the procedure was difficult and a recognized ureteral perforation occurred, an indwelling type of stent is fluoroscopically placed over the guidewire. If the procedure was atraumatic (Fig. 15–17), either the angled end-hole ureteral catheter, which was initially used to perform the retrograde pyelogram, or an indwelling stent with a suture attached may be used. The indwelling stent allows for earlier discharge of the patient, while the suture allows for easy stent removal without cystoscopy. Large perforations are stented for 4 to 6 weeks. If the procedure has been atraumatic, the stent is removed in 24 to 48 hours. Preoperative antibiotics are continued until all catheters are removed. A follow-up excretory urogram is obtained 6 to 8 weeks after removal of the ureteral catheter (Fig. 15–18).

RESULTS

Politis and Griffith reviewed the world's literature through 1986, and of a total of 1571 attempted ureteroscopic stone extractions, 1274 were successful (81 per cent).[27] The majority of treated stones were in the distal ureter (71 per cent). Successful ureteroscopic stone removal of distal stones ranged from 60 to 98 per cent (overall, 90 per cent). Stones in both the mid and the proximal ureter were successfully removed 68 per cent of the time (range of 22 to 100 per cent). More recently, Blute and associates[28] reviewed the Mayo Clinic experience in managing

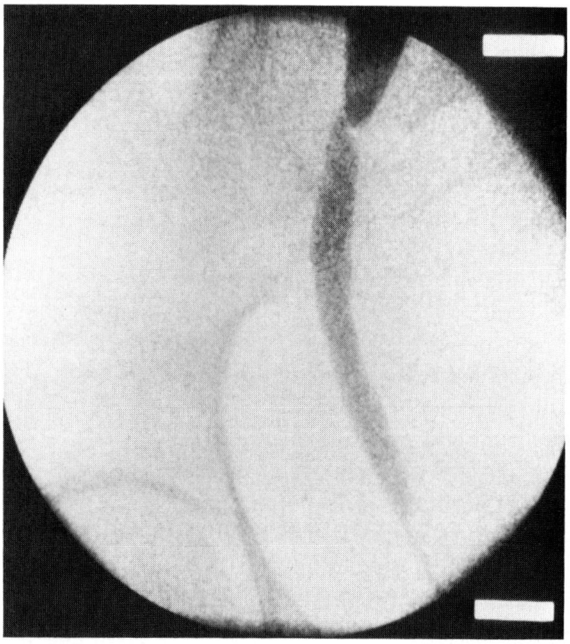

FIGURE 15–17. Final retrograde pyelogram after successful ureteroscopic stone removal performed using the Finlayson ureteral access system. Note the absence of extravasation.

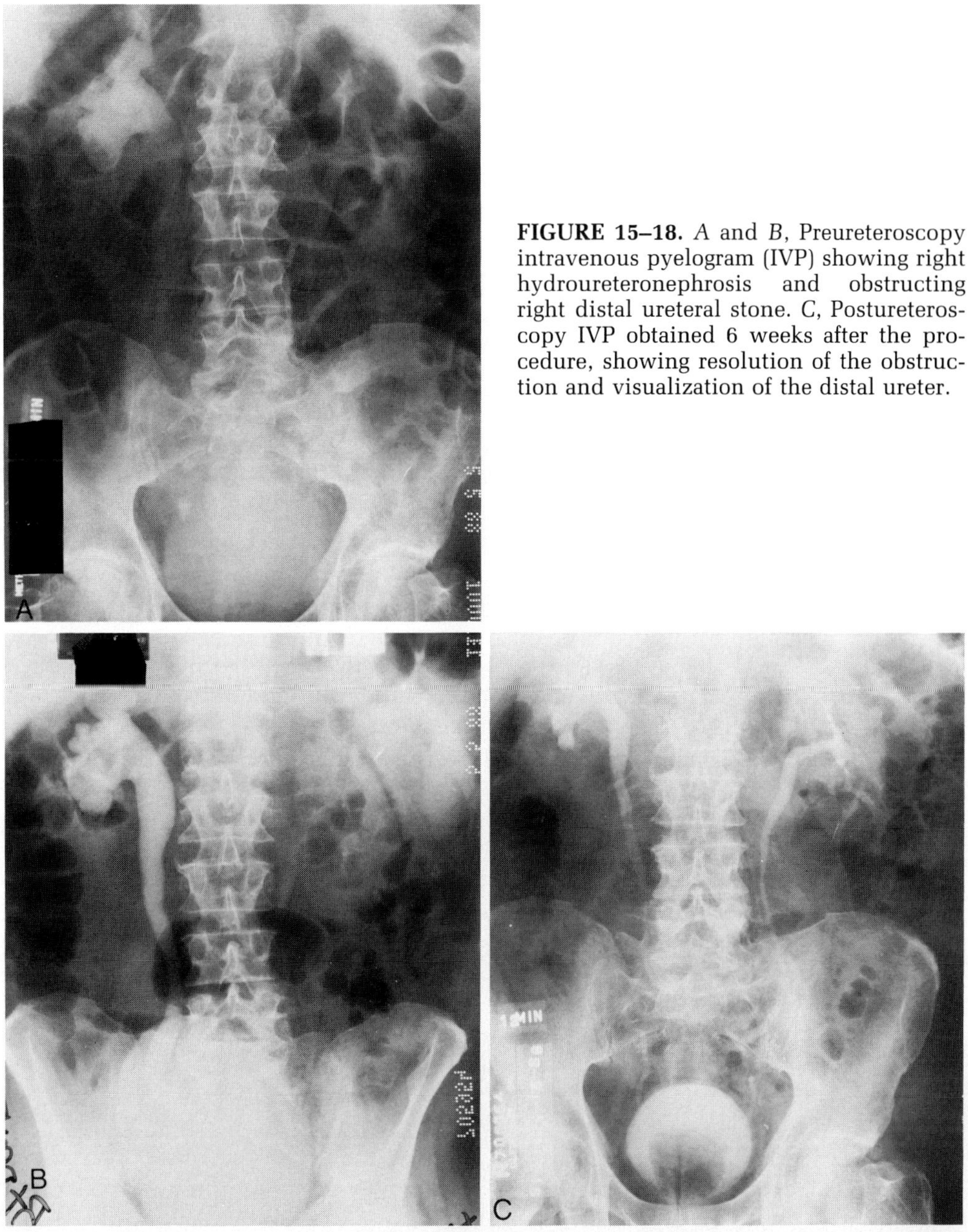

FIGURE 15–18. *A* and *B*, Preureteroscopy intravenous pyelogram (IVP) showing right hydroureteronephrosis and obstructing right distal ureteral stone. *C*, Postureteroscopy IVP obtained 6 weeks after the procedure, showing resolution of the obstruction and visualization of the distal ureter.

274 ureteral stones in 264 patients. They reported an overall 89 per cent success rate. When stratified according to location, lower ureteral stones were removed successfully 95 per cent of the time, whereas mid and upper ureteral stones had a 72 per cent success rate. Similar findings were reported by Lingeman and associates.[56] They had an overall success rate of 87 per cent. Stones below the pelvic brim had a 94 per cent success rate, while those above had a 62 per cent success rate. Daniels and associates[29] reported the Northwestern University experience in managing 99 ureteral stones. They had an overall success rate of 79 per cent. Calculi below the pelvic brim had an 83 per cent success rate, while those above the pelvic brim had a 68 per cent chance of being successfully

removed. When stratified according to stone size, calculi larger than 7 mm had a 67 per cent success rate, while those smaller than 7 mm had an 85 per cent success rate. Similar success rates have been reported by Schultz from Denmark[57] and Ekman from Saudi Arabia.[58] In summary, the majority of ureteral stones may be successfully managed using ureteroscopic techniques; however, results are related to stone size, location, and experience of the operator. Distal stones have about a 90 per cent chance of being successfully removed, while more proximal stones have a 60 to 70 per cent chance.

COMPLICATIONS

Ureteroscopy is a highly successful and safe means to eradicate stones in all levels of the ureter. However, minor (those responding to conservative or ureteral catheter drainage) and major complications (those requiring immediate or delayed surgical intervention) may occur. The reported incidence of minor complications ranges from 0 to 35 per cent, and these complications include hematuria, fever, mild ureteral trauma responsive to stent drainage, and proximal stone migration.[59–63] Although proximal stone migration was considered undesirable prior to the widespread availability of ESWL, it is now considered to be the treatment of choice for many ureteral stones and is followed in preference by ESWL.[56] Major complications include acute ureteral perforation deemed too large to be safely managed by stent or percutaneous tube drainage (Fig. 15–19), ureteral avulsion, ureteral necrosis, and ureteral stricture. These complications have been reported to occur in up to 8 per cent of all ureteroscopic procedures.[29] Ureteral perforation, in many series, is the most common complication of rigid ureteroscopy[27, 45, 56, 61, 64–66] and has been reported to occur in up to 28 per cent of all procedures.[60] Ureteral trauma may occur during ureteral dilation, passage of the ureteroscope, or stone manipulation and fragmentation. The severity of the injury may range from an inconsequential mucosal tear, identified at the

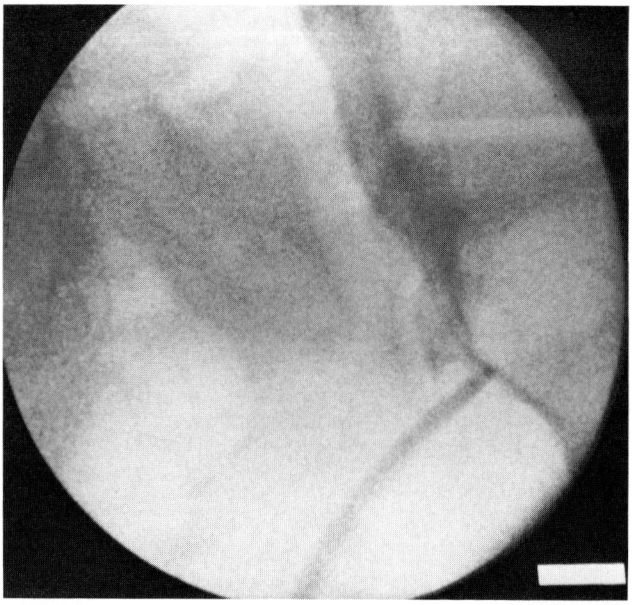

FIGURE 15–19. Urinary extravasation resulting from ureteral perforation at the level of the pelvic brim. This patient underwent ureterolithotomy under the same anesthetic.

time of ureteroscopy and requiring no further evaluation or treatment, to complete ureteral avulsion, necessitating prompt surgical correction. Lacerations associated with extravasation are managed by stent drainage (2 to 6 weeks) and, in many cases, will heal without incident. If a stent cannot be placed beyond the traumatized area, a percutaneous nephrostomy tube should be placed. Strictures that may develop are initially treated by retrograde balloon dilation and ureteral stenting. Should retrograde access be impossible, an attempt is made in an antegrade fashion. Should all endourologic techniques fail, open repair is indicated.

To minimize ureteral trauma, strict attention must be paid to a gentle technique, and one must set aside sufficient time so that there is no urgency to complete the procedure. Ureteroscopic stone removal is generally considered to be more time consuming than open ureterolithotomy.[63] It is not unusual to require 3 to 4 hours for successful removal of a large impacted proximal ureteral calculus. A number of different techniques are available to dilate the ureteral orifice and intramural ureter. Perforation may occur with any technique, although Seeger has reported no failures in 90 patients dilated with a high-pressure balloon.[63] To minimize trauma and the incidence of false passage, the dilators are passed over a guidewire under direct vision. When sequential dilation is used, the initial dilation is performed under direct vision, and the passage of the larger dilators (>12F) is performed under fluoroscopic guidance. If the dilators cannot be passed without resorting to force, then either a different type of dilator should be used or a stent should be placed and the procedure repeated in several days.

Ureteral trauma may also occur while passing the ureteroscope. To minimize trauma, the scope should be passed only under direct vision, either over or alongside a guidewire. It should never be advanced if the proximal ureteral lumen is not clearly seen. Bladder distention may cause bowing of the distal ureter, making it difficult to pass the ureteroscope. A small ureteral catheter passed alongside the ureteroscope will decompress the bladder. Ureteral rings or congenital areas of narrowing[67] in the distal ureter may also impede passage of the instrument. Forceful passage of the instrument beyond these areas of narrowing risks telescoping of the ureteral mucosa and ureteral avulsion. These areas are balloon dilated before further advancement of the instrument is attempted. I have found that the use of the ureteral access sheath fluoroscopically placed at the level of the stone diminishes the incidence of perforation during passage of the instrument.[46]

A high incidence of ureteral perforation can be expected in patients with large stones requiring either electrohydraulic or ultrasonic fragmentation.[29, 61] Stone fragmentation must be performed only when the stone is clearly seen and the probe is able to be directly placed on its surface. The electrohydraulic lithotripsy unit must not be discharged when the probe is in direct contact with the ureteral wall. In the future, the use of smaller 3F electrohydraulic lithotripsy probes may help diminish the incidence of ureteral trauma.[68]

Ureteral perforation associated with retroperitoneal stone displacement has also been reported.[45, 69] Depending on the degree of trauma, stent drainage alone may prove therapeutic. There is no need to pursue stone removal aggressively in those patients with sterile calculi effectively managed by stent drainage, as no complications resulting from stone displacement have been reported.[69]

Postoperative fever (>100°F or 38°C) is commonly seen following ureteroscopy and has been reported by Seeger as occurring in 35 per cent of his patients.[63] In large series reported by Weinberg[45] and Blute,[28] postoperative fever was the most common complication. Although fever is common, urosepsis is rarely seen.[63] Patients should have a sterile urine at the time of the procedure, and prophylactic antibiotics are routinely used. The height of the irrigation should be kept as low as possible to limit pyelovenous backflow, and, finally, ureteral stents are routinely used to avoid postprocedure obstruction. Strict attention must also be paid to sterile technique.

Although the incidence of delayed complications is low, ureteral stricture[28, 61, 66, 70] and reflux have been reported.[61, 71] Kramolowsky[66] has reported the largest experience in managing ureteral perforation. Of 142 ureteroscopic procedures, 24, or 17 per cent, sustained a perforation. Twenty patients were managed conservatively, and 7 (or 5 per cent) of 142 patients developed ureteral obstruction requiring additional intervention. All seven patients, or 3.5 per cent of those managed conservatively, demonstrated stricture formation within 6 weeks of the procedure, four had stents placed (1 to 5 days) as the initial method of managing the perforation, and six of the seven strictures involved the pelvic ureter. Thus, it would appear that short-term ureteral stenting did not affect the outcome of stricture formation and that distal ureteral trauma is more likely to result in stricture formation. Perhaps a longer period of stenting would have improved the outcome. The 5 per cent incidence of stricture formation does not differ from that reported following ureterolithotomy.[72]

Vesicoureteral reflux has been reported rarely following ureteral dilation and ureteroscopy. Experimentally, Ford dilated the ureters of rabbits approximately three-fold from a diameter of 0.55 mm (1.5F) to a diameter of 1.7 mm (5.1F) and obtained intravenous pyelograms at 8 weeks, which were normal in all cases.[73] Similarly, histologic evaluation of the vesicoureteral junction at 8 weeks appeared to be normal with no evidence of anatomic disruption or fibrosis. The ureters of four animals were dilated to a diameter of 7F (2.3 mm). At 2 weeks, all four animals showed gross upper tract dilation, which was histologically associated with disruption and fibrosis of the vesicoureteral junction. Thus, it would appear that acute ureteral dilation is well tolerated up to a certain point (three times in the rabbit), and further dilation beyond that point may be associated with ureteral disruption, fibrosis, and stricture formation. Green[42] dilated dog ureters to 14F to 16F, which he equated with 20F to 24F in humans and noted ureteral hypertonicity and a functional obstruction that resulted in pyelectasis and ureterectasis, findings not associated with moderate dilation to 14F to 16F. Dretler[73] has reported no adverse effects in more than 100 consecutive ureteroscopic procedures performed after dilating the ureter to 18F.

Stackl and Marberger[61] evaluated 35 patients 19 to 20 months following ureteral dilation (12F) and ureteroscopy and identified two patients with low-grade (1 Grade I, 1 Grade II) reflux (6 per cent). Both patients were clinically asymptomatic and required no further intervention. Ford[71] also reported 1 patient with mild reflux of 10 evaluated 3 months after ureteral dilation and ureteroscopy. Others have not reported reflux. Thus, both clinical and experimental studies indicate that the ureter tolerates acute dilation to 18F without long-term complications. On the basis of animal studies, overly aggressive dilation may be associated with ureteral trauma and chronic stricture formation.

FLEXIBLE URETEROPYELOSCOPY

Because of the limitation in the size of the working channel, flexible ureteroscopy has been primarily used for diagnostic purposes. Refinements in

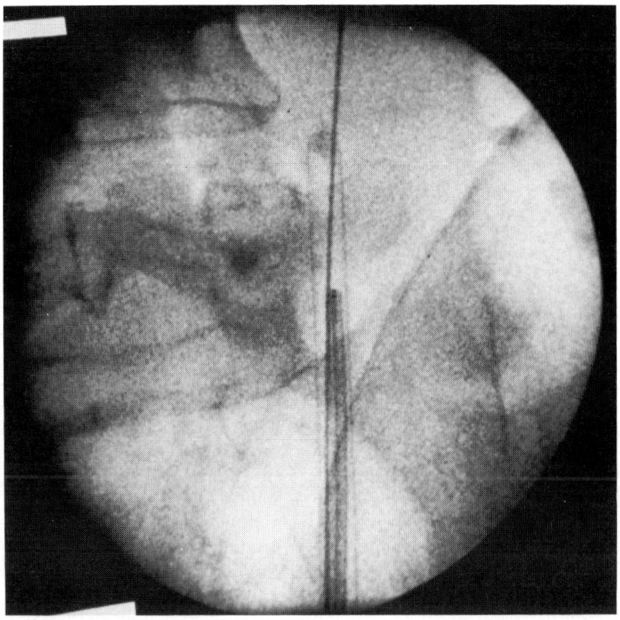

FIGURE 15–20. Flexible ureteroscope advanced through the Finlayson sheath to a midureteral stone.

fiberoptic instrumentation and the development of flexible instruments with an irrigation channel separate from the working channel now allow for successful stone removal.[22, 74, 75] Nine French instruments currently exist that, in many cases, may obviate ureteral dilation. These smaller instruments are passively passed through the working port of a cystoscope similar to the way a ureteral catheter is placed. Two 0.038-inch floppy tip guidewires are placed up the ureter and fluoroscopically positioned beyond the stone. One guidewire serves as a safety wire and will remain throughout the procedure. The instrument is passed over the second working wire. If the ureteroscope does not readily pass through the ureteral orifice, it is dilated to 10F. The ureteroscope is fluoroscopically positioned at the level of the stone, and the working wire is removed. Depending on the size, it is either removed with a basket or forceps or fragmented with electrohydraulic lithotripsy. Where available, laser lithotripsy may also be used. The instrument is removed, and a ureteral catheter is placed over the safety guidewire.

The larger flexible ureteroscope (10F to 14F), which allows active deflection of the tip, is also available. When used for stone removal, these instruments offer no real advantage over the rigid instruments, as ureteral dilation is still required (Fig. 15–20).

THE FUTURE OF URETEROSCOPY

The success rates for ureteroscopic stone removal have steadily improved. This can be attributed to both improvement in instrument design and the availability of smaller grasping forceps and electrodes capable of fragmenting large calculi. In the future, one can expect additional refinements in currently available rigid instruments. Smaller diameters and shorter instruments designed specifically for distal ureteral stone manipulation will further improve the surgical results. The development of smaller flexible ureteroscopes that can be actively deflected and the more widespread availability of laser lithotripsy can also be expected to improve clinical results.

REFERENCES

1. Murphy LJT: The History of Urology. Springfield, IL, Charles C Thomas, 1972, p 180.
2. Wickham JEA, Miller RA: Nephroscopy: Endoscopic instruments and their accessories. *In* Wickham JEA, Miller RA (eds): Percutaneous Renal Surgery. Edinburgh, Churchill-Livingstone, 1983, pp 45–74.
3. Hopkins HH, Kapany NS: A flexible fiberscope, using static scanning. Nature 173:39, 1954.
4. Hopkins HH: British patent 954, 629 and US patent 3, 257, 902, 1960.
5. Hopkins HH: The modern urological endoscope. *In* Gow JA, Hopkins HH (eds): A Handbook of Urological Endoscopy. Edinburgh, Churchill-Livingstone, 1978, p 29.
6. Curtiss LE, Hirschowitz BI, Peters CW: A long fiberscope for internal medical examination. J Opt Soc Am 46:1030, 1956.
7. Hirschowitz BI, Curtiss LE, Peters CW, Pollard HM: Demonstration of a new gastroscope, the "fiberscope." Gastroenterology 35:50, 1958.
8. Van Heel ACS: A new method of transporting optical images without aberrations. Nature 173:39, 1954.
9. Young HH, McKay RW: Congenital valvular obstruction of the prostatic urethra. Surg Gynecol Obstet 48:409, 1929.
10. Marshall VF: Fiberoptics in urology. J Urol 91:110, 1964.
11. Goodman TM: Ureteroscopy with pediatric cystoscope in adults. Urology 9:394, 1977.
12. Lyon ES, Kyker JS, Schoenberg HW: Transurethral ureteroscopy in women: A real addition to the urologic armamentarium. J Urol 119:35, 1978.
13. Lyon ES, Banno JJ, Schoenberg HW: Transurethral ureteroscopy in men using juvenile cystoscopy equipment. J Urol 122:152, 1979.
14. Perez-Castro EE, Martinez-Pineiro JA: Transurethral ureteroscopy—a current urological procedure. Arch Esp Urol 33:445, 1980.
15. Das S: Transurethral ureteroscopy and stone manipulation under direct vision. J Urol 125:112, 1981.
16. Huffman JL, Bagley DH, Lyon ES: Extending cystoscopic techniques into the ureter and renal pelvis—experience with ureteroscopy and pyeloscopy. JAMA 250:2004, 1983.
17. Takagi T, Go T, Takayasu H, Hioki R: Small caliber fiberscope for visualization of the urinary tract, biliary tract and spinal canal. Surgery 64:1033, 1968.
18. Takagi T, Go T, Takayasu H, Aso Y: Fiberoptic pyeloureteroscope. Surgery 70:661, 1971.
19. Bush IM, Goldberg E, Javadpour N, et al: Ureteroscopy and renoscopy: A preliminary report. Chicago Med School Q 30:46, 1970.
20. Weinberg JJ, Snyder JA, Smith AD: Mechanical extraction of stones with rigid ureteroscopes. Urol Clin North Am 15:339, 1988.
21. Tolley DA: Endoscopic ureteric stone extraction: Experience with the short ureteroscope. Br J Urol 59:401, 1987.
22. Bagley DH: Active versus passive deflection in flexible ureteroscopy. J Endourol 1:15, 1987.
23. O'Flynn JD: The treatment of ureteric stones. Br J Urol 52:436, 1980.
24. Sandegard E: Prognosis of stone in the ureter. Acta Chir Scand [Suppl] 219:1, 1956.
25. Ueno A, Kawamura T, Ogawa A, et al: Relationship of spontaneous passage of ureteral calculi to size. Urology 10:544, 1977.
26. Spirnak JP, Resnick MI: Urinary stones. *In* Tanagho EA, McAninch JW (eds): Smith's General Urology. Norwalk, CT, Appleton and Lange, 1988, pp 275–301.
27. Politis G, Griffith DP: Ureteroscopy in management of ureteral calculi. Urology 30:39, 1987.
28. Blute ML, Segura JW, Patterson DE: Ureteroscopy. J Urol 139:510, 1988.
29. Daniels GF, Garnett JE, Carter MF: Ureteroscopic results and complications: Experience with 130 cases. J Urol 139:710, 1988.
30. Perez-Castro E: Ureteromat: Method to facilitate ureteroscopy and avoid dilation. Urol Clin North Am 15:315, 1988.
31. Motola JA, Shahon RS, Smith AD: Anatomy of the ureter. Urol Clin North Am 15:295, 1988.
32. Eshghi M: Dilation of ureteral orifice for ureterorenoscopy. Urol Clin North Am 15:301, 1988.
33. Newman RC, Hunter PT, Hawkins IF, Finlayson B: A general ureteral dilator-sheathing system. Urology 25:287, 1985.
34. Newman RC, Hunter PT, Hawkins IF, Finlayson B: The ureteral access system: A review of the immediate results in 43 cases. J Urol 137:380, 1987.
35. Humble L, Venable DD: Perioperative use of indwelling ureteral catheter as an adjunct to ureteroscopic stone manipulation. J Endourol 1:165, 1987.

36. Perez-Castro E, Mancebo JM, Massarra J: Method to obviate dilation in ureterorenoscopy: Uromat J Endourol 1:223, 1987.
37. Lewis B: Report of operative work in the ureter through the author's catheterizing and operative cystoscope. Am J Urol 1:134, 1905.
38. Buerger L: A new method of facilitating the passage of ureteral calculi. Am J Surg 27:151, 1913.
39. Illievitz AB: A new method for the removal of stones in the ureter, a preliminary report. Surg Gynecol Obstet 40:575, 1925.
40. Ravitch A: New irrigating ureteral bougie. J Urol 20:517, 1928.
41. Dourmashkin RL: Cystoscopic treatment of stones in the ureter with special reference to large calculi based on the study of 1550 cases. J Urol 54:245, 1945.
42. Greene LF: The renal and ureteral changes induced by dilating the ureter. J Urol 52:505, 1944.
43. Hunter PT, Newman RC, Finlayson B: Acute mechanical dilation of the ureter: An experimental study. J Urol 138:161, 1987.
44. Clayman RV, Elbers J, Palmer JO, Wassynger W: Experimental extensive balloon dilation of the distal ureter: Immediate and long term effects. J Endourol 1:19, 1987.
45. Weinberg JJ, Ansong K, Smith AD: Complications of ureteroscopy in relation to experience: Report of survey and author experience. J Urol 137:384, 1987.
46. Spirnak JP: The Finlayson ureteral access system: Is it a suitable alternative to other ureteral dilating techniques? North Central Section AUA 62nd meeting, Orlando, November 13–19, 1988, p 77.
47. Newman RC: Ureteral access system: Technique and results. Urol Clin North Am 15:323, 1988.
48. Keating MA, Heney NM, Young HH II, et al: Ureteroscopy: The initial experience. J Urol 135:689, 1986.
49. Clayman RV, McMurtry JM: Complications of ureteroscopic lithotripsy. Probl Urol (calculus disease) 1:593, 1987.
50. Segura J: Ureteroscopy, including lithotripsy and the stone basket. *In* Stephen Rous (ed): Stone Disease: Diagnosis and Management. Orlando FL, Grune and Stratton, 1987, pp 213–222.
51. Howard SS, Merrill E, Harris S, Cohn J: Ultrasonic lithotripsy. Invest Urol 11:273, 1974.
52. Reuter HJ, Kern E: Electronic lithotripsy of ureteral calculi. J Urol 110:181, 1973.
53. Watson GM, Wickham JEA: Initial experience with a pulsed dye laser for ureteric calculi. Lancet 1:1357, 1986.
54. Dretler SP, Watson G, Parrish JA, Murray S: Pulsed dye laser fragmentation of ureteral calculi: Initial clinical experience. J Urol 137:386, 1987.
55. Coptcoat MJ, Ison KT, Watson G, Wickham JEA: Lasertripsy for ureteric stones in 120 cases: Lessons learned. Br J Urol 61:487, 1988.
56. Lingeman JE, Sonda LP, Kahnoski RJ, et al: Ureteral stone management: Emerging concepts. J Urol 135:1172, 1986.
57. Schultz A, Kristensen JK, Bilde T, Eldrup J: Ureteroscopy: Results and complications. J Urol 137:865, 1937.
58. Ekman P, Uasain I, Sharma ND, Al-Faqih SR: Transurethral ureteroscopy: Safety guide wire as an aid to a more aggressive approach. Br J Urol 60:23, 1987.
59. Lyon ES, Huffman JL, Bagley DH: Ureteroscopy and pyeloscopy. Urology [Suppl 5] 23:29, 1984.
60. Hosking DH, Ramsey EW: Rigid transurethral ureteroscopy. Br J Urol 58:621, 1986.
61. Stackl W, Marberger M: Late sequelae of the management of ureteral calculi with the ureteroscope. J Urol 136:386, 1986.
62. El-Faqih SR, Husain I, Ekman PE, et al: Primary choice of intervention for distal ureteric stone: Ureteroscopy or ESWL. Br J Urol 62:13, 1988.
63. Seeger AR, Rittenberg MH, Bagley DH: Ureteropyeloscopic removal of ureteral calculi. J Urol 139:1180, 1988.
64. El-Kappany H, Gaballah MA, Ghoneim MA: Rigid ureteroscopy for the treatment of ureteric calculi: Experience in 120 cases. Br J Urol 58:499, 1986.
65. Chang R, Marshall FF: Management of ureteroscopic injuries. J Urol 137:1132, 1987.
66. Kramolowsky EV: Ureteral perforation during ureteroscopy: Treatment and management. J Urol 138:36, 1987.
67. Lytton B: Complications of ureteroscopy. Semin Urol 4:183, 1986.
68. Begun FP, Jacobs SC, Lawson RK: Use of a prototype 3F electrohydraulic electrode with ureteroscopy for treatment of ureteral calculous disease. J Urol 139:1188, 1988.
69. Lytton B, Weiss RM, Green DF: Complications of ureteral endoscopy. J Urol 137:649, 1987.
70. Biester R, Gillenwater JY: Complications following ureteroscopy. J Urol 136:380, 1986.
71. Ford TF, Parkinson MC, Wickham JEA: Clinical and experimental evaluation of ureteric dilation. Br J Urol 56:460, 1984.
72. Amar AD, Das S, Bulusu NV: Ureteral strictures following ureterolithotomy. J Urol 125:416, 1981.
73. Dretler SP: Management of ureteral calculi. AUA Update Series 7:42, 1988.
74. Preminger GM, Kennedy TJ: Ureteral stone extraction utilizing nondeflectable flexible fiberoptic ureteroscopes. J Endourol 1:31, 1987.
75. Aso Y, Ohtawara Y, Fukuta K, et al: Operative fiberoptic nephroureteroscopy: Removal of upper ureteral and renal calculi. J Urol 137:629, 1987.

16

Percutaneous Management

J. Patrick Spirnak
Martin I. Resnick

HISTORICAL REVIEW

Prior to the development and widespread acceptance of percutaneous technique, patients with symptomatic renal stone disease required open surgical lithotomy. It was not until 1941, when Rupel and Brown[1] reported the first successful percutaneous stone removal performed through a surgically established nephrostomy tract, that an alternative became available. This technique was largely overlooked by the urologic community, and a review of both the German and the English literature from 1941 to 1980 revealed only 11 reported cases.[2] In all 11 cases, the stone was removed via a surgically established nephrostomy tract.

In 1953, Seldinger[3] described a percutaneous technique that allowed access to the femoral artery without the need for a formal surgical incision. The Seldinger technique of placing manipulative catheters over a previously placed guidewire, when expanded to the urinary tract, allowed ready access to the collecting system without the need for a surgical incision. In 1955, Goodwin[4] reported the first percutaneous nephrostomy tube placed using the Seldinger technique. Although percutaneous access to the urinary tract held great promise, widespread acceptance of this technique was slow to occur. In 1973, Stables[5] reviewed the available literature and reported 516 cases of percutaneous nephrostomy tube placement. Soon thereafter, both radiologists and urologists recognized the importance of achieving percutaneous access to the collecting system, and in 1979, Smith, Lange, and Fraley[6] coined the term "endourology" to refer to the closed, controlled manipulation of the entire urinary tract. Since the initial reports, application of the basic technique first described by Seldinger has been limited only by the imagination and expertise of the clinician.

In 1976, Fernström and Johansson[7] reported the first percutaneous stone extraction performed via a nephrostomy tract established solely for that purpose. Three years later, Smith and associates[8] reported the first American series of five patients undergoing percutaneous stone removal. Early reports limited attempted percutaneous stone extraction to small stones generally less than 1.5 cm in their largest diameter and to patients considered poor surgical risks.[7, 8] Stone extraction was generally performed under fluoroscopic control using a variety of techniques (grasping, flushing, and basketing) and equipment already familiar and readily available to urologists.

Although early attempts at percutaneous stone removal were limited by the size of the stone, the technology to fragment stones already existed. In 1975, Raney and Handler[9] reported successful electrohydraulic renal stone disintegration in a patient with a preexisting nephrostomy tract. In 1977, Kurth and associates[10] reported successful atraumatic disintegration of a staghorn calculus using ultrasound. In 1981, Alken and associates[11] reported the initial experience in using ultrasound to fragment stones successfully via a percutaneously established nephrostomy tract. Since the initial clinical reports, both electrohydraulic and ultrasonic stone fragmentation procedures have become an integral and widely accepted part of percutaneous nephrolithotomy and have been successfully used to remove complex renal stones.

As it became obvious that percutaneous nephrolithotomy was a suitable alternative to open surgical techniques, emphasis was placed on developing new instrumentation designed specifically for use via a nephrostomy tract. Prior to this time, only intraoperative nephroscopy had been available. Trattner[12] in the late 1940s developed the initial rigid nephroscope. This 24F instrument was straight and was designed to use available telescopes. It was constructed without an operative port and was difficult to use. Leadbetter[13] recognized the limitations of the Trattner instrument and designed a 22F one-piece right-angled instrument (Fig. 16–1). The right-angled design allowed for complete viewing of the renal collecting system while minimizing manipulative renal trauma. In the early 1970s, both the Storz Company (Culver City, CA) and the Wolf Company (Rosemont, IL) developed fiberoptic right-angled nephroscopes with built-in instrument channels that allowed for the intraoperative removal of stones under direct vision[14] (Fig. 16–2). No further changes in nephroscope design occurred until the late 1970s, when Marberger,[15] with support from the Richard Wolf Corporation, developed a rigid instrument with a 12F instrument channel designed specifically for percutaneous use. The 24F instrument had a side arm viewing piece that articulated with the shaft of the instrument at a 90-degree angle (Fig. 16–3). By utilizing right-angled construction, the center of the

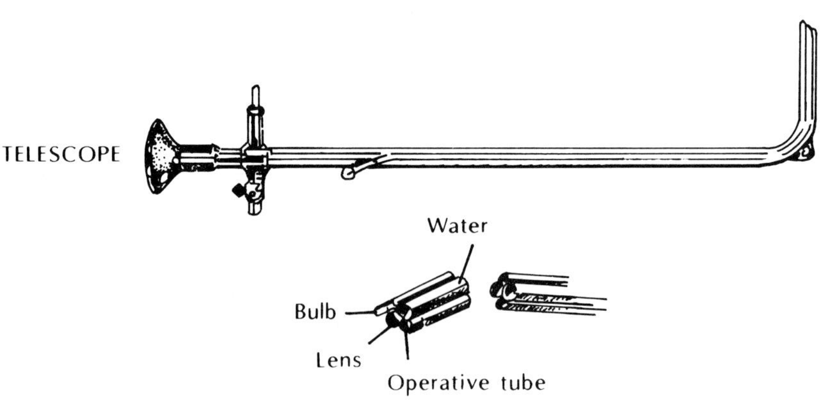

FIGURE 16–1. Leadbetter right-angled nephroscope designed for intraoperative use.

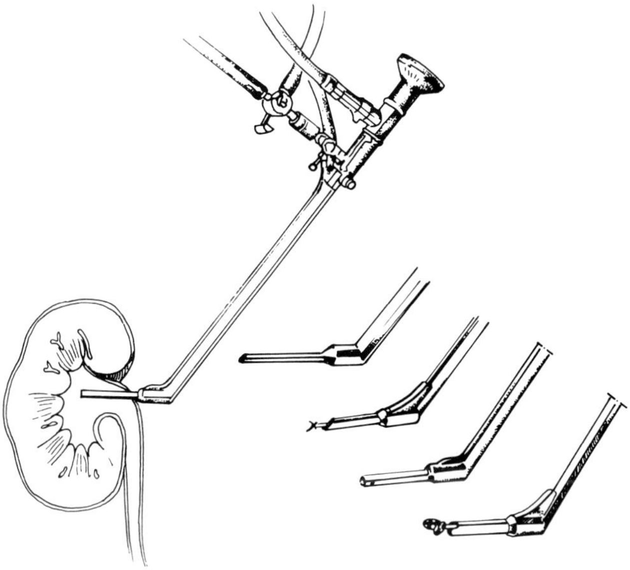

FIGURE 16–2. Operative nephroscope with add-on instrument tips designed to aid in the identification and removal of residual calculi at the time of open stone removal.

instrument was free to accept a rigid ultrasound probe. In 1979, American Cystoscope Makers (ACMI, Stamford, CT) introduced a 16F flexible fiberoptic nephroscope that was steerable and capable of viewing the entire renal collecting system.[16] The entire intrarenal collecting system was now accessible via a percutaneously established access tract.

Initial attempts at percutaneous nephrolithotomy were limited to high-risk patients with multiple medical problems or to those who had undergone prior renal surgery.[7, 8] Rupel and Brown[1] performed the first successful stone removal through a 26F nephrostomy tract, which accepted a panendoscope without requiring additional tract dilation. In 1974, Bissada and colleagues[17] reported successful stone removal via a surgically created percutaneous tract which was dilated to 30F over 4 days. Alken and coworkers[11] reported successful stone removal in 34 patients. In 19 patients, percutaneous nephrostomy tube drainage was established, and the tract was slowly dilated to 26F over 1 week. The 26F nephrostomy tract was allowed to mature for 5 days prior to stone manipulation. Although excellent clinical results were achieved using this deliberate technique

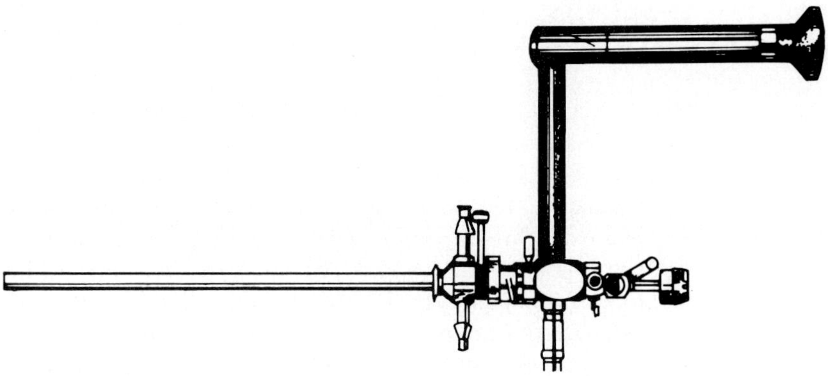

FIGURE 16–3. Percutaneous nephroscope designed for use with ultrasound probe.

of tract dilation, the lengthy hospitalization and prolonged treatment period negated many of the potential benefits when compared with open surgery. In 1982, Segura and associates[18] reported successful stone removal in 15 patients in a single session. For the first time, it was possible to demonstrate clear advantages in terms of length of hospital stay, cost of treatment, and decreased loss of working days when compared with open stone removal. Similar reports followed from other centers,[15, 19, 20–23] and percutaneous nephrolithotomy became the procedure of choice for most uncomplicated renal stones.

As the available instrumentation continued to evolve and clinicians gained experience in percutaneous techniques, the indications for attempted percutaneous stone removal expanded to include more complex renal stones. In 1983, Clayman and associates[24] reported successful removal of branched renal stones with minimal morbidity. Although their initial experience was limited to patients who had undergone multiple previous renal operations or who were considered poor surgical risks, corroborative results reported by other clinical investigators expanded the indications to include all patients with complex stones.[25, 26] Thus, as of 1983, the indications for percutaneous nephrolithotomy were limited only by the clinical expertise of the surgeon and the ability to achieve intrarenal access. Stones contained in a nondilated collecting system continued to represent a relative contraindication to percutaneous stone removal, as the process of gaining intrarenal access was often time consuming, fraught with frustration, and traumatic to the kidney. In December of 1983, clinical investigators working independently in Milwaukee, Wisconsin, and Gainesville, Florida, described the technique of achieving retrograde percutaneous renal access.[27, 28] Initial clinical reports using these techniques were favorable, particularly in patients with nondilated collecting systems.[29–32] By combining both the antegrade and the retrograde techniques, it was now possible to achieve atraumatic renal access in nearly all patients.

In just a few short years, percutaneous nephrolithotomy had become the procedure of choice for nearly all renal stones. The popularity of this approach, however, was short lived, as the technology for shock wave lithotripsy was being developed by Chaussy and associates[33] at the same time that percutaneous techniques were evolving. In 1984, the golden age of percutaneous stone surgery effectively ended as Lingeman and associates[34] treated the first American patients with shock wave therapy. The urologic community had entered the shock wave era.

PRINCIPLES

Successful percutaneous nephrolithotomy implies the completion of three separate yet interdependent procedures. Anything short of complete success in performing any of these three procedures will result in failure to remove the targeted stone. First, percutaneous access to the collecting system must be obtained. This can be achieved by using antegrade or retrograde techniques. There are advantages and disadvantages to each approach, and the two techniques are best thought of as being complementary rather than as alternatives to achieving the same goal. The retrograde approach is best suited for achieving access in the nondilated collecting system and in those cases with large stone bulk with little room to negotiate wires and catheters between the stone and the wall of the collecting system. Under these circumstances, the retrograde approach allows precise atraumatic access with a guidewire securely positioned from the urethra through the flank. Once access has been achieved, the tract must be dilated sufficiently (26F to 34F) to allow stone manipulation. Finally, the stone must be visualized and removed. Success rates approaching 100 per cent are possible, depending on the experience of the operator.

INSTRUMENTS

As the benefits of percutaneous nephrolithotomy became obvious, the major manufacturers of urologic endoscopic equipment (Storz, Wolf, and ACMI) focused on developing rigid and flexible instruments suitable for use in the kidney. Rigid instruments manufactured by the Karl Storz and Richard Wolf Corporations measured 26F and 24F, respectively. These instruments were similar in design to available cystoscopes in that they utilized a rigid metal sheath through which an operating telescope could be placed (Fig. 16–4). Both initial telescopes utilized fiberoptics and had the eyepiece offset at 90 degrees from the body of the telescope. By utilizing right-angled construction, the 12F working channel passed straight through the nephroscope sheath and allowed passage of a variety of straight rigid instruments (Fig. 16–5). Early design was such that the irrigating port was made part of the nephroscope sheath. The design of the irrigating port was later modified, and it was positioned on the operating telescope. This slight modification facilitated use of the instrument by not requiring passage of the metal sheath. Further changes in instrument design were introduced by Thackray Ltd. (Orlando, FL) and Richard Wolf. The viewing lens in both instruments was redesigned to be oriented at an acute angle to the shaft of the instrument rather than at 90 degrees (Fig. 16–6). The proposed advantage of this modification was an improvement in instrument balance.[35]

A variety of rigid baskets and grasping instruments are available for use with the rigid nephroscope (Fig. 16–7). In general, stones less than 1 cm in their greatest diameter may be removed intact through a 30F nephrostomy tract. Larger stones are fragmented using electrohydraulic, ultrasound, or laser energy.

Of the three techniques currently available to fragment calculi percutaneously, ultrasound is used most frequently[36] (Fig. 16–8). Ultrasonic lithotripsy is based on the piezoelectric effect first demonstrated by Curie in 1880. When

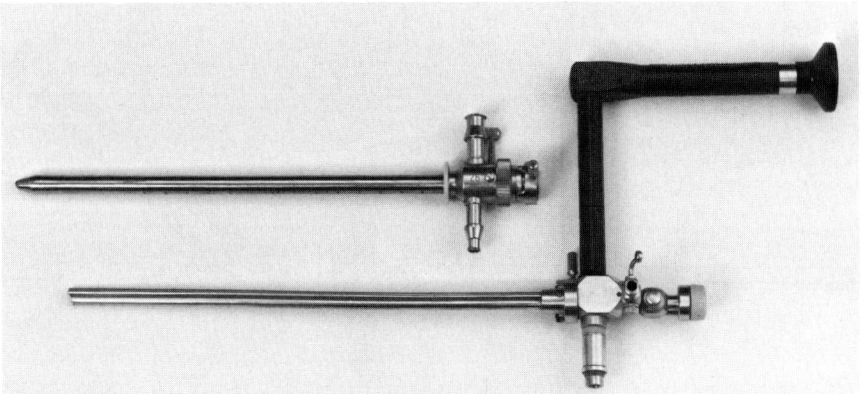

FIGURE 16–4. A 26F Storz nephroscope and sheath.

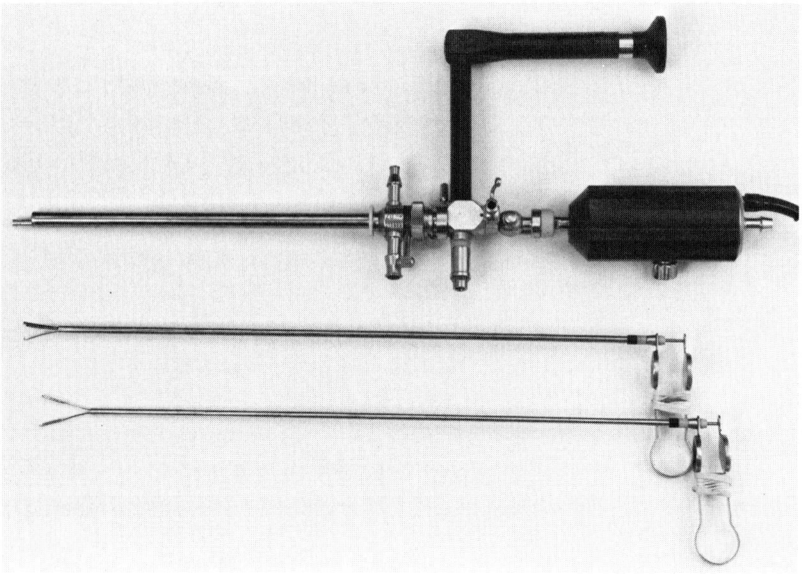

FIGURE 16–5. A 26F Storz nephroscope with ultrasound probe in place. Grasping forceps are also shown.

an electrical charge is applied to a piezoceramic crystal, vibrations occur at a specific frequency (23,000 to 27,000 Hz). The vibrations of the crystal produce ultrasound waves, which, when transmitted to the end of a hollow metal probe, cause it to vibrate. It is the rapid (several thousand times per second) mechanical vibration of the probe tip that is responsible for the stone fragmentation. To be effective, the tip of the probe must be in close contact with the stone.

In 1953, Mulvaney[37] was the first to attempt stone fragmentation using ultrasound energy. Coates, 3 years later, applied ultrasound to stones in cadaveric kidneys and noted no tissue damage.[38] The absence of tissue-damaging effects was corroborated by other investigators.[10, 39] Terhorst and associates[40] reported mucosal edema as the only discernible tissue alteration in rabbit bladders even after exposure of up to 5 minutes of ultrasonic vibration. It has been shown that the tissue-sparing effect is related to the high elasticity of the soft tissue, which preferentially absorbs the ultrasound energy.[40, 41] One potential tissue complica-

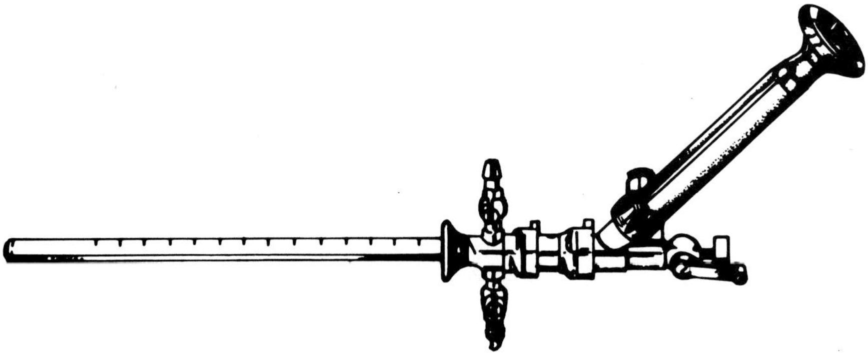

FIGURE 16–6. Rigid nephroscope with viewing lens at acute angle to the shaft.

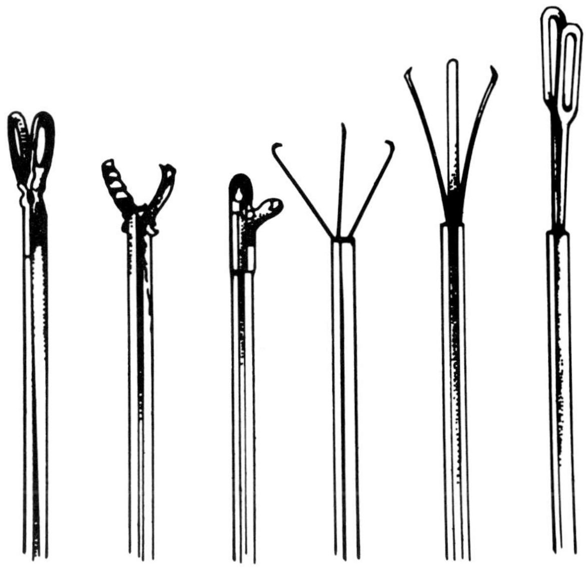

FIGURE 16–7. Various instruments available for use with rigid nephroscope.

tion is related to excessive heat buildup at the probe tip. However, Marberger has shown that the maintenance of an irrigation rate of 30 ml/min will limit the increased temperature at the probes tip to a maximum of 1.4°C.[42] In vitro studies have shown that all urinary stones may be fragmented using this technology.[43, 44] Although all stones may be successfully fragmented, the density of the calculus is the most important variable in determining the ease of fragmentation.[42] Calculi with rounded, smooth surfaces, such as uric acid or calcium oxalate monohydrate

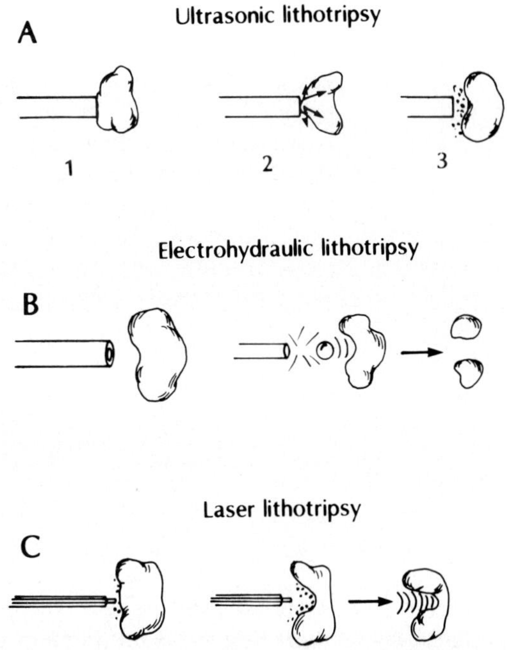

FIGURE 16–8. Current techniques available to fragment urinary stones.

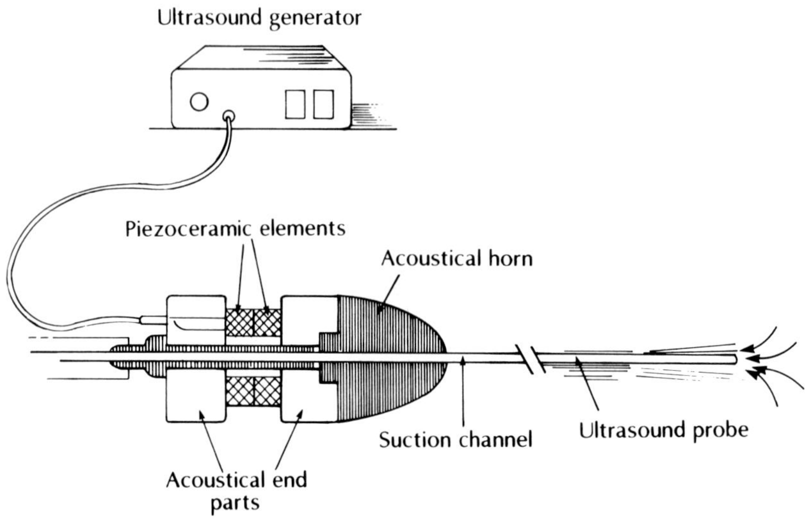

FIGURE 16–9. Diagram of ultrasonic probe.

stones, fragment poorly, while stones with a rough, crystalline surface, such as struvite stones, are readily fragmented. Size is not a limiting factor. However, larger stones require a longer treatment time.

Early clinical use of ultrasound was limited to fragmenting bladder stones, and it was not until 1982 that Alken reported the first series of patients in whom ultrasonic lithotripsy was used in the kidney.[11] Since then, ultrasonic lithotripsy has been shown to be a safe and effective way to fragment large stones in the ureter and kidney.

The instrumentation necessary to fragment urinary stones ultrasonically is manufactured by the largest providers of urologic instruments (Storz, Wolf, and ACMI), and the models are similar in their basic design. The ultrasonic lithotrite (sonotrode) consists of a 10F to 12F hollow steel probe that is attached to a transducer at one end (Fig. 16–9). The transducer forms the handle of the sonotrode and houses the piezoceramic crystal. The high-frequency sound waves generated by exciting the piezoceramic crystal are transmitted to the hollow probe via an acoustical horn. The Storz probe detaches from the transducer and is available in two sizes (Fig. 16–10). The short probe exits only 1.5 cm from the sheath of the nephroscope, while the longer probe exits about 4 cm from the tip. The Wolf sonotrode is constructed as a fixed single unit, which increases the cost of probe replacement. Attached to the tip of the Storz probe is a ragged-edged drill bit, which may enhance stone disintegration by providing a rotational effect (Fig. 16–11). The lumen of the probe is attached to a standard suction

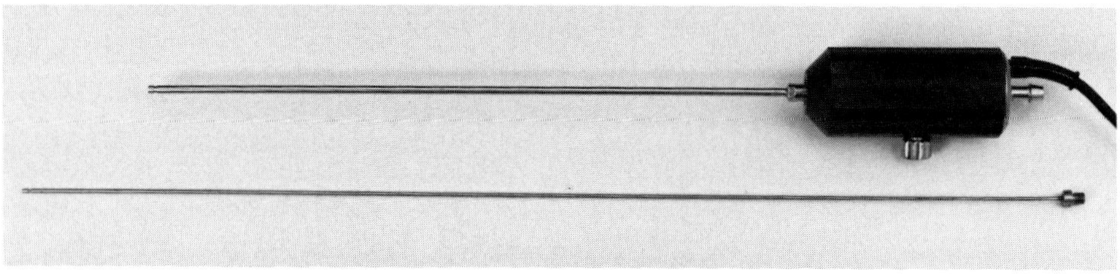

FIGURE 16–10. Storz detachable ultrasonic probes with transducer.

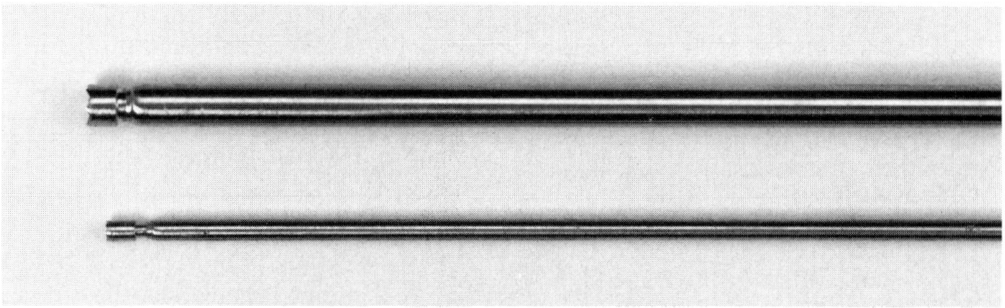

FIGURE 16–11. Tip of Storz ultrasound probe.

device at the transducer end of the sonotrode. Persistent application of suction helps hold the tip of the probe in direct contact with the stone while aspirating all of the stone debris as it is being formed. The generator is activated by depressing a foot pedal (Fig. 16–12). Pumps capable of delivering the irrigation fluid while simultaneously providing suction are commercially available; however, these may prove difficult to use, and standard bottle irrigation, combined with wall suction is adequate. The sonotrode is placed through the instrument channel of the rigid nephroscope, and the irrigation is attached. Under direct vision, the tip of the sonotrode is placed firmly against the surface of the stone, and the generator is activated. The space between the telescope and working sheath allows sufficient drainage of the irrigant to maintain a low-pressure system even at maximal inflow rates (Fig. 16–13). Controlled visual fragmentation of the stone is performed until it is reduced sufficiently to be grasped and removed (Fig. 16–14) (usually 6 to 10 mm, depending on the extent of tract dilation and the size of the working sheath.

Continuous irrigation is required to maintain visibility throughout the procedure. Patients undergoing ultrasonic lithotripsy are thus at risk for complications similar to those that may occur during transurethral resection and are directly related to excessive fluid absorption.[45, 46] Since electroresection is not a

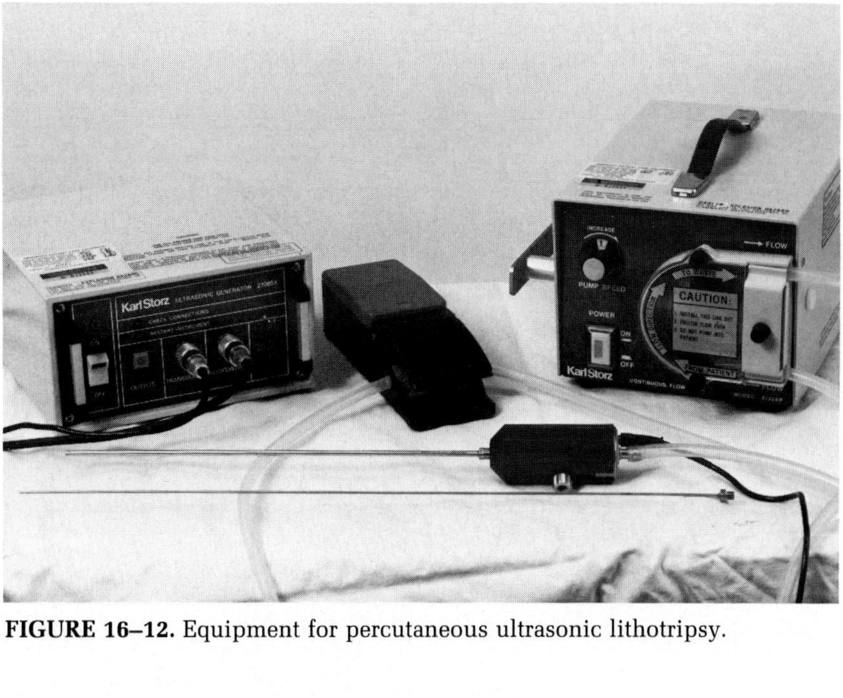

FIGURE 16–12. Equipment for percutaneous ultrasonic lithotripsy.

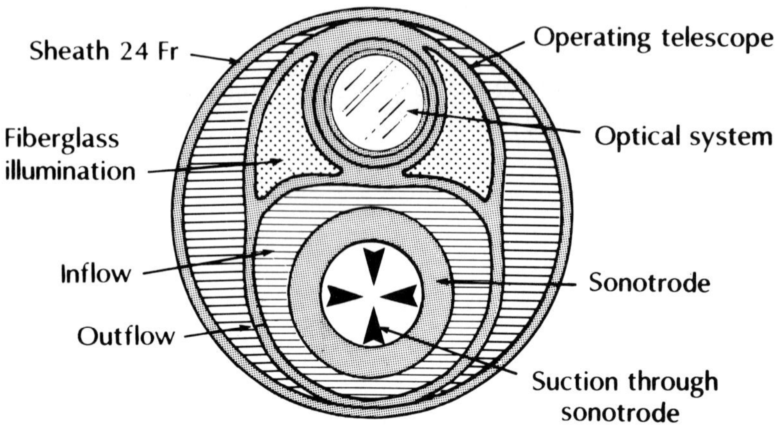

FIGURE 16–13. Cross-section of rigid nephroscope with the ultrasound probe in place.

routine part of this procedure, it is recommended that a warmed physiologic saline solution be used as the irrigant.[47] The use of saline will avoid the potential complication of hyperammonemia that has been associated with excessive glycine absorption.[48]

Electrohydraulic lithotripsy (EHL) may also be used to fragment urinary stones. Yutkin in the 1950s was the first to describe the destructive effects of electrohydraulic energy.[49] Rose developed the first EHL unit that could be used to fragment bladder calculi,[49] and in 1960, Goldberg reported the first use of EHL to fragment a bladder stone.[50] It was not until 1975 that Raney and Handler first applied this technology to fragment renal stones,[9] and in 1983, Clayman and associates[24] reported success in percutaneously fragmenting renal stones with EHL. Since then, EHL has been used to fragment stones in the ureter and at present is used to complement the use of ultrasound in fragmenting stones throughout the urinary tract. The mechanism by which electrohydraulic energy acts to fragment stones is similar to the effects of extracorporeal lithotripsy in that both are dependent on shock wave generation occurring as a result of an

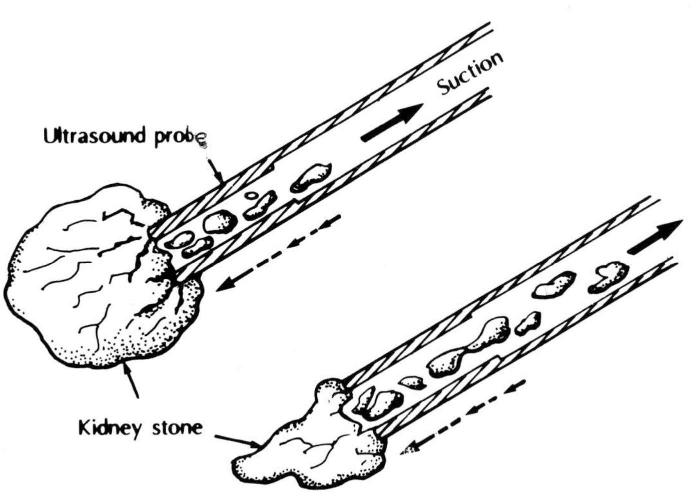

FIGURE 16–14. The stone is fragmented, and the pieces are removed by suction applied to the hollow center of the ultrasound probe.

underwater electrical discharge. The high energy discharge results in intense heat and vaporization of water at the electrode tip, which causes a cavitation bubble and the generation of a compression (shock) wave (Fig. 16–15). The shock wave radiates spherically in all directions and will damage air-containing tissue or those tissues of densities markedly different from that of water, such as a urinary stone. As it strikes the stone, it is reflected at the front and back, as well as by faults existing within the stone. Fragmentation occurs when the stresses acting on the stone are greater than the forces holding the stone intact. The initial compression wave is typically followed by two and as many as four bubble waves, which have as much destructive potential as the initial compression wave.[51] The entire sequence of shock wave generation occurs during 0.08 second.[52] If the initial compression or subsequent bubble waves contact stone fragments with sufficient energy, these fragments may become embedded in the tissue. In addition, thermal tissue damage will occur if the probe is discharged while in contact with the urothelium.

The use of EHL is best viewed as being complementary rather than competing with ultrasonic lithotripsy. There are advantages and disadvantages to each mode of therapy. In general, the initial cost of EHL is less.[53] It is also more successful in fragmenting extremely hard or dense stones (uric acid, calcium oxalate monohydrate) than is ultrasonic energy. The use of flexible EHL probes (3F, 5F, and 9F) allows stones located in calyces remote from the percutaneous tract to be successfully accessed and fragmented using flexible instruments (Fig. 16–16). Disadvantages include the following: the short life span of the EHL probes (<60 seconds and is related to the strength and duration of each discharge), which necessitates having several backup probes available for large stone cases; the need to remove all stone fragments manually; and the tissue-damaging effect that occurs if the probe is discharged while in contact with the urothelium.

EHL works best when used with an irrigant solution of one-sixth to one-seventh normal saline and is ineffective in a standard saline solution. For maximal efficiency, the tip of the probe must be 1 mm or less away from the stone surface when the generator is activated. To prevent damaging the lens of the telescope, the tip of the probe must project at least 5 mm from the end of the endoscope (see Fig. 16–15). The goal of EHL is to fragment the stone into several pieces, which are then manually removed. In an effort to limit the number of stone fragments generated with EHL, it is best to start at a low discharge voltage (75 V to 85 V) and to limit the number of discharges per second to 30 to 50.[52] If the stone is refractory to fragmentation at these settings, the voltage and number of discharges per second are increased.

With the stone clearly in view and after changing the irrigant to one-sixth saline, the tip of the probe is placed on or less than 1 mm from the surface of the stone. The probe is discharged by depressing the foot pedal. A single

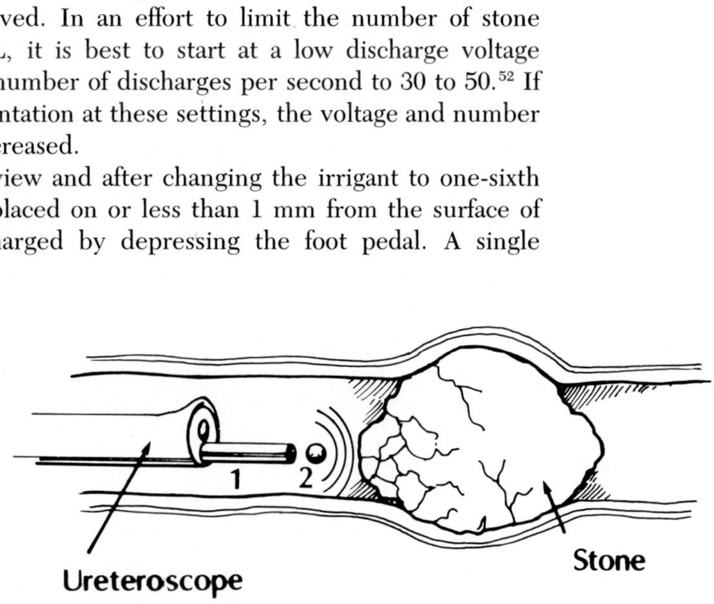

FIGURE 16–15. Diagrammatic representation of electrohydraulic lithotripsy (EHL). Note (1) EHL probe and (2) cavitation bubble.

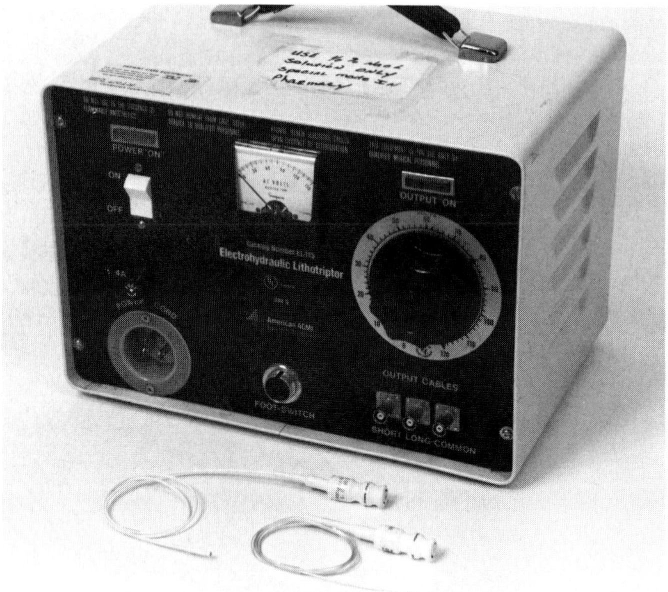

FIGURE 16–16. EHL generator and flexible probes.

prolonged firing of the probe is preferable to multiple short firings.[52] The procedure is continued until the stone fragments. As the procedure progresses, the probe must be intermittently inspected for signs of wear. A worn probe does not fire efficiently, and persistent use may result in separation of the central metal core from the rest of the probe, resulting in a retained foreign body. Probe wear is easily detected endoscopically and is identified by the peeling back of the outer layer of insulation to reveal the inner concentric ring of metal. The fragments are manually removed as they are formed.

The primary role of EHL is in fragmenting stones refractory to ultrasonic disintegration (uric acid and calcium oxalate monohydrate) or in fragmenting calculi accessible only with the flexible instruments.

Laser lithotripsy is another alternative available to fragment urinary stones. Mulvaney and Beck were the first to describe the effects of laser energy on calculi.[54] They applied laser energy from carbon dioxide and ruby lasers directly onto stones and noted minimal vaporization but no fragmentation. In 1982, Tanahashi and associates[51] used the neodymium-yttrium-aluminum-garnet (Nd YAG) laser set at 70 W to fragment canine vesical calculi. The laser energy was delivered through an optical fiber placed in direct contact with the stone. The procedure required such high energy levels that thermal damage to surrounding tissue occurred.

It is now known that continuous-wave lasers cannot be effectively used to fragment stones. When continuous-wave laser energy is applied, stone fragmentation occurs only by vaporization, which requires the melting point of the stone to be reached. The melting point for oxalate and phosphate stones is higher than 2500°C, a temperature that is unrealistic in vivo.[55] In 1977, Fair[56] demonstrated the potential use of lasers to fragment stones when he produced a high-amplitude shock wave as a result of a plasma produced when a Q-switched laser was pulsed onto solid material surfaces. Fair's work laid the foundation for additional studies utilizing this photoacoustic effect, which resulted in the production of rapidly expanding shock waves, which, when focused on the surface of a stone, could result in mechanical damage. Subsequent animal studies by Watson showed that a wavelength of 504 nm is selectively absorbed by the stone and is poorly absorbed by the urothelium. Tissue damage did not occur unless laser energy was applied for a minimum of 15 seconds.[55]

The Candela Corporation (Wayland, MA) manufactures the only pulsed dye laser that has been approved for urologic use. The laser energy is delivered to the stone surface via a 250-μm quartz laser fiber (Fig. 16–17). In contrast to other surgical lasers, which rely on thermal energy to achieve their desired effect, the Candela laser uses the photoacoustic effect to fragment stones. The pulsed dye laser is a flash lamp green dye laser that emits energy at a wavelength (504 nm) that is selectively absorbed only by the stone, thereby avoiding thermal damage to the adjacent soft tissue. The laser energy is emitted in short bursts with brief pulse durations. As the laser energy is absorbed by the stone, a plasma forms at the surface. This plasma, composed of ions and electrons, continues to absorb laser energy. The plasma, confined by surrounding liquid, is raised to very high pressures and produces a shock wave that fragments the stone. By repeating the process, additional stress fractures occur that will eventually cause the stone to fragment.

The degree of stone fragmentation is directly related to the stone composition and crystal lattice structure of the calculus. Coptcoat[57, 58] has noted that both calcium oxalate dihydrate and phosphate calculi readily fragment into small particles (<1 mm), while calcium oxalate monohydrate and mixed stones fragment less readily and into larger particles.

To be effective, the laser fiber must be placed directly on the stone. To facilitate passage of the 250-μm fiber through the large working channels of currently available endoscopic instruments, the fiber is first passed through the

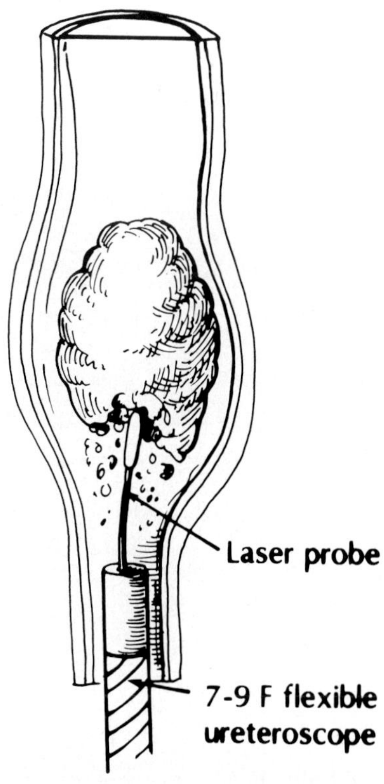

FIGURE 16–17. Laser probe in contact with stone.

lumen of a 4F or 5F end-hole ureteral catheter. A 7.2F semirigid ureteroscope has recently become available. This instrument has a 1F instrument channel, which allows direct placement of the laser fiber. Segura[59] recommends starting with a power setting of 30 mJ. If no effect is seen, the power is increased to a maximum of 60 mJ. Others have suggested starting with a power setting of 60 mJ.[60] The laser frequency may be set at 5 or 10 Hz. The laser is activated by stepping on a foot pedal. Treatment is continued either until the stone is reduced entirely into fragments (<1 mm), which will pass spontaneously, or until the stone is reduced sufficiently in size so that it may be safely grasped and removed.

The first flexible nephroscope was introduced in 1979 by the ACMI Corporation. The initial instrument was designed specifically for intraoperative use and measured only 11 cm in length. Since the average distance from the skin to the renal pelvis is about 10 cm, this instrument proved inadequate for most percutaneous procedures. The flexible choledochoscope originally designed for the intraoperative examination of the biliary tree was used for percutaneous nephroscopy. Its usefulness was hindered by its short length (30 cm), which limited its use to the intrarenal collecting system and proximal ureter. Soon after percutaneous procedures gained widespread acceptance, the flexible choledochoscope was redesigned to meet the needs of the endourologists. These instruments are typically 15F in diameter, measure at least 60 cm in length, have 5F or 6F working channels, and are fully immersible in sterilizing solutions[61] (Fig. 16–18). Most of the currently available instruments are capable of manual deflection, usually between 100 and 180 degrees in a single plane. A variety of 4F and 5F accessory instruments are available for use with the flexible nephroscope (Fig. 16–19). One drawback to the use of the flexible instrument is the relatively poor flow through the irrigation port that occurs when an instrument is in place. Flow may be improved by raising the height of the irrigation fluid or by increasing the delivery pressure by placing the irrigation bag in a pressurized blood pump.

INDICATIONS

From 1979 to 1984, percutaneous nephrolithotomy replaced open surgical lithotomy as the treatment of choice for the majority of urinary stones. Specific

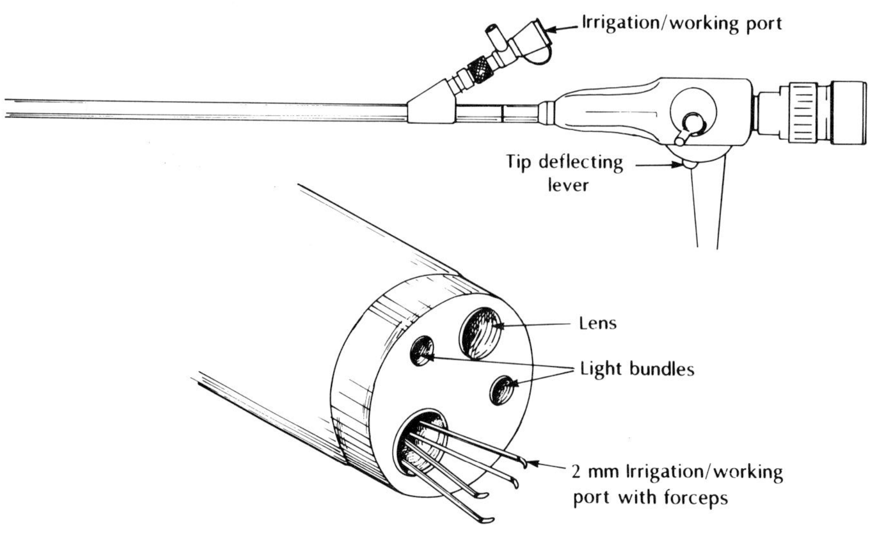

FIGURE 16–18. Diagrammatic representation of typical flexible nephroscope.

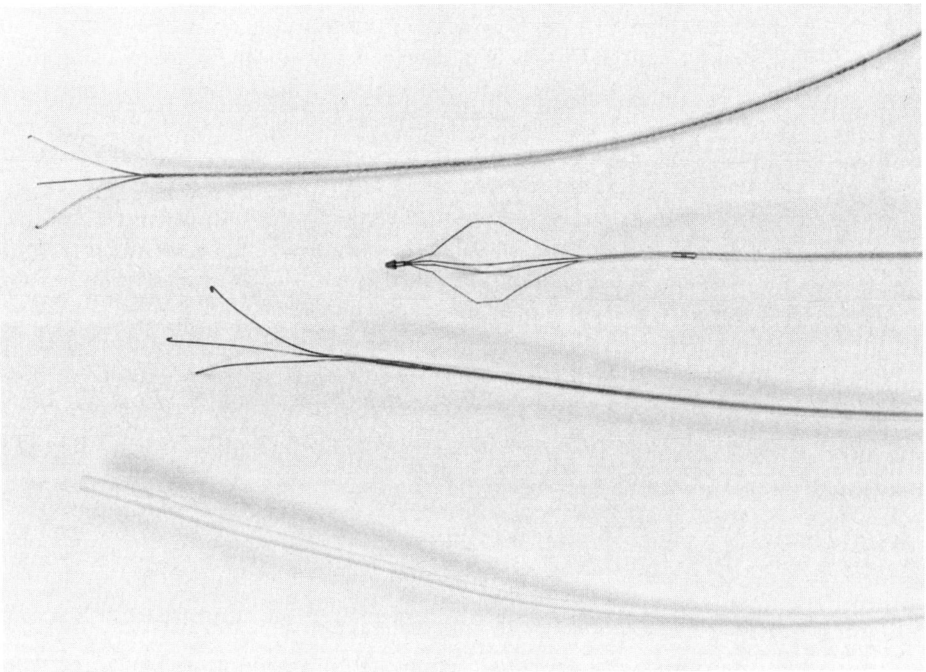

FIGURE 16 10. Instruments for use with flexible nephroscope.

indications for stone removal include obstruction, progressive loss of renal function, pain, infection, recurrent gross hematuria, and the patient's occupation.[62] Indications specifically related to ureteral stones include size, degree of obstruction, and failure to progress down the ureter.[63]

It was recommended that initial attempts at percutaneous stone removal be limited to small (<1.5 cm) renal pelvic stones present in a dilated collecting system. As experience was gained, it became apparent that nearly any stone with a surgical indication could be successfully removed using the percutaneous approach. Clinical results were most often determined by the experience of the operating surgeon and not solely on the basis of stone location or composition. Medical centers with extensive expertise in percutaneous techniques were capable of successfully managing nearly all urinary stones. Contraindications to percutaneous nephrolithotomy were based primarily on the surgeon's ability to achieve intrarenal access and to visualize and remove all of the calculus. The only absolute contraindication to attempting the percutaneous approach is an irreversible coagulopathy.

As experience was gained in extracorporeal shock wave lithotripsy (ESWL) techniques, it became apparent that many stones formerly treated by the percutaneous approach were now better managed using ESWL. At centers where both techniques are currently available, specific indications for percutaneous stone removal still exist. The percutaneous approach is preferred in patients with renal stones associated with anatomic obstruction of the ureteropelvic junction. Favorable results may be obtained by performing an endopyelotomy[64] at the same time the stone is removed. Patients with renal stones associated with significant infundibular stenosis for calyceal diverticula may not be candidates for ESWL if it is thought that the fragments may not pass beyond the obstruction. In these cases, a percutaneous approach may successfully treat both problems.[65]

Massively obese patients (>300 lb) or those with severe kyphoscoliosis are not candidates for ESWL and may be successfully managed using the percutaneous approach.[66] Cystine stones for which dissolution fails may be more readily destroyed using the percutaneous approach and the ultrasonic or electrohydraulic lithotrite. Patients with large (>3 cm) or branched calculi are at a high risk for obstructive complications and a high residual stone rate following ESWL; therefore, the percutaneous approach may be preferred either alone or in combination with ESWL.[67] Finally, about 1 per cent of all patients undergoing ESWL will fail to demonstrate adequate stone fragmentation.[68] The percutaneous approach is then indicated.

Whereas prior to ESWL most ureteral stones were successfully managed by either a ureteroscopic or a percutaneous approach, most are today treated by either ESWL or ureteroscopy. The percutaneous approach is reserved for those ureteral stones for which ESWL has failed and ureteroscopy is either unsuccessful or contraindicated.

PROCEDURE

Successful percutaneous nephrolithotomy implies the completion of three separate yet interdependent procedures:

1. Percutaneous access or nephrostomy tube placement.
2. Tract dilation to a size sufficient for insertion of the nephroscope.
3. Percutaneous stone removal.

Failure to complete successfully any of the three procedures will result in treatment failures. In experienced hands, success rates approaching 100 per cent are possible.

Candidates for percutaneous stone removal should have sterile urine prior to the procedure. The presence of a urinary tract infection represents a relative surgical contraindication. Patients with complex struvite calculi are admitted 48 hours prior to the procedure and are administered intravenous culture-specific antibiotics prior to the procedure. Standard preoperative blood testing and a type and screen are routinely obtained. Patients taking aspirin on a chronic basis or receiving nonsteroidal antiinflammatory types of drugs must have the medication stopped a suitable length of time prior to the procedure. An excretory urogram (intravenous pyelogram [IVP]) with oblique views is the only standard radiologic study obtained routinely and is considered essential in planning the appropriate access site. Nephrotomograms may be helpful in identifying isolated, poorly calcified calculi but are not routinely obtained. In general, renal pelvic calculi, as well as polar calculi, are approached through the lower pole of the kidney. Stones in the midportion of the kidney or in selected isolated calyces are approached directly. Ureteral stones are best accessed through the mid or upper pole of the kidney (Fig. 16–20).

There are two techniques of achieving intrarenal access: (1) antegrade or (2) retrograde. At most centers where the antegrade approach is preferred, the procedure is performed under the auspices of the urologist with the full cooperation of the invasive radiologist, who typically achieves intrarenal access and in some situations helps in tract dilation. Unfortunately, in many clinical situations, a radiologist skilled and interested in percutaneous techniques may not be readily available to assist in the procedure. Under those circumstances, the urologist must be capable of performing the entire procedure. For the

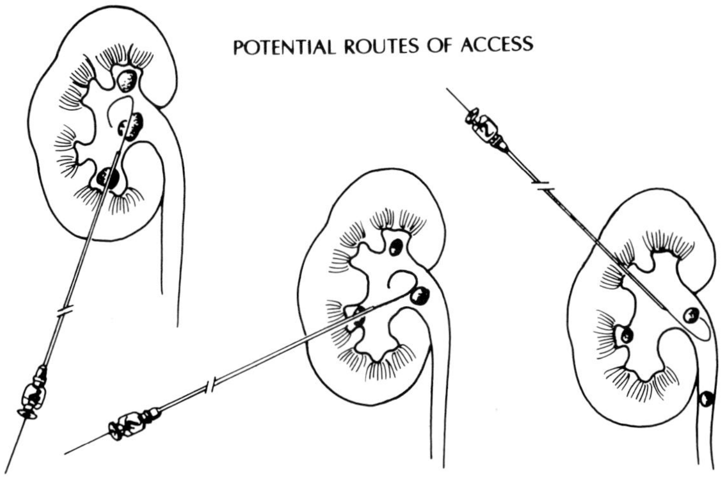

FIGURE 16–20. Renal puncture site is selected based on the location of the stone.

clinician inexperienced in percutaneous techniques, the process of establishing an adequate nephrostomy tract may be frustrating, time consuming, and traumatic to the kidney. In addition, a surgical stone not associated with a dilated collecting system may represent a relative contraindication to the percutaneous approach. The technique of achieving intrarenal access using the retrograde approach, as initially described independently by Lawson[28] and Hunter,[27] represents a suitable alternative to the classic antegrade approach. It utilizes skills and techniques familiar to all trained urologists and may minimize renal trauma while enhancing initial success rates. It is essential that prior to attempting percutaneous stone manipulation the endourologist have an excellent understanding of the intrarenal anatomy and adjacent viscera.

Percutaneous access may be achieved with the patient under local anesthesia, with supplementation of intravenous analgesics as necessary. However, the process of tract dilation and stone removal may be tedious and quite painful; therefore, it is recommended the procedure be performed with the patient under either general or epidural anesthesia.

Percutaneous Access

All of the equipment necessary to achieve successful retrograde access is available in prepackaged kit form from Cook Urological (Spencer, IN). The Lawson retrograde access set is routinely used. The Hawkins-Hunter set provides a stiffer puncture wire and is reserved for patients who have excessive perinephric scarring from prior surgical procedures or for situations in which the calculus completely fills the targeted calyx and infundibulum or in those patients in whom the Lawson approach has failed.

The entire procedure is performed in a standard operating room on an operating table that allows the use of the portable C-arm fluoroscope. After suitable anesthesia has been achieved, the patient is positioned in the lithotomy position. An initial retrograde pyelogram is obtained to delineate the entire ureter and renal collecting system. Under fluoroscopic guidance, the 0.038-inch in diameter, 145-cm-long flexible tip guidewire (Lawson retrograde nephrostomy set; Cook Urological No. 08700) is advanced into the renal pelvis (Fig. 16–21*A*). The 7F polyethylene ureteral catheter is advanced over the guidewire and into the renal pelvis. The guidewire is removed, and the pelvis is filled with contrast medium (Fig. 16–21*B*). The 0.045-inch in diameter deflecting wire is backloaded

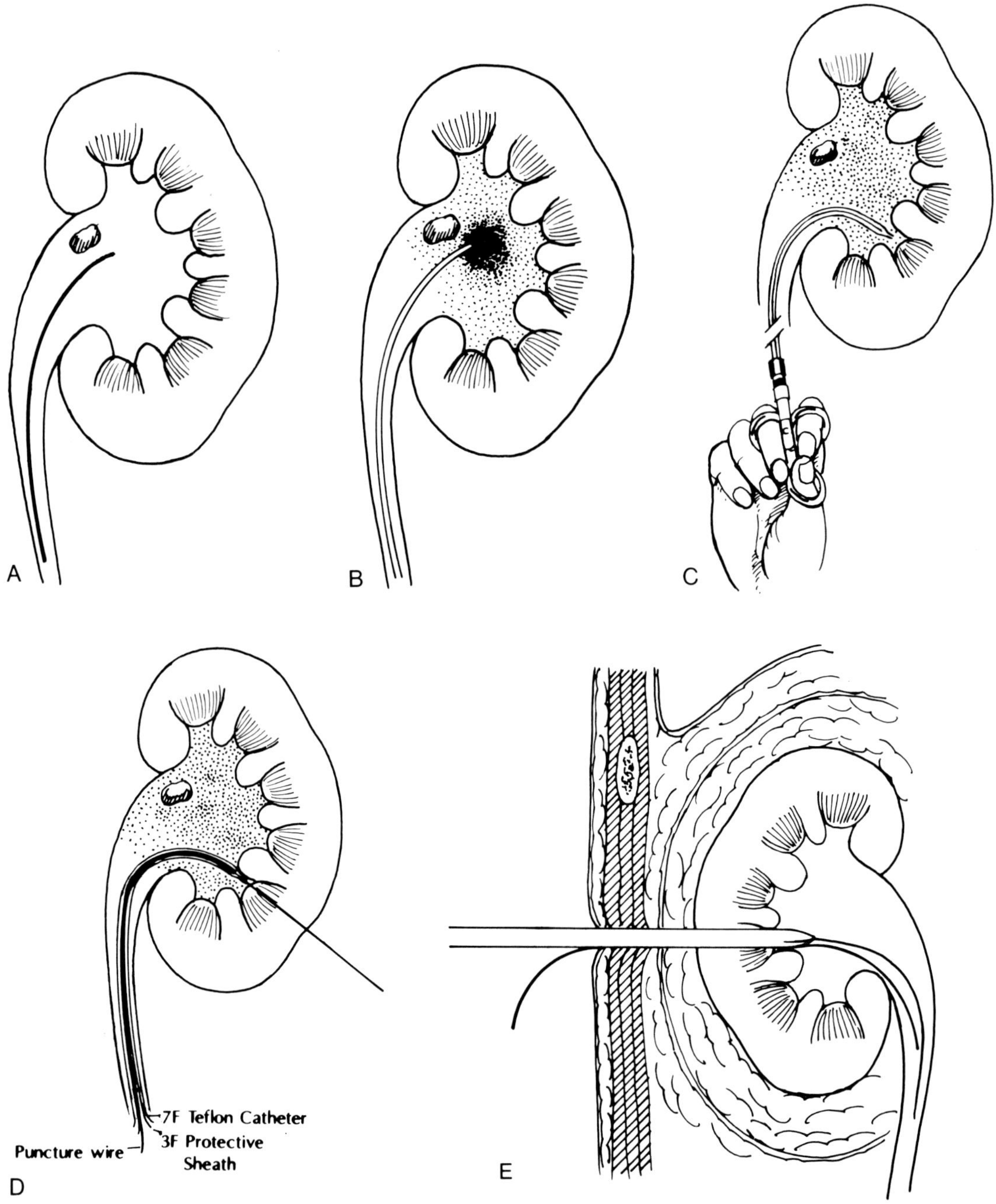

FIGURE 16–21. *A*, Initial guidewire in place. *B*, Retrograde pyelogram is performed through the 7F catheter. *C*, A 7F ureteral catheter is positioned in selected calyx. *D*, Cutting wire is advanced until it is seen exiting the skin. *E*, Dilation performed with Amplatz-type dilators.

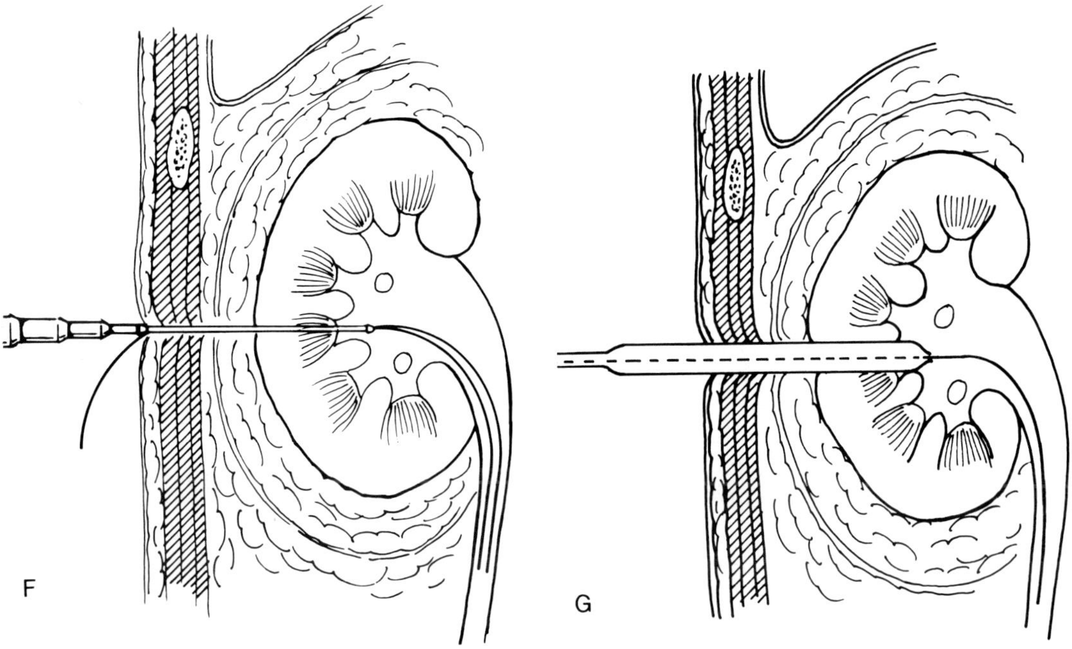

FIGURE 16–21 *Continued F,* Dilation performed with rigid metal coaxial-type dilators. *G,* Dilation performed with a balloon dilator.

through the 7F catheter until both can be twist locked into position. By manipulating the three-ring handle attached to the deflecting wire, the catheter is manually maneuvered under fluoroscopic guidance into the desired infundibulum and embedded in the selected calyx (Fig. 16–21*C*). The deflecting wire is unlocked from the 7F catheter and is carefully removed so as not to dislodge it. The 145-cm-long 0.017-inch in diameter puncture wire encased in its protective 3F Teflon sheath is advanced through the ureteral catheter until both are twist locked into position.

After ensuring that the ureteral catheter has remained in the chosen position, the puncture wire is unlocked and advanced fluoroscopically through the renal parenchyma, renal capsule, perinephric fat, and muscles of the back or flank until it is seen to exit the skin (Fig. 16–21*D*). On occasion, the puncture wire will not penetrate the skin, and a small incision is required to retrieve the puncture wire.

In most instances, either the lower pole calyx or a middle posterior calyx is selected for needle puncture. When access is achieved through a posterior calyx, the nephrostomy tract is shorter and more posterior than is the tract developed through a lower pole calyx. However, as long as the puncture needle exits posterior to the midaxillary line, tract dilation is not more difficult or dangerous to neighboring viscera. If the puncture wire exits anterior to the midaxillary line, it is withdrawn, repositioned more posteriorly, and once again advanced. Complications have not occurred as a result of these aberrant needle sticks.

The puncture wire is advanced from below until the distal end is completely ensheathed in the 7F ureteral catheter. The protective 3F Teflon sheath is unlocked and removed from the 7F ureteral catheter. The hub on the ureteral catheter is cut off, and the cystoscope is removed. Under fluroscopic guidance, the proximal end of the ureteral catheter is withdrawn into the proximal ureter, and the distal end is fixed to a Foley catheter. The ureteral catheter now serves a dual purpose. It is used to administer contrast to aid in tract dilation, and should significant extravasation occur, it may be positioned in the renal pelvis to facilitate drainage. A hemostat is used to stabilize the puncture wire at the skin level, and the patient is placed prone. The 0.017-inch puncture wire is used as the guidewire over which tract dilation is performed. The long 18-gauge needle provided with the nephrostomy set serves as the first fascial dilator and is fluoroscopically positioned in the renal pelvis. Tract dilation continues using the dilators and technique of choice (Fig. 16–21*E–G*). The puncture wire serves as both the working and the safety wires. Passage of a second safety wire is not routinely performed, as it is extremely difficult to dislodge the working wire, which traverses the entire urinary tract and exits the urethra.[69] To avoid lacerating the renal parenchyma, the puncture wire is never pulled from the flank without first placing either a protective fascial dilator or a ureteral catheter over it and into the renal pelvis. Various modifications of this technique have been reported.[28, 29, 31, 70–72]

Alternatively, the nephrostomy tract may be established using the antegrade approach as initially described by Seldinger.[3] The patient is placed in the prone oblique position with the ipsilateral flank elevated approximately 20 degrees[73] (Fig. 16–22*A*). Ultrasonographic, fluoroscopic, or computerized tomographic (CT) guidance may be used to insert the access needle into the collecting system.[74] The optimal puncture site is in the posterior axillary line beneath the twelfth rib. On occasion, it may be necessary to obtain access through the upper pole, which may require a nephrostomy tract above the twelfth rib.[75] By approaching the kidney laterally, the tract will traverse the renal parenchyma before entering the collecting system and thus help hold the catheter in place. This approach will also avoid traumatizing adjacent viscera and will be more comfortable for the patient. When the antegrade approach is used, the needle puncture is performed in the operating room under fluoroscopy. In other clinical settings, renal access is achieved by the radiologist in the radiology suite, with the patient under local anesthesia with intravenous sedation. The collecting system is visualized by the retrograde instillation of contrast. Although the contrast may be given intravenously, opacification of the collecting system may be less than desirable. In the nondilated system, a balloon ureteral occlusion catheter with a central lumen may be used to administer contrast and acutely dilate the collecting system. A 21-gauge needle is introduced into the collecting system (usually a depth of 8 to 10 cm). Aspiration of urine confirms entry into the renal pelvis. Ideally, the needle will enter the collecting system through the calyx of a posteriorly selected infundibulum. Puncture directly into the infundibulum risks significant bleeding from intralobular vessels and is best avoided. Once the position of the needle has been confirmed in the collecting system, a 0.018-inch guidewire is advanced through the needle and positioned in the pelvis (Fig. 16–22*B*). The 21-gauge needle is removed and replaced with a 6.3F dilator. The 0.018-inch guidewire is replaced with a floppy tip 0.038-inch guidewire, which is advanced into the distal ureter (Fig. 16–22*C*). If the guidewire cannot be passed down the ureter, it may be coiled in the renal pelvis or in a dilated calyx. Tract dilation proceeds using the dilators and technique of choice. When the antegrade approach is used, it is desirable to place a second safety wire, which is held in reserve and used only if the working wire becomes dislodged (Fig. 16–22*D*). Prior to proceeding with additional tract dilation, either 20 mg of furosemide (Lasix) or 12.5 gm of mannitol is given intravenously to induce a diuresis,

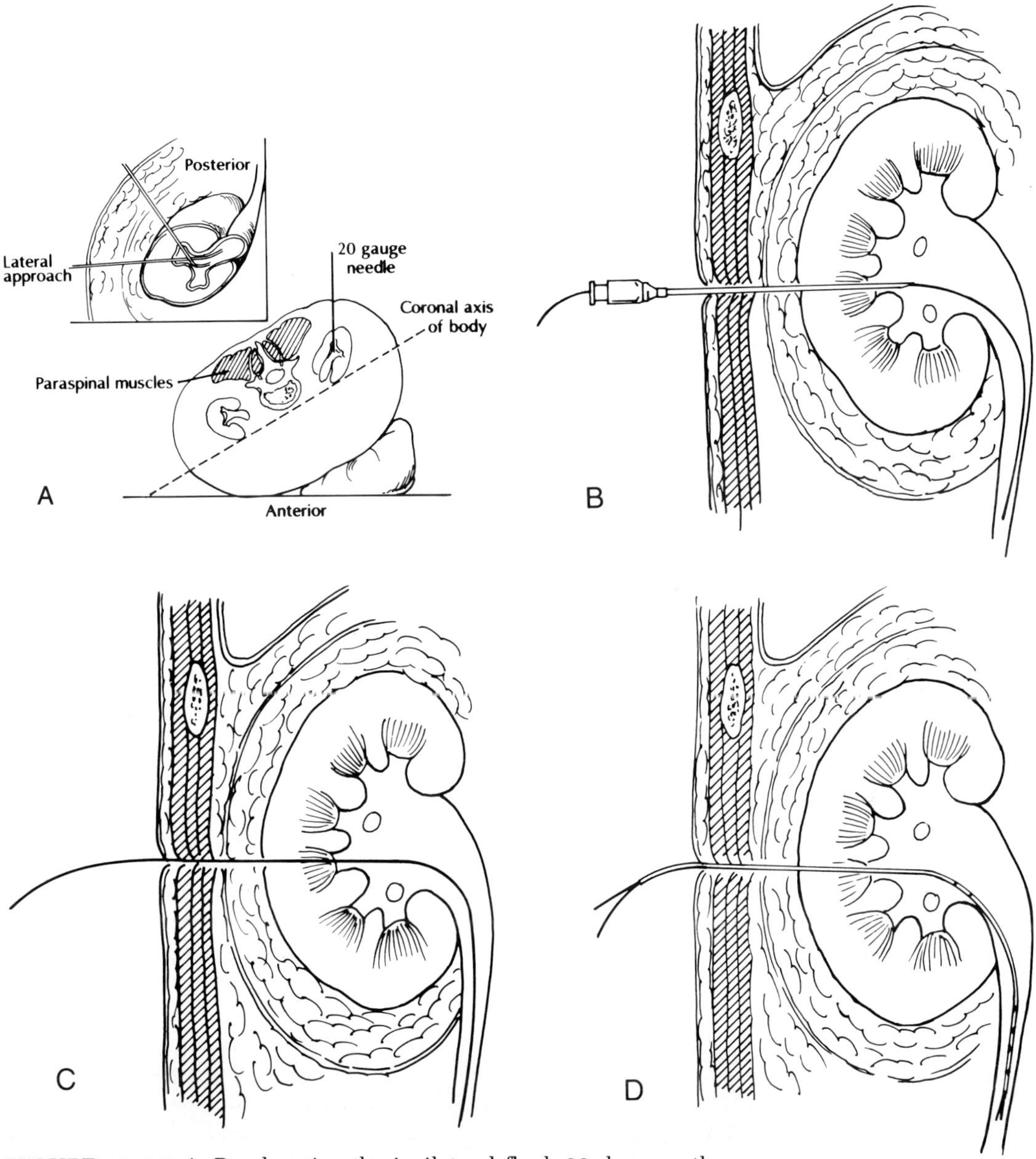

FIGURE 16–22. *A*, By elevating the ipsilateral flank 20 degrees, the targeted posterior calyx lies on end. *B*, A 21-gauge needle is positioned in the renal pelvis, and a 0.018-inch guidewire is passed down the ureter. *C*, A 0.038-inch guidewire is positioned down the ureter. *D*, A second safety wire is positioned in the ureter.

which helps limit blood clot formation and may limit pyelovenous backflow and excessive fluid absorption.

Tract Dilation

The nephrostomy tract is dilated under fluoroscopic guidance, usually to 24F to 36F. There are three basic types of dilators: rigid (metal), semirigid (polyethylene), and balloon (Fig. 16–23). Although each individual has his or her own preference, clinical situations will arise in which use of a specific type of

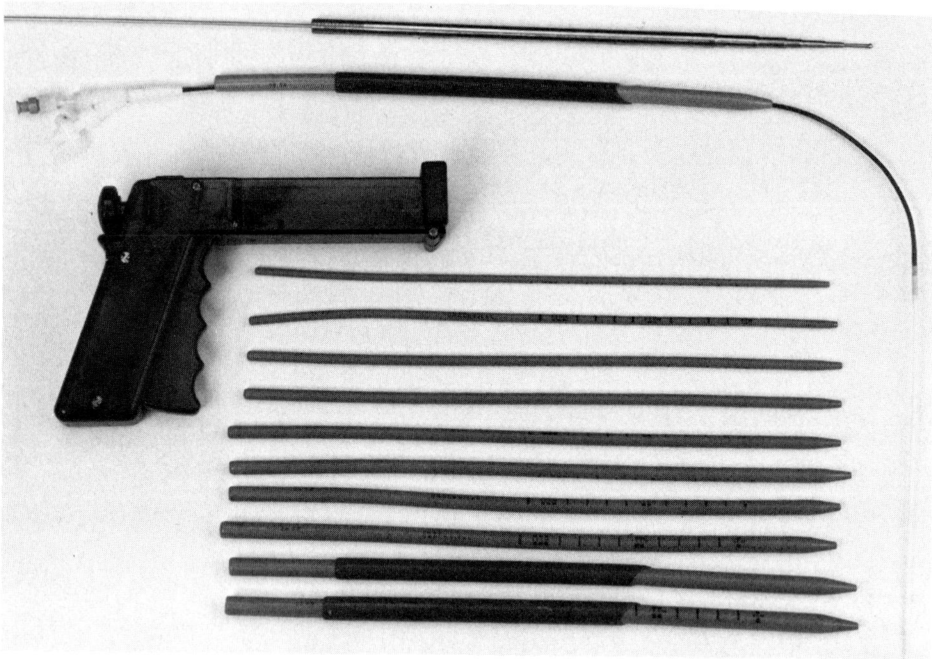

FIGURE 16–23. Three types of fascial dilators: metal (*top*), balloon (*middle*), and semirigid (*bottom*).

dilator is indicated. Therefore, it is recommended that more than one dilator be available.

The rigid metal dilators are preferred in patients who have dense scar from previous renal surgery (Fig. 16–24). They are coaxial in design and consist of a central 8F metal guide over which concentrically larger metal telescoping dilators are passed (12F to 24F). The coaxial telescoping design, similar to that of an antenna, saves time by not requiring each dilator to be removed before passage of the next size and minimizes bleeding by providing a continuous tamponading effect. One disadvantage is that it is easy to perforate the collecting system if the 8F metal guide is advanced too far into the renal pelvis. In addition, if the tract is even slightly curved, the metal guide may not follow the guidewire into the collecting system.

The semirigid (polyethylene) fascial dilators (Amplatz) range in size from 8F

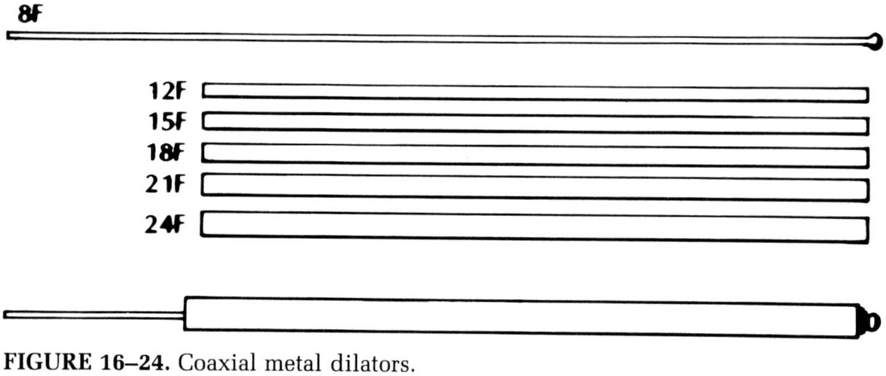

FIGURE 16–24. Coaxial metal dilators.

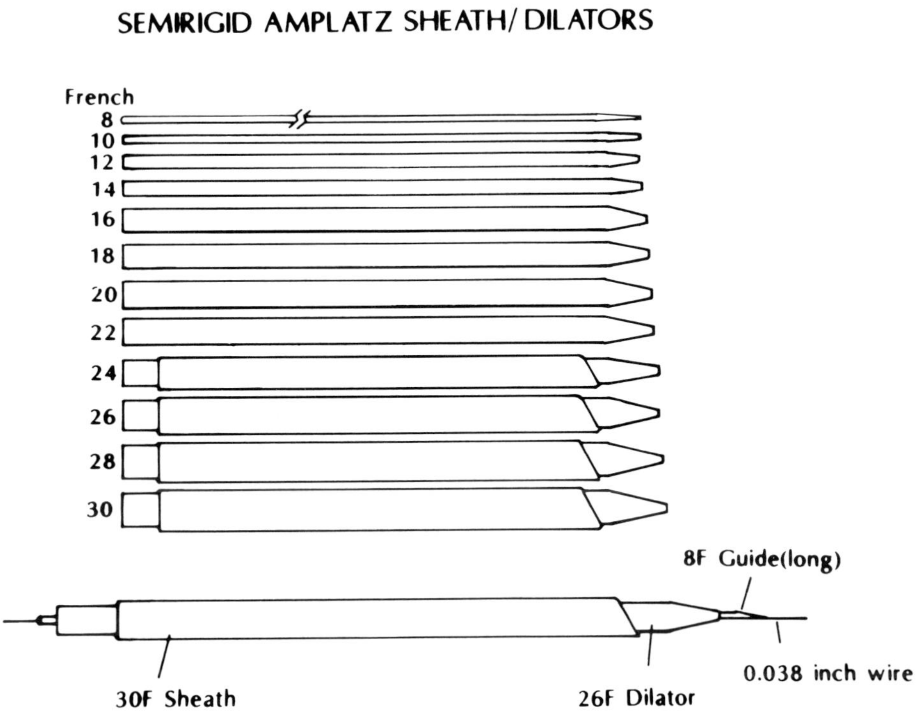

FIGURE 16–25. Semirigid Amplatz-type dilators.

to 30F (Fig. 16–25). The tip of the smaller dilators (8F and 10F) are tapered to fit over a 0.038-inch guidewire, while the larger dilators are tapered to fit snugly over an 8F central guide catheter (long 8), which is passed over the guidewire and down the ureter. This design decreases the chance of buckling the guidewire, which is likely to occur if the larger dilators are passed solely over a guidewire. In addition, the larger dilators (24F to 30F) are equipped with a snugly fitting Teflon working sheath, which may be passed directly over the dilator and into the collecting system. Advantages of the working sheath include continuous tamponade of bleeding vessels, maintenance of the nephrostomy tract during stone manipulation, maintenance of a low-pressure system by allowing ready egress of irrigating fluid, and facilitation of nephrostomy tube placement at the end of the procedure. The Amplatz system takes longer to use than the metal telescoping dilators and probably results in more bleeding from the nephrostomy tract, as each dilator must be removed prior to placing a larger one. Advantages include the low cost and the semirigid construction, which allows tract dilation to proceed even if the path of the guidewire is slightly curved.

The third method of tract dilation is with a balloon dilator (Fig. 16–26). The catheter shaft is 7F to 9F in diameter, with a tapered tip that fits over a 0.038-

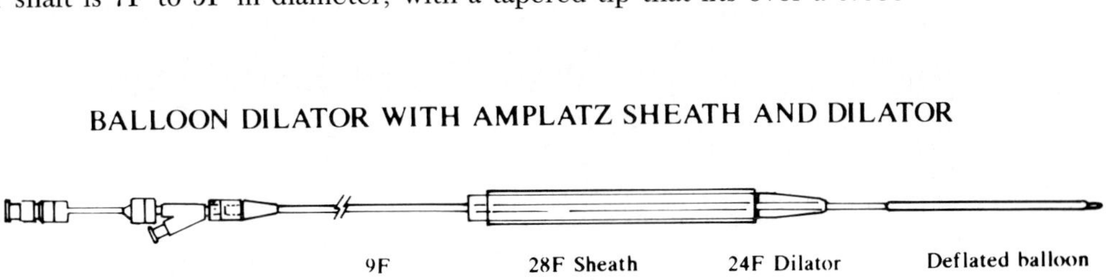

FIGURE 16–26. Balloon dilator.

inch guidewire. The balloon measures 10 to 15 cm in length, can be inflated to 24F to 36F, and is reinforced to withstand 12 to 18 atm of pressure. The radiopaque marker at the distal end of the balloon allows precise placement. Current balloon dilators come equipped with a backloaded 28F or 30F Amplatz dilator and sheath, which may be passed directly over the deflated balloon and into the collecting system once the tract has been dilated. When the balloon dilator is used, the tract must be initially dilated to 12F. The balloon dilator is then fluoroscopically positioned, and with use of the inflation pistol the balloon is maximally inflated. The balloon is deflated, and the backloaded dilator and sheath are positioned in the renal pelvis. The deflated balloon and fascial dilator are then removed. Theoretic advantages include the speed and ease of dilation and decreased bleeding from the tract. A major disadvantage is the cost.[76]

After the tract has been dilated (24F to 30F) and the Amplatz sheath is in position, the operating telescope is placed alongside the puncture wire and into the renal pelvis. A physiologic solution of either normal saline or Ringer's lactate prewarmed to 37°C is used as the irrigant. The height of the irrigant is kept at 40 cm or less above the patient. An attempt is made to visualize the stone. If blood clots obscure the operator's vision, they may be removed by adjusting the flow of irrigant and flushing them with mild suction or manually removing them with a grasping device. The size of the stone that may be removed intact depends on the size of the Amplatz sheath that is being used. Generally, stones up to 1 cm in largest diameter may be removed intact through a 30F sheath (Fig. 16–27). Once the stone is visualized, either it is grasped using one of the many currently available endoscopic forceps or it may be basketed. The stone is extracted under vision by removing it and the operating telescope through the Amplatz sheath. Stones larger than 1 cm are fragmented using the ultrasonic lithotrite (Fig. 16–28). Calyceal or infundibular stones lying at right angles to the nephrostomy tract may be visualized and removed using the flexible nephroscope

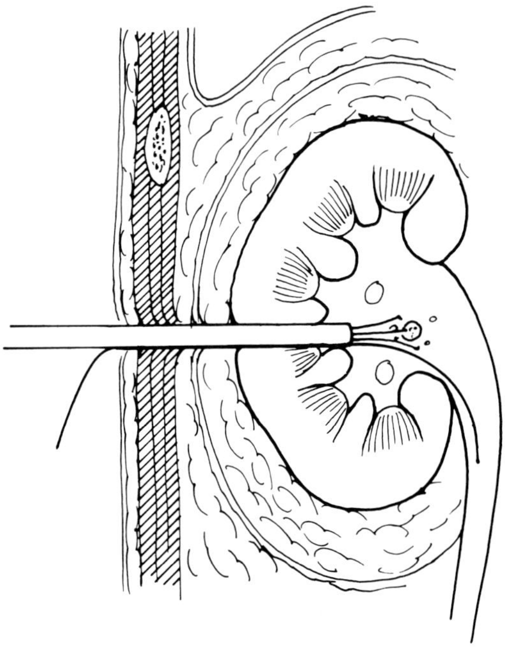

FIGURE 16–27. Small stones are grasped under vision.

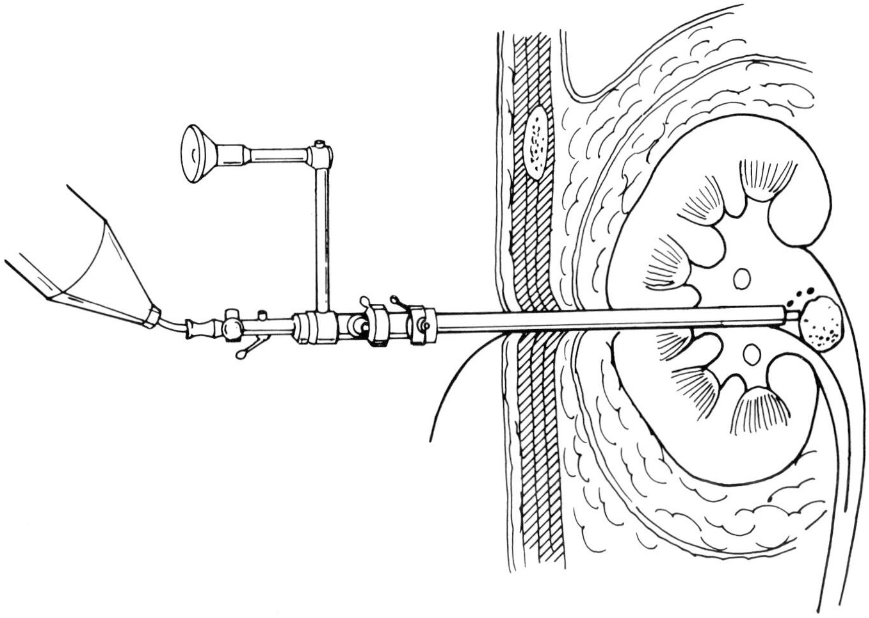

FIGURE 16–28. Large stones are fragmented using the ultrasonic lithotrite.

(Fig. 16–29). If the stone can be seen with the flexible endoscope, it may be grasped or basketed and removed intact. Larger stones may be fragmented with either the 5F electrohydraulic lithotrite or the pulsed dye laser.

Visualization of the stone usually ensures its removal, as evidenced by the Mayo Clinic experience. Segura has reported failure to fragment a visualized stone in only 2 cases out of more than 1400 percutaneous procedures.[77]

After the stone has been removed, a 20F Councill catheter is fluoroscopically

FIGURE 16–29. Stones located at right angles to the nephrostomy tract are removed using the flexible nephroscope.

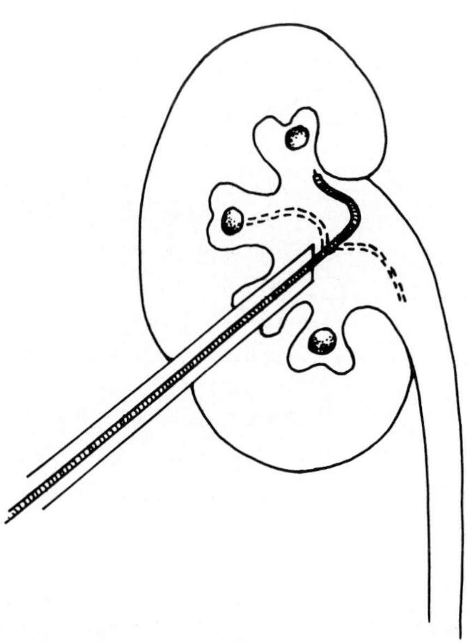

placed through the working sheath over the guidewire. The balloon is inflated with 3 to 5 ml of dilute contrast, and the working sheath is removed by splitting it with heavy scissors. The 0.017-inch puncture guidewire is removed after a nephrostogram has confirmed the proper position of the nephrostomy tube. If extravasation is minimal and the nephrostomy tube is well positioned, the ureteral catheter is also removed. If a second session is required, it is helpful to leave a reentry catheter (either the long 8 or a second end-hole ureteral catheter) down the ureter and brought out as a second access site alongside the nephrostomy tube. The nephrostomy tube and reentry catheter are sutured securely to the skin with nylon suture, and a protective dressing is applied.

The urine is typically bloody for the first 12 to 24 hours. To prevent blood clots from forming and obstructing the catheters, intravenous furosemide (20 mg) is given to promote and maintain a diuresis. Broad-spectrum intravenous antibiotics are continued for the first 24 hours, after which oral antibiotics are continued until all the catheters have been removed. A nephrostogram is performed on postoperative day 2. If all of the stone has been removed and there is free flow of contrast down the ureter without extravasation, the nephrostomy catheter is clamped overnight and removed the following day. The nephrostomy tract site generally closes in 12 to 24 hours. In uncomplicated situations, the patient is discharged on postoperative day 4 or 5. A follow-up IVP is performed 4 to 6 weeks after the procedure. Patients may return to work 1 week after their discharge.

Percutaneous Extraction of Ureteral Stones

The majority of surgical ureteral stones are today managed either by ESWL or by ureteroscopic techniques. However, prior to the widespread availability of ESWL, percutaneous techniques were routinely used to remove stones in both the upper ureter and the midureter. An attempt at percutaneous extraction is still indicated for those stones for which ESWL or ureteroscopic extraction or both fail.[78, 79] The retrieval rate of ureteral stones will be enhanced if the calculus can first be manipulated back into the renal pelvis and then percutaneously extracted (push-pull technique).[80]

In the cystoscopic suite, with the patient in lithotomy position, a floppy tip guidewire is placed under fluoroscopic guidance, and a 6F or 7F end-hole ureteral catheter is advanced over the guidewire to the level of the stone. With the patient in a Trendelenburg position, an attempt is made to push the stone physically back into the renal pelvis by gently manipulating the guidewire while simultaneously pushing the ureteral catheter against the calculus. If this preliminary maneuver fails to dislodge the stone, an attempt is made to flush it back into the renal pelvis using lidocaine jelly.[81] The wire is removed from the ureteral catheter, and under fluoroscopic guidance, 5 to 7 ml of 2 per cent lidocaine jelly diluted with radiographic contrast is vigorously injected through the end-hole catheter. If this procedure fails to reposition the stone in the pelvis, a second attempt is made 3 to 5 minutes later. Lyon has reported 94 per cent (44 of 47 stones) success in repositioning ureteral stones using undiluted lidocaine jelly injected through an 8F to 10F Van Andle catheter.[81] Sterile water,[80] carbon dioxide,[82] saline,[83] dilute radiopaque dye,[82] and 2 per cent lidocaine jelly diluted with saline[84] have all been reported as being useful adjuncts to aid in the repositioning of ureteral stones with varying degrees of success (23 to 94 per cent).[82, 85–88] Lingeman has reported an 86.5 per cent success rate in manipulating proximal ureteral stones back into the kidney using a 6F or 7F balloon occlusion catheter with or without retrograde flushing.[87] Evans and associates[88] attempted to determine the best irrigant for flushing ureteral stones back into the renal pelvis. Seventy-five patients were randomized in a blinded prospective manner to receive instillation of saline, 2 per cent viscous lidocaine, or dilute surgical lubricant. In all patients, an initial attempt to dislodge the stone by catheter manipulation alone had failed. The average stone size in the three groups was slightly greater than 0.9 cm. Nineteen of the 25 patients who received saline irrigation had their stone successfully displaced into the renal pelvis (76 per cent), while 60 per cent of the lidocaine group (15 of 25) and only 48 per cent (12 of 25) of the surgical lubricant group had their stones successfully repositioned. These findings were not statistically significant. Stones in the proximal one third of the ureter had an 80 per cent success rate, while 54 per cent of midureteral stones and only 30 per cent of distal stones were successfully repositioned. In regard to size, stones less than 0.5 cm had a 77 per cent success rate, while stones between 0.6 and 1.0 cm had a 72 per cent success rate and stones larger than 1.0 cm had only a 38 per cent success rate. On the basis of current experience, one can conclude that there is no technique universally accepted by all or no one that has been shown to be significantly better than any other.

After the stone has been repositioned in the renal pelvis, and with the patient still in lithotomy position, a nephrostomy tract is established using the retrograde approach, and the calculus is endoscopically removed (Fig. 16–30). If the stone proves recalcitrant to all attempts at repositioning and remains impacted in the ureter, the patient is placed prone and antegrade access is established. In contrast to renal stones, ureteral stones are best approached through a nephrostomy tract placed through the mid or upper pole of the kidney. Stones impacted in the proximal ureter may be visualized with the rigid nephroscope and removed under vision. Large stones may be fragmented using ultrasound, while smaller stones are either grasped or basketed. Stones that are not accessible with use of the nephroscope may be visualized with flexible instruments. Electrohydraulic or laser lithotripsy is used to fragment large calculi, while smaller stones are grasped or basketed. If the stone is unable to be visualized, an attempt to basket the calculus fluoroscopically may prove successful.

COMPLICATIONS

Although success rates approaching 100 per cent have been reported for percutaneous nephrolithotomy, the procedure is not without morbidity. Complications may occur while obtaining intrarenal access, during nephrostomy tract dilation, or during stone manipulation. Complications unique to each phase of the procedure have been reported. In 1978, Stables and associates[5] reviewed the available literature (516 cases) and published the first large review of patients undergoing percutaneous nephrostomy tube placement for a variety of medical reasons. The procedure was successfully performed in 94 per cent of patients with a major complication rate of only 4 per cent. Related infectious complications were the most frequently encountered and constituted nearly 60 per cent (12 of 21) of all reported major complications. Since many of these patients had preexisting infections not associated with renal stones, the incidence of symptomatic infection should be much less in a stone population and was reported by LeRoy[89] as occurring in only 3 of 716 (0.4 per cent) nephrostomies placed for

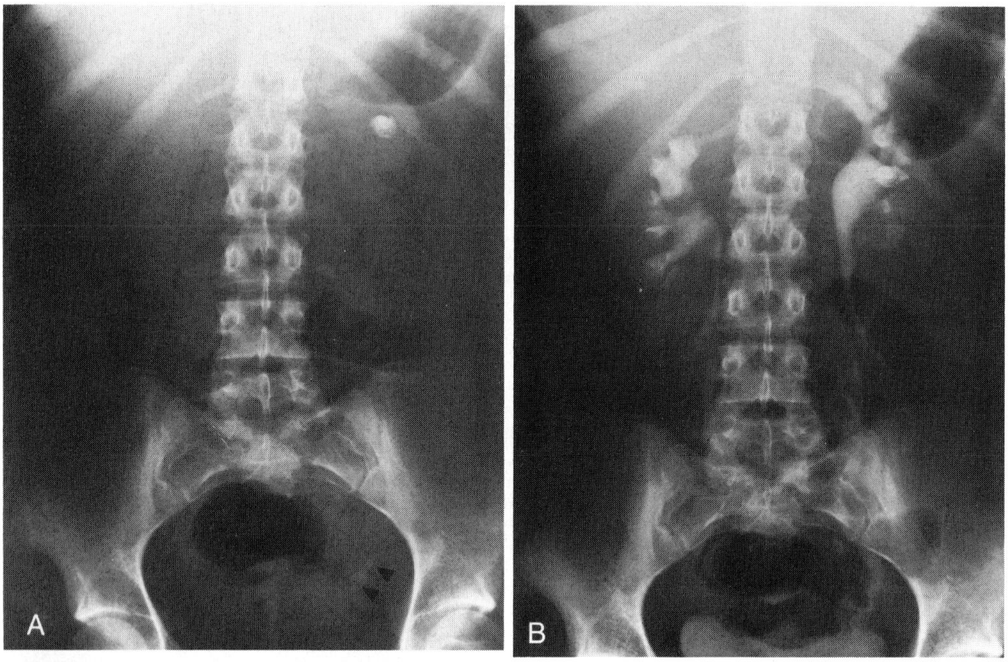

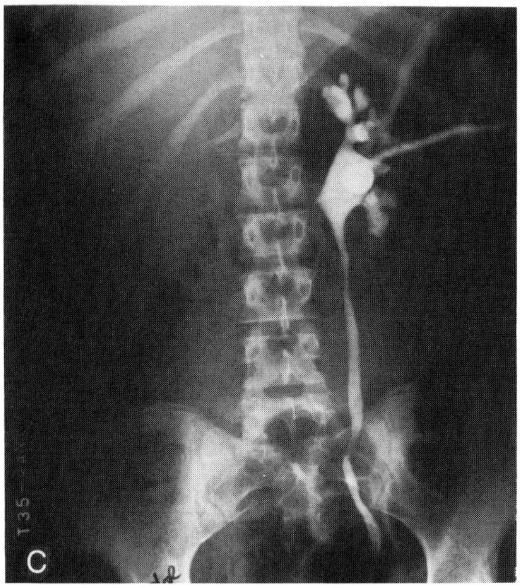

FIGURE 16–30. *A*, Preoperative kidney, ureter, and bladder (KUB) film showing calculus in left kidney and two distal ureteral stones (*arrows*). *B*, Intravenous urogram. *C*, Final nephrotomogram following percutaneous extraction of all stones.

stone disease. Complications of clinically significant bleeding were reported in six patients, and only two required blood transfusions. Although all patients had temporary hematuria, no patient in the LeRoy series required a blood transfusion. No patient in either series died as a direct result of nephrostomy tube placement. Since that initial review, several deaths[4] have been reported.[74] Each death resulted from hemorrhage in a patient with a coagulopathy. The 0.2 per cent mortality compares favorably with the reported 1.3 to 6.0 per cent mortality following surgical nephrostomy placement.[90, 91] Although deaths have occurred in patients with stones who have undergone percutaneous nephrolithotomy, in no instance was the death specifically related to the initial nephrostomy tube placement.[92, 93] Pneumothorax and extravasation from the collecting system were the other major complications reported in the Stables series. Minor complications occurred in 16 per cent of reported patients and were usually related to poor catheter drainage or catheter dislodgment.[5] Improvements in catheter design have all but eliminated these problems.

Failure to access the collecting system is the leading cause of treatment failure and is directly related to the experience of the operator.[92, 94] In a large multiinstitutional survey summarizing over 8000 percutaneous procedures, there was a 1 to 6 per cent failure rate to enter the collecting system.[92] When stratified according to experience, the failure rate was 10 per cent among operators who had performed fewer than 20 procedures. After their first 20 procedures, the failure rate decreased to less than 1 per cent. Similar results have been reported by others.[21, 22] A surgical stone present in a nondilated collecting system is perhaps the most common cause of failure to access the collecting system. Under these circumstances, access rates can be improved by using the retrograde approach or by creating an artificial hydronephrosis by placing a ureteral balloon catheter to obstruct the proximal ureter and injecting saline or contrast into the collecting system (Fig. 16–31). LeRoy and associates[89] have reported a 99.4 per cent success rate in achieving intrarenal access (716 of 720 patients). In their series, more than 50 per cent of all patients had a normal collecting system. All four failures had tightly adherent calyceal stones associated with a hydrocalyx. Clearly, in experienced hands, the failure to access the collecting system percutaneously is rarely a cause of treatment failure.

Bleeding complications associated with percutaneous nephrolithotomy may range from being clinically insignificant to causing hypotension, anuria, perinephric hematoma with risk of abscess formation, and/or emergency nephrectomy.[5, 95–97] Bleeding may occur during initial nephrostomy tube placement or during tract dilation or stone manipulation. Delayed bleeding may occur after

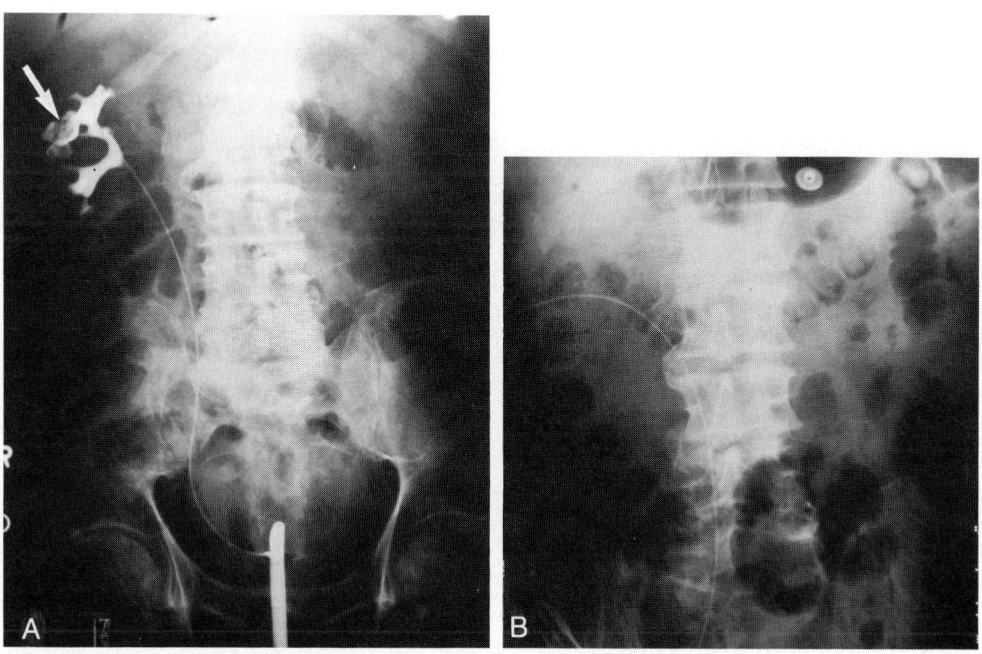

FIGURE 16–31. *A*, Initial retrograde pyelogram showing calyceal stone (*arrow*) in a nondilated collecting system. *B*, Renal access achieved using the retrograde approach.

hospital discharge. Clinically unimportant bleeding occurs in nearly all cases of percutaneous nephrolithotomy and usually clears in 24 to 48 hours. Segura and LeRoy[98] have reported an average change in hemoglobin of about 1.2 gm (1 unit) even in uncomplicated stone cases. Transfusion rates as high as 11 per cent[93] and 53 per cent[26] have been reported and are usually associated with complex stone removal. Clinically significant bleeding has been reported to occur in 0.8 to 3.0 per cent of all stone cases.[96] Acute bleeding may occur from damage to small vessels in the skin of subcutaneous tissue and is usually controlled by final placement of the nephroscope or Amplatz sheath and is seldom responsible for a large blood loss. Clinically insignificant bleeding will also occur from an unavoidable trauma to small cortical renal vessels. The major cause of clinically significant bleeding results from injury to a posterior or an anterior major segmental vessel[97] (Fig. 16–32). To minimize this complication, renal access is best achieved through a posterolateral approach, with the needle directed toward the calyx of a middle or lower pole infundibulum. This path is most likely to traverse Brödel's avascular line and will avoid traumatizing the major intrarenal vessels. The number of needle punctures should likewise be kept to a minimum. The retrograde approach ensures precise needle placement directly through the chosen calyx and minimizes the likelihood of major renal vascular injury occurring from needle puncture. Rarely, significant bleeding may occur from needle damage to an intercostal vessel.

An insignificant amount of bleeding always occurs during tract dilation and stops when the working sheath or nephroscope sheath has been placed into the collecting system. If bleeding persists, making visualization difficult, it is prudent to terminate the procedure and place a large nephrostomy tube. A repeat procedure is delayed for 3 to 5 days to allow the vessel to heal and the tract to mature. If the bleeding persists even after the nephrostomy tube has been placed, the Kaye nephrostomy balloon catheter, designed specifically to tamponade the nephrostomy tract, is placed.[99] Persistent bleeding in spite of these measures requires angiographic evaluation with embolization of the bleeding vessel. If all these measures fail to control the bleeding, surgical exploration is

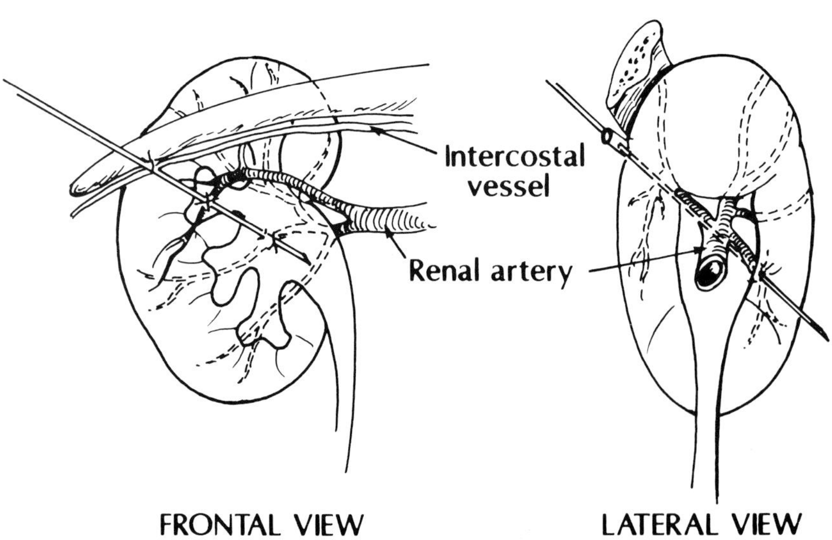

FIGURE 16–32. Vessels susceptible to injury while percutaneous access is being achieved.

indicated. Delayed bleeding reported as long as 12 weeks following stone removal[100] suggests the possibility of an arteriovenous fistula and is evaluated by angiography and treated by selective embolization. The incidence is less than 1 per cent in patients undergoing percutaneous nephrostomy with or without stone removal.[93]

Extravasation of contrast from the collecting system is a common finding on the final nephrostogram performed at the end of the procedure (31 per cent in some series)[94] and in most instances does not represent a true complication, as the majority of these heal without sequelae. Large perforations occurring early in the procedure are best managed by nephrostomy tube placement and termination of the procedure. Complications seldom occur, providing the drainage is adequate, and in most instances a repeat nephrostogram will be normal in 24 to 36 hours. The intraperitoneal accumulation of irrigating fluid has been reported and represents the most serious sequela of an unrecognized intraperitoneal perforation.[101]

Because of the kidney's intimate anatomic relationship with the colon, duodenum, liver, spleen, and pleura, these organs are susceptible to trauma during initial nephrostomy tube placement.[92] Transcolonic stone manipulation is a rare but increasingly reported complication, with a reported incidence of 0.2 to 0.5 per cent.[65, 102, 103] Although operative intervention has been reported,[104] conservative treatment consisting of parenteral antibiotics and nephrostomy tube removal will be therapeutic, provided the injury is confined to the retroperitoneum. The staged removal of the tube,[94, 98] as advocated by some, does not appear to be essential for a satisfactory outcome. Variations in the normal anatomic relationship of the colon to the kidney may increase the risk of colon injury. A posterolateral colon has been reported in 3 to 19 per cent of individuals, and a retrorenal colon has been reported in about 0.5 per cent of the population.[105, 106] In the absence of anatomic variants, colonic injuries may be avoided by positioning the nephrostomy tract posterior to the posterior axillary line.

The risk of pleural injury is slight when percutaneous access is obtained below the twelfth rib. However, in certain clinical situations, it is desirable or essential to achieve access above the twelfth rib. In those situations, there is a higher risk of pleural injury with subsequent pneumothorax, hydrothorax, or hemothorax. These complications have been reported in 0.1 to 3.0 per cent of patients undergoing percutaneous nephrolithotomy and will respond to chest tube placement.[92, 93, 107]

Splenic, hepatic, and duodenal injuries, although reported, are exceptionally rare.[92, 108] In clinically stable patients, conservative management of these injuries may be therapeutic.[95] Surgical intervention is obviously indicated if the patient is clinically unstable.

Death is a regrettable complication of any surgical procedure and, as one would expect, has been reported in association with percutaneous nephrolithotomy. Lang reported four deaths out of a total of 8595 attempted stone procedures (0.046 per cent).[92] Three deaths were attributable to hemorrhage: two renal artery tears and one venous laceration. The fourth death was due to overwhelming gram-negative septicemia. Deaths attributable to pulmonary and cardiac complications have also been reported.[93]

Postprocedural temperature elevation ($\geq$38.5°C) is common and has been reported in nearly 25 per cent of all patients.[93] In spite of this relatively common febrile response, the incidence of sepsis and other infectious complications (e.g., perinephric abscess) is low ($\leq$1.0 per cent).[92, 94, 107] An active urinary tract infection represents a relative contraindication to percutaneous stone manipulation. All patients with sterile urine are given prophylactic antibiotics prior to the procedure. Individuals with complex struvite calculi are at high risk for septic complications because of the liberation of bacteria from the stone and the absorption of infected irrigant. These patients are hospitalized 2 days prior to the procedure and are treated with intravenous culture-specific antibiotics. An aminoglycoside and synthetic penicillin (usually mezlocillin) are given prophylactically and continued for 24 to 36 hours after the procedure. In spite of these precautions, patients with complex calculi are at high risk for the development of urosepsis, with an incidence as high as 26.6 per cent being reported.[26]

Although a number of concerns have been raised regarding the long-term side effects of percutaneous stone removal on both the patient and the operator, long-term complications have not been reported.

Animal studies designed to evaluate the effects of nephrostomy tube placement and tract dilation on renal function have shown the procedure to be safe and to result in no significant change in renal function. Webb and Fitzpatrick[109] performed open nephrostomy tube placement and tract dilation in dogs. Intravenous urography at 48 hours either was normal or showed a faint linear parenchymal defect. The microscopic appearance of the kidneys was normal except for a small capsular defect at the site of nephrostomy insertion. On gross section, the site of the nephrostomy tract was hemorrhagic, but the rest of the kidney appeared normal. At 6 weeks, only a small dimple was noted on the renal surface. On gross section, the nephrostomy site had healed to a fine linear scar. Ex situ arteriograms and casts of the collecting systems were normal or showed minimal peripheral small vessel damage. No major renal vessel damage was identified. Creatinine clearance studies at 48 hours and 6 weeks showed no significant changes compared with the normal contralateral kidney. One criticism of this study was that the initial nephrostomy tracts were established at open surgery using a 6F dilator and not a nephrostomy needle. Boyd and Boyce[110] established retrograde access in porcine kidneys and studied casts of the vascular system. They reported a 1 to 2 per cent loss of vascularity and attributed it to vascular trauma induced at the time of needle puncture. Clayman[111] performed antegrade access in pigs using the same technique applied to patients with stones and dilated the nephrostomy tract either to 24F with Amplatz dilators or to 36F with a balloon dilator and noted renal damage estimated at 0.15 per cent of the total cortical surface. There was no significant difference in the amount of renal damage caused by the two techniques.

Clinical investigators have reported similar findings in patients with stones. Marberger[112] studied 82 patients from 1.0 to 3.5 years (mean, 22 months) after percutaneous lithotripsy and noted no significant morphologic changes based on serial CT scans. Functional studies showed no adverse effects and were actually improved in some instances in which preoperative obstruction had been present. Corroborative findings have been reported by others.[113–115] Similarly, Lang reported no change in renal function in 19 of 20 patients who required two or more nephrostomy tracts for stone removal.

Initial concern over hearing damage[116] induced by frequent use of the ultrasound probe and exposure to sound levels that may exceed 90 decibels has proved unwarranted. Audiograms performed on operating personnel not protected by ear plugs remained unchanged from baseline studies.[112]

The amount of fluoroscopy time for percutaneous nephrolithotomy is generally longer than that required for most other radiologic procedures. Therefore, the significance of radiation exposure to patient and operator has been questioned (Fig. 16–33). Standard fixed fluoroscopy or portable C-arm units typically have

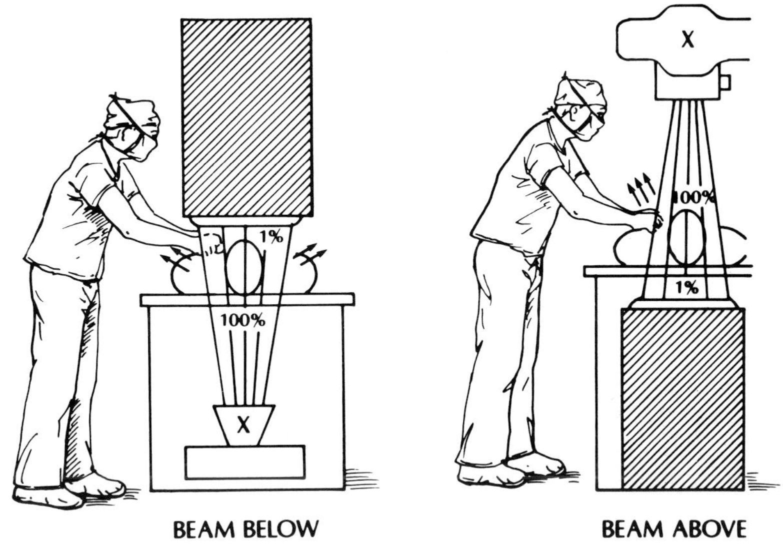

FIGURE 16–33. Common configuration of available fluoroscopy units. *Left*, Recommended x-ray tube position under the patient minimizes the operator's radiation exposure. *Right*, Excessive scattering will occur when the x-ray tube is positioned above the patient.

the x-ray tube beneath the table, with the image intensifier above the patient. This arrangement minimizes the exposure to the operator. Ninety-five per cent of the radiation beam is absorbed as it traverses the patient's body, 3 per cent is lost or scattered, and only 2 per cent strikes the image intensifier. This x-ray arrangement minimizes significantly the risk to the operator when compared with x-ray units that deliver the beam from above the patient. Scatter radiation can be further reduced by positioning the image intensifier close to the patient's back. In spite of the limited exposure, it is recommended that certain precautions be taken. Lead glasses, thyroid shield, and lead aprons are mandatory for all operators performing more than 90 procedures per year.[53] By taking these precautions, it has been estimated that about 400 examinations per year could be safely performed without exceeding the safety standards prescribed by the National Council on Radiation Protection.[53] Clinical studies by Rao[117] and Bush[118] have confirmed the safety of percutaneous procedures in regard to radiation exposure.

RESULTS

The primary objective of renal stone surgery has always been a stone-free patient. A testimonial to this goal is the number of different surgical stone procedures, each designed to facilitate the removal of a specific type or configuration of calculus. In addition, a number of intraoperative and postoperative adjunctive procedures have been employed to help identify and remove residual fragments. In spite of this goal, residual stone rates ranging from 5 to 45 per cent have been reported.[119–122] Why has there been such an intense effort to render the patient stone free, and why is a low residual stone rate used to measure the success of a specific surgical approach? Residual stones represent a potential source for both immediate and delayed patient morbidity, the most

TABLE 16–1. ANTEGRADE PERCUTANEOUS

FIRST AUTHOR (REF. NO.)	TIME SERIES COMPILED (YR. PUB.)	SELECTION CRITERIA	NO. PTS.	NO. STONES
Wickham (21)	NA (1983)	Consecutive	50 20	NA NA
White (126)	NA (1984)	NA First 200	200	235
Clayman (127)	1/79–12/82 (1984)	Branched/staghorns excluded	82	105
Streem (125)	13 mo (1985)	NA	91	NA
Segura (107)	10/81–6/84 (1985)	NA	805	NA
Bass (128)	11/82–2/84 (1985)	Limited to ≤2 cm	43	NA
Brannen (22)	11/82–11/84 (1985)	Consecutive	250	345
Reddy (65)	12/82–NA (1985)	Consecutive	332	602
Goldwasser (130)	NA (1986)	NA First 210	210/221 kidneys	
Lingeman (129)	6/83–10/84 1987	NA	74	NA

NA = not available; KUB = kidney, ureter, and bladder; X-R = X-ray; OR = operating room.

serious of which is the need for reoperation. Stone fragments may become dislodged in the immediate postoperative period and cause pain, obstruction, sepsis, and/or urinary extravasation. Residual fragments of struvite calculi represent a continued source of bacteriuria, a prerequisite essential for stone growth or new stone formation.[123, 124] For metabolic stones (calcium, cystine, and uric acid), the significance of the residual fragment is less clear. It has never been

TABLE 16–2. RETROGRADE PERCUTANEOUS

FIRST AUTHOR (REF. NO.)	TIME SERIES COMPILED (YR. PUB.)	SELECTION CRITERIA	TECHNIQUE	NO. PTS./ KIDNEYS
Hunter (30)	2/83–10/83 (1985)	Consecutive	Hunter-Hawkins	30/NA
Hosking (29)	11/84–NA (1986)	Consecutive	Lawson Hunter-Hawkins (6)	47/51*
Spirnak (32)	8/84–9/85 (1987)	26 consecutive 2 failed antegrade	Lawson	28/30
Morrisseau (71)	22 mo (1988)	Consecutive	Lawson Hunter-Hawkins (2)	71/71
Leal (70)	982–7/86 (1988)	Consecutive (2 staghorns excluded)	Hunter-Hawkins (78) Antegrade (7)	78/NA

NEPHROLITHOTOMY (RESULTS)

Success/ Attempted (%)	Residual Stone Rate	Method to Detect Residual Stones	Failure (%)	No. Procedures	Comments
30/50 (60) 18/20 (90)	NA	NA	22/70 (31)	Repeat 17/30	Stone size not listed
226/235 (96)	NA	NA	Stratified 10/20 (50) 4/82 (5) 3/98 (3)	11/15 staghorns ≥2	10% transfusion Learning curve emphasized
98/105 (93)	2%	Tomograms	(7)	≈2	Results stratified by experience
86/91 (94)	NA	NA	(6)	NA	—
791/805 (98.3)	Fragments of targeted stones 8.1%	KUB ± tomograms	(1.7)	Repeat 12.5%	—
33/43 (77)	2.5%	KUB	(23)	NA	Community series
243/250 (97)	NA	Tomograms	(3)	33 (13% in X-R) 20 (8% in OR)	No mention as to how many of 345 stones removed
328/332 (99)	(1%)	Tomograms	All kidneys accessed	Repeat—54% ≥3—13%	Includes branched calculi—best results in literature based on residual stone rate
160/221* (72.4)	(25%)	Plain film ± tomograms	(2.7)	NA	*Success = complete removal of all stones
64% at discharge* 86% at 3 mo	NA	NA	NA	Repeat 17%	*Success = stone free or asymptomatic fragments ≤4 mm and not struvite; staghorn calculi excluded from this series

clearly shown that residual fragments are associated with new stone formation, provided the underlying metabolic cause has been elucidated and corrected. The need for repeat operation for renal stones is associated with a much higher rate of complication and nephrectomy. Therefore, prior to the availability of less invasive stone procedures (i.e., percutaneous nephrolithotomy, ESWL), heroic attempts to achieve a stone-free status were indicated.

NEPHROLITHOTOMY (RESULTS)

Nephrostomy Success (%)	Stone Removal Success/Attempted (%)	Overall Success (%)	Residual Stone (%)	Comments
28/31 (90)	25/28 (89)	25/30 (83)	NA	—
49/51 (96)	46/46 (100)	46/48 (90)	NA	*3 nephrostomy tubes placed for irrigation; Hunter-Hawkins used when Lawson failed
28/30 (93)	26/28 (93)	26/30 (87)	2/28 (7)	Failed access, 2 staghorns; all stones removed in 1 session; transfusions—0
71/71 (100)	61/71 (86)	61/71* (86)	NA	Multiple procedures; 100% success (8–2 procedures; 2–3 procedures) transfusions—0
76/78 (97)	*85/85	85/85†	11/85 (13)	*Results not stratified based on access technique. †Multiple procedures (15–2 procedures; 1–4 procedures)

NA = not available.

TABLE 16–3. PERCUTANEOUS COMPLEX

First Author (Ref. No.)	Time Series Compiled (Yr. Pub)	No. Pts.	Success	Residual Stone Rate
Snyder (26)	7/83–NA (1986)	75	86.7% stone free	10 (13.3%)*
White (126)	NA (984)	15	87% stone free	2 (13%)*
Winfield (131)	10/84–11/85 (1988)	23 (16 partial, 7 complete)	86% stone free	3/22 (14%)*
LeRoy (132)	4/85–4/86 (1987)	143	143 (100)*	60 (42%)

With the emergence of less invasive stone procedures as successful alternatives to open surgical removal for all but the most complex renal stones came the realization that multiple or repeat percutaneous (or ESWL) procedures were not necessarily associated with the significant morbidity found in repeat open stone procedures. In addition, aggressive efforts to reach peripheral asymptomatic metabolic calculi percutaneously could only increase patient morbidity while not necessarily enhancing the surgical outcome (in terms of recurrent stone formation). Therefore, the concept of targeted stone emerged as a measure of surgical success and replaced a stone-free status as the primary objective for all but struvite calculi.

Success rates approaching nearly 100 per cent have been reported in large series using either antegrade or retrograde percutaneous techniques to remove renal calculi (Tables 16–1 and 16–2). When stratified according to stone size, higher success rates are associated with smaller stones (≤1 cm), which do not require fragmentation but may be removed intact. The more complex the configuration, the greater the chance of failure and the higher the residual stone rate (Table 16–3). Regardless of the technique or the size of the stone, residual stone rates ranging from less than 1 per cent to 42 per cent have been reported.

TABLE 16–4. PERCUTANEOUS REMOVAL OF URETERAL STONES (RESULTS)

First Author (Ref. No.)	Time Series Compiled (Yr. Pub.)	No. Pts. (No. Stones)	Success (%)	Failure (%)	Comment
White (126)	NA (1984)	49	38 (78)	11 (22)	Stones in all levels of ureter
Clayman (127)	1/79–12/82 (1984)	(44)	(63)	(37)	—
Segura (107)	10/81–6/84 (1985)	195	172 (88)	23 (11.8)	Primary reason for failure: unable to engage stone in basket
Reddy (65)	12/82–NA (1985)	68 (72)	64 (94.5)	(5.5)	—
Kahn (86)	9/82–3/84 (1986)	60	57 (95)	(5)	Stones throughout ureter Success in proximal 35/37; in mid, 20/20, in distal, 2/3
Lingeman (129)	6/83–10/84 (1987)	36	34 (94)	(6)	—

RENAL STONE REMOVAL (RESULTS)

No. Procedures	Comments
Average, 1.24; 16 (21.4%) required multiple procedures	All patients had staghorn calculi Stone volume not estimated *All asymptomatic <5 mm Renacidin used
11 (70%) ≥2 procedures	*No mention how determined Stone volume not determined Renacidin used
Average, 2.7	*Based on tomograms and/or CT Renacidin used
59 (42%) required multiple procedures	*Targeted stone All patients deemed not candidates for ESWL (>3 cm)

These results are comparable to those following open surgical removal. Success rates approaching nearly 95 per cent have been reported for ureteral stones (Table 16–4). Stones located in the proximal ureter and midureter are associated with higher success rates than are distal stones.

Another concept that emerged during the percutaneous era is that of learning curve. This concept implies that initial success rates will be lower while the operators become familiar with a new technique (20 to 50 cases), and it was substantiated by the less than favorable initial results reported in a number of reviews.[21, 92] The retrograde approach utilizes techniques familair to all urologists and in some reports was thought to minimize the learning curve.

REFERENCES

1. Rupel E, Brown R: Nephroscopy with removal of stone following nephrostomy for obstructive calculous anuria. J Urol 46:177, 1941.
2. Alken P: Percutaneous ultrasonic destruction of renal calculi. Urol Clin North Am 9:145, 1982.
3. Seldinger SI: The Seldinger technique—catheter replacement of the needle in percutaneous arteriography. AJR 142:5, 1984.
4. Goodwin WE, Casey WC, Woolf W: Percutaneous trocar (needle) nephrostomy in hydronephrosis. JAMA 157:891, 1955.
5. Stables DP, Ginsberg NJ, Johnson ML: Percutaneous nephrostomy: A series and review of the literature. AJR 130:75, 1978.
6. Smith AD, Lange PH, Fraley EE: Application of percutaneous nephrostomy: New challenges and opportunities in endo-urology. J Urol 121:382, 1979.
7. Fernström I, Johansson B: Percutaneous pyelolithotomy. Scand J Urol Nephrol 10:257, 1976.
8. Smith AD, Reinke DB, Miller RP, et al: Percutaneous nephrostomy in the management of ureteral and renal calculi. Radiology 133:49, 1979.
9. Raney AM, Handler J: Electrohydraulic nephrolithotripsy. Urology 6:86, 1975.
10. Kurth KH, Hohenfellner R, Altwein JE: Ultrasound litholapaxy of a staghorn calculus. J Urol 117:242, 1977.
11. Alken P, Hutschenreiter G, Günther R, Marberger M: Percutaneous stone manipulation. J Urol 125:463, 1981.
12. Trattner HR: Instrumental visualization of the renal pelvis and its communications: Proposal of a new method. J Urol 60:817, 1948.
13. Leadbetter WF: Instrumental visualization of the renal pelvis at operation as an aid to diagnosis: Presentation of a new instrument. J Urol 63:1006, 1950.
14. Gittes RF: Nephroscopy. Urol Clin North Am 6:555, 1979.

15. Marberger M, Stackl W, Hruby W: Percutaneous litholapaxy of renal calculi with ultrasound. Eur Urol 8:236, 1982.
16. Clayman RV, Miller RP, Reinke DB, Lange PH: Nephroscopy: Advances and adjuncts. Urol Clin North Am 9:51, 1982.
17. Bissada NK, Meacham KR, Redman JF: Nephroscopy with removal of renal pelvic calculi. J Urol 112:414, 1974.
18. Segura JW, Patterson DE, LeRoy AJ, et al: Percutaneous removal of kidney stones. Mayo Clin Proc 57:615, 1982.
19. Kahn RI: Nonsurgical technique for removal of upper urinary tract stones. Contemp Surg 22:35, 1983.
20. Smith AD, Lee WJ, Benderev T: Percutaneous management of urinary calculi: Clinical status of a new approach. Intern Med Specialist 4:1, 1983.
21. Wickham JEA, Kellett MJ, Miller RA: Elective percutaneous nephrolithotomy in 50 patients: An analysis of the technique, results and complications. J Urol 129:904, 1983.
22. Brannen GE, Bush WH, Correa RJ, et al: Kidney stone removal: Percutaneous versus surgical lithotomy. J Urol 133:6, 1985.
23. Preminger GM, Clayman RV, Hardeman SW, et al: Percutaneous nephrostolithotomy vs. open surgery for renal calculi. JAMA 254:1054, 1985.
24. Clayman RV, Surya V, Miller RP, Castaneda-Zuniga WR, et al: Percutaneous nephrolithotomy: An approach to branched and staghorn renal calculi. JAMA 250:73, 1983.
25. Elder JS, Gibbons RP, Bush WH: Ultrasonic lithotripsy of a large staghorn calculus. J Urol 131:1152, 1984.
26. Snyder JA, Smith AD: Staghorn calculi: Percutaneous extraction versus anatrophic nephrolithotomy. J Urol 136:351, 1986.
27. Hunter PT, Hawkins IF, Finlayson B, et al: Hawkins-Hunter retrograde transcutaneous nephrostomy: A new technique. Urology 22:583, 1983.
28. Lawson RK, Murphy JB, Taylor AJ, Jacobs SC: Retrograde method for percutaneous access to kidney. Urology 22:580, 1983.
29. Hosking DH: Retrograde nephrostomy: Experience with 2 techniques. J Urol 135:1146, 1986.
30. Hunter PT, Finlayson B, Drylie DM, et al: Retrograde nephrostomy in percutaneous calculus removal in 30 patients. J Urol 133:369, 1985.
31. Spirnak JP, Resnick MI: Retrograde percutaneous stone removal using modified Lawson technique. Urology 30:551, 1987.
32. Spirnak JP: Retrograde percutaneous nephrostolithotomy: An acceptable alternative to antegrade techniques. J Urol 137:841, 1987.
33. Chaussy C, Brendel W, Schmiedt E: Extracorporeally induced destruction of kidney stones by shock waves. Lancet 2:1265, 1980.
34. Lingeman JE, Newman D, Mertz JHO, et al: Extracorporeal shock wave lithotripsy: The Methodist Hospital of Indiana experience. J Urol 135:1134, 1986.
35. Miller RA, Wickham JEA: Percutaneous nephrolithotomy: Advances in equipment and endoscopic techniques. Urology [Suppl] 23:2, 1984.
36. Segura JW: Endourology. J Urol 132:1079, 1984.
37. Mulvaney WP: Attempted disintegration of calculi by ultrasonic vibration. J Urol 70:704, 1953.
38. Coates CE: The application of ultrasound energy to urinary and biliary calculi. J Urol 75:865, 1956.
39. Goodfriend R: Disintegration of ureteral calculi by ultrasound. Urol Int 28:260, 1973.
40. Terhorst B, Cichos M, Versin F, et al: Der Einfluss von electrohydraulischer Schlagwelle und Ultraschall auf das Uroepithel. Urologe A14:41, 1975.
41. Howard SS, Merill E, Harris S, et al: Ultrasonic lithotripsy: Laboratory evaluations. Invest Urol 11:273, 1974.
42. Marberger M: Disintegration of renal and ureteral calculi with ultrasound. Urol Clin North Am 10:729, 1983.
43. Lutzeyer W, Pohlmann R, Terhorst B, et al: Die Zerstörung von Harnsteinen durch Ultraschall. Urol Int 25:47, 1970.
44. Gasteyer KH: Eine neue Methode der Blasensteinzert Rummerung: Die Ultraschall Lithotripsie. Urologe A10:30, 1971.
45. Marx GF, Orkin LR: Complications associated with transurethral surgery. Anesthesiology 23:802, 1962.
46. Carson CC, Nesbitt JA: Peritoneal extravasation during percutaneous lithotripsy. J Urol 134:725, 1985.
47. Schultz RE, Hanno PM, Wein AJ, et al: Percutaneous ultrasonic lithotripsy: Choice of irrigant. J Urol 130:858, 1983.
48. Spirnak JP, Resnick MI: Hyperammonemia induced coma: A potential complication of transurethral prostatic resection. *In* Proceedings of the Annual Meeting of the North Central Section of the American Urological Association, Detroit, September 17, 1987, p 59.
49. Bülow H, Frohmüller HGW: Electrohydraulic lithotripsy with aspiration of the fragments under vision—304 consecutive cases. J Urol 126:454, 1981.
50. Rouvalis P: Electronic lithotripsy for vesical calculus with "Urat-1": An experience of 100 cases

and an experimental application of the method to stones in the upper urinary tract. Br J Urol 42:486, 1970.
51. Watson GM: Laser fragmentation of urinary calculi. *In* Smith JA (ed): Lasers in Urologic Surgery. Chicago, Year Book Medical Publishers, 1985, pp 120–137.
52. Clayman RV: Techniques in percutaneous removal of renal calculi. Urology [Suppl] 23:11, 1984.
53. Clayman RV: Endourology. Mongr Urol 6:50, 1985.
54. Mulvaney WP, Beck CW: The laser beam in urology. J Urol 99:112, 1968.
55. Coptcoat MJ: Lasertripsy: Candela pulsed dye laser. *In* Coptcoat MJ, Miller RA, Wickham JEA (eds): Lithotripsy II. London, BDI Publishing, 1985, pp 151–164.
56. Fair HD: In vitro destruction of urinary calculi by laser induced stress waves. Med Instrum 12:100, 1978.
57. Coptcoat MJ, Ison KT, Watson G, Wickham JEA: Lasertripsy for ureteral stones: 100 clinical cases. J Endourol 1:119, 1987.
58. Coptcoat MJ, Ison KT, Watson G, Wickham JEA: Lasertripsy for ureteric stones in 120 cases. Lessons learned. Br J Urol 61:487, 1988.
59. Segura JW: Pulsed dye laser for treatment of ureteral calculi. Urol Clin North Am 15:257, 1988.
60. Dretler SP: Techniques of laser lithotripsy. J Endourol 2:123, 1988.
61. Kahn RI: Flexible nephroscopy and electrohydraulic lithotripsy. *In* Carson CC, Dunnick NR (eds): Endourology. New York, Churchill Livingstone, 1985, pp 107–125.
62. Spirnak JP, Resnick MI: Kidney stone surgery. *In* Gillenwater JG, Grayhack JT, Howards SS, Duckett JW (eds). Adult and Pediatric Urology. Chicago, Year Book Medical Publishers, 1987, pp 555–578.
63. Spirnak JP, Resnick MI: Urinary stones. *In* Tanagho EA, McAninch JW (eds): Smith's General Urology. Norwalk, CT, Appleton and Lange, 1988, pp 275–301.
64. Badlani G, Eshghi M, Smith AD: Percutaneous surgery for ureteropelvic junction obstruction (endopyelotomy): Technique and early results. J Urol 135:26, 1986.
65. Reddy PK, Hulbert JC, Lange PH, et al: Percutaneous removal of renal and ureteral calculi: Experience with 400 cases. J Urol 134:662, 1985.
66. Carson CC III, Danneberger JE, Weinerth JL: Percutaneous lithotripsy in morbid obesity. J Urol 139:243, 1988.
67. Streem SB, Geisinger MA, Risius B, et al: Endourologic "sandwich" therapy for extensive staghorn calculi. J Endourol 1:253, 1987.
68. Patterson DE, Segura JW: Endourology—requiem or renaissance? Urol Ann 1:29, 1987.
69. Spirnak JP, Resnick MI: Retrograde percutaneous nephrostomy. Urol Clin North Am 15:393, 1988.
70. Leal JJ: Percutaneous removal of renal and ureteral stones with and without concomitant transurethral manipulation by a urologist using antegrade and retrograde techniques without a radiologist's assistance. J Urol 139:1184, 1988.
71. Morrisseau PM, Trotter SJ: Retrograde percutaneous nephrolithotomy: Urological treatment of a urological problem. J Urol 139:1163, 1988.
72. Newman RC, Finlayson B: Retrograde percutaneous nephrostomy: The Hunter-Hawkins method. Endourology 2:8, 1987.
73. Kaye KW, Goldberg ME: Applied anatomy of the kidney and ureter. Urol Clin North Am 9:3, 1982.
74. Stables DP: Percutaneous nephrostomy: Techniques, indications and results. Urol Clin North Am 9:15, 1982.
75. Young AT, Hunter DW, Castaneda-Zuniga WR, et al: Percutaneous extraction of urinary calculi: Use of the intercostal approach. Radiology 154:633, 1985.
76. Clayman RV: Percutaneous removal of renal calculi: Use of the backloaded balloon catheter for rapid dilation and instrumentation of the nephrostomy tract. Br J Urol [Suppl] 1:19, 1983.
77. Segura JW: Percutaneous nephrolithotomy and ureterolithotomy. *In* Rous SN (ed): Stone Disease Diagnosis and Management. Orlando, FL, Grune and Stratton, 1987, pp 227–242.
78. Lingeman JE, Sonda LP, Kahnoski RJ, et al: Ureteral stone management: Emerging concepts. J Urol 135:1172, 1986.
79. Dretler SP, Weinstein A: A modified algorithm for the management of ureteral calculi: 100 consecutive cases. J Urol 140:732, 1988.
80. Kellett MJ, Wickham JEA, Payne SR: Combined retrograde and antegrade manipulations for percutaneous nephrolithotomy of ureteric calculi: "Push-pull" technique. Urology 25:391, 1985.
81. Chadbourne DM, Lyon ES: Lidocaine jelly push-back of ureteral stones. Urology 31:395, 1988.
82. Hulbert JC, Reddy PK, Hunter DW, et al: Percutaneous management of ureteral calculi facilitated by retrograde flushing with carbon dioxide or radiopaque dye. J Urol 134:29, 1985.
83. Pollack HM, Banner MP: Percutaneous extraction of renal and ureteral calculi: Technical considerations. AJR 143:778, 1984.
84. Lupu AN, Fuchs GJ, Chaussy CG: A new approach to ureteral stone manipulation for ESWL. Endourology 1:13, 1986.
85. Carson CC: Percutaneous antegrade approach to ureteral calculi. Urol Clin North Am 15:399, 1988.

86. Kahn RI: Endourological treatment of ureteral calculi. J Urol 135:239, 1986.
87. Lingeman JE, Shirrell WL, Newman DM, et al: Management of upper ureteral calculi with extracorporeal shock wave lithotripsy. J Urol 138:720, 1987.
88. Evans RJ, Wingfield DD, Morollo BA, Jenkins AD: Ureteral stone manipulation before extracorporeal shock wave lithotripsy. J Urol 139:33, 1988.
89. LeRoy AJ, May GR, Bender CE, et al: Percutaneous nephrostomy for stone removal. Radiology 151:607, 1984.
90. Gonzales-Serva L, Weinerth JL, Glenn JF: Minimal mortality of renal surgery. Urology 9:253, 1977.
91. Holden S, McPhee M, Grabstald H: The rationale of urinary diversion in cancer patients. J Urol 121:19, 1979.
92. Lang EK: Percutaneous nephrostolithotomy and lithotripsy: A multi-institutional survey of complications. Radiology 162:25, 1987.
93. Lee WJ, Smith AD, Cubelli V, et al: Complications of percutaneous nephrolithotomy. Am J Radiol 148:177, 1987.
94. Brannen GE, Bush WH: Complications and morbidity of endourology. AUA Update Series 4:2, 1985.
95. Roth RA, Beckmann CF: Complications of extracorporeal shock wave lithotripsy and percutaneous nephrolithotomy. Urol Clin North Am 15:155, 1988.
96. Carson CC, Brown MW, Weinerth JL: Vascular complications of percutaneous renal surgery. J Endourol 1:181, 1987.
97. Clayman RV, Surya S, Hunter D, et al: Renal vascular complications associated with the percutaneous removal of renal calculi. J Urol 132:228, 1984.
98. Segura JW, LeRoy AJ: Complications from percutaneous stone removal. *In* Marshall FM (ed): Urologic Complications. Chicago, Year Book Medical Publishers, 1986, pp 155–163.
99. Kaye KW, Clayman RV: Tamponade nephrostomy catheter for percutaneous nephrostolithotomy. Urology 27:441, 1986.
100. Gavant ML, Gold RE, Church JC: Delayed rupture of renal pseudoaneurysm: Complication of percutaneous nephrostomy. AJR 138:948, 1982.
101. Dunnick NR, Carson CC, Braun SD, et al: Complication of percutaneous nephrostolithotomy. Radiology 157:51, 1985.
102. LeRoy AJ, Williams HJ, Bender CE, et al: Colon perforation following percutaneous nephrostomy and renal calculus removal. Radiology 155:83, 1985.
103. Morse RM, Spirnak JP, Resnick MI: Iatrogenic colon and rectal injuries associated with urological intervention: Report of 14 patients. J Urol 140:101, 1988.
104. Vallancien G, Capdoville R, Veillon B, et al: Colonic perforation during percutaneous nephrolithotomy. J Urol 134:1185, 1986.
105. Skoog SJ, Reed MD, Gaudier FA, Dunn NP: The posterolateral and the retrorenal colon: Implication in the percutaneous stone extraction. J Urol 134:110, 1985.
106. Sherman JL, Hopper KD, Greene AJ, Johns JT: The retrorenal colon on computed tomography: A normal variant. J Comput Assist Tomogr 9:339, 1985.
107. Segura JW, Patterson DE, LeRoy AJ, et al: Percutaneous removal of kidney stones: Review of 1,000 cases. J Urol 134:1077, 1985.
108. Culkin DJ, Wheeler JS, Canning JR: Nephro-duodenal fistula: A complication of percutaneous nephrolithotomy. J Urol 134:528, 1985.
109. Webb DR, Fitzpatrick JM: Percutaneous nephrolithotripsy: A functional and morphological study. J Urol 134:587, 1985.
110. Boyd JC, Boyce WH: Find significant vascularity loss in percutaneous nephrostomies. Urology Times, September 1984, p 1.
111. Clayman RV, Elbers J, Miller RP, et al: Percutaneous nephrostomy: Assessment of renal damage associated with semi-rigid (24F) and balloon (36F) dilation. J Urol 138:203, 1987.
112. Marberger M, Stackl W, Hruby W, Kroiss A: Late sequelae of ultrasonic lithotripsy of renal calculi. J Urol 133:170, 1985.
113. Thomas R, Roberts JA, Lewis RW, Ulkers EE: Effect of percutaneous removal of urinary calculi on kidney function. J Urol 131:135A, 1984.
114. Mayo ME, Krieger JN, Rudd TG: Effect of percutaneous nephrostolithotomy on renal function. J Urol 133:167, 1985.
115. Ekelund L, Lindstedt E, Lungquist SB, et al: Studies on renal damage from percutaneous nephrolitholapaxy. J Urol 135:682, 1986.
116. Miller RA, Wickham JEA, Kellett MJ: Percutaneous destruction of renal calculi: Clinical and laboratory experience. Br J Urol [Suppl] 51, 1983.
117. Rao PN, Faulkner MK, Sweeney JK, et al: Radiation dose to patient and staff during percutaneous nephrostolithotomy. Br J Urol 59:508, 1987.
118. Bush WH, Brannen GE, Gibbons RP, et al: Radiation exposure to patient and urologist during percutaneous nephrostolithotomy. J Urol 132:1148, 1984.
119. Sutherland JW: Recurrence following operations for upper urinary tract stone. Br J Urol 26:22, 1954.
120. Boyce WH, Elkins IB: Reconstructive renal surgery following anatrophic nephrolithotomy: Followup of 100 consecutive cases. J Urol 115:505, 1976.

121. Rous SN, Turner WR: Retrospective study of 95 patients with staghorn calculus disease. J Urol 118:902, 1977.
122. Redman JF, Bissada NK, Harper DL: Anatrophic nephrolithotomy: Experience with complications of the Smith and Boyce technique. J Urol 122:595, 1979.
123. Sleight MW, Wickham JE: Long-term follow-up of 100 cases of renal calculi. Br J Urol 49:601, 1977.
124. Fowler JE: Bacteriology of branched renal calculi and accompanying urinary tract infection. J Urol 131:213, 1984.
125. Streem SB, Zelch MG, Risius B, Geisinger MA: Percutaneous extraction of renal calculi. Urol Clin North Am 12:381, 1985.
126. White EC, Smith AD: Percutaneous stone extraction from 200 patients. J Urol 132:437, 1984.
127. Clayman RV, Surya V, Miller RP, et al: Percutaneous nephrolithotomy: Extraction of renal and ureteral calculi from 100 patients. J Urol 131:868, 1984.
128. Bass RB, Beard JH, Cooner WH, et al: Percutaneous ultrasonic lithotripsy in the community hospital. J Urol 133:586, 1985.
129. Lingeman JE, Coury TA, Newman DM, et al: Comparison of results and morbidity of percutaneous nephrostolithotomy and extracorporeal shock wave lithotripsy. J Urol 138:485, 1987.
130. Goldwasser B, Weinerth JL, Carson CC, Dunnick NR: Factors affecting the success rate of percutaneous nephrolithotripsy and the incidence of retained fragments. J Urol 136:358, 1986.
131. Winfield HN, Clayman RV, Chaussy CG, et al: Monotherapy of staghorn renal calculi: A comparative study between percutaneous nephrolithotomy and extracorporeal shock wave lithotripsy. J Urol 139:895, 1988.
132. LeRoy AJ, Segura JW, Williams HJ, Patterson DE: Percutaneous renal calculus removal in an extracorporeal shock wave lithotripsy practice. J Urol 138:703, 1987.

17

Extracorporeal Shock Wave Lithotripsy

J. Patrick Spirnak
Martin I. Resnick

Extracorporeal shock wave lithotripsy (ESWL) has, for the first time, provided a completely noninvasive technique for the management of renal and ureteral calculi. The procedure has been in use for nearly 10 years and has revolutionized the management of urinary stone disease. It is currently available world wide and, when used in conjunction with other endourologic procedures, can be used to manage nearly all urinary calculi safely. Short-term complications appear to be related primarily to stone volume and to the chosen method of anesthesia. Long-term complications have not been identified. Recent developments with alternative ways of shock wave generation have, in many cases, all but eliminated the morbidity associated with anesthesia.

HISTORICAL ASPECTS

Initial interest in the study of shock wave physics began in Germany in the 1960s and was initiated by researchers employed by the Dornier Laboratories who had noticed "pitting" as a common phenomenon in aircraft following supersonic flight. Investigators revealed the cause of the pitting to be due to the generation of shock waves that occurred when the spacecraft collided with rain drops or micrometeorites. It was determined that the shock waves generated by these supersonic collisions followed the basic principles and laws of acoustical physics. The basic principle that explains the destructive force of shock waves is related to the buildup of a pressure gradient that occurs when the shock wave encounters two materials that differ significantly in their acoustical properties (e.g., liquid and metal). Under those circumstances, a strong tensile force is generated at the surface of the solid material. Breakdown occurs when the tensile forces become greater than the comprehensive forces holding the material intact.[1]

Soon after these initial observations, collaborative efforts were established between scientists working at the Dornier System and researchers and physicians at the Institute of Surgical Research, University of Munich, West Germany, to assess the feasibility of employing shock wave principles to the fragmentation of urinary stones. Many individuals, including Professor E. Schmidt, Professor F. Eisenberger, and Professor C. Chaussy, were involved in the early research and development conducted from 1974 to 1980. Once a safe means of generating shock waves was identified, animal studies were conducted to determine the effects of shock waves on the various body tissues. These early clinical studies showed that shock waves generated in water could be safely transmitted into and through the body without appreciable loss of energy because of the similarities in the acoustical impedances (densities) of water and the body tissues. The lung proved to be the only body organ damaged extensively by the effects of the shock waves. This finding may be attributed to the large difference in acoustical properties the shock waves encounter at the alveolar surface (tissue-air interface).[2] Clinically, this did not pose a problem, since the shock waves could be focused precisely on the stone.[3] The experimental work culminated in 1979 with the development of the "HM-1" (human model) prototype.

The first clinical ESWL procedure was performed in Munich on February 20, 1980, using the Dornier HM-1 lithotripter. By May of 1982, more than 200 patients had been treated, and the HM-2 model was introduced. In October of 1983, a second stone center was established in Stüttgart that used an HM-3 model. After treating more than 1000 patients at the two centers, the HM-3 lithotripter became commercially available in 1984. The Food and Drug Administration (FDA) approved the experimental use of ESWL at six American centers, and on February 23, 1984, physicians at the Methodist Hospital of Indiana performed the first ESWL in this country. In December of that year, after more than 2000 treatments, ESWL was approved by the FDA for the treatment of urinary stones. The technology was approved by the Japanese Ministry of Public Welfare in November of 1985. During that same year, experimental trials with second-generation lithotripters were being conducted, and the first patient with gallstones was treated on the HM-3 lithotripter. By February of 1986, more than 130 Dornier machines were operational world wide, and more than 90,000 patients had been treated. By 1989, the number of patients treated had increased to more than 500,000 and there were more than 250 HM-3 lithotripters operational in 23 countries.[4] In addition, there are more than 12 mobile units currently operational in the United States. At present, there are at least nine other manufacturers involved in the development of second-generation machines, and it is anticipated that the lithotripter of the future will be office based, have multiple functions, and will not require anesthesia.

TECHNIQUE OF SHOCK WAVE GENERATION

To be successful, any lithotripter must be capable of generating and then focusing a shock wave on the stone's surface (Fig. 17–1). Shock waves are characterized by a high-energy pressure front of multiple low-frequency waves that rise sharply, to peak in nanoseconds, and then slowly decay (Fig. 17–2). The attenuation coefficient (i.e., loss of energy as the wave is propagated through tissue) is related to the square of its frequency. Since shock waves are of low frequency, they are capable of penetrating tissues with little loss of energy when

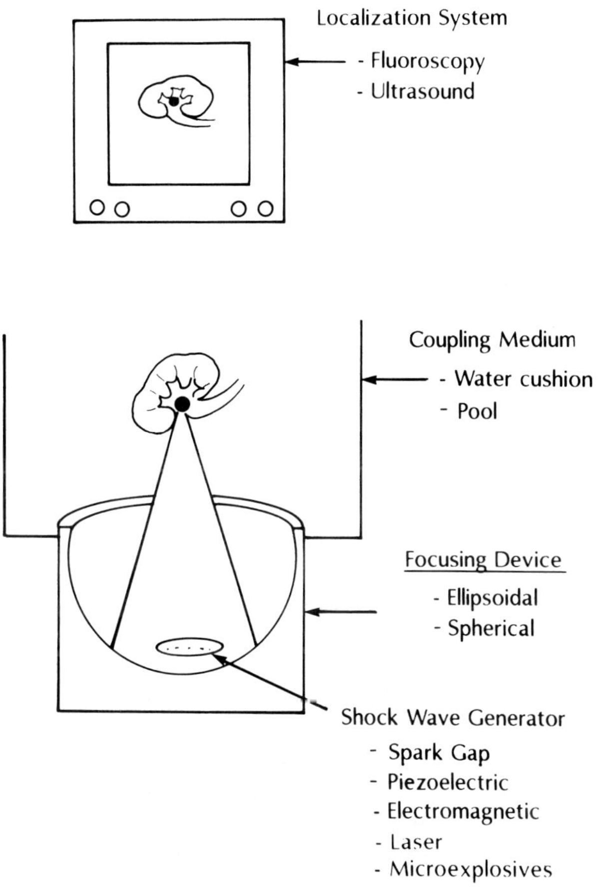

FIGURE 17–1. Diagrammatic representation of the four primary components essential to any functional lithotripter.

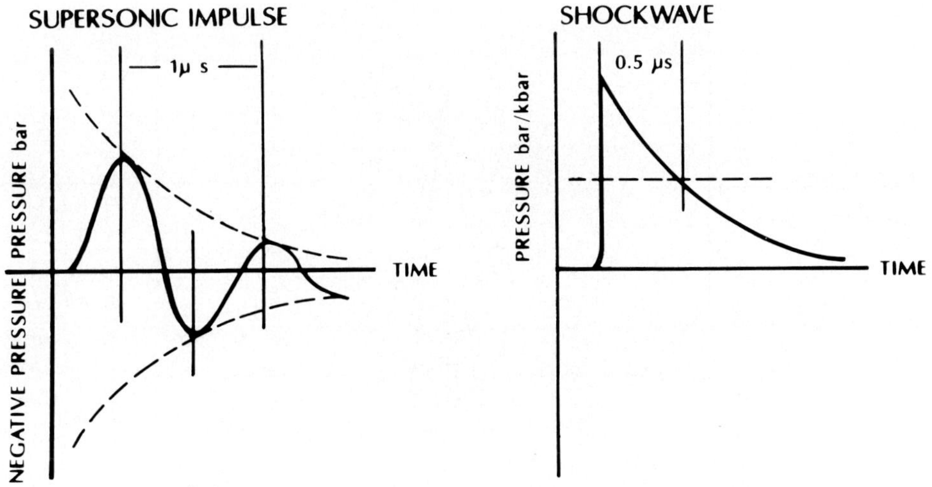

FIGURE 17–2. Schematic representation of pressure-time diagram for shock waves and ultrasound waves.

compared with higher frequency shock waves, such as ultrasound. Shock waves may be generated by any mechanism that provides for an abrupt release of energy in a small space. The Dornier HM-3 system employs spark gap technology and is therefore the most widely utilized technique of shock wave generation today.

The Dornier system uses an underwater electrode placed in the center of a semiellipsoid reflector (F_1) to generate the shock wave (Fig. 17–3). When the electrode is discharged with 16 to 30 kV, a spark lasting approximately 1 msec is generated between the two points of the electrode. The intense heat generated by the underwater discharge of the electrode causes vaporization of the surrounding fluid, and a pressure wave is generated. The initial ellipsoid reflector measures approximately 15.2 cm in diameter. Its geometric properties are such that the majority of shock waves generated at F_1 are reflected and focused at a second focal point (F_2) located about 12.5 cm above the top of the ellipsoid. F_2 represents the site of maximal energy density. The acoustical properties of water and body tissues are similar; therefore, the shock waves are propagated with little loss of energy. However, it has been estimated that as shock waves travel through 6 cm of tissue, there is a 10 to 20 per cent damping effect.[2] This can be overcome by increasing the kilovoltage. Approximately 10.5 per cent of the shock waves are unreflected by the ellipsoid and are nontherapeutic.[5] The reflected shock wave front reaches F_2 in about 29 μsec. When the shock wave reaches the stone surface (a medium that differs considerably in its acoustical characteristics from the soft tissues), a portion of the wave energy is reflected back into the body tissue, a portion is absorbed, and the remainder is transmitted through the stone (Fig. 17–4). Shock waves result in a compressive force when moving from an area of low (body tissue) to high (stone) acoustic impedance and a tensile force when moving from areas of high to low impedance.[6] The greater the impedance gradient between two tissues, the greater is the force generated. When the compressive forces at the front side of the stone become greater than the comprehensive forces holding the stone intact, fragmentation occurs.

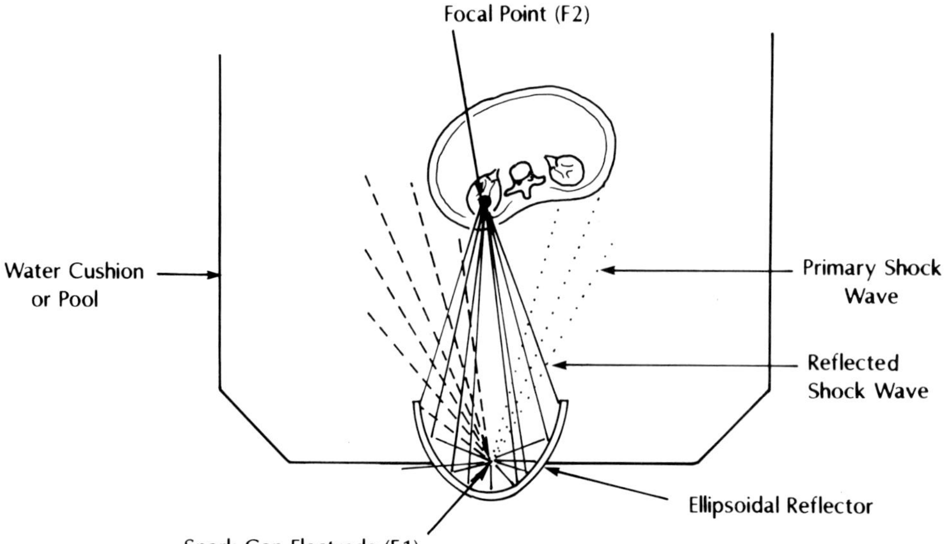

FIGURE 17–3. Schematic diagram of the essential components found in spark gap lithotripters, such as the Dornier HM-3.

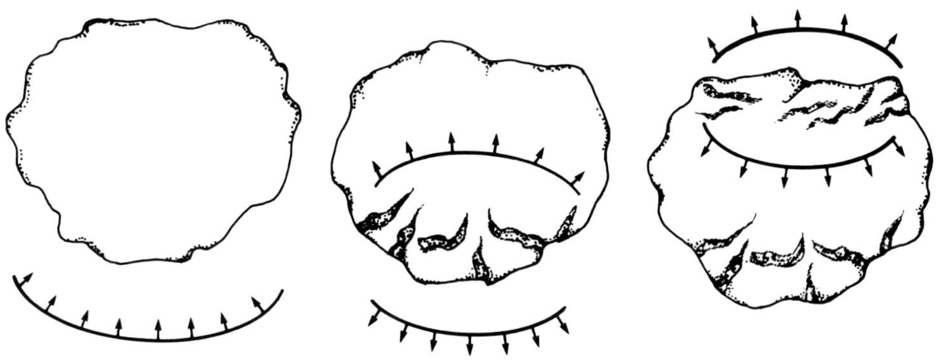

FIGURE 17–4. Fragmentation occurs when the shock wave front encounters tissue of a different acoustic density (*middle*). Stone fragmentation on the front side is due to compressive forces. Fragmentation on the back side of the stone is due both to compressive and to reflected tensile forces.

As the transmitted shock wave reaches the back surface of the stone, it once again encounters tissue of a significantly different density (acoustical impedance), and a portion of the compressive wave is reflected back into the stone as a tensile pulse wave while the remaining shock wave is transmitted through the body to exit anteriorly into the water medium. Maximal tensile stress is created by the interaction between tensile and compressive pulses near the back of the stone.[4] Fragmentation occurs at the back side of the stone when the tensile forces are greater than the comprehensive forces holding the stone intact. If the tensile portion of the reflected wave encounters faults within the stone, the wave will again be reflected, and the stone fragments as the comprehensive forces are overcome. The stone is continually bombarded with shock waves until fragmentation is complete.

The stone must be positioned at F_2 if maximal clinical benefit is to be derived. Shock waves generate pressures of up to 1000 atm at F_2. Pressures dissipate rapidly as one moves away from the focal point. Pressures measured only 2 cm away from F_2 are approximately 20 per cent of the maximal pressure recorded at the focal point.[7] The measured size of the focal point is 1.5 cm^3. A stone positioned outside this area will likely receive insufficient energy to fragment the stone adequately. The "blast path," as described by Finlayson, represents the lone exception to this general concept and may be used to fragment successfully stones that cannot be positioned precisely within the F_2 focal point. The axis of the "blast path" extends from the lower outer quadrant of each video monitor up and into the upper medial quadrant (Figs. 17–5 and 17–6). The blast path can be precisely located by drawing a line at a 25-degree angle to the x-axis on the medial half of each screen.[8] As the shock wave approaches F_2, its vector forces are primarily compressive, whereas after passing F_2, the major forces are tensile. Studies by Watanabe and associates have shown the compressive strength of renal calculi to vary from 19.2 to 1750.0 atm, whereas the tensile strength varies from 0.8 to 34.3 atm.[9] Owing to the low tensile strength of most calculi, stones positioned in the "blast path" are subjected primarily to tensile forces and should fragment. Studies performed by Finlayson have shown the degree of fragmentation not only to be material dependent but also to decrease as the distance from F_2 increases.[10] Effective fragmentation has occurred in stones positioned 10 cm from F_2 along the "blast path."[8] The "blast

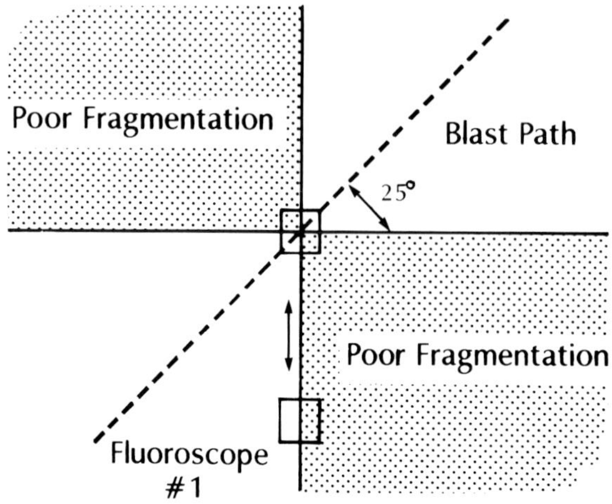

FIGURE 17–5. Diagrammatic representation of blast path, as defined by Finlayson.

path" may be used to treat patients who otherwise might not be considered as candidates for ESWL because of an inability to locate the stone precisely at F_2. It may also prove helpful in inducing fragmentation in stones refractory to standard treatment at F_2. Fragmentation may be further enhanced by increasing the number of shocks or the voltage or both.[10]

The size of F_2 can be altered by changing the curvature of the ellipsoid, a principle that has been employed in second-generation lithotripters to allow anesthesia-free treatment. As the diameter of the ellipsoid is increased, the size of the focal point is decreased and the surface penetration area of the shock wave is increased. The amount of energy reaching F_2 can also be altered by increasing the amount of voltage discharge and by changing the distance between the electrode tips. Experimental studies have shown that repeated exposure to shock waves ranging in pressure from 700 to 900 bar resulted in smaller fragments when compared with the effect of shock waves ranging from 3000 to 4000 bar.[11]

Regardless of how the shock wave is generated, the basic principles of shock wave therapy remain constant. The amount of pressure generated at the stone surface must be greater than the comprehensive forces holding the stone intact if fragmentation is to be successful. To date, there are two basic types of energy sources with proven usefulness in generating clinically effective shock waves: point sources and extended sources. The point sources include spark gap and

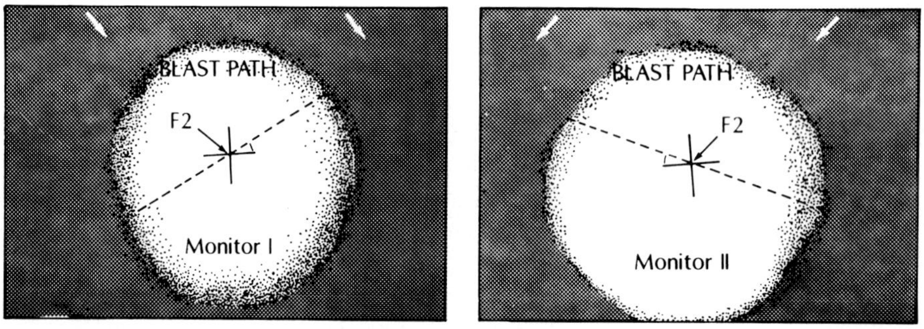

FIGURE 17–6. Diagram depicting blast path as it appears on the fluoroscopic screen. Use of the blast path will facilitate stone fragmentation when it is impossible to position the stone at F_2.

laser technology. Spark gap technology is currently the most widely utilized. It is used in the Dornier as well as in the Direx, Medstone, Northgate, and Technomed lithotripters (Dornier, Marietta, GA; Direx, Tikva, Israel; MedStone, Costa Mesa, CA; Northgate, Arlington Heights, IL; Technomed, Bay Shore, NY). The extended sources include piezoelectric (EDAP, Wolf, Diasonics [Wolf, Rosemont, IL; Diasonics, San Francisco, CA]) and electromagnetic (Siemens, Iselin, NJ; Storz, Kennesaw, GA) technology (Table 17–1).

The Siemens Lithostar is the only FDA-approved lithotripter using the electromagnetic technique of shock wave generation (Fig. 17–7). A shock wave is generated when an electrical impulse moves a metallic membrane housed in a "shock tube." The shock wave is focused by an acoustic lens and is transmitted to the body surface by means of a water cushion. The shock waves are coordinated to the patient's respiratory rate, thus improving treatment efficiency by delivering a greater percentage of the shock waves to the stone surface. Peak pressure delivered to the focused area is estimated at 1200 bar.[12] Proposed advantages of the Siemens machine include a built-in endoscopy table, which allows simultaneous stone manipulation and is capable of generating hard-copy radiographs during treatment. In addition, anesthesia requirements are less when compared with those of the HM-3 machine. The shock wave tube and electromagnetic source are quite durable and require changing every 50 to 100 patients. Wilbert and Clayman and their associates have reported favorable initial experience using this machine.[13, 14] The Storz Modulith also uses an electromagnetic source but offers the advantage of generating a more powerful shock wave (Fig. 17–8).

Piezoelectric shock waves are generated by the sudden expansion of a ceramic (piezoelectric) element excited by a high-frequency, high-voltage pulse. This slight movement generates an ultrasonic wave that produces a shock wave directed to the focal point. There are a number of these piezoelectric elements (330 in the EDAP machine compared with 3000 in the Wolf machine) mounted on the surface of a concave dish. Each of these elements can be excited simultaneously. Because of the spherical shape of the disc, all elements are

TABLE 17–1. CHARACTERISTIC FEATURES OF VARIOUS LITHOTRIPTERS

Lithotripter	Shock Wave Generation	Focusing	Coupling	Localization	Year Introduced
Diasonics	Piezoelectric	Spherical	Water cushion	Fluoro/US	1989
Direx Tripter X_7	Spark gap	Ellipsoid	Water cushion	C-arm fluoro/US	1987
Dornier					
HM-3	Spark gap (80 nF)	Ellipsoid (14 cm)	Water bath	Fluoro (biplane)	1980
HM-3 modified	Spark gap (40 nF)	Ellipsoid (17 cm)	Water bath	Fluoro (biplane)	1980
HM-4	Spark gap (40 nF)	Ellipsoid (17 cm)	Water cushion	Fluoro (biplane)	1986
MPL 9000	Spark gap (60 nF)	Ellipsoid (21 cm)	Water cushion	US	1987
MPL 5000	Spark gap (40 nF)	Ellipsoid (17 cm)	Water cushion	Fluoro	1988
EDAP LT01	Piezoelectric (300 elements)	Spherical (aperture, 54 cm)	Water cushion	US	1986
MedStone 1000	Spark gap	Ellipsoid	Water cushion	Plain x-ray	1987
Nitech Lithotripter	Spark gap	Ellipsoid	Water cushion	US	1987
Northgate SD-3	Spark gap	Ellipsoid	Water cushion	US	1987
Storz Modulith	Electromagnetic	Parabola	Water cushion	C-arm fluoro/US	1989
Siemens Lithostar	Electromagnetic	Acoustic lens (aperture, 12 cm)	Water cushion	Fluoro (biplane)	1986
Technomed Sonolith 3000	Spark gap	Ellipsoid (14 cm/ 20.5 cm)	Partial bath	US	1985
Wolf Piezolith	Piezoelectric (3000 elements)	Spherical (aperture, 30 cm)	Partial bath	US	1987
Yashiyoda	Chemical explosion (lead azide pellet)	Ellipsoid	Water bath	C-arm fluoro	1986

US = Ultrasound; Fluoro = Fluoroscopy.

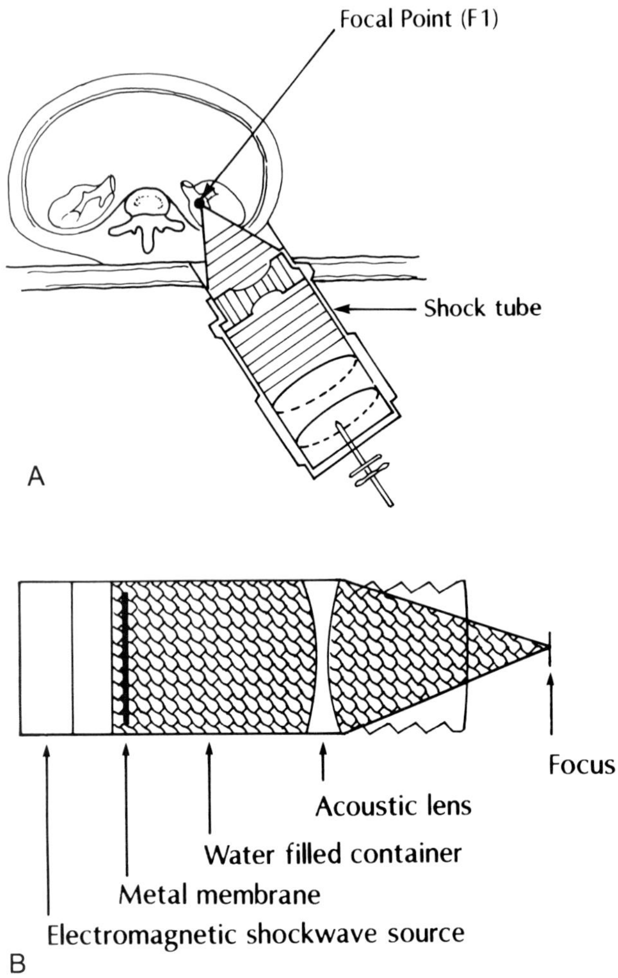

FIGURE 17–7. *A*, Diagrammatic components of electromagnetic shock wave lithotripter as used in the Siemens Lithostar. *B*, Shock wave tube that combines the shock wave source and acoustic lens and allows direct coupling to the patient, thus avoiding the cumbersome water bath used in the HM-3 lithotripter.

focused to a single point (Fig. 17–9). The Wolf machine has an aperture of about 300 mm. As the aperture increases, the shock wave pressure at the skin surface is decreased owing to the increase in skin surface area penetrated by the shock waves. The very small focal zone (6 × 10 mm in the Wolf machine compared with 60 × 12 mm in the standard HM-3)[15] and the wide area of shock wave entry at the skin surface, combined with the lower maximal pressures generated at F_1 (900 to 1000 bar), allow for anesthesia-free treatment.[16, 17] Unlike shock waves induced by spark gap techniques, the shock waves generated by the piezoelectric method do not induce cardiac arrhythmias and thus do not require electrocardiographic triggering. The stone is localized by an ultrasound sector scanner positioned at the center of the concave dish. The shock wave is transmitted to the patient using either a water cushion (EDAP) or a small exposed pool of water (Wolf). Advantages of piezoelectric lithotripsy include lower startup and maintenance cost, ability to treat without anesthesia, and absence of a cumbersome water bath. Disadvantages include difficulties in localizing small renal stones (<3 mm) and ureteral calculi. Clinical results comparable to those achieved with the Dornier technique have been reported by Marberger, Vallancien, and Ryan and their associates.[16–18]

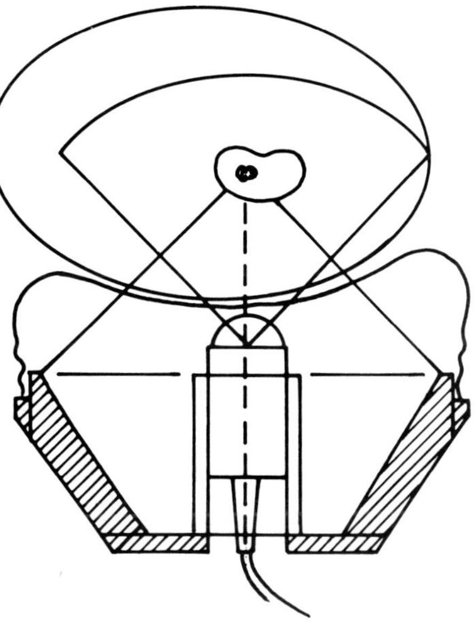

FIGURE 17–8. Diagrammatic representation of Storz Modulith. Cylindrical source within a parabola allows for focusing of the shock wave.

Shock Wave Focusing

Shock waves that are generated by a point source, such as the Dornier HM-3, require focusing to be effective. Spark gap electrodes generate shock waves that are propagated in a circular fashion. All lithotripters employing this technique use ellipsoid reflectors to focus the shock wave at a second focal point. As the diameter of the ellipsoid reflector increases, so, too, does the skin surface area penetrated by the shock waves, while the focal zone is decreased. Second-generation lithotripters typically have larger reflectors, which reduce pain by dispersing the shock waves at the skin surface and reducing the pressures at the level of the kidney. Anesthesia-free treatment is thus possible.

The piezoelectric technique utilizes the concave spherical dish on which is

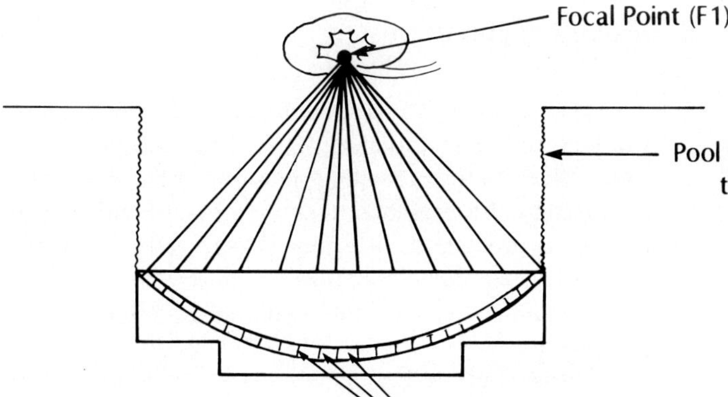

FIGURE 17–9. Diagrammatic representation of the shock wave source focusing device and coupling medium found in piezoelectric lithotripters. Note the presence of only one focal point.

mounted the piezoelectric elements to focus the shock wave effectively. The Siemens electromagnetic device uses an acoustical lens built into the shock tube to focus the shock wave.

Coupling Medium

Since the shock waves are generated extracorporeally, a suitable medium must be employed to allow transmission of the shock wave to the patient. Water and human tissues have similar acoustical properties; therefore, shock waves may be propagated in a water medium with little loss of energy. The Dornier HM-3 system utilizes a stainless steel tank filled with 1000 liters (about 211 gallons) of degassed (distilled) water. If regular tap water is used, transmission of the shock wave to the patient may be unpredictable owing to the phenomenon of pseudocavitation. Carbon dioxide gas bubbles in tap water create air-water interfaces, which partially absorb the shock wave energy and thus reduce the amount of energy reaching F_2. The temperature of the water bath is maintained between 36 and 37°C to prevent potential hemodynamic changes due to peripheral vessel dilation and pseudocavitation. The higher the water temperature, the higher the partial pressure of dissolved gases and the greater the probability that bubbles will form to interfere with shock wave transmission.

The water bath system, although effective, is quite cumbersome and represents a major source of added expense to the overall cost of the unit. The weight of the water bath often requires expensive reinforcing of the floor beneath the machine. The gantry required to move the patient in and out of the tub is expensive and requires extra height in the room. A floor drain is essential to rid the room of water spilled during the transfer of the patient out of the tub. In addition to the cost concerns, the water bath represented a new challenge for the anesthesiologist. For these reasons, second-generation machines have turned to alternative coupling techniques. Current models use an enclosed water cushion, a partial water bath, or a totally contained shock tube.

Stone Localization

The Dornier HM-3 system uses biplanar fluoroscopy to identify and locate the targeted stone precisely at F_2 (Fig. 17–10). Second-generation lithotripters use either C-arm or ceiling-mounted retractable fluoroscopy units or biplanar fluoroscopy. Fluoroscopic techniques are familiar to most urologists and do not require a prolonged "learning curve." Disadvantages include the expense, an inability to visualize radiolucent stones, the risk of radiation exposure to the patient and staff, and the inability to obtain hard x-ray copies during the procedure.

Ultrasound is the alternative to fluoroscopy (Fig. 17–11). Sonographic techniques are less familiar to practicing urologists and require a learning period. Additional drawbacks to the use of ultrasound include difficulties in visualizing small 2- to 3-mm calculi in both the kidney and the ureter and problems in identifying when adequate fragmentation has occurred. Reduced cost, the capability to be used for gallstone lithotripsy, and the ability to visualize radiolucent stones represent advantages over standard radiographic techniques.

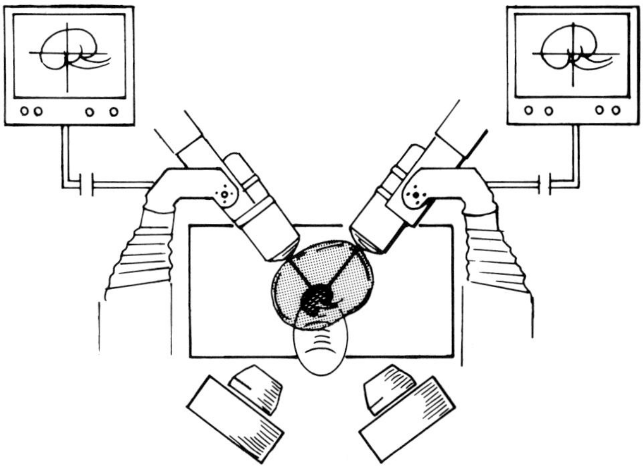

FIGURE 17–10. Diagrammatic representation of biplanar fluoroscopy utilized in Dornier HM-3 system.

INDICATIONS AND CONTRAINDICATIONS

The indications for extracorporeal shock wave lithotripsy include the standard indications for surgical stone removal: pain, obstruction, progressive loss of renal function, infection, recurrent gross hematuria, and occupation of the patient.[19] Indications specifically related to ureteral stones include size, degree of obstruction, and failure to progress down the ureter.[20] In some stone centers, patients with asymptomatic calculi are also considered suitable candidates for ESWL therapy.[21–23]

Initial clinical trials limited the use of ESWL to patients with solitary uninfected renal stones measuring less than 2 cm in diameter.[24] Patients were required to be of reasonably good health, could not weigh more than 300 lbs, and could not be shorter than 1.2 meters (4 feet) or taller than 2 meters (6 feet, 6 inches). After the initial clinical experience was reviewed and the technology was approved by the FDA, indications were expanded to include all patients

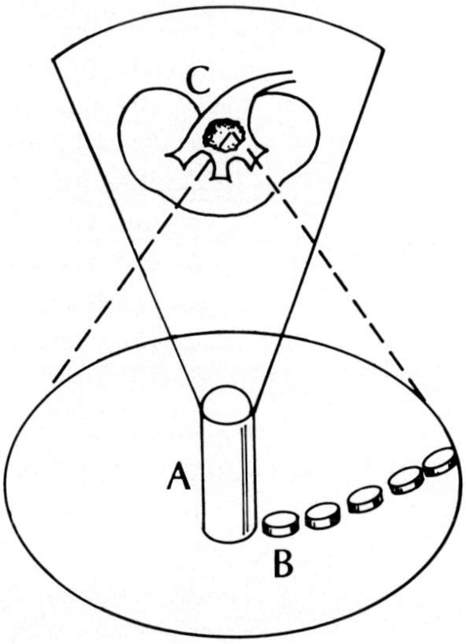

FIGURE 17–11. Diagrammatic representation of ultrasonic localization (A) in piezoelectric lithotripsy. Piezoelectric elements (B) and F_1 (C) are shown.

with stones above the bony pelvis, with the exception of staghorn calculi. With time, it became apparent that any stone contained in the urinary tract could be treated, provided it could be positioned at F_2 and there were no overlying bony projections. By modifying the gantry, children may also be treated.[25] Stones located in the midureter or overlying the bony pelvis may be treated with the patient prone.[26, 27] Similarly, distal ureteral stones may be visualized with the patient in a modified sitting position.[28] Stones in both the midureter and distal ureter may be first manipulated into a more desirable proximal location, thereby avoiding gantry modifications. The management of large ($\geq$3.0 cm) and branched renal stones remains controversial; however, even these complex calculi may be managed by combining ESWL with percutaneous techniques and the judicious use of chemolysis. It is estimated that in experienced hands more than 95 per cent of all urinary stones may be managed without a surgical incision. The remaining indication for open surgical lithotomy is a stone associated with an anatomic abnormality not amenable to advanced percutaneous techniques.

Prior to the advent of less invasive techniques of surgical stone removal, it was generally accepted that patients with nonobstructing calyceal stones did not require surgical intervention. This belief was based on sound urologic principles:

1. Nonobstructing stones are not associated with pain.
2. The intraoperative localization of small peripheral stones was difficult and often resulted in significant surgical trauma.
3. Twenty per cent of patients with flank incisions complained of chronic wound irritability.[29]

As less invasive techniques became available, many patients with calyceal stones and chronic flank pain were considered candidates for stone removal, and many became pain free following removal.[30, 31] It is now accepted by many that nonobstructing calyceal stones may be associated with intermittent symptoms either related to the stone's shifting position, with intermittent calyceal obstruction, or resulting from chronic mucosal irritation.[21] In addition, a number of calyceal stones will drop into the ureter and become symptomatic at a later time. For these reasons, many urologists have expanded the indications for ESWL to include calyceal calculi.[21–23]

During the initial clinical experience, there were a number of contraindications to ESWL that were unrelated to stone size, type, or position. Contraindications included the following:

1. The presence of a cardiac pacemaker.
2. Renal artery calcification.
3. Creatinine value greater than 3.
4. Bleeding diathesis.
5. Severe orthopedic deformities.
6. Urinary tract infection.
7. Obstruction distal to the stone.
8. Pregnant females.
9. Children.

With experience, the list of absolute contraindications has been reduced to include only those patients with uncorrectable coagulopathies, pregnant females, and patients weighing over 300 lbs. (The machine warranty is not effective if weight is >297.6 lbs). Patients with distal obstruction are candidates, provided the obstruction may be bypassed with a ureteral catheter. Individuals with severe kyphoscoliosis and spinal cord–injured patients are candidates, provided they may be safely positioned on the gantry and their stones positioned at F_2.[32] Prior to scheduled stone treatment, it is best to simulate the procedure with these patients to be certain that their stone can be adequately positioned. Active urinary tract infection remains a contraindication to any urologic procedure and is best treated before ESWL treatment. Patients with struvite calculi are admitted to the hospital 2 days before scheduled treatment and receive culture-specific systemic antibiotics.[33] The judicious use of ureteral stents and nephrostomy tubes will further reduce treatment-associated sepsis.

Individuals with cardiac arrhythmias controlled with medication are also candidates for the procedure. Patients with stable calcified aneurysms of the aorta or renal artery may be treated, provided the calcified vessel is not at the focal point when the stone is positioned at F_2.

During the early clinical trials, the presence of an implanted cardiac pacemaker represented a contraindication to ESWL therapy.[34] Reasons for this included concern that the shock waves might damage the device and the fear that the shock discharge might interfere with pacemaker activity. Since then, both laboratory and clinical studies have shown that these patients may be treated with no adverse effects on pacemaker function.[35–37] However, it is recommended that these patients be forewarned of possible deleterious effects on pacemaker function and that the procedure be performed in the presence of a cardiologist capable of reprogramming the device or providing a temporary transvenous pacemaker, should it become necessary to do so.

The presence of vascular clips does not represent a contraindication. Studies conducted by Abber and associates showed that vascular clips placed on vessels exposed to a high mean arterial pressure and placed directly at F_2 were not dislodged or affected by the pressure and shearing forces generated by ESWL.[36]

PROCEDURE

Preparation of Patients

ESWL performed with the standard nonmodified Dornier HM-3 lithotripter requires an anesthetic; therefore, preparation of the patient is similar to the evaluation performed prior to any urologic procedure requiring anesthesia. A preoperative history and physical examination are routine. Particular attention is directed at detecting any medication that can prolong the blood-clotting mechanisms. All aspirin and aspirin-containing compounds, in addition to the nonsteroidal antiinflammatory agents, may cause platelet dysfunction and bleeding problems. Aspirin-containing compounds are stopped 2 weeks before treatment, while the nonsteroidal antiinflammatory agents are stopped 1 week before the procedure. Complete blood count, serum chemistry profile, and urinalysis are routinely obtained. Clotting parameters, urine culture, chest film, and electrocardiogram are selectively ordered. Type and screen are not necessary. Antiflatulents are selectively started 1 to 2 days before scheduled treatment in an attempt to limit the bowel gas that may obscure the stone and make fluoroscopic localization impossible. This practice is particularly important in spinal cord–injured patients with poorly calcified stones, who are prone to gaseous bowel distention. The shock waves also have the potential to cause mucosal bleeding of the gastrointestinal tract, which may be related to gaseous distention.[38, 39] This bleeding is rarely of any clinical significance.

Anesthetic Considerations

Although one discharge of the lithotripter is well tolerated and may be felt as nothing more than a mild slap, the repeated discharge of up to 3000 shocks will be quite painful at the shock wave entry point and will necessitate some form of analgesia. Stone fragmentation is dependent on being able to localize the stone at the point of maximal energy density, F_2. Rapid and uncontrolled respirations cause excessive stone movement, thereby minimizing the effect of the shock waves. Adequate anesthesia with controlled respirations limits stone movement and enhances the therapeutic effectiveness of the procedure. ESWL may be successfully performed with the patient under regional (spinal or epidural), general endotracheal, or local, anesthesia and, in selected cases (e.g., spinal cord–injured patients), with the patient receiving intravenous sedation alone.

Anesthetic Considerations Unique to ESWL

Cardiovascular System. The induction of either general or regional anesthesia is often accompanied by peripheral vasodilation and hypotension. General anesthesia is also known to reduce cardiac stroke volume. As the anesthetized patient undergoing ESWL is transferred to the semisitting position, gravitational forces favor the additional pooling of blood in the extremities and a further reduction in blood pressure. Weber monitored cardiac parameters in 46 patients undergoing ESWL and confirmed an initial fall in central venous pressure and hypotension immediately prior to water immersion.[40] Arborelius and associates[41] studied the hemodynamic changes associated with water immersion and reported an average increase in central blood volume of 700 ml, with a concomitant increase in central venous pressure of 12 mm Hg. Mean cardiac output increased by 32 per cent, while mean stroke volume increased by 35 per cent. Systemic vascular resistance decreased, while right atrial and pulmonary artery transmural pressure gradients increased. The redistribution of blood volume is primarily mediated by an immersion-induced increase in hydrostatic pressure, which acts to squeeze the blood from the vessels of the lower extremities and increase venous return. Weber confirmed findings in fully submersed patients underoing ESWL by documenting an increase in right atrial pressure (RAP) (3.0 to 16.5 mm Hg), pulmonary capillary wedge (PCW) (6.5 to 17.5 mm Hg), and cardiac index (20.5 to 24.8 liters/min) and a decrease in mean arterial pressure (MAP) (85 to 80.5 mm Hg).[40] He also studied the effects of gradual water immersion on patients undergoing ESWL while under general anesthesia and noted an increase in the central venous pressure to baseline levels when the patient was immersed to the level of the umbilicus. Complete immersion to the level of the clavicles further increased the central venous pressure. In general, the blood pressure rose slightly. Patients with a history of valvular heart disease or congestive heart failure may not be able to compensate for the increase in preload associated with the water immersion process. In these high-risk patients, the use of inotropes and peripheral vasodilators will help reduce the risk of congestive heart failure. Heating the water temperature higher than 37°C will cause peripheral vasodilation and a reduction in blood pressure.

Pulmonary System. General anesthesia, unlike regional anesthesia, tends to decrease the functional residual capacity of the lungs, which may lead to a decrease in arterial oxygenation. Water immersion increases the hydrostatic pressure on the submerged chest and abdomen and may further decrease the functional residual capacity by approximately 35 per cent.[41] Although the pulmonary mechanics are impaired in virtually all submerged patients, major pulmonary problems rarely occur except in those with severe preexisting pulmonary disease.

Regional Anesthesia. The kidney derives its nerve supply from spinal segments T10–T12 and the ureters from T10–L2. The shock wave entry site is supplied by T11–L1. Production of a regional block extending from T6–L2 will provide adequate analgesia.

Excellent results have been reported using regional anesthesia (epidural or spinal), and in many centers epidural anesthesia is considered to be the anesthetic of choice.[42] Contraindications to this approach include a bleeding diathesis, progressive neurologic disease, congenital deformities of the back or a history of back trauma, infection, or massive obesity. Patients who are extremely anxious or uncooperative are poor candidates for this approach, as in all likelihood they will find it difficult to control their respirations satisfactorily and limit stone movement.

The site where the epidural catheter exits the skin is covered with an occlusive waterproof dressing. Although the dressing frequently becomes dislodged during treatment, infection has not been a problem.[43] An adequate epidural anesthetic offers several advantages over spinal anesthesia:

1. Spinal headache should not occur if the dura has not been entered.
2. The use of indwelling catheter allows for the administration of more anesthetic, should the procedure be prolonged.
3. In high-risk cardiac patients, the administered anesthetic dose may be more easily titrated to maintain a stable blood pressure.

Advantages of regional anesthesia when compared with general anesthesia include the following:

1. Full cooperation by the patient as he or she is being positioned on the gantry.
2. The need for less intense postoperative recovery room monitoring.
3. Less gastrointestinal upset.
4. The need for less postoperative narcotics.

Disadvantages include the following:

1. Poor or no control of the patient's respirations, which could cause excessive stone movement and less efficient treatment.
2. Prolonged preparation and recovery room times.

General Anesthesia. General endotracheal anesthesia is also satisfactory for ESWL treatment and, in many centers, is the technique of choice. It offers the obvious advantages of complete respiratory control, which theoretically should improve treatment efficiency. It also allows for a more rapid turnover of patients, which may be of significance in a busy stone center.

Tidal volumes during general anesthesia usually range from 10 to 15 ml/kg. A 1000-ml breath is likely to move the diaphragm a considerable distance. With the use of standard ventilatory techniques, maximal stone movement has been measured on the fluoroscopy monitor to be greater than 30 mm.[44] Excessive stone movement theoretically leads to less efficient ESWL therapy, as the targeted stone spends less time at F_2.[45] More time is necessary for radiologic imaging (increased radiation exposure), and more shock waves are required for stone disintegration. Delivery of lower tidal volumes (4 to 6 ml/kg) at a more rapid rate (12 to 20 per minute) helps minimize stone movement.[43]

High-frequency jet ventilation (rates, 100 to 200 breaths per minute), with tidal volumes 80 to 140 ml/min, minimizes stone movement while maximizing treatment efficiency.[46] The mechanism of action of high-frequency jet ventilation is controversial. Two theories exist:

1. There is coaxial flow of gas, with fresh gas flowing in through the center of the endotracheal tube while exhaled gas flows simultaneously out along the periphery of the tube.
2. The constant molecular motion of oxygen and carbon dioxide, rather than bulk flow, accounts for gas exchange.[47]

Although it has been definitely shown that high-frequency jet ventilation reduces stone movement to 2 to 3 mm, it has not been clearly demonstrated to offer distinct economical or clinical advantages when compared with conventional anesthetic techniques.[8] The advantages of the improved treatment efficiency—that is, an additional 30 per cent of shock waves hit the stone—and savings because fewer electrodes are used are offset by the need for more costly equipment.[42]

Local Anesthesia. Although the use of local anesthesia offers many advantages over general or regional anesthesia, initial clinical experience with patients undergoing ESWL was disappointing. Malhotra reported success in treating 100 patients using a regional block technique combined with an intercostal nerve block.[48] Intravenous sedation with diazepam or fentanyl is helpful in relieving anxiety and limiting movement by the patient. Stone movement is minimized by encouraging a rapid but shallow breathing pattern, which helps limit diaphragmatic excursion. Selection of patients is important, and the use of local anesthesia is best suited for highly motivated and cooperative patients with uncomplicated renal stones. The treatment was successfully completed in all patients, and only four required posttreatment recovery room monitoring. Similarly favorable results were reported by Loening and associates using only a regional block technique.[49] Obvious advantages include reduced cost, more rapid turnover of patients, and improved safety to the patient. Spinal cord–injured patients who lack pain sensation may be selectively managed with only intravenous analgesia.[32]

Shock Wave Treatment

The anesthetized patient is catheterized, placed on the gantry, and secured with adjustable straps. The patient is hydraulically lifted and immersed in the water bath up to the clavicles. It is important to keep both the shock wave entry and exit sites covered with water to avoid excessive skin bruising.[50] The image intensifiers are positioned against the anterior abdominal wall, and with the use of fluoroscopy, the targeted stone is positioned at the F_2 of both x-ray monitors. The F_2 is marked on the fluoroscopy screens by two cross-hair targets (see Fig. 17–10).

There are two x-ray tubes fixed to the bottom of the tank on either side of the ellipsoid. These tubes are aimed at their corresponding image intensifiers and offer opposite oblique views, which allows precise positioning of the targeted stone at the F_2 focal point. The x-ray tubes are covered with inflatable balloons. When these balloons are inflated with air during stone localization, less attenuation and scattering of the x-ray beam give a better fluoroscopic image. The balloons are deflated during stone treatment to avoid possible distortion of the shock wave. The x-ray system allows the stone to be visualized in both "real-time" fluoroscopy and "hard-copy" snapshots.

Once the stone has been positioned between the cross-hairs on both fluoroscopy screens, treatment is begun by depressing the hand-held switch. Small stones (>1 cm) are placed entirely within the cross-hairs of the fluoroscopic screens for the duration of the treatment. Larger stones require a treatment strategy (Fig. 17–12). In general, the stone portion occupying the ureteropelvic junction is first treated. If one assumes a limit of 2000 to 2400 shocks, 600 to 800 are administered to this portion. Kilovoltage is initially set at 18 and increased to maximum of 24 kV, as needed. Dependent calyces are next treated with 300 to 400 shocks. The renal pelvic portion is then treated, followed by the upper pole calyces. Treatment is stopped at 2000 to 2400 shocks. When treating

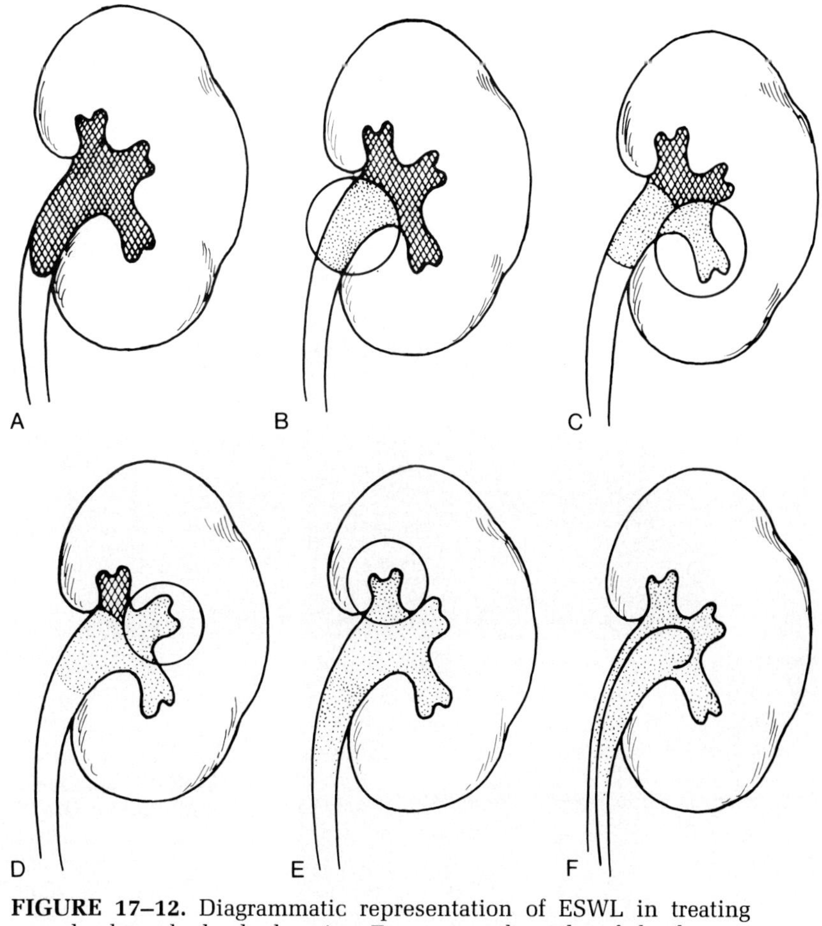

FIGURE 17–12. Diagrammatic representation of ESWL in treating complex branched calculus. A to F represent the order of shock wave administration. Note the placement of the double **J** catheter (F) at the end of the procedure. Alternatively, this may be placed at the beginning of the procedure.

complex stones located throughout the kidney, the number of shock waves is arbitrarily set at 2400, since multiple areas of the kidney are treated. The amount of energy (power) that can be safely delivered to the stone is still unknown. The FDA established guidelines during the initial clinical trials that limited the number of shocks to 2000, and the allowable kilovolts ranged from 18 to 24. Although at the present time no known complications have been directly related to the number of shocks delivered to the kidney, and in spite of reports in which more than 2000 shocks have been safely used,[39, 51, 52] it is recommended that the established limits be adhered to.[34] Treatment progression is fluoroscopically assessed after every 200 to 300 shocks (Fig. 17–13). Successful fragmentation may be difficult to assess. Fluoroscopically, the stone may appear to enlarge and spread out. The image may also appear less dense when compared with pretreatment images. Gross hematuria typically occurs after as few as 200 shocks and is due to either shock wave–induced renal trauma or trauma to the epithelium caused by the movement of the stone or its fragments. A diuretic (furosemide [Lasix]) is usually administered during the procedure to avoid fluid overload and to limit blood clot formation. A forced diuresis may also aid in dispersement and passage of stone fragments. A diuretic also increases renal blood flow, which may help protect the kidney from shock wave–induced trauma.

Repeated discharge of the electrode causes widening of the spark gap, which generates ineffective shock waves. Electrode wear is directly related to the voltage of spark discharge. The manufacturer initially recommended changing the electrode after every 700 shock waves.[8] For large stones, three electrodes were required. Finlayson has since shown that measured pressures at F_2 can be maintained out to 4000 shocks on a single electrode if the voltage is increased by 1 or 2 kV at the time the electrode is heard to misfire.[53] The sound of a new

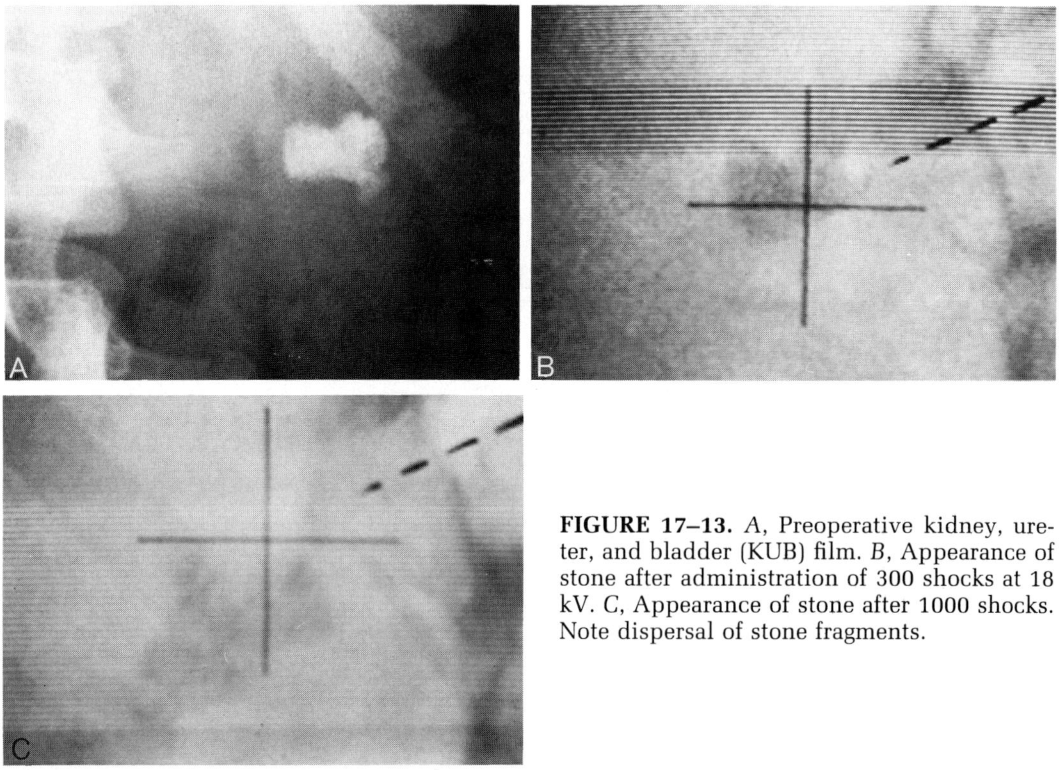

FIGURE 17–13. *A*, Preoperative kidney, ureter, and bladder (KUB) film. *B*, Appearance of stone after administration of 300 shocks at 18 kV. *C*, Appearance of stone after 1000 shocks. Note dispersal of stone fragments.

electrode is easy to detect, as it is sharp and crisp compared with the duller and softer sound generated by a worn electrode. The Finlayson method of gradually increasing the discharge voltage will increase the life of the electrode and make the treatment more cost effective. The Dornier Company has improved on the initial electrode design and now provides an electrode capable of delivering 1500 shocks at 18 to 20 kV. When the kilovoltage is increased to 22 and 24, it is recommended that the electrode be replaced every 1200 and 800 shocks, respectively.

The treatment is ended when either the allotted number of shocks has been administered (2000 to 2400) or when the stone has been adequately fragmented. Since pain and obstruction are major potential problems and may be related to inadequate stone fragmentation and since "adequate" fragmentation is difficult to assess during treatment, an additional several hundred shocks are administered to the fragments once fragmentation has been thought to be complete. Treatment time varies, depending on the complexity of the stone. In the initial clinical trials conducted in Munich from 1980 to 1983, treatment time averaged 45 minutes and 1350 shocks were administered.[54]

When treatment has been completed, the patient is lifted from the water bath, unstrapped, and transferred to the hospital bed. The Foley catheter is removed once the patient is fully awake and recovered from anesthesia. A plain abdominal film is obtained to assess the adequacy of fragmentation (Fig. 17–14). In some clinical settings, the abdominal film is immediately obtained, and if the treatment is judged to be inadequate, the patient may be immediately returned to the bath for additional therapy.

After the patient is fully recovered, he or she is either transferred to the hospital room or discharged to home. During the initial FDA trials, it was

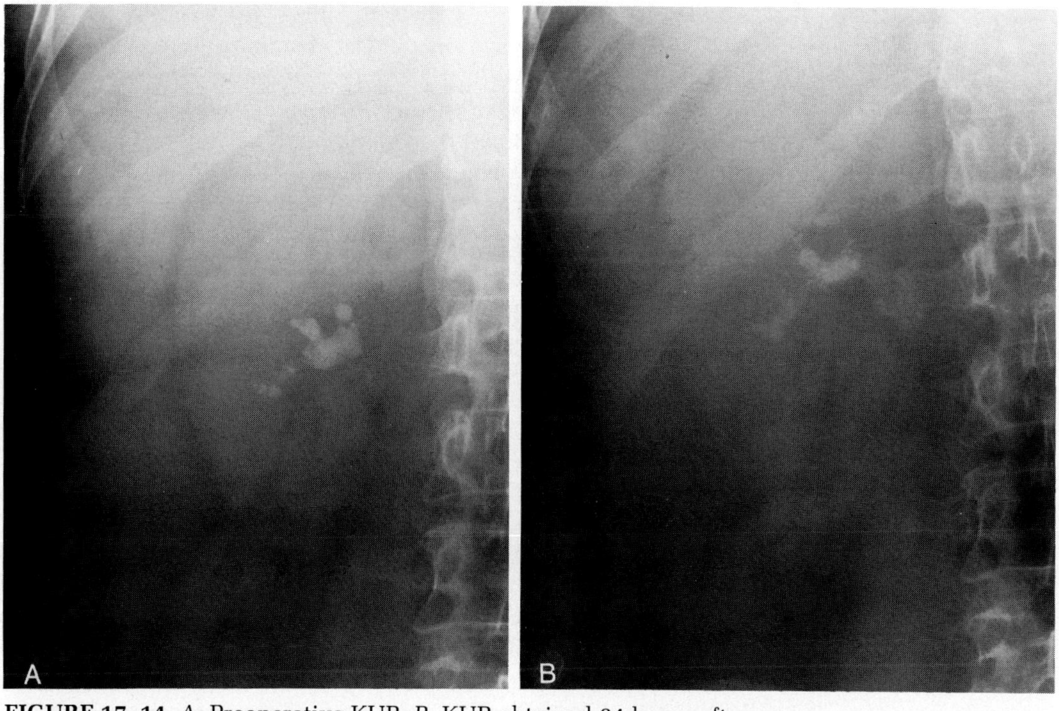

FIGURE 17–14. *A*, Preoperative KUB. *B*, KUB obtained 24 hours after treatment.

mandatory for all patients to be hospitalized for several days following the procedure. Results of these initial studies attested to the safety of the procedure[34, 55] and raised the possibility of performing ESWL as an outpatient procedure.[56] A number of stone centers consider outpatient ESWL preferable to hospitalization, with more than 90 per cent of all patients managed on an ambulatory basis.[51, 56] The ideal candidate for outpatient lithotripsy lives in close proximity to the stone center (<1 hour) and is healthy, with uncomplicated stone disease. Absolute contraindications to ambulatory ESWL include the presence of infectious stones and significant medical problems that require in-hospital care by a physician.

For hospitalized patients, intravenous fluids are continued and a diuresis is maintained. Nausea is common and may be due to a reflex ileus secondary to obstructed hydronephrosis or to treatment-associated retroperitoneal irritation. Antiemetics are administered as required. Pain is a subjective sensation that is difficult to quantitate. The majority of patients experience moderate-to-severe pain, which may be related to the number of shocks and voltage used. The pain may be superficial and localized to the area of shock wave entry or may be deeper and more visceral in origin.[57] Parenteral narcotics are routinely prescribed. Patients with pain that persists for more than 24 hours or seems out of proportion to the treatment should be evaluated to rule out obstruction or perirenal hematoma. The gross hematuria typically clears in a matter of hours. The urine is strained and the fragments are collected and sent for qualitative analysis. The majority of patients begin to pass stone fragments within 12 hours of treatment. The higher the level of the patient's activity, the more rapid and complete the stone passage.[58] Ambulation is therefore encouraged. Most patients are discharged within 48 hours after the procedure.

The process of stone passage must be carefully monitored on an outpatient basis, as silent obstruction leading to complete loss of renal function may occur.[59] Plain films of the abdomen are obtained to check for residual fragments. Ultrasound is used to check for hydronephrosis. Duration of stone passage is related to stone volume. Patients with large stones may continue to pass fragments for 8 to 12 weeks or longer after treatment. Stone-free rates at 3 months have been reported to range from 65 to 90 per cent[3, 55] and are related to stone size. A final intravenous pyelogram is obtained when the plain film shows passage of the majority of fragments, usually 6 to 8 weeks after the treatment.

EXTRACORPOREAL SHOCK WAVE LITHOTRIPSY FOR THE PEDIATRIC POPULATION

Urinary stone disease is relatively uncommon in the pediatric population and accounts for only 2 to 3 per cent of all stone formers.[60] The initial HM-3 Dornier lithotripter limited the treatment of children to those taller than 120 cm (4 feet). Patients smaller than this could not be positioned on the patient support and were thus considered ineligible for treatment. Newman and associates were the first to report successful stone fragmentation in the pediatric population.[25] By modifying the patient support system, ESWL was performed successfully in children shorter than 120 cm. Similar reports soon followed from other stone centers.[61–63] Because of the close proximity of the lung to the kidney and the potential pulmonary complications that may occur if the lung is inadvertently included in the field of treatment, special precautions must be taken to shield the lung from the shock wave. Sheets of styrofoam strategically placed to cover the lung will absorb any misdirected shock waves and protect the patient from pulmonary complications.[62] In addition, when treating pediatric patients, the tub must be only partially filled, or the child will be completely submersed when the stone is in focus. To prevent hematoma formation at the shock wave exit site, a liter bag of intravenous fluid is placed on the child's abdomen if the exit site is not completely covered by the water bath. Complications and success rates mirror those of the adult population.

RESULTS

Renal Stones

The initial German experience showed that successful stone fragmentation was possible in 97 to 99 per cent of all renal stones.[64] Cystine stones are especially recalcitrant to the effects of shock wave treatment, presumably because of their uniform crystalline structure and organic composition.[65, 66] Cystine is the only major stone group composed of organic material. The acoustical properties of the stone may not differ enough from the surrounding body tissues to generate sufficient forces to overcome the comprehensive forces keeping the stone intact.[65] When fragmentation does occur, the pieces are generally larger (5 to 7 mm) than those of other stones and may be too large to pass.[67] Cystine stones greater than 1 to 2 cm in diameter are perhaps better treated by percutaneous techniques. Dretler has shown that the success of fragmentation and the size of the fragments may be predicted on the basis of the composition of the stone.[68] Struvite, uric acid, and apatite stones and stones composed predominately of calcium oxalate dihydrate fragment readily, whereas calcium phosphate dihydrate (brushite) and calcium oxalate monohydrate stones break into small chunks, which may prove too large to pass without difficulty. In general, "harder" calculi will require more shocks generated at a higher voltage to achieve the same degree of fragmentation when compared with more fragile calculi. In addition, patients with hard calculi are more likely to require multiple ESWL sessions and may be more prone to obstructive complications.

Chemical composition is not the only stone characteristic of importance when preoperatively trying to assess the feasibility of performing ESWL. Stone size and location must also be considered. Riehle and associates have studied the voided stone fragments following ESWL in 200 patients and found the most common particle size to be 0.85 to 1.4 mm in diameter.[69] The largest fragment in each sample was usually between 1.4 and 2.0 mm. Fifteen per cent of patients passed fragments between 2.8 and 5.6 mm in size. The largest fragments (>4 mm) were from patients with uric acid or struvite calculi. These stones are typically larger than are those of other composition, and the larger fragments may be a reflection of stone size and inadequacy of treatment rather than composition. When large stones are treated, if the fragments cannot disperse and fall away from the main calculus, new surface area will not be exposed to the shock wave, thus resulting in incomplete fragmentation and larger than desired stone fragments.

The primary goal of open stone surgery is a stone-free patient. Stone surgeons had to be familiar with a variety of different techniques, each designed specifically to remove calculi of a particular size or shape. Although ESWL will fragment the vast majority of calculi, many patients will not become stone free. The initial German experience reported a stone-free rate of 90 per cent 3 months following successful ESWL.[70] The 10 per cent residual stone rate compares favorably with other, more invasive techniques.[71–73] The initial favorable results were accrued in a highly select group of patients with small renal pelvic stones. As the indications were expanded to include more complex calculi, the stone-free rates decreased to 84 per cent at 6-month follow-up.[3] The initial FDA study yielded a stone-free rate of 66 per cent at the time of 3-month follow-up.[55] When stratified by size alone, patients with stones less than 1 cm had a stone-free rate of 82 per cent, while patients with stones greater than 2 to 3 cm had only a 52.5 per cent stone-free rate at 3-month follow-up. Similarly, patients with multiple stones had a higher residual stone rate compared with those with a single stone. Only 29 per cent of patients with more than four stones were stone free at 3 months compared with 77.4 per cent of those with a single stone. Initial results reported by Lingeman were similar, with a 28 per cent residual stone rate reported at the time of 3-month follow-up.[24] Similar results have been reported by others.[74–77] In general, the larger the stone volume, the higher the incidence of retained fragments.

Stone location also influences the treatment outcome.[78, 79] Patients with dependent calyceal stones have a higher residual stone rate compared with individuals having a similar-sized pelvic or upper pole calyceal stone.[80] Marked dilation of the stone-containing collecting system has also been shown to be associated with a high residual stone rate.[78, 79, 81]

The true significance of retained ESWL fragments has yet to be determined. Liedl and associates have reported an 8 per cent recurrent stone rate in patients followed 5 years after ESWL.[82] Unfortunately, the stone recurrence rate was not stratified into those who were stone free and then formed stones and those who formed additional stones in the face of persistent stone fragments. Newman and associates evaluated more than 600 patients at 1 and 2 years from the time of ESWL.[78] At 1-year follow-up, there was an 8.4 per cent recurrent stone rate in patients who had previously achieved a stone-free status. At 2-year follow-up, there was a 10.6 per cent recurrent stone rate. Patients who did not achieve a stone-free status demonstrated a 22 per cent rate of new stone growth. When stratified according to stone composition, the recurrent stone rate was less than the residual fragment growth rate in all stone categories.[78] Unfortunately, in neither of the two studies was metabolic evaluation a routine part of the patients' stone management. The growth of residual stone fragments is not surprising. It is well accepted that residual stone fragments will continue to grow in an abnormal metabolic or stone-forming environment. If metabolic abnormalities are detected and medically corrected, fragment growth does not usually occur. The 8 per cent incidence of new stone formation is comparable to the known 10 to 14 per cent incidence of new stone formation in patients with untreated calcium stone disease.[83, 84] These two studies emphasize and reinforce the importance of obtaining a metabolic evaluation in the stone-forming patient.

Infected renal calculi are caused by urinary tract infection with urease-producing organisms. As the struvite stone forms and grows, bacteria are incorporated into the calculus, forming a nidus for chronic bacteriuria resistant to conventional antibiotic therapy.[85, 86] If stone removal is incomplete, persistent bacteriuria and recurrent stone growth are likely. The Mayo Clinic experience in percutaneously treating struvite calculi confirms this belief.[87] Patients who were rendered stone free had a much lower rate of metabolic stone activity (9 per cent) compared with those having residual stone fragments (63 per cent). It has been assumed that the persistence of residual struvite fragments following ESWL will act as a nidus for chronic recurrent infection and will result in new stone growth. Since struvite calculi tend to be associated with a large stone volume that frequently extends into the peripheral calyceal system, a high residual stone rate is common following ESWL. A high residual stone rate is generally considered to be unacceptable in these patients. Combination therapy—that is, percutaneous debulking followed by ESWL—used in conjunction with chemolysis has yielded results comparable to open stone removal.[33, 77, 88] Michaels and associates have recently studied 15 patients with struvite stones treated by ESWL. All patients had documented *Proteus* infection prior to treatment.[89] In all 15 patients, the stone was completely fragmented to fragments less than 2 mm in diameter. All patients received culture-specific perioperative antibiotics and were followed for an average of 13 months. Stone fragments collected after ESWL were cultured in 11 patients. *Proteus* was cultured from only 3 of 11 stone specimens. Of the 12 patients with residual stone fragments, only 3 experienced persistent *Proteus* infections. No patient demonstrated new stone growth. The authors suggested an increased susceptibility of the pulverized stone material to sterilization with antibacterials as the most reasonable explanation for this finding. Sonda has also reported sterile cultures in several patients following ESWL of struvite calculi with residual fragments.[90] At present, the persistence of residual struvite fragments must be considered undesirable; however, further evaluation is needed to confirm or refute the possibility that pulverization of struvite calculi into minute particles may allow antibiotics to sterilize the residual debris.

Approximately 4 to 16 per cent of all patients will require repeat ESWL treatment.[34, 55, 75, 76] Retreatment rates are directly related to stone size, number of stones, and stone location. Although some stone centers will repeat ESWL within several days of the initial treatment, others have found it advantageous to wait several weeks to allow adequate dispersion of the stone fragments before deciding on the need for retreatment.

Ureteral Stones

Following the initial favorable results in treating renal calculi with the Dornier HM-1 lithotripter, two patients with ureteral stones underwent attempted ESWL treatment. Both stones had been in the ureter for a considerable length of time. In both patients the treatment failed, and they required ureterolithotomy.[70] At the time of surgery, it was noted that although the stones had fragmented, the pieces were unable to disperse, presumably owing to inflammation and ureteral wall edema. As a result of the initial treatment failures, patients with ureteral stones were not considered good candidates for ESWL.

In 1982, with the introduction of the HM-2 lithotripter came a renewed interest in treating ureteral stones.

The ureter is traditionally classified into proximal, mid, and distal segments. When discussing ESWL treatment of ureteral stones, it is helpful to classify the ureter into upper and lower segments. The upper ureter extends from the ureteropelvic junction to the top of the sacroiliac joint. The lower ureter includes the ureteral segment, which passes over the sacroiliac joint and the distal pelvic ureter. Initial attempts at treating stones were limited to those calculi residing in the upper ureter. Recently, favorable results have been reported in treating lower ureteral stones. At this time, it is possible to extend the indications for ESWL therapy to include both upper and lower ureteral calculi.

The results of treating ureteral stones in situ are generally less favorable than those obtained when treating renal pelvic stones. Riehle has proposed both anatomic and technical considerations that contribute to the difficulty in treating upper ureteral calculi[91]:

1. The ureter runs along the psoas muscle, which places it more anterior than the renal pelvis. Since more tissue is interposed between the stone and shock wave electrode, theoretically at least, one would expect increased attenuation of the shock were energy. This problem can be overcome by increasing both the kilovoltage and the number of shocks.
2. The proximity of the vertebral bodies requires rotation of the patient to avoid overlying bony projections that may interfere with stone localization and shock wave transmission.
3. Stones require an expansion chamber, that is, surrounding fluid, for fragmentation to be successful. Stones present in the ureter for prolonged periods are frequently impacted and tightly adherent to the ureteral wall, making dispersion of fragments impossible.
4. Ureteral stones are frequently difficult to visualize fluoroscopically, and thus it is difficult to determine when adequate fragmentation has occurred.

As a result of these considerations, upper ureteral stones in general require more shocks, and higher kilovoltage, than comparably sized renal stones.[27, 45, 54, 91, 92] In addition, treatment failure and retreatment rates are increased.[92, 93]

Stones overlying the sacroiliac joint are refractory to in situ fragmentation using conventional treatment techniques. In the majority of cases, as the shock waves encounter the bony pelvis, sufficient loss of energy occurs to prevent stone fragmentation. Similarly, patients with distal ureteral stones are frequently unable to be positioned at F_2. By modifying positioning of the patient, stone localization and treatment are possible.[26–28, 94]

Upper Ureteral Stones

Following the initial treatment failure in 2 patients, Chaussy reported success in treating 30 patients with ureteral stones. In contrast to the two failures, these stones had become lodged in the ureter only 2 to 4 weeks prior to ESWL therapy.[50, 95] Initial results reported by Lingeman were not as encouraging. Twenty-eight per cent required either retreatment or some other ancillary procedure.[96, 97] Success rates ranging from 60 to 85 per cent have been reported by others treating upper ureteral stones in situ.[98–102]

On the basis of these early clinical results, it was obvious that in situ treatment of ureteral stones was much less successful than treating similar-sized renal pelvic stones. Mueller and colleagues experimentally studied the effects of shock waves on a stone placed in an artificial ureter (Penrose drain) under simulated clinical conditions that varied from a stone that was lying freely in the water-filled ureter to a stone tightly adherent to the wall of the Penrose drain.[99] For fragmentation to be successful, a water-filled space (expansion chamber) surrounding the stone was necessary to allow the fragments to fall away and expose new stone surface to the effects of the shock waves. They concluded that for best clinical results ureteral stones should be displaced back into the pelvis, or at least a ureteral catheter should be placed alongside the stone. This concept was clinically corroborated by Fuchs and associates, who retrospectively reviewed their patients with ureteral stones who underwent attempted ESWL. The presence of an expansion space surrounding the stone was the single most important determinant of a sucessful outcome.[103] Today the presence of an expansion chamber is generally considered to be essential if ureteral fragmentation is to be successful[93, 100, 104] (Fig. 17–15). Stones that are not tightly impacted will demonstrate a natural expansion chamber on intravenous pyclography and may be treated in situ with a reasonable chance of success (70 to 83 per cent).[93, 103, 105] Radiographically, contrast should be seen to flow around the stone and fill the distal ureter. There should be no significant delay in visualization of the collecting system compared with the contralateral side. The naturally present expansion chamber may be increased in size, with a concomitant improvement in treatment results to about 90 to 95 per cent, by placing a ureteral stent alongside the stone[103, 105] (Fig. 17–16).

Success rates approaching 100 per cent are possible after the stone has been repositioned back into the renal pelvis—the "push and bang" technique.[93, 97, 103] In the absence of significant ureteral narrowing around the stone, the simple passage of a ureteral catheter may prove sufficient to dislodge the stone back into the pelvis. If the stone is refractory to stent dislodgment, irrigation with saline or lidocaine may prove beneficial (see Chapter 16). If a catheter cannot be passed beyond the stone and the stone cannot be dislodged, an end-hole ureteral catheter is placed next to the stone and either manual or continuous irrigation is provided during the treatment to create an artificial fluid space around the stone and to dislodge any fragments.[105]

Lower Ureteral Stones

The initial investigative studies conducted by the FDA limited the treatment of urinary stones to those in the kidney or upper ureter. Patients with lower ureteral stones were managed primarily by either stone basketing or ureteroscopic

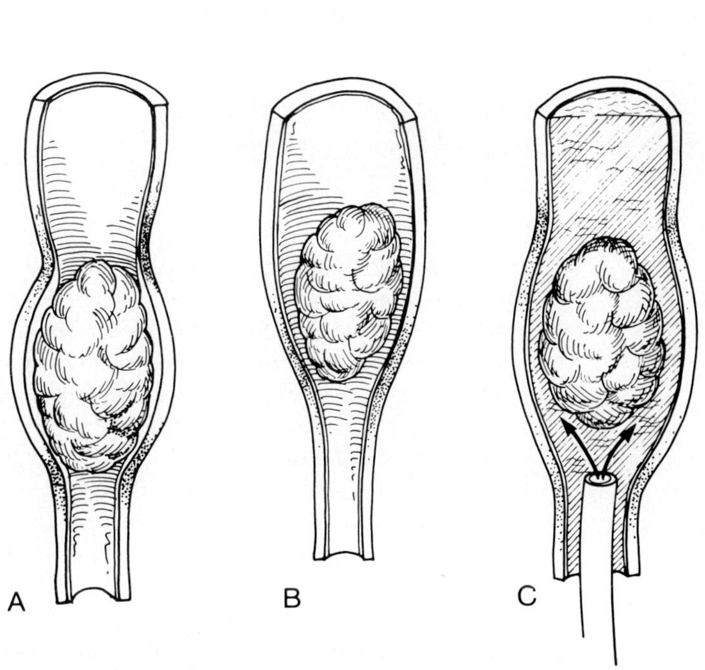

FIGURE 17–15. Diagrammatic representation of ureteral stone (*A*) and concept of both natural (*B*) and artificially created (*C*) expansion chambers.

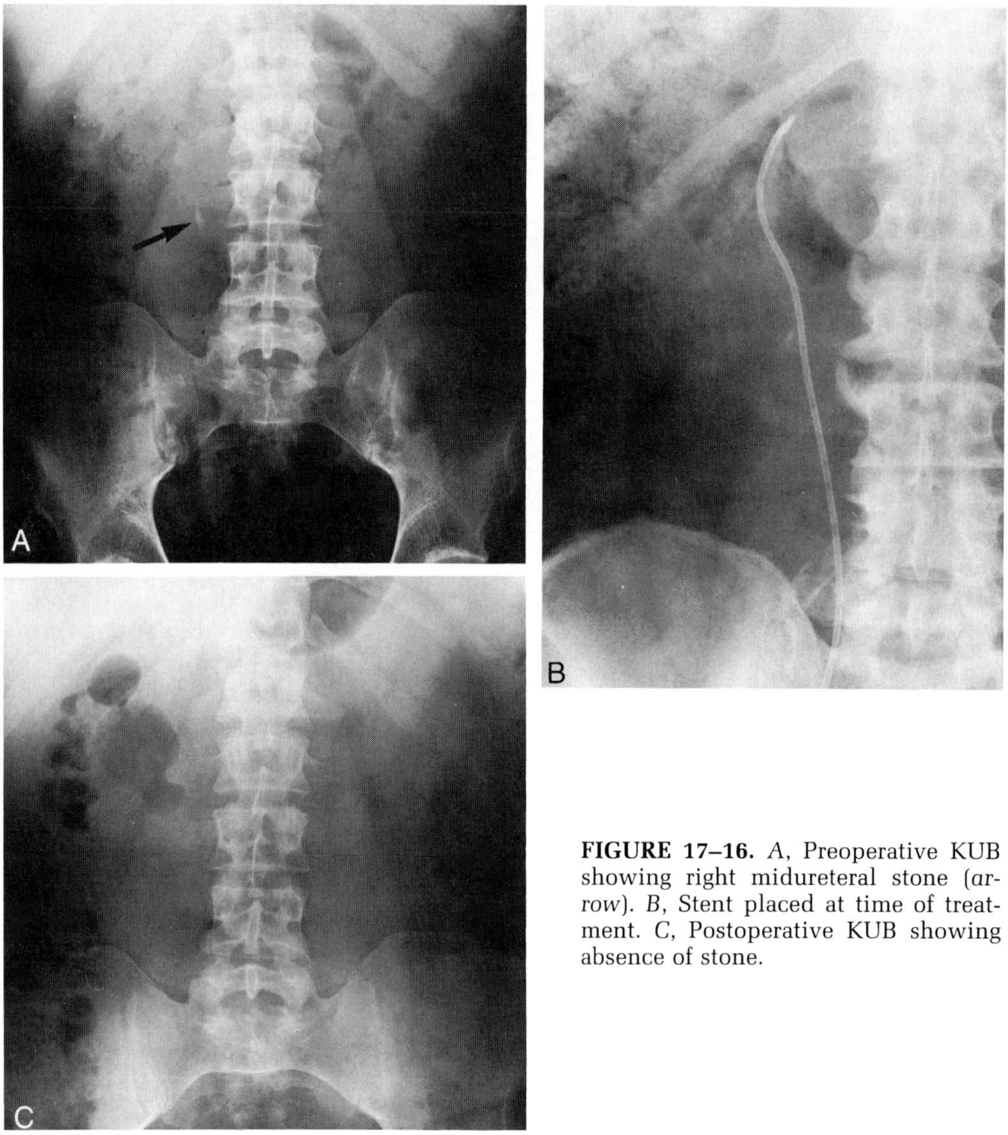

FIGURE 17–16. *A*, Preoperative KUB showing right midureteral stone (*arrow*). *B*, Stent placed at time of treatment. *C*, Postoperative KUB showing absence of stone.

stone extraction. ESWL was limited to those stones that could be repositioned into the upper ureter or renal pelvis. Although the FDA has not officially approved the use of ESWL for the treatment of lower ureteral stones, ESWL has been shown to be effective in treating many lower ureteral calculi[28, 94, 96, 105–107] and is less traumatic than other treatment options.

Miller and associates were the first to report the successful ESWL treatment of lower ureteral calculi.[96] By altering the gantry, the patient is placed in a modified sitting position[94] (Fig. 17–17). The shock wave passes through the buttock and utilizes the bony pelvic outlet as a suitable window through which the shock waves may be directed to the prevesical ureter. Active cooperation by the patient is required to maintain the sitting position. A regional anesthetic is recommended. Becht and associates reported a 95 per cent success rate in treating 39 patients with prevesical calculi.[28] Patients were placed more horizontal than the traditional position for upper tract calculi. The shock waves entered

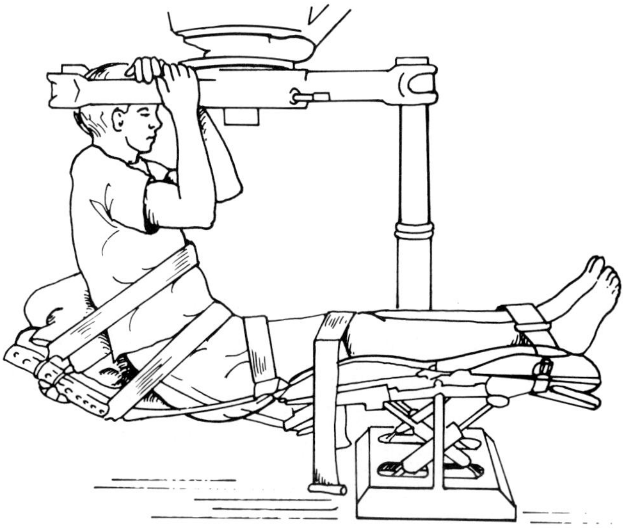

FIGURE 17–17. Modified sitting position useful in treating lower ureteral stones.

through either the obturator foramen or the greater sciatic notch. Success rates of 89 and 94 per cent have been reported by other investigators.[94, 107]

Patients with ureteral stones located over the sacroiliac joint have until recently not been considered candidates for ESWL. There is no current evidence to suggest that the bone is damaged by shock wave treatment. However, sufficient loss of energy occurs to render the treatment ineffective. Jenkins and Miller and their colleagues have reported success in treating these stones with the patient in the prone position[26, 27] (Fig. 17–18). The prone position is also useful in treating calculi in pelvic kidneys and in obese patients in whom the stone cannot be placed at F_2 using the traditional treatment position.

COMPLICATIONS

In spite of the noninvasiveness of ESWL therapy, complications may occur. As in any surgical procedure, problems may arise during the procedure, immediately postoperative, or in the long term.

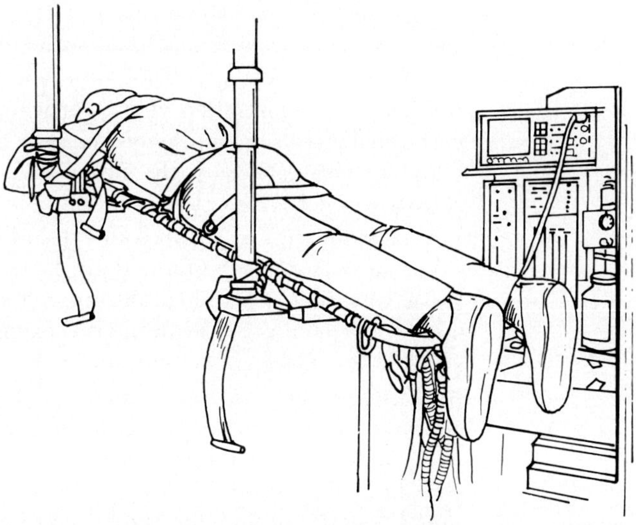

FIGURE 17–18. Prone position useful for treating lower ureteral stones.

Procedural complications are related primarily to the anesthetic or to the tissue effects of the shock wave. Anesthetic-related complications are similar to those reported during any surgical procedure. Mechanical malfunctions are rare. Perhaps the most serious of these malfunctions is a failure of the shock wave to be delivered during the refractory period of the cardiac cycle. Initial experience by Chaussy showed a high (80 per cent) incidence of dysrhythmias when the shock wave was manually triggered.[23] To avoid this problem, shock wave discharge is timed to occur outside the period of the cardiac cycle during which serious arrhythmias may occur. Each shock is timed to be delivered only during the period of ventricular refractoriness (<10 msec after the onset of the R wave). A heart rate of 120 beats per minute or less will allow for this critical timing. It is recommended that if the shock waves are not being delivered during the refractory period, the procedure be terminated.

Transient gross hematuria occurs in nearly all patients during the procedure and usually resolves within 24 hours. Clinically significant bleeding with the need for blood transfusion is rare. Charig and associates reviewed more than 300 consecutive patients and reported no blood transfusions.[108] Riehle and colleagues reported the need for a blood transfusion in only 1 of 518 consecutive patients.[74] Lingeman and coworkers noted an average fall in hematocrit of only 2 per cent.[24] Of all the many techniques available to remove urinary calculi surgically, ESWL is associated with the lowest rate of blood transfusion.

Two theories have been proposed to explain the generalized occurrence of gross hematuria. First, it may be due to local urothelial trauma caused by the shifting of the stone fragments in the renal pelvis. In vitro studies performed independently by Eisenberger and Jaeger have failed to show significant urothelial trauma resulting from the fragmentation of calculi.[109, 110] Canine kidneys without stones subjected to shock wave treatment all developed gross hematuria. In addition, hematuria has been reported to occur in all patients subjected to biliary lithotripsy. These last two observations by Jaeger implicate intrinsic renal trauma as the most likely cause of hematuria.[109] Rubin studied 50 patients before and after ESWL with computerized tomography (CT) and noted a 15 per cent incidence of subcapsular hematoma and a 4 per cent incidence of intrarenal hematomas.[111] Magnetic resonance imaging (MRI) findings suggestive of blunt renal trauma and consisting of subcapsular hemorrhage, loss of corticomedullary junction demarcation, and perirenal fluid collection were reported after ESWL by Kaude and associates in 29 per cent of 38 treated kidneys.[112] Baumgartner and coworkers reported MRI abnormalities in 29 of 39 kidneys (74 per cent) studied after ESWL.[113] The most common MRI abnormality (63 per cent) consisted of an alteration of the corticomedullary junction, a finding consistent with renal contusion and hemorrhage or edema. The severity of the changes was found to correlate with the number of shock waves administered, a finding substantiated by Newman and colleagues, who reported a correlation between histologic findings in canine kidneys and the number of shocks administered.[114]

Canine studies performed by Jaeger in which kidneys treated with 1500 shock waves were histologically studied at 1 hour, 24 to 36 hours, 7 to 11 days, and 3 to 6 months following ESWL exposure confirmed the traumatic nature of shock wave therapy.[115] Findings at 1 hour consistently showed bleeding foci primarily at the corticomedullary junction and extending into the medulla. Rupture of the glomerular capsule, veins, arteries, peritubular vessels, and juxtaglomerular apparatus with perivascular hemorrhage was seen in many areas. Bleeding into ruptured arterial walls and subcapsular hemorrhage were also noted. Significant findings 24 to 36 hours after treatment consisted of the presence of vacuolated tubule cells, signifying the start of tubular necrosis and fibrin deposition consistent with early encapsulation. At 7 to 11 days, encapsulation of the hemorrhagic foci was noted. At 3 months after ESWL, the histologic findings were minimal and consisted of streaky interstitial fibrosis at the site of previous hemorrhage. Similar experimental findings have been reported by Newman, who used a Dornier lithotripter, and Abrahams, who used a Medstone machine.[114, 116] There was no evidence of ESWL-induced loss of renal function, as measured by serum creatinine, creatinine clearance, or renal scintigraphy. Enzyme changes—that is, changes in *N*-acetylglucosaminidase (NAG) and lactate dehydrogenase (LDH)—indicative of renal tubular damage have been reported.[117] In addition, cell cultures placed at the focal point have demonstrated both morphologic and functional changes, the extent of which may be correlated with the number of shock waves administered.[118, 119] It has been speculated that the traumatic effects of shock waves are due to cavitation bubbles produced in the wake of the passing shock wave.[120, 121] Experimental and clinical evidence suggests that the hematuria associated with ESWL is related primarily to shock wave–induced parenchymal trauma, which is usually self-limiting and rarely requires blood transfusions.

Pain is a subjective sensation, the severity of which is difficult to evaluate clinically. Pain in various degrees of severity is present in nearly all patients being treated with the HM-3 lithotripter.[55] The pain may be perceived as superficial and localized to the site of shock wave entry and exit or may be more visceral in nature. Approximately 40 per cent of patients will have pain severe enough to require narcotics.[122] Those treated as outpatients tend to require fewer analgesics. Pain severity has been shown to be related to stone size. In the United States Cooperative Study, approximately 40 per cent of patients with stones less than 1 cm experienced no pain, while 2.5 per cent of those patients reported severe pain. Of the patients with staghorn calculi, 20 per cent reported no pain, whereas approximately 10 per cent reported severe pain.[55] Patients with severe pain that persists for more than 24 hours or those in whom the pain seems out of proportion to the extent of treatment should be evaluated for either obstruction or hematoma formation.

The earliest clinical studies by Chaussy showed the lung to be extremely susceptible to the effect of shock wave therapy. The tissue-damaging effect is presumably due to the wide differences in acoustical impedance between the air-filled alveoli and soft tissue. The danger is more theoretic than actual, as hemoptysis has rarely been a problem. Patients with low-lying lung fields and high-riding kidneys are at high risk for this complication, as are patients with severe spinal deformities. When indicated, a CT scan to evaluate the position of the stone in relationship to the lung field should be performed. Styrofoam has proved effective in shielding the lung from the tissue-damaging effects of the shock wave and should be used in children and adults when the lung field is thought to project into the line of treatment.

Although the renal tissue–damaging effect of shock waves is irrefutable, seldom does it lead to major clinical complications. The incidence of clinically significant perirenal or subcapsular hematoma is less than 1 per cent (about 1 in 450 patients in the Cooperative Study[54]). Knapp and colleagues reviewed 3620 ESWL treatments and identified 24 perirenal hematomas (incidence, 0.66 per cent).[123] All hematomas were discovered by renal ultrasound and confirmed by either CT or MRI (Fig. 17–19). Coagulation studies were normal in all patients, and there was no correlation between the kilovoltage or number of shock waves used. Preexisting hypertension, especially when poorly controlled (diastolic

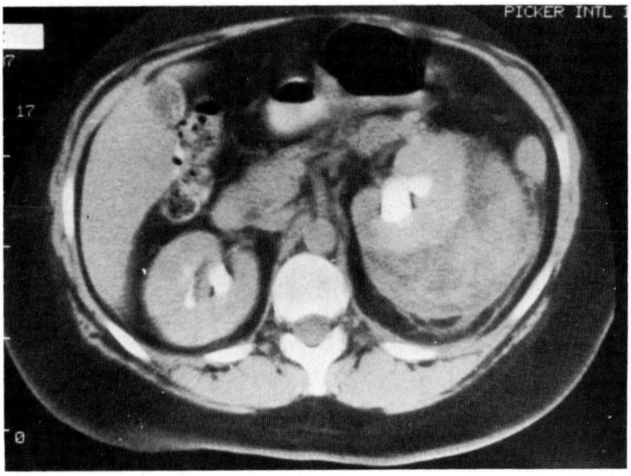

FIGURE 17–19. CT demonstrating left perirenal hematoma after ESWL.

pressure >90 mm Hg), and infection before ESWL were significant risk factors. Conservative management consisting of bedrest and blood transfusions as needed was successful in all but one patient, who required selective embolization of a bleeding vessel. All patients experienced significant post-ESWL pain, with 90 per cent requiring parenteral narcotics. Owing to the risk of intrarenal and perirenal bleeding, all patients should have stopped taking anticoagulants and any medication known to affect the clotting mechanism 1 to 2 weeks before scheduled treatment.

Urinary tract infection and sepsis are potential complications of any invasive urologic procedure and have been reported in 0.1 to 5.0 per cent of patients undergoing ESWL.[101, 124] Patients with complex struvite calculi are at high risk for urosepsis, owing to the liberation of bacteria as the stone is fragmented. These patients are admitted 48 hours prior to treatment and receive culture-specific broad-spectrum parenteral antibiotics. The antibiotics are continued for a minimum of 24 hours after ESWL, at which time the patient is started on an oral antibiotic. The judicious use of nephrostomy tubes and indwelling ureteral stents will help promote drainage and avoid obstruction and further limit the incidence of urosepsis. The use of prophylactic perioperative antibiotics in patients with uncomplicated calculi and sterile urine is controversial. Roth has recommended prophylaxis with a first-generation cephalosporin administered intravenously at the time of the procedure and then followed by an orally administered cephalosporin for 2 days.[101]

Urinary tract obstruction has been reported in up to 31 per cent of patients undergoing ESWL.[34, 125] The incidence of obstruction is related to size, stone location, and number of calculi. Patients with stones greater than 2 to 3 cm appear at high risk for developing post-ESWL obstruction, with a reported incidence of partial obstruction being 50 per cent.[34] In the same study, stones less than 1 cm in diameter had an incidence of obstruction of 24 per cent, while stones 1 to 2 cm in diameter produced partial obstruction in 34 per cent of cases. The obstruction may be due to a single large fragment (>5 mm) that has become lodged in the ureter, or it may be due to the accumulation of multiple small fragments (a condition known as *Steinstrasse*, or "stone street") (Fig. 17–20). The onset of obstruction is usually heralded by colicky pain, nausea, and vomiting. If the obstruction is detected on routine follow-up and kidney, ureter, and bladder

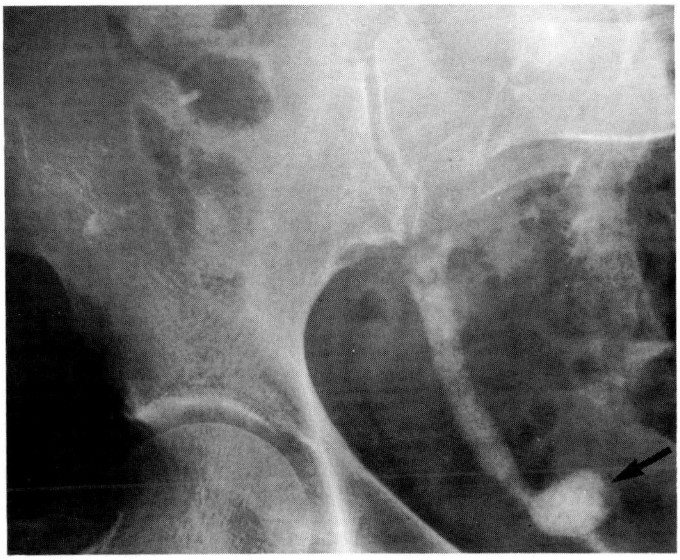

FIGURE 17–20. KUB demonstrating typical appearance of distal *Steinstrasse*. Note fragment accumulation in bladder (*arrow*).

(KUB) film and the patient is asymptomatic, a trial of observation is appropriate. The indications for intervention are similar to those for patients presenting with obstruction due to ureteral calculi and are as follows:

1. Pain.
2. Complete obstruction.
3. Significant obstruction in a solitary kidney, as evidenced by rising creatinine levels.
4. Urosepsis.
5. Failure to pass fragments after a reasonable time.

Large series have shown the incidence of post-ESWL intervention for obstruction to range from 6 to 12 per cent, with obstruction directly related to stone size.[34, 126, 127] Chaussy has reported a 39 per cent incidence of percutaneous tube placement in patients with partial staghorn calculi.[54]

Intervention for obstruction should proceed in an orderly manner from the least invasive to more invasive procedures. Patients with a single large obstructing fragment undergo cystoscopy and attempted indwelling stent placement under attended local anesthesia. Solitary distal fragments may be fluoroscopically basketed or removed with the ureteroscope. Upper ureteral fragments may respond to repeat ESWL. If passage of a ureteral catheter is impossible, a nephrostomy tube is placed. If the stone fragment fails to pass with proximal diversion repeat ESWL, a percutaneous manipulation is then indicated. Open surgical procedures are seldom indicated.

The management of *Steinstrasse* varies only slightly from that of a solitary obstructing fragment. Symptomatic *Steinstrasse* typically involves the distal ureter. Attempted stent placement is usually ineffective in bypassing the obstruction owing to the tight packing of the fragments in the ureter. Percutaneous nephrostomy tube palcement with the patient under local anesthesia will provide symptomatic relief. With proximal diversion, the *Steinstrasse* often passes spontaneously. If obstruction persists, endoscopic intervention is indicated. Rarely is stone basketing successful. Dretler has reported success in clearing the distal ureter of fragments by manually pulsing saline through a ureteral catheter.[65] Once the distal ureter has been cleared, ureteroscopy with ultrasonic clearance of the fragments may be performed. Proximal *Steinstrasse* may respond to repeat ESWL, especially if there is a lead fragment as a source of the obstruction. If this is ineffective, a percutaneous antegrade approach should be considered. It is best to avoid this complication. The judicious use of ureteral stents in the perioperative period will help avoid obstruction by maintaining ureteral patency as the fragments pass alongside the stent. Ureteral stents placed prior to ESWL and removed at the time of treatment have been shown to dilate the ureter[128] and facilitate fragment passage.[52, 125] The current indications for the perioperative use of indwelling stents are controversial.[129–133] The decision for stent placement is based on stone location, size (>2.5 cm), clinical circumstances (outpatient therapy), stone composition (struvite), and the patient's body habitus (spinal cord–injured patient). When treating large complex calculi, the stent is best left until the majority of fragments have cleared the urinary tract (usually 6 to 8 weeks).

The use of indwelling ureteral stents is not without complication and should not give the treating physician a false sense of security, as ureteral obstruction may still occur.

Death is a potential complication of any procedure requiring general anesthesia. In 1987, the American Urological Association Lithotripsy Committee reported a mortality of 0.02 per cent in patients undergoing ESWL.[134] Of the 13 reported deaths, only 3 appeared to be directly related to the ESWL procedure. The causes of death included pulmonary emboli (2), myocardial infarction (3), retroperitoneal hemorrhage (1), cerebrovascular accident (1), suicide (1), sepsis (1), mesenteric thrombosis (1), respiratory arrest after a fall (1), complication of solvent irrigation (1), and gallbladder cancer (1).

LONG-TERM COMPLICATIONS

Although both morphologic and radiographic studies have shown ESWL to cause renal parenchymal changes similar to those seen following significant blunt renal trauma, no long-term side effects directly attributable to ESWL have been reported. However, Lingeman has suggested the possibility of hypertension developing in patients following ESWL.[135] Two hundred and ninety-five patients who were followed a minimum of 1 year after ESWL were reviewed retrospectively. He reported an 8.2 per cent onset of newly diagnosed hypertension that required medical treatment, and an additional 15.2 per cent of patients demonstrated an elevation in diastolic blood pressure that did not require drug therapy. The proposed mechanism is related to the morphologic changes that have been reported following ESWL, that is, subcapsular hematoma and other subtle changes thought to be due to the intraparenchymal extravasation of blood or urine or both. It is proposed that these changes could lead to chronic fibrosis with compression of the kidney, an increase in renin release, and hypertension, a scenario not unlike that reported with the Page kidney.[136, 137] Reports by others have not substantiated Lingeman's findings. Liedl reviewed 487 patients followed 40 months after ESWL and reported only a 3.1 per cent (9 patients) incidence of hypertension (<160/95 mm Hg).[82] The expected incidence of developing hypertension in an age-related population followed for 40 months is 2.8 per cent. The slight difference was not statistically significant. Chaussy prospectively studied 124 patients and found that only 1 patient became hypertensive following ESWL (incidence, 0.9 per cent).[134] Lingeman, in a follow-up to his initial report, reviewed more than 1000 patients and concluded that "if there is an effect of ESWL on blood pressure it is a very small one."[138] Sandlow reviewed 112 patients who underwent repeated ESWL (two to five procedures), a group of patients one would suspect as being at high risk for developing hypertension, and reported 17 patients as having an increase in mean blood pressure of at least 10 mm Hg, while 19 had a decrease of at least 10 mm Hg. On the basis of their findings, ESWL was not found to cause hypertension.[139, 140] Similar findings have been reported by others.[141, 142] Zwergel identified 12 of 208 patients who developed hypertension following ESWL. Peripheral and central plasma renin values were studied, and no significant correlation was found to exist between renin activity and postoperative hypertension.[142]

At this time, one cannot implicate ESWL as a direct cause of hypertension. Additional prospective studies are required, as are studies to determine the incidence of hypertension in patients with stones who are managed by alternative surgical techniques.

Chaussy has reported no ill effects on renal function (based on I-131 hippurate scans) following ESWL in patients followed for 4 years.[54] Gilbert and associates have reported proteinuria in the nephrotic range following ESWL, which returned to normal in 3 to 6 months.[143] They also reported improvement in glomerular filtration rates following ESWL in patients previously obstructed. Patients not obstructed showed no significant change in glomerular filtration rates before and after ESWL. Treated kidneys maintained their ability to dilute urine and conserve sodium.

The Dornier system uses biplanar fluoroscopy both to localize and to monitor the effects of shock wave therapy. The amount of radiation delivered to the patient is determined by a number of variables, including size, location, and composition of the stone. In addition, the operator's experience, degree of balloon inflation, size of the patient, and number of spot films also determine the amount of radiation exposure.[144, 145] Calculated doses of radiation delivered to the operating room personnel and the treating urologist have been shown to be minimal and of no consequence.[146] Measurements taken 1 meter from the tub showed the level of radiation to be less than one thirtieth of that measured at the tub's rim.[147]

Radiation exposure to the patient has been shown by many to compare favorably with other standard radiographic studies[141–150] and to be considerably less than the amount of radiation delivered to the patient during percutaneous nephrolithotomy.[147, 148, 150]

Pollack has defined a number of strategies to help reduce the amount of radiation exposure[151]:

1. Always keep the image intensifier as close to the patient as possible. This reduces the amount of surface exposed to radiation and increases the image clarity, thus reducing the need for extended fluoroscopy to localize the stone.
2. Resist the temptation to use continuous fluoroscopy.
3. Avoid using fluoroscopy with the balloons deflated. The poor image quality will undoubtedly require prolonged fluoroscopy time.
4. Limit the use of video images or snapshots to those situations in which the improved image quality is essential. Each snapshot delivers the equivalent of 8 seconds of fluoroscopy time.
5. View fluoroscopic screens in subdued light.

6. Use ureteral catheters to help localize poorly calcified stones or in those patients in whom localization is anticipated as being difficult.
7. Avoid using fluoroscopy while attendants are leaning over the tub.

Concerns regarding hearing loss in operating room personnel exposed daily to ESWL have been raised. Patients are exposed to sound impulses of 112 dB levels.[152] Sound intensity of this degree is sufficient to cause noise-induced sensorineural hearing loss. Since the hazardous effects of noise depend also on the number of exposures to the high-intensity sound, the risk of hearing loss to the patient is minimal. Operating room personnel are exposed to sounds of less intensity, but of greater duration and on a daily basis, thereby increasing the risk of hearing loss. Further studies are required to assess the risk of hearing loss in ESWL personnel. Until those studies are performed, noise protection is recommended.[153]

Damage to Surrounding Organs

Shock waves unequivocally cause renal parenchymal damage, as documented by radiographic and histologic animal studies. In addition, serum enzyme elevation of *N*-acetyl-β-glucosaminidase and lactic dehydrogenase confirms the damaging effect to the kidney. Trauma to adjacent organs—that is, liver, pancreas, and skeletal muscle—also occurs during ESWL. Studies have shown transient elevation in the following serum and urine values after treatment: bilirubin, serum glutamic oxaloacetic transaminase, creatinine phosphokinase, β-galactosidase, and glutamyl transpeptidase.[80] Myocardial damage due to the direct effects of shock wave energy has not been reported.[153] Pancreatitis, with elevation in amylase and lipase levels, has also been reported.[80] To date, no long-term side effects have been reported in any of the adjacent organs following ESWL. Studies have failed to show any deleterious effect of shock wave on either the spinal cord[124] or the ovary[154] of experimental animals in spite of their being exposed to energy levels greater than those delivered in clinical practice. Studies in rats to determine the effect of shock waves on developing bone have shown that shock waves focused directly on the growth plate of immature bone can affect future bone growth.[155] The clinical significance of this finding is still unknown. There have been no reports of skeletal or other bony abnormalities occurring after stone therapy. In addition, it is difficult to extrapolate the experimental animal findings to the clinical setting. The animals were exposed to higher shock wave energy levels than used in clinical practice, and the growth plate was placed directly at F_2, a situation that is not likely to occur in clinical practice.

INPATIENT AND OUTPATIENT EXTRACORPOREAL SHOCK WAVE LITHOTRIPSY

The advantages of outpatient surgery include financial savings and increased convenience to the patient. The ideal procedures suited for an ambulatory setting are those that are relatively short, are associated with minimal perioperative pain, and have a low incidence of perioperative complications. Patients with multiple medical problems or a history of severe cardiac disease are not candidates for outpatient procedures. Many common urologic procedures are performed routinely on an outpatient basis; recently, lithotripsy, both percutaneous and extracorporeal, has been added to that list.

ESWL is a procedure that fulfills the criteria for an outpatient procedure. Operative time varies, depending on the size and composition of the stone, but generally lasts from 30 to 90 minutes. Chaussy reported an average treatment time of 45 minutes (range, 20 to 60 minutes).[54] Operative complications are minimal and related primarily to anesthesia. The incidence of perioperative blood transfusions is less than 1 per cent. Charig and colleagues reviewed more than 300 consecutive patients and reported no blood transfusion.[108] Riehle and associates reported the need for transfusions in only 1 of 518 treated patients.[74] Lingeman and coworkers reported an average postoperative fall in hematocrit of only 2 per cent.[24] Renal and perirenal bleeding may be life threatening but occurs in fewer than 1 per cent (0.66 to 0.10 per cent) of all patients. This complication can be minimized by stopping all medications that affect the blood-clotting mechanism 1 to 2 weeks prior to therapy; in addition, hypertension must be well controlled and the urine must be sterile. Of 15 subcapsular hematomas identified by Jocham and colleagues (1836 patients), only 3 required blood transfusions.[149]

The incidence of urosepsis is also low (0.3 per cent).[101] Patients with infectious complex calculi must be treated perioperatively with culture-specific antibiotics. The use of nephrostomy tubes or indwelling stents or both further limits this complication.

Reported success with ambulatory ESWL is encouraging[51, 156] and, in some stone centers, represents the preferred approach to management of patients, with 90 to 97 per cent of all patients being successfully treated on an outpatient basis.[56] The use of indwelling ureteral stents to limit perioperative obstruction ranges from 30 to 80 per cent of patients managed as outpatients.[56]

Contraindications to outpatient treatment include complex struvite calculi, a history of poorly controlled cardiac arrhythmias, significant cardiac disease, and the presence of other medical problems that require in-hospital care by a physician other than a urologist.

FUTURE CONSIDERATIONS

Many questions regarding the safety of ESWL remain unanswered. How many shocks may be safely administered to the kidney in one treatment session? The arbitrary figure of 2000 was selected during the initial clinical trials and has remained in spite of reports using more than 3000 shocks per treatment without immediate complications.[156] Can the kidney tolerate more shocks if administered over multiple areas of the kidney? Is it safer to administer 3000 shocks to the kidney in a single session or divide the dose into two treatment sessions? How many days should separate multiple treatment sessions? What is the maximal voltage that can be safely used? Are the alternatives to spark gap technology less traumatic to the kidney and surrounding tissues? These are all clinical questions regarding safety that only careful studies can answer.

It is estimated that at least 70 per cent of all stones may be treated solely by ESWL. Owing to the noninvasiveness of the procedure, it is expected that stones will be treated earlier, and perhaps even when asymptomatic, to limit future morbidity. One can expect to see fewer large complex calculi that require open surgical intervention. As improvements in the current technology continue and tubless, anesthesia-free lithotripters become more readily available, it is anticipated that even patients with complex renal calculi will be managed by staged ESWL sessions rather than by more invasive techniques.

In an attempt to limit the need for anesthesia, the Dornier HM-3 lithotripter has undergone several modifications. The modified HM-3 is equipped with a low-pressure generator (40 nF compared with 80 nF). The generator modification reduces by 30 per cent the pressures in F_2 compared with the standard system. A generator voltage of 18 kV will yield a pressure of 600 bars at F_2 compared with 900 bars with the standard system.[157] With the low-pressure generator, patients may be comfortably treated using a long-acting anxiolytic combined with a centrally acting analgesic. More shocks and a prolonged treatment time are usually required.[157, 158] By increasing the aperture of the focusing ellipsoid from 15.6 cm to 17.2 cm, the focal area at F_2 may be reduced, while the pressures are slightly increased. In addition, the penetrating surface of the shock waves increased, thus diminishing the peak pressure per square inch of skin, a modification that, theoretically at least, should decrease the surface pain. When a twin-pulse technique is used whereby two shocks are sequentially timed to a single R wave, treatment results comparable to those achieved with the standard HM-3 have been reported.[15] The incidence of postoperative ancillary procedures, the number of shocks, and the time of treatment did not differ significantly from the results using the standard HM-3 lithotripter. The incidence of skin bruising was lower, suggesting that perhaps the modified HM-3 caused less tissue damage to surrounding tissue.

REFERENCES

1. Forssman B, Hepp W, Chaussy C, et al: Eine Methode, 2 UR berührungsfreien Zertrümmerung von Nierensteinen durch Stosswellen. Biomed Tech (Berlin) 22:164, 1977.
2. Chaussy C, Schmiedt E, Jocham D, et al: In vitro and in vivo studies on biological systems. *In* Chaussy C (ed): Extracorporeal Shock Wave Lithotripsy. Basel, S. Karger, 1982, pp 21–35.
3. Chaussy C, Schmiedt E, Schuller J, et al: Extracorporeal shock wave lithotripsy (ESWL) for treatment of urolithiasis. Urology [Suppl] 23:5, 1984.
4. Ison KT: Physical and technical introduction to lithotripsy. *In* Coptcoat MJ, Miller RA, Wickham JEA (eds): Lithotripsy II. London, BDI Publishing, 1987, pp 7–14.
5. Griffin AS, Kandel LB, Harrison LH: Electrohydraulic (Dornier) Lithotripter. *In* Kandel LB, Harrison LH, McCullough DL (eds): Extracorporeal Shock Wave Lithotripsy. Mount Kisco, NY, Futura Publishing Company, 1987, pp 37–71.
6. Hunter PT: Principles of Extracorporeal Shock Wave Lithotripsy. New York, Churchill Livingstone, 1987, pp 13–17.
7. Hunter PT, Finlayson BJ, Hirko RI, et al: Measurement of shock wave pressures used for lithotripsy. J Urol 136:733, 1986.
8. Newman RC, Finlayson B: New developments in ESWL. AUA Update Series 7:50, 1988.
9. Kaneko H, Watanabe H, Takahashi T, et al: Studies on the application of microexplosion to medicine and biology. IV. Strength of wet and dry urinary calculi. Nippon Hinyokika Gakkai Zasshi 70:61, 1979.
10. Whelan JP, Finlayson B, Welch J, et al: The blast path: Theoretical basis, experimental data and clinical application. J Urol 140:401, 1988.
11. Chaussy C, Schmiedt E, Jocham D, et al: Shock wave generation apparatus arrangement and in vitro testing of the prototype—methods and results. *In* Chaussy C (ed): Extracorporeal Shock Wave Lithotripsy. Basel, S. Karger, 1982, pp 8–19.
12. Saltzman B: Second-generation shock wave lithotripters. Urol Clin North Am 15:385, 1988.
13. Wilbert DM, Reichenberger H, Noske E, et al: New generation shock wave lithotripsy. J Urol 138:563, 1987.
14. Clayman RV, McClennan BL: Extracorporeal shock wave lithotripsy with an electromagnetic acoustic source. (Lithostar): Preliminary report. J Endourol 2:177, 1988.
15. Rassweiler J, Gumpinger R, Mayer R, et al: Extracorporeal piezoelectric lithotripsy using the Wolf-lithotriptor versus low energy lithotripsy with the modified Dornier HM-3: A cooperative study. World J Urol 5:218, 1987.

16. Marberger M, Tuck C, Steinkogler I: Painless piezoelectric extracorporeal lithotripsy. J Urol 139:695, 1988.
17. Vallancien G, Aviles J, Munoz R, et al: Piezoelectric extracorporeal lithotripsy by ultrashort waves with the EDAP LT01 device. J Urol 139:689, 1988.
18. Ryan PC, Butler MR: EDAP LT01 lithotripter. J Endourol 2:181, 1988.
19. Spirnak JP, Resnick MI: Kidney stone surgery. *In* Gillenwater JG, Grayhack JT, Howard SS, Duckett JW (eds): Adult and Pediatric Urology. Chicago, Year Book Medical Publishers 1987, pp 555–578.
20. Spirnak JP, Resnick MI: Urinary stones. *In* Tanagho EA, McAninch JW (eds): Smith's General Urology. Norwalk, CT, Appleton and Lange, 1988, pp 275–301.
21. Mee SL, Thuroff JW: Small caliceal stones: Is extracorporeal shock wave lithotripsy justified? J Urol 139:908, 1988.
22. Brannen GE, Bush WH, Lewis GP: Caliceal calculi. J Urol 135:1142, 1986.
23. Riehle RA: Extracorporeal shock wave lithotripsy. Prob Urol 1:608, 1987.
24. Lingeman JE, Newman D, Mertz JHO, et al: Extracorporeal shock wave lithotripsy: The Methodist Hospital of Indiana experience. J Urol 135:1134, 1986.
25. Newman DM, Coury T, Lingeman JE, et al: Extracorporeal shock wave lithotripsy experience in children. J Urol 136:238, 1986.
26. Miller K, Bachor R, Hautmann R: Extracorporeal shock wave lithotripsy in the prone position: Technique, indications, results. J Endourol 2:113, 1988.
27. Jenkins AD, Gillenwater JY: Extracorporeal shock wave lithotripsy in the prone position: Treatment of stones in the distal ureter or anomalous kidney. J Urol 139:911, 1988.
28. Becht E, Moll V, Neisius D, et al: Treatment of prevesical ureteral calculi by extracorporeal shock wave lithotripsy. J Urol 139:916, 1988.
29. Brannen GE, Bush WH, Correa RJ, et al: Kidney stone removal: Percutaneous versus surgical lithotomy. J Urol 133:6, 1985.
30. Anderson L, Sylven M: Small renal caliceal calculi as a cause of pain. J Urol 130:752, 1983.
31. Brannen GE, Bush WH, Lewis GP: Caliceal calculi. J Urol 135:1142, 1986.
32. Spirnak JP, Bodner D, Udayashankar S, et al: Extracorporeal shock wave lithotripsy in traumatic quadriplegic patients: Can it be safely performed without anesthesia. J Urol 139:18, 1988.
33. Spirnak JP, DeBaz BP, Green HY, et al: Complex struvite calculi treated by primary extracorporeal shock wave lithotripsy and chemolysis with hemiacidrin irrigation. J Urol 140:1356, 1988.
34. Report of American Urological Association Ad Hoc Committee to Study the Safety and Clinical Efficacy of Current Technology of Percutaneous Lithotripsy and Noninvasive Lithotripsy. Baltimore, American Urological Assocation, 1986.
35. Langberg J, Abber J, Thuroff JW, et al: The effects of extracorporeal shock wave lithotripsy on pacemaker function. PACE 10:1142, 1987.
36. Abber JC, Langberg J, Mueller SC, et al: Cardiovascular pathology and extracorporeal shock wave lithotripsy. J Urol 140:408, 1988.
37. Cooper D, Wilkoff B, Masterson M, et al: Effects of extracorporeal shock wave lithotripsy on cardiac pacemakers and its safety in patients with implanted cardiac pacemakers. PACE 11:1607, 1988.
38. Al Karawi MA, Mohamed ARE, El-Etaibi KE: Extracorporeal shock wave lithotripsy (ESWL) induced erosions in upper gastrointestinal tract. Urology 30:224,1987.
39. Cass AS, Onstad G: Colonic mucosal ecchymoses after extracorporeal shock wave lithotripsy for upper ureteral calculus. J Urol 140:1012, 1988.
40. Weber W, Madler C, Keil B, et al: Cardiovascular effects of ESWL. *In* Gravenstein J, Peter K (eds): Extracorporeal Shock Wave Lithotripsy for Renal Stone Disease. Boston, Butterworths, 1986, pp 101–112.
41. Arborelius M, Balldin UI, Lilja B, et al: Hemodynamic changes in man during immersion with the head above water. Aerospace Med 43:592, 1972.
42. Bub P, Rohs M, Rassweiler J, et al: The efficacy of epidural catheter anesthesia for extracorporeal shock wave lithotripsy. Endourology 2:9, 1987.
43. London RA, Kudlak T, Riehle RA: Immersion anesthesia for extracorporeal shock wave lithotripsy. Urology 28:86, 1986.
44. Whelan JP, Gravenstein N, Welch JL, et al: Simulation of ventilatory-induced stone movement and its effect on stone fracture during extracorporeal shock wave lithotripsy. J Urol 140:405, 1988.
45. Carlson CA, Boysen PG, Banner MJ, et al: Stone movement during ESWL: Conventional and high frequency jet ventilation. *In* Gravenstein JS, Peter K (eds): Extracorporeal Shock Wave Lithotripsy for Renal Stone Disease. Boston, Butterworths, 1986, pp 77–86.
46. Warner MA, Warner ME, Buck CF, et al: Clinical efficacy of high frequency jet ventilation during extracorporeal shock wave lithotripsy of renal and ureteral calculi: A comparison with conventional mechanical ventilation. J Urol 139:486, 1988.
47. Banner MJ: Technical aspects of high frequency ventilation. Curr Rev Respir Ther 7:91, 1985.
48. Malhotra V: The use of regional block technique for extracorporeal shock wave lithotripsy. Endourology 1:7, 1986.

49. Loening S, Kramalowsky EV, Willoughby B: Use of local anesthesia for extracorporeal shock wave lithotripsy. J Urol 137:626, 1987.
50. Chaussy C, Schmiedt E: Extracorporeal shock wave lithotripsy (ESWL) for kidney stones: An alternative to surgery? Urol Radiol 6:80, 1984.
51. Nisonson I, Witus WS, Madorsky ML, et al: Ambulatory extracorporeal shock wave lithotripsy. Urology 28:384, 1986.
52. Libby JM, Meacham RB, Griffith DP: The role of silicone ureteral stents in extracorporeal shock wave lithotripsy of large renal calculi. J Urol 139:15, 1988.
53. Hunter PT, Finlayson B, Newman RC, et al: Geometry of and pressures with ESWL. *In* Gravenstein JS, Peter K (eds): Extracorporeal Shock Wave Lithotripsy for Renal Stone Disease. Boston, Butterworths, 1986, pp 19–28.
54. Chaussy CG, Fuchs GJ: Extracorporeal shock wave lithotripsy. Monogr Urol 4:80, 1987.
55. Drach GW, Dretler S, Fair W, et al: Report of the United States Cooperative Study of Extracorporeal Shock Wave Lithotripsy. J Urol 135:1127, 1986.
56. Spirnak JP, Resnick MI: Inpatient versus outpatient ESWL. *In* Kandell B, Harrison LH, McCullough DL (eds): Extracorporeal Shock Wave Lithotripsy. Mount Kisco, NY, Futura Publishing Company, 1987, pp 375–381.
57. Roth RA, Beckman CF: Complications of extracorporeal shock wave lithotripsy and percutaneous nephrolithotomy. Urol Clin North Am 15:155, 1988.
58. Riehle RA: Extracorporeal shock wave lithotripsy. Bull NY Acad Med 62:291, 1986.
59. Hardy MR, McLeod DG: Silent renal obstruction with severe functional loss after extracorporeal shock wave lithotripsy: A report of 2 cases. J Urol 137:91, 1987.
60. Sinno K, Boyce WH, Resnick MI: Childhood urolithiasis. J Urol 121:662, 1979.
61. Kramolowsky EV, Willoughby BL, Loening SA: Extracorporeal shock wave lithotripsy in children. J Urol 137:939, 1987.
62. Sigman M, Laudone VP, Jenkins AD, et al: Initial experience with extracorporeal shock wave lithotripsy in children. J Urol 138:839, 1987.
63. Kroovand RL, Harrison LH, McCullough DL: Extracorporeal shock wave lithotripsy in children. J Urol 138:1106, 1987.
64. Chaussy CG, Fuchs GJ: Extracorporeal shock wave lithotripsy (ESWL) for the treatment of upper urinary stones. *In* Gillenwater JY, Grayhack JT, Howards SH, Duckett JW (eds): Adult and Pediatric Urology. Chicago, Year Book Medical Publishers, 1987, pp 605–619.
65. Dretler SP: Extracorporeal shock wave lithotripsy: A review of its first two years of operation in the United States. Urol Annu 1:1, 1987.
66. Kahn SR, Hackett RL, Finlayson B: Morphology of urinary stone particles resulting from ESWL treatment. J Urol 136:1367, 1986.
67. Riehle RA: Extracorporeal shock wave lithotripsy: Patient selection and results. Probl Urol 1:608, 1987.
68. Dretler SP: Stone fragility—a new therapeutic distinction. J Urol 139:1124, 1988.
69. Riehle RA, Carter H, Vaughan E: Quantitative and crystallographic analysis of stone fragments voided after extracorporeal shock wave lithotripsy. J Endourol 1:37, 1987.
70. Chaussy C, Schmiedt E, Jochman D, et al: First clinical experience with extracorporeally induced destruction of kidney stones by shock waves. J Urol 131:417, 1982.
71. Blandy JP, Singh M: The case for a more aggressive approach to staghorn stones. J Urol 115:505, 1976.
72. Boyce WH, Elkins IB: Reconstructive renal surgery following anatrophic nephrolithotomy: Follow-up of 100 consecutive cases. J Urol 111:307, 1974.
73. Redmon JF, Bissada NK, Harper DL: Anatrophic nephrolithotomy: Experience with complications of the Smith and Boyce technique. J Urol 122:595, 1979.
74. Riehle RA, Fair WD, Vaughan D: Extracorporeal shock wave lithotripsy for upper urinary tract calculi. JAMA 255:2043, 1986.
75. Sofras F, Karayannis A, Kostakopoulos A, et al: Methodology, results and complications in 2000 extracorporeal shock wave lithotripsy procedures. Br J Urol 61:9, 1988.
76. Nesbitt JA, Drago JR, Wise HA, et al: Extracorporeal shock wave lithotripsy: First year experience with 1360 patients. J Endourol 2:235, 1988.
77. Miller K, Bachor R, Hautman R: Percutaneous nephrolithotomy and extracorporeal shock wave lithotripsy versus ureteral stent and ESWL for the treatment of large renal calculi and staghorn calculi—a prospective randomized study: Preliminary results. J Endourol 2:131, 1988.
78. Newman DM, Scott JW, Lingeman JE: Two-year follow-up of patients treated with extracorporeal shock wave lithotripsy. J Endourol 2:163, 1988.
79. Pode D, Lenkovsky Z, Shapiro A, et al: Can extracorporeal shock wave lithotripsy eradicate persistent urinary infection associated with infected stones? J Urol 140:257, 1988.
80. Lingeman JE, Woods J, Toth PD, et al: The role of lithotripsy and its side effects. J Urol 141:793, 1989.
81. Fuchs GJ, Chaussy CG, Royce PL: Staghorn stones: Emerging treatment strategies. Endourology 2:1, 1987.
82. Liedl B, Jocham D, Lunz C, et al: Five-year follow-up of urinary stone patients treated with extracorporeal shock wave lithotripsy. J Endourol 2:157, 1988.

83. Marshall V, White RH, Chaput de Saintonge M, et al: The natural history of renal and ureteral calculi. Br J Urol 47:117, 1975.
84. Ettinger B: Recurrent nephrolithiasis: Natural history and effect of phosphate therapy. Am J Med 61:200, 1976.
85. Thompson RB, Stamey TA: Bacteriology of infected stones. Urology 2:627, 1973.
86. Fowler JE: Bacteriology of branched renal calculi and accompanying urinary tract infections. J Urol 131:213, 1984.
87. Patterson DE, Segura JW, LeRoy AJ: Long-term follow-up of patients treated by percutaneous ultrasonic lithotripsy for struvite calculi. J Endourol 1:171, 1987.
88. Tiselius HG, Hellgren E, Wall I: Infected staghorn stones treated with extracorporeal shock wave lithotripsy and hemiacidrin. J Endourol 2:137, 1988.
89. Michaels EK, Fowler JE, Mariano M: Bacteriuria following extracorporeal shock wave lithotripsy of infectious stones. J Urol 140:254, 1988.
90. Sonda LP, Wang S, Ellis J, et al: Resolution of bacteriuria with infectious stones: Comparison of results employing newer treatment modalities. J Endourol 2:151, 1988.
91. Riehle RA: Extracorporeal shock wave lithotripsy of ureteral stones. Semin Urol 4:175, 1986.
92. Lingeman JE: ESWL for ureteral stones above the pelvic brim. Prob Urol 1:630, 1987.
93. Graff J, Pastor J, Funke PJ, et al: Extracorporeal shock wave lithotripsy for ureteral stones: A retrospective analysis of 417 cases. J Urol 139:513, 1988.
94. Chaussy CG, Fuchs GJ: Extracorporeal shock wave lithotripsy of distal ureteral calculi: Is it worthwhile? J Endourol 1:1, 1987.
95. Chaussy C, Schmiedt E: Shock wave treatment for stones in the upper urinary tract. Urol Clin North Am 10:743, 1983.
96. Lingeman JE, Sonda LP, Kahnoski RJ, et al: Ureteral stone management: Emerging concepts. J Urol 135:1172, 1986.
97. Lingeman JE, Shirrell WL, Newman DM, et al: Management of upper ureteral calculi with extracorporeal shock wave lithotripsy. J Urol 138:720, 1987.
98. Dretler SP, Keating MA, Riley J: An algorithm for the management of ureteral calculi. J Urol 136:1190, 1986.
99. Mueller SC, Wilbert D, Thucroff JW, et al: Extracorporeal shock wave lithotripsy of ureteral stones: Clinical experience and experimental findings. J Urol 135:831, 1986.
100. Riehle RA, Näslund EB, Fair W, et al: Impact of shock wave lithotripsy on upper ureteral calculi. Urology 28:261, 1986.
101. Riehle RA, Näslund EB: Treatment of calculi in the upper ureter with extracorporeal shock wave lithotripsy. SGO 164:1, 1987.
102. Miller K, Fuchs G, Rassweiler J, et al: Treatment of ureteral stone disease: The role of ESWL and endourology. World J Urol 3:53, 1985.
103. Fuchs GJ, Chaussy CG, Stenzl A: Current management concepts in the treatment of ureteral stones. J Endourol 2:107, 1988.
104. Jenkins AD: Dornier extracorporeal shock wave lithotripsy for ureteral stones. Urol Clin North Am 15:377, 1988.
105. Manzone DJ, Chiang B: Extracorporeal shock wave lithotripsy of stones in the upper, mid and lower ureter. J Endourol 2:107, 1988.
106. Cole RS, Shuttleworth KED: Is extracorporeal shock wave lithotripsy suitable treatment for lower ureteric stones? Br J Urol 62:525, 1988.
107. El-Faqih SR, Husain I, Ekman PE, et al: Primary choice of intervention for distal ureteric stone: Ureteroscopy of ESWL. Br J Urol 62:13, 1988.
108. Charig CR, Webb DR, Payne SR, et al: Comparison of treatment of renal calculi by open surgery, percutaneous nephrolithotomy and extracorporeal shock wave lithotripsy. Br Med J 292:879, 1986.
109. Jaeger P, Redha F, Uhlschmid G, et al: Morphologic changes in canine kidneys following extracorporeal shock wave treatment. J Endourol 2:205, 1988.
110. Eisenberger F, Chaussy C, Wanner K: Extracorporale Anwendung von rochenergetischen Stosswellen: Ein neuer Aspekt in der Behandlung des Harnstein Leidens. Akt Urol 8, 1977.
111. Rubin JI, Arger PH, Pollack HM, et al: Kidney changes after extracorporeal shock wave lithotripsy: CT evaluation. Radiology 162:21, 1987.
112. Kaude JV, Williams CM, Millner MR, et al: Renal morphology and function immediately after extracorporeal shock wave lithotripsy. AJR 145:305, 1985.
113. Baumgartner BR, Dickey KW, Ambrose SS, et al: Kidney changes after extracorporeal shock wave lithotripsy: Appearance on MR imaging. Radiology 163:531, 1987.
114. Newman R, Hackett R, Senior D, et al: Pathologic effects of ESWL on canine renal tissue. Urology 29:194, 1987.
115. Jaeger P, Redha F, Uhlschmid G: Morphological changes in canine kidneys following extracorporeal shock wave treatment. Urol Res 16:161, 1988.
116. Abrahams C, Lipson S, Ross L: Pathologic changes in the kidneys and other organs of dogs undergoing extracorporeal shock wave lithotripsy with a tubeless lithotriptor. J Urol 140:391, 1988.
117. Ruiz Marcellan FJ, Ibarz Servio L: Evaluation of renal damage in extracorporeal lithotripsy by shock waves. Eur Urol 12:73, 1986.

118. Russo P, Stephenson RA, Mies C, et al: High energy shock waves suppress tumor growth in vitro and in vivo. J Urol 135:626, 1986.
119. Russo P, Mies C, Huryk R, et al: Histopathologic and ultrastructural correlates of tumor growth suppression by high energy shock waves. J Urol 137:338, 1987.
120. Fischer N, Muller HM, Gulhan A, et al: Cavitation effects: Possible causes of tissue injury during extracorporeal shock wave lithotripsy. J Endourol 2:215, 1988.
121. Delius M: This month in investigative urology: Effect of extracorporeal shock waves on the kidney. J Urol 140:390, 1988.
122. Newman RC, Bezirdjian L, Steinbock G, et al: Complications of extracorporeal shock wave lithotripsy: Presentation and treatment. Semin Urol 4:170, 1986.
123. Knapp PM, Kulb TB, Lingeman JE, et al: Extracorporeal shock wave lithotripsy—induced perirenal hematomas. J Urol 139:700, 1988.
124. McCullough DL: Complications of ESWL. Prob Urol 1:604, 1987.
125. Steinbock GS, Bezirdjian L, Newman RC, et al: Extracorporeal shock wave lithotripsy. Surgical Rounds, July 1986, p 45.
126. Chaussy CG, Fuchs GJ: World experience with extracorporeal shock wave lithotripsy (ESWL) for the treatment of urinary stones: An assessment of its role after 5 years of clinical use. Endourology 1:7, 1986.
127. Van Arsdalen KV: Adjunctive procedures for extracorporeal shock wave lithotripsy. AUA Update Series 6:2, 1987.
128. Ramsay JWA, Payne SR, Gosling PT, et al: The effects of double J stenting in unobstructed ureters: An experimental and clinical study. Br J Urol 57:630, 1985.
129. Segura JW: Use and abuse of stents in the management of upper tract calculus disease. Prob Urology 1:649, 1987.
130. Bregg K, Riehle RA: Morbidity associated with indwelling internal ureteral stents after shock wave lithotripsy. J Urol 145:510, 1989.
131. Saltzman B: Ureteral stents: Indications, variations and complications. Urol Clin North Am 15:481, 1988.
132. Shabsigh R, Gleeson MJ, Griffith DP: The benefits of stenting on a more-or-less routine basis prior to extracorporeal shock wave lithotripsy. Urol Clin North Am 15:493, 1988.
133. Riehle RA: Selective use of ureteral stents before extracorporeal shock wave lithotripsy. Urol Clin North Am 15:499, 1988.
134. Chaussy CG: ESWL: Past, present and future. J Endourol 2:97, 1988.
135. Lingeman JE, Kulb TB: Hypertension following extracorporeal shock wave lithotripsy (abstract). J Urol 137:45A, 1987.
136. Masson GMC, Kashii C, Matsunaga M, et al: Hypertensive vascular disease induced by heterologous renin circulation. Circ Res 18:219, 1966.
137. Page IH: The production of persistent arterial hypertension by cellophane perinephritis. JAMA 113:3046, 1939.
138. Lingeman J, Newman D, Mosbaugh et al: Blood pressure changes following ESWL (abstract). *In* Proceedings of the 62nd Annual Meeting of North Central Section of the American Urological Association, Orlando, 1988, p 59.
139. Sandlow J, Winfield HN, Loening SA: Blood pressure changes in patients treated with repeated extracorporeal shock waves (abstract). *In* Proceedings of the 62nd Annual Meeting of North Central Section of the American Urological Association, 1988, p 23.
140. Sandlow JI, Winfield HN, Loening SA: Blood pressure changes related to extracorporeal shock wave lithotripsy (ESWL). J Urol 141:242A, 1989.
141. Germinale F, Puppo P, Bottino P, et al: ESWL and hypertension: No evidence for causal relationship. J Urol 141:241A, 1989.
142. Zwergel T, Neisius D, Zwergel U, et al: Hypertension in patients with extracorporeal lithotripsy of urinary stones—incidence in first and second generation lithotriptor treatment. J Urol 141:242A, 1989.
143. Gilbert BR, Riehle RA, Vaughan D: Extracorporeal shock wave lithotripsy and its effect on renal function. J Urol 139:482, 1988.
144. Daniels C, MacKay J, MacGregor JH, et al: Variations in fluoroscopic and spot film techniques during extracorporeal shock wave lithotripsy. J Urol 141:489, 1989.
145. Carter HB, Näslund EB, Riehle RA: Variables influencing radiation exposure during extracorporeal shock wave lithotripsy. Urology 30:546, 1987.
146. Lin PP, Hrejsa AF: Patient exposure and radiation environment of an extracorporeal shock wave lithotripsy system. J Urol 138:712, 1987.
147. Bush WH, Jones D, Gibbons RP: Radiation dose to patient and personnel during extracorporeal shock wave lithotripsy. J Urol 138:716, 1987.
148. Van Swearingen FL, McCullough DL, Dyer R, et al: Radiation exposure to patients during extracorporeal shock wave lithotripsy. J Urol 138:18, 1987.
149. Jocham D, Brandl H, Chaussy C, et al: Treatment of nephrolithiasis with ESWL. *In* Gravenstein JS, Peter K (eds): Extracorporeal Shock Wave Lithotripsy for Renal Stone Disease. Boston, Butterworths, 1986, pp 35–60.
150. Griffith DP, Gleeson MJ, Politis G, et al: Effectiveness of radiation control program for Dornier HM-3 lithotriptor. Urology 33:20, 1989.

151. Pollack HM: Radiation exposure and extracorporeal shock wave lithotripsy. J Urol 138:850, 1987.
152. Lusk RP, Tyler RS: Hazardous sound levels produced by extracorporeal shock wave lithotripsy. J Urol 137:1113, 1987.
153. Assimos DG, Boyce WH, Furr WH, et al: Urinary enzyme levels after extracorporeal shock wave lithotripsy (abstract 157A). J Urol 137:143A, 1987.
154. McCullough DL, Yeaman LD, Bo WJ, et al: Effects of shock waves on the rat ovary. J Urol 141:666, 1989.
155. Yeaman LD, Jerome CP, McCullough DL: Effects of shock waves on the structure and growth of the immature rat epiphysis. J Urol 141:670, 1989.
156. Breaux E, Burns JR: Outpatient extracorporeal shock wave lithotripsy. Urology 29:131, 1987.
157. Graff J, Pastor J, Herberhold D, et al: Technical modifications of the Dornier HM-3 lithotriptor with an improved anesthesia technique. World J Urol 5:202, 1987.
158. Graff J, Schmidt A, Pastor J, et al: New generator for low pressure lithotripsy with the Dornier HM-3: Preliminary experience of 2 centers. J Urol 139:904, 1988.

Index

Note: Page numbers in *italics* refer to illustrations; page numbers followed by (t) refer to tables.